Administrative Medical Assisting

Sixth Edition

Marilyn T. Fordney, CMA-AC

Formerly, Instructor of Medical Insurance,
Medical Terminology, Medical Machine Transcription,
and Medical Office Procedures
Ventura College, Ventura, California

Linda L. French, CMA-C, NCICS, CPC

Formerly, Instructor and Business Consultant,
Administrative Medical Assisting,
Medical Terminology, and Medical Insurance Billing and Coding
Simi Valley Adult School and Career Institute, Simi Valley, California
Ventura College, Ventura, California
Oxnard College, Oxnard, California
Santa Barbara Busines College, Ventura, California

Joan J. Follis, BS

Formerly, Instructor of Business Education and Medical Office Procedures
Ventura College, Ventura, California

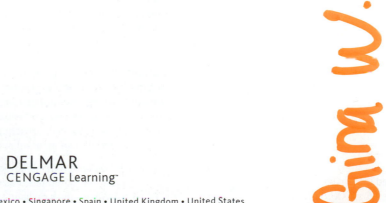

DELMAR
CENGAGE Learning™

Australia • Brazil • Japan • Korea • Mexico • Singapore • Spain • United Kingdom • United States

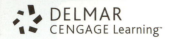
DELMAR
CENGAGE Learning™

Administrative Medical Assisting, Sixth Edition
Marilyn T. Fordney, Linda L. French, Joan J. Follis

Vice President, Health Care Business Unit:
William Brottmiller

Director of Learning Solutions:
Matthew Kane

Senior Acquisitions Editor:
Rhonda Dearborn

Product Manager:
Sarah Prime

Marketing Director:
Jennifer McAvey

Technology Product Manager:
Mary Colleen Liburdi

Technology Project Manager:
Ben Knapp

Production Director:
Carolyn Miller

Content Project Manager:
Brooke Greenhouse

Senior Art Director:
Jack Pendleton

Printed in Canada
1 2 3 4 5 6 7 XXX 10 09 08 07

For product information and technology assistance, contact us at
Professional & Career Group Customer Support, 1-800-648-7450

For permission to use material from this text or product, submit all requests online at **www.cengage.com/permissions**
Further permissions questions can be emailed to
permissionrequest@cengage.com

ExamView® and ExamView Pro® are registered trademarks of FSCreations, Inc. Windows is a registered trademark of the Microsoft Corporation used herein under license. Macintosh and Power Macintosh are registered trademarks of Apple Computer, Inc. Used herein under license.

© 2007 Cengage Learning. All Rights Reserved. Cengage Learning WebTutor™ is a trademark of Cengage Learning.

Library of Congress Control Number: 2007940728
ISBN-10: 1-4180-6411-4
ISBN-13: 978-1-4180-6411-2

Delmar Cengage Learning
5 Maxwell Drive
Clifton Park, NY 12065-2919
USA

Cengage Learning products are represented in Canada by Nelson Education, Ltd.

For your lifelong learning solutions, visit **delmar.cengage.com**

Visit our corporate website at **www.cengage.com**

Notice to the Reader

Publisher does not warrant or guarantee any of the products described herein or perform any independent analysis in connection with any of the product information contained herein. Publisher does not assume, and expressly disclaims, any obligation to obtain and include information other than that provided to it by the manufacturer. The reader is expressly warned to consider and adopt all safety precautions that might be indicated by the activities described herein and to avoid all potential hazards. By following the instructions contained herein, the reader willingly assumes all risks in connection with such instructions. The publisher makes no representations or warranties of any kind, including but not limited to, the warranties of fitness for particular purpose or merchantability, nor are any such representations implied with respect to the material set forth herein, and the publisher takes no responsibility with respect to such material. The publisher shall not be liable for any special, consequential, or exemplary damages resulting, in whole or part, from the reader's use of, or reliance upon, this material.

Current Procedural Terminology only © 2006 American Medical Association. All rights reserved. No fee schedules, basic unit relative values, or related listings are included in *CPT*. The AMA assumes no liability for the data contained therein.

DEDICATION

I am honored, but awestruck to be taking on this project as its sole author while my coauthor, Marilyn "Winkie" Fordney, retires after having given birth to it many years ago with retired coauthor Joan Follis and having cradled it close to her heart for five editions.

How special is it to have someone in your life who is in your corner and roots you on in each endeavor you pursue? I am blessed to have three such people. I dedicate this book to the memory of my late mother, Eleanor Campbell Barnes, who despite her sight impairment always strived to learn more. Who always cheered me on, thought whatever I was doing was wonderful, and who listened with great interest when I told her about my current endeavors. To my husband Dick, who day in and day out supported my efforts to make this project the best it could be so that students and instructors would benefit from its use in the classroom. His unfaltering belief in me and my efforts is what spurred me on through many difficult moments. And, to my mentor and friend, Winkie Fordney, who patiently walked me through all the delicate steps of creating a publication such as this and encouraged me to fly solo saying, "You can do this, I know you can." I am forever grateful for this support and my hope is that you will LEARN as you **L**isten **E**nthusiastically **A**nd **R**eceive **N**ew information. It is my privilege to stand in *your* corner and cheer you on as you pursue the exciting world of administrative medical assisting.

—Linda L. French, CMA-C, NCICS, CPC

CONTENTS

UNIT 1 Professional and Career Responsibilities / 1

UNIT 2   Interpersonal Communications / 99

Chapter 7   Appointments / 189

UNIT 3   Records Management / 225

Chapter 8   Filing Procedures / 226

Chapter 9   Medical Records / 261

Chapter 10   Drug and Prescription Records / 299

UNIT 4   Written Communications / 333

Chapter 11   Written Correspondence / 334

Chapter 12   Processing Mail and Telecommunications / 370

UNIT 5   Financial Administration / 411

UNIT 6   Managing the Office / 569

UNIT 7   Employment / 653

Comprehensive List of

PROCEDURES and JOB SKILLS

The following Procedures appear in the text and Job Skills appear in the *Workbook*:

Chapter 1 A Career As an Administrative Medical Assistant

Performance Objectives (Procedures) in This Textbook

- Procedure 1-1 Interpret and accurately spell medical terms and abbreviations

Performance Objectives (Job Skills) in the *Workbook*

- Job Skill 1-1 Interpret and accurately spell medical terms and abbreviations
- Job Skill 1-2 Use the Internet to obtain information on certification and/or registration
- Job Skill 1-3 Use the Internet to test your knowledge on anatomy and physiology or medical terminology
- Job Skill 1-4 Develop a medical practice survey

Chapter 2 The Health Care Environment: Past, Present, and Future

Performance Objectives (Procedures) in This Textbook

- Procedure 2-1 Direct patients to specific hospital departments
- Procedure 2-2 Refer patients to the correct physician specialist

Performance Objectives (Job Skills) in the *Workbook*

- Job Skill 2-1 Direct patients to specific hospital departments
- Job Skill 2-2 Refer patients to the correct physician specialist
- Job Skill 2-3 Define abbreviations for health care professionals
- Job Skill 2-4 Determine basic skills for the administrative medical assistant

Chapter 3 Medicolegal and Ethical Responsibilities

Performance Objectives (Procedures) in This Textbook

- Procedure 3-1 Release patient information
- Procedure 3-2 Accept a subpoena

Performance Objectives (Job Skills) in the *Workbook*

- Job Skill 3-1 Compose letter of withdrawal

Chapter 4 The Art of Communication

Performance Objectives (Procedures) in This Textbook

- Procedure 4-1 Demonstrate active listening by following guidelines

Performance Objectives (Job Skills) in the *Workbook*

- Job Skill 4-1 Demonstrate body language
- Job Skill 4-2 Name unique qualities of other cultures

Chapter 5 The Receptionist

Performance Objectives (Procedures) in This Textbook

- Procedure 5-1 Open the medical office
- Procedure 5-2 Assist patients with in-office registration procedures
- Procedure 5-3 Assist patient in preparing an application form for a disabled person placard
- Procedure 5-4 Develop a patient education plan for diseases/injuries related to the medical specialty
- Procedure 5-5 Close the medical office

Performance Objectives (Job Skills) in the *Workbook*

- Job Skill 5-1 Prepare a patient registration form
- Job Skill 5-2 Prepare an application form for a disabled person placard
- Job Skill 5-3 Research materials for in-office resources and/or patient education

Chapter 6 Telephone Procedures

Performance Objectives (Procedures) in This Textbook

- Procedure 6-1 Prepare and leave a voice mail message
- Procedure 6-2 Take messages from an answering service
- Procedure 6-3 Answer incoming telephone calls
- Procedure 6-4 Place outgoing telephone calls
- Procedure 6-5 Identify and manage emergency calls
- Procedure 6-6 Handle a complaint from an angry caller

List of
TABLES

FOREWORD

When I began writing in 1975, little did I envision that the journey would lead me to write several books on many topics allied to the field of medical assisting, and that I would have a writing career that would last well over 30 years. But indeed this has happened, and it has been enjoyable work—doing the research, traveling to medical assisting conventions, and meeting the many individuals whose lives have been touched by the books.

I will continue to write in the field of health insurance, billing, coding, and compliance, but I have decided to retire from this project. It will be in the good, capable hands of an author/educator who is a true perfectionist, knowledgeable, dedicated to medical assisting, and one that I have known for about 30 years.

Thank you, Linda, for tackling this massive project. Best wishes and continued success and happiness as you meet the new challenges of each edition.

Also thank you to the readers and users of the past for allowing me to come into your lives. May the students of the future receive the benefits and rewards from using this tool to enhance their careers.

—Marilyn Takahashi Fordney-Havasi, CMA-AC
Oxnard, California

PREFACE

The sixth edition of *Administrative Medical Assisting* features numerous content updates and additions as well as new photographs, figures, tables, and examples. It focuses on competencies for medical assisting programs outlined by the Commission on Accreditation for Allied Health Education Programs (CAAHEP) and the Accrediting Bureau of Health Education Schools (ABHES) as well as certification test parameters set forth by the American Association of Medical Assistants (AAMA) and the American Medical Technologists (AMT). An emphasis has been placed on step-by-step procedures for various job skills and the development of critical thinking presented in real-life scenarios to help with the development of problem-solving skills.

The textbook material is designed for the learner who plans to work as an administrative (front office) medical assistant in a private physician's office, single- or multi-specialty clinic, or hospital setting; however, the skills presented also apply to other technicians and assistants who perform clerical functions similar to that of an administrative medical assistant. The book can be used in community colleges, vocational and commercial educational institutions, welfare-to-work programs, and in-service training in the private medical office. It is an appropriate textbook for a one- or two-semester course. It may be used for self-study if no formal classes are available in the community or if a medical assistant wants to increase his or her skills but is unable to attend classes. Finally, the book serves as a reference for the working medical assistant, featuring the most up-to-date methods of performing medical office tasks.

The textbook and workbook chapters are arranged to better facilitate learning with legal and computer information integrated throughout. The chapters are divided into seven units that progress from professional and career responsibilities, interpersonal communications, records management, written communications, financial administration, and managing the medical office to the final unit, where the learner prepares for employment.

NEW CONTENT FEATURES

▌ **Chapter content** is updated to reflect changes in technology, job responsibilities, insurance regulations, legal requirements, and compliance mandates. The order of some chapters has been changed to assist the presentation of topics, focusing the reorganization within each chapter on better flow of content.

▌ **Objectives** are divided into (1) Learning Objectives that state chapter goals, (2) Performance Objectives in the textbook that contains a numbered list of step-by-step procedures, and (3) Performance Objectives for the Workbook containing a numbered list of Job Skills, provided as an opportunity for practice.

▌ **Customer service** is emphasized at the beginning of each chapter in a section titled "Heart of the Health Care Professional."

▌ **Key terms** introduce the student to basic terminology at the beginning of each chapter and are listed throughout the chapter in bold, colored type, with expanded definitions in the glossary at the end of the textbook.

▌ **Photographs** visually support textual content and give the learner a better perspective of the office duties and situations mentioned.

■ **Icons** give quick reference to Customer Service applications, Compliance issues, Patient Education boxes, Procedures, Stop and Think Case Scenarios, Summary of Certification Topics, Exam-Style Review Questions, Workbook Assignments, Computer Assignments, and Resources.

■ **Compliance issues** mandated by the federal government are emphasized by a color screened box with an icon for quick identification. Many site HIPAA regulations.

■ **Patient Education boxes** describes how the medical assistant should keep the patient informed.

■ **Figures, tables, and examples,** enhanced in full color, present information in a succinct, easy-to-understand format. Each is numbered for easy reference, and is referred to throughout each chapter to clarify concepts, illustrate graphics, and depict realistic scenarios.

■ **New Chapter 4**, The Art of Communication, which has been developed to include all elements of communication as experienced in a medial office setting. Elements that interfere with and influence communication (e.g., cultural differences, special needs patients) are also included, and the Communication Skills section from Chapter 1 has been incorporated to maximize its focus.

NEW INSTRUCTIONAL FEATURES

■ **Procedures**, previously called "Job Skills," are step-by-step guidelines for completing tasks in the medical office. Each are numbered and listed at the beginning of each chapter, and many are cross-referenced to be referred to while completing Job Skills in the *Workbook*.

■ **Critical Thinking Component** is presented in Stop and Think Case Scenarios, which have been expanded and moved to the end of each chapter. These questions help stimulate the thought process and exercise reasoning skills.

■ **Focus on Certification** summarizes the key areas of study for students who are preparing to take the CMA, RMA, or CMAS certification exams.

■ **Exam-Style Review Questions** offer a quick review of key points in the same multiple-choice format as seen on certification examinations.

■ **Workbook Assignments** are divided into (1) Review Questions, which have been expanded to include all major topics, (2) Critical Thinking Exercises, which have been developed to stimulate reasoning capabilities, and (3) Job Skills, which offer step-by-step directions and hands-on practice for all major tasks an administrative medical assistant performs.

■ **Computer Competency** exercises in the *Workbook,* which utilize Medical Office Simulation Software (MOSS), version 2.0, and compliment the topical material in the text. These exercises are found in the Online Companion, at www.delmarlearning.com/companions. Select Allied Health from the left navigational bar and then click on this book's title.

■ **Resources** listed at the end of each chapter have been updated and expanded to include booklets, books, Internet sites, medical directives, newsletters, professional magazines, and organizations pertinent to each chapter topic.

■ **Revised CMS-1500 Claim Form Instructions and Templates** are in Appendix A for quick reference. Each field is listed, with specific instructions for commercial payers, Medicare (Medicare/Medicaid, Medicare/Medigap, MSP), and TRICARE.

PRACTICE SOFTWARE

A Practice Software CD-ROM accompanies this book, which contains StudyWARE interactive software and the Critical Thinking Challenge. These activities challenge you to apply content, think critically, develop competency in skills, and improve your knowledge base.

StudyWARE interactive software includes learning activities and quizzes to help study key concepts and test your comprehension. The activity and quiz content correspond with each chapter of the book. You can take the quizzes in both "Practice Mode" and "Quiz Mode." Activities include Flashcards, Concentration, Hangman, and Crossword Puzzles.

In the Critical Thinking Challenge, you are on a 3-month externship in a medical office. You will be confronted with a series of situations in which you must use your critical thinking skills to choose the most appropriate action in response to the situation.

MEDICAL ASSISTING AREAS OF COMPETENCE

Appendix B contains numbered lists for each of the following, and tables with reference numbers from these lists correlate text and assignments by chapter for the following:

- CAAHEP Curriculum Competencies
- ABHES Curriculum Competencies
- CMA Certification Examination Content
- RMA Certification Examination Competencies
- CMAS Examination Specifications
- AAMA Role Delineation Study

LEARNING PACKAGE SUPPLEMENTS

Workbook

The workbook is an essential resource available for use with this text. A realistic approach is experienced as the student assumes that he or she is employed by two physicians who are married to each other and who share a professional corporation. Through job skill exercises, the student, assuming the role of the administrative medical assistant, performs a variety of duties that are a realistic part of the day-by-day activities in the joint office of a general practitioner and a family practitioner. Following is a list of features. New features are preceded by an asterisk (*).

Part I

- **Objectives** are clearly stated for all Job Skill exercises.
- ***Focus on Certification** outlines key points to study in preparation for the CMA, RMA, and CMAS examinations.
- **Abbreviation and Spelling Review** incorporates medical terminology into a short chart note for each chapter, giving learners an opportunity to write definitions for abbreviations and spell medical terms.

- **Review Questions** cover key points in chapters, address areas not covered in the Exam-Style Review Questions in the text and are presented in various formats to increase learning (answers are found in the Instructor's Manual).
- **Critical Thinking Exercises** offer learners an opportunity to address situations and solve problems that are realistic to an office setting (answers are found in the Instructor's Manual).
- ***Job Skill** exercises offer students experience as they practice job skills realistic to the medical office. Step-by-step directions now incorporate *Performance Evaluation Checklists* so students and instructors have both detailed directions and the checklist in the same area. The student has three attempts to complete each job skill and points have been assigned proportionate to the time and effort the student spends completing the exercise and performing the job skill.

Part II

- **Blank forms** are realistic and similar to those found in medical offices; they are easily removable and require completion for a variety of job skill exercises.

Part III

- ***Competency Grids**, with reference numbers, correlates text and assignments by chapter to:
  1. CAAHEP Competency Standards for Medical Assisting Educational Programs
  2. ABHES Competencies for Medical Assisting Programs
  3. AAMA Certification Examination Content Outline for the CMA
  4. AMT Competencies and Construction Parameters for the RMA
  5. AMT Competencies and Examination Specifications for the CMAS
  6. AAMA Role Delineation Study

Part IV

- **Appendix** for Practon Medical Group, Inc., lists references for the simulated medical practice and states office policies to be followed while completing exercises and making decisions that relate to the operations of a medical office. A mock fee schedule with procedure codes, description of services, and fees are included as well as *CPT* modifiers and a small selection of *HCPCS Level II* codes with descriptions and fees.

Part V

▌ **List of Abbreviations** includes all abbreviation tables found in the text in one location.

Pegboard Bookkeeping

Although most medical practices have converted to computerized accounting, it is necessary for students to have basic knowledge of how to trace where figures originate, make computations, and determine where and how they should be posted before tackling a sophisticated computerized financial system. To gain experience in step-by-step bookkeeping procedures, this text incorporates the same forms used in *Medical Office Procedures with Medical Pegboard* (ISBN 0-7668-1645-1). Students can use Chapter 15, Bookkeeping, textbook and *Workbook* exercises for a basic introduction to medical pegboard theory and activities. If more extensive knowledge of the pegboard is desired, they can also use the medical pegboard procedures kit. This allows for an even better understanding of this complex aspect of financial practices.

Instructor's Manual

An *Instructor's Manual* is available for use with this textbook. It contains the following features. New features are preceded by an asterisk.

▌ **General Instructions** cover materials and equipment, audiovisual aids, student software, online companion, Electronic Classroom Manager, pegboard bookkeeping kit, *competency-based learning, *competency checklists, grading and correcting, grading software programs, *competency grids outline and contents of the course, student evaluation, and evaluation of course and instructor.

Section I

Each chapter contains:

▌ ***CAAHEP and ABHES Areas of Competence** listed with reference numbers as they pertain to each chapter.

▌ **Lesson Plan** suggestions that offer ideas of topics to discuss and list activities to assign.

▌ **Additional Activities** suggested for each chapter and could be adopted to enhance class time and motivate students or assigned as extra credit.

▌ ***Stop-and-Think Case Scenario Answer Key** included to aid the instructor with possible answers to problems presented in realistic office situations.

▌ ***Exam-Style Review Question Answers** included for end of chapter multiple-choice questions.

▌ **Review Questions and Answers** listed for easy reference during class discussion or independent assignment correction.

▌ **Critical Thinking Exercises and Answers** listed for easy reference during class discussion or independent assignment correction.

▌ **Job Skill Answer Keys** listed with rationals and illustrated for various forms to assist the instructor with correction.

Section II

▌ **Medical Terminology and Abbreviation Tests** offered as a review of terms and abbreviation definitions.

Instructors' feedback and comments on the textbook and all ancillary materials are welcome and should be e-mailed or addressed to the publisher or authors using the addresses listed in the *Instructor's Manual*.

Electronic Classroom Manager

The **Electronic Classroom Manager** is a CD-ROM loaded with content to provide instructors with complete support in the classroom. Deliver powerful lectures, create total lesson plans, customize exams, and monitor student progress throughout the course with the following tools:

▌ Customize the **electronic Instructor's Manual files** to individual class needs

▌ Deliver effective presentations with chapter **PowerPoint presentations** that include visuals and video clips

▌ Create quizzes and tests to monitor student progress with the **Computerized Test Bank** in ExamView with more than 1000 questions

- Pick out important visuals from the **Image Library** to incorporate into your own class presentations

Web Tutor Advantage

Use the **Web Tutor** on either Blackboard or WebCT to help manage your course.

- **Course management tools** include course calendar, chat, e-mail, threaded discussions, web links, and a white board
- Loaded with **content related to each chapter,** such as objectives, frequently asked questions, glossary term flash cards, and web links
- Features **critical thinking case studies** that include video assets and assessment quizzes
- Uploaded with **PowerPoint presentations** and a **Computerized Test Bank**

Online Companion Website

The **Online Companion** contains extra content for both students and instructors. To access, go to www.delmarlearning.com/companions, select Allied Health from the left navigational bar, and click on the title of this book. The site includes:

- Password-protected complete **Curriculum,** including detailed lesson outlines for each Unit
- **Editable forms** to fill out and print
- **Performance Evaluation Checklists** from the *Workbook to Accompany Administrative Medical Assisting* allow the instructor easy access for printing and record keeping.

- **Correlation grids** compare *Administrative Medical Assisting,* sixth edition, and the primary competitive titles to assist instructors in changing from one of these titles to the sixth edition of *Administrative Medical Assisting* for classroom use.
- **Crossover grid** compares the fifth and sixth editions of *Administrative Medical Assisting* to assist instructors in modifying lesson plans to make the transition to the sixth edition.

SUMMARY

One of the things that makes medical assisting such an exciting field is its ever-changing nature; nothing stays the same. As technology increases, health care costs rise, and our population grows, government agencies address security, safety issues, standardization, and the increase of the uninsured population. Thus, it is essential that all medical personnel attend workshops and continue to update their knowledge by reading newspapers, federal bulletins and booklets, and professional newsletters and journals as supplied in the expanded Resources section at the end of each chapter. It is my hope that this learning package will assist in patient care by helping to educate competent, service-oriented medical assistants and will be a stepping stone to new knowledge, understanding, appreciation, and advancement in the medical assisting profession.

ACKNOWLEDGMENTS

This book made its first appearance in 1981 and many students, physicians, friends, colleagues, and instructors have contributed valuable suggestions and interesting material throughout the years. I wish to express my thanks to all of them.

A special thank you to former coauthors Marilyn T. Fordney and Joan J. Follis, who dedicated more than 25 years to write, research, and accumulate materials to make the previous five editions top-quality educational and instructional information.

I am indebted to many individuals on the staff of Delmar Learning for encouragement and guidance. I express particular appreciation to Sarah Prime, Product Manager/Developmental Editor, who was always there to answer questions and motivate me along the way. I want to thank Rhonda Dearborn, senior acquisitions editor, who allowed me to "fly solo" on this project and whose insight and vision I greatly admire. Special thanks go to Brooke Baker, content project manager; Ben Knapp, technology project manager; and Jack Pendleton, senior art director, for their special gifts and diligent attention to detail.

Deepest gratitude is extended to Barbara Warfield and Ted Hernandez of Rhino Graphics in Port Hueneme, California, for designing the Practon Medical Group, Inc., letterhead, business card, envelope, and form heads for use in this project.

Several medical office supply companies were kind enough to cooperate by providing forms and descriptive literature of their products and their names will be found throughout the text and workbook figures.

But colleagues, production staff, and editors working alone do not quite make a book; there are others to whom I am deeply indebted.

Special thanks to Evie O'Nan and Susan Royce, who created the content for the new Study-WARE interactive software; Robin Berenson, who wrote the WebTutor materials; and Annette Hoffman, who developed the computerized test bank and the PowerPoint slides for this edition. All of these ancillaries enhance learning and make the instruction process easier. I would also like to express my gratitude to Cindy Correa who shared her expertise of the Medical Office Simulation Software and developed exercises to incorporate the computerized medical office into the *Workbook* so students will be trained in both hands-on skills and computerized skills.

I would like to acknowledge Tom Stock of Stock Studios Photography, Saratoga Springs, New York, cameraman and chief photographer, and his assistant Jonathan McKee for the new photographs appearing in the sixth edition. I appreciate the staff at Delmar Learning who correlated this effort and former coauthor, Marilyn T. Fordney, who acted as the technical consultant. A special note of appreciation is extended to the Urgent Care of Southern Saratoga, Clifton Park, New York, for the use of their facility and to the following professionals who were models: Karlin Antoine, Jenna Carroll, Martha Cason, John Kevin Landy III, Matt McGuire, Meaghan O'Brien, Scott Royael, and Todd Duthaler, M.D.

I also wish to state my deepest gratitude to the people and organizations who so willingly and enthusiastically contributed to the contents of this book. I take great pride in listing the following people who acted as consultants and assisted in reviewing various parts of the manuscript. Without their expertise, comments, and suggestions, this work would not be as complete as it is.

Kay C. Bertrand, EdM
Vice President of Education Development
National Center for Competency Testing
Overland Park, Kansas

Hal Buntley, LVN, CMA, EMT
Administrative Medical Assisting Instructor
San Antonio College
San Antonio, Texas

George S. Conomikes and Staff
President
Conomikes Associates, Inc.
Los Angeles, California

Maria D'Addario, MS
Certified Genetic Counselor
Genzyme Genetics
Orange, California

Deborah Sue Emmons, CMA
President
S.T.A.T. Transcription Service
Port Hueneme, California

Dr. William Fisher and Staff
Urgent Care of Southern Saratoga
Clifton Park, New York

Cynthia Hotta
Executive Senior Managed Care Representative
GlaxoSmithKline
Pittsburgh, Pennsylvania

Joanne Kennedy, MSLS
Health Sciences Librarian
St. John's Regional Medical Center
Oxnard, California

Janet LaMacchia
Travel Consultant
Camarillo Travel
Camarillo, California

Lucille M. Loignon, MD, FACE
Diplomate American Board of Ophthalmology
Oxnard, California

Jim Nonn, CFO
Accountant
Pemko Manufacturing Company
Ventura, California

Cecelia C. Rice, MBA, CQA
Contract Operations Division
TRICARE Management Activity
Aurora, Colorado

John Skovmand, Pharm.D.
Seebers Pharmacy
Santa Paula, California

Dr. and Mrs. William E. Starr
Channel Islands Plastic and Reconstructive Surgery
Medical Group, Inc.
Oxnard, California

Sue Stratton
Director, Marketing
Medical Administrative Consultants
Calabasas, California

Carolyn Talesfore
Advertising and Promotion Manager
Bibbero Systems, Inc.
Petaluma, California

Ivy Young, CCMA-AC
Phlebotomist for Daryoush Jadali, MD
Ventura, California

REVIEWERS

A special thanks to the following individuals who graciously reviewed this edition:

Ursula Cole, MEd, CMA, CCS-P
Medical Program Coordinator/Medical Curriculum
Chair
Indiana Business College
Terre Haute, Indiana

Mary Gjernes, MLT (ASCP), CLT, CMA
MA Program Director
MT Program Director
Presentation College
Aberdeen, South Dakota

Constance L. Lieseke, CMA, MLT (ASCP)
Medical Assistant Program Coordinator
Olympic College
Bremerton, Washington

Wilsetta McClain, NRCMA, NCICS, RMA, MBA
Program Director
Baker College of Auburn Hills
Auburn Hills, Michigan

Michelle C. McCranie, CPhT
Pharmacy/Medical Assisting Instructor
Ogeechee Technical College
Statesboro, Georgia

Pat Gallagher Moeck, PhD, MBA, BA, CMA
Director, Medical Assisting Program
El Centro College
Dallas, Texas

Everlee O'Nan, RMA
Director of Health Care Education
National College
Florence, Kentucky

Donna Otis, LPN
Medical Instructor
Metro Business College
Rolla, Missouri

Alma D. Philpott, NCRMA, Phlebotomist, EMT-Basic
Medical Program Chair
Kaplan Career Institute
Brooklyn, Ohio

Pratima Sampat-Mar
Corporate Curriculum Coordinator
Pima Medical Institute
Mesa, Arizona

David Lee Sessoms, Jr. M.Ed., CMA
Miller-Motte Technical College
Medical Assisting Program Director
Wilmington, North Carolina

Lynn G. Slack, BS, CMA
Medical Programs Director
ICM School of Business and Medical Careers
Pittsburgh, Pennsylvania

Stephanie Suddendorf, CMA
Medical Assisting Program Director
Minnesota School of Business
Oakdale, Minnesota

Gayla Taylor
Instructor & Assistant Director of Education
Dallas, Texas

Tracy A. Thomas
Medical Assistant Lead Instructor
St. Louis College of Health Careers
St. Louis, Missouri

Fifth Edition Reviewers

Lisa Cook, CMA
Medical Assistant Program Director
Eton Technical Institute
Port Orchard, Washington

Julayne Masterman, MA, BSBA, CMA
Program Chair—Medical Assisting
Ivy Tech State College
Muncie, Indiana

Cris McTighe, CMA
Director of Education
Bryman College
Hayward, California

Ethel Morikis, BSN, RNC, CMA
Program Director—Medical Assisting
Ivy Tech State College
Michigan City, Indiana

Donna Otis, LPN
Medical Instructor
Metro Business College
Rolla, Missouri

Linda Scarborough, RN, CMA, CMBS, BSM
Medical Assisting Program Director
Lanier Technical College
Oakwood, Georgia

Geraldine M. Todaro, MSTE, CMA, CLPIb
Associate Professor
Stark State College of Technology
Canton, Ohio

ABOUT THE AUTHORS

MARILYN T. FORDNEY, CMA-AC

Marilyn Takahashi Fordney worked as a medical assistant performing administrative and clinical duties for 14 years. She taught at community colleges and in adult education for 19 years. In the mid-1970s she became a Certified Medical Assistant, Administrative and Clinical, and from 1979 to 2007 she was also a Certified Medical Transcriptionist.

In 33 years she has authored and co-authored more than 50 books for two major publishers. With Harcourt General (now Reed Elsevier), her books include *Insurance Handbook for the Medical Office, Medical Insurance Billing and Coding: An Essentials Worktext, Medical Keyboarding: Typing and Transcribing Techniques and Procedures, Medical Transcription Guide Do's and Don'ts,* and *Saunders Manual of Medical Transcription.* With Delmar, she has published *Administrative Medical Assisting, Workbook to Accompany Administrative Medical Assisting,* and *Instructor's Manual to Accompany Administrative Medical Assisting.*

In 1977 she received the Outstanding Woman of the Year award from the Business and Professional Women's Club of Oxnard, California. She is listed in a number of Who's Who books. In 2002 the seventh edition of *Insurance Handbook for the Medical Office* won the William Holmes McGuffey Award. In 2003 she and her coauthor, Linda French, won the Text Excellence Award for *Medical Insurance Billing and Coding: An Essentials Worktext,* and in 2004 they won the William Holmes McGuffey Award in Life Sciences for *Administrative Medical Assisting*—both awards from the Text and Academic Authors Association. In June 2005, she was inducted into the Council of Fellows by the Text and Academic Authors Association as a recognition by her peers. She continues to give professional lectures and is a member of a number of national professional associations.

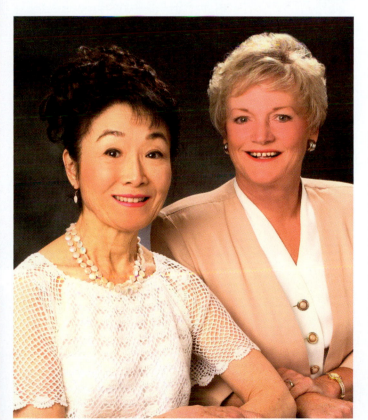

LINDA L. FRENCH, CMA-C, NCICS, CPC

Linda French worked in a physician office setting for 15 years as a clinical and administrative medical assistant, medical insurance biller, and office manager. The practices included chiropractic medicine, obstetrics and gynecology, internal medicine, cardiology, and orthopedics. Certifications she holds are Certified Medical Assistant—Clinical Specialist through the American Association of Medical Assistants, Nationally Certified Insurance Coding Specialist through the National Center for Competency Testing, and Certified Professional Coder through the American Academy of Professional Coders. She is a member of a number of national professional organizations.

She has recently retired from the Medical Insurance Billing and Coding Program at Simi Valley Adult School and Career Institute and has taught a variety of medically related courses at community colleges, private post-secondary institutions, and at private corporations through the University of California at Santa Barbara's UCSB–Extend for the past twelve years.

She has contributed to a number of textbooks, including *Understanding Medical Coding: A Comprehensive Guide* (by Sandra L. Johnson, Delmar, 2000), and is coauthor of *Medical Insurance Billing and Coding: An Essentials Worktext* (W. B. Saunders, 2003). She lectures on occasion, does private consulting work for physicians, and has performed customized employee training for a private billing service.

HOW TO USE THE TEXT

CHAPTER OPENER

Each chapter begins with a list of the objectives to be met through a study of the chapter content and completion of the assignments and exercises in the *Workbook*.

Learning Objectives state the chapter goals; **Performance Objectives in the Textbook** list the step-by-step procedures presented in the text and **Performance Objectives in the** *Workbook* list the exercises that allow learners to practice the job skills.

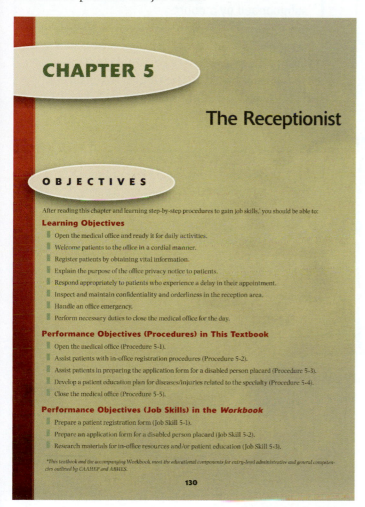

An **Outline** is provided as a roadmap for each chapter, and includes space to write notes as you learn about each topic.

KEY TERMS

biohazard
face sheet
hazardous waste
infectious waste
patient instruction form

patient/practice infor
professionalism
reception room
registration form
universal precautions

The **Key Terms** identify the new vocabulary for the chapter. Each term appears in **color** the first time it is used in the chapter. Each key term is defined in the glossary at the back of the book.

ICONS AND BOXED ELEMENTS

Icons and boxes quickly identify content highlighting critical areas, including Heart of the Health Care Professional, Compliance issues, and Patient Education.

HEART OF THE HEALTH CARE PROFESSIONAL

Service

Patients appreciate a medical assistant who can expedite their care by performing behind-the-scenes tasks. Having information at your fingertips and being able to locate documents quickly are a great service to patients.

Heart of the Health Care Professional emphasizes the customer service responsibilities of the medical practice.

COMPLIANCE

Disclosure of data from a medical record is allowed only after written permission is given by the patient, by the guardian in the case of a minor, or if subpoenaed by a court.

Compliance boxes draw attention to the issues surrounding the protection of personal medical information as mandated by the Health Insurance Portability and Accountability Act (HIPAA).

STOP AND THINK CASE SCENARIOS

Practice Mail Security

Scenario: You are opening mail for Practon Medical Group, Inc., and come across a piece of mail that looks like it has been opened and resealed with tape.

Critical Thinking: How would you proceed? List several things that you might do to verify the safety of the mail.

1. _____
   _____
2. _____
   _____
3. _____
   _____

Stop and Think Scenarios promote critical thinking by asking the learner to exercise reasoning skills in response to scenarios.

PROCEDURES AND EXAMPLES

These elements provide the practical information needed to develop the day-to-day skills required in the medical office.

EXAMPLE 4-4

Avoid "Why" Questions

No: Why are you calling?

Yes: What may I help you with today?

No: Why are you upset?

Yes: Please describe what has upset you.

No: Why don't you call back later?

Yes: Please call back this afternoon.

Example boxes clarify concepts in an easy-to-understand format.

STEP 1 2 3

PROCEDURE 10-3

Record Medication in a Patient's Chart and on a Medication Log

Objective: To record medication in a patient's medical record and on a medication sheet.

Equipment/Supplies: Patient's medical record, progress sheet, medication log sheet, and pen.

Directions: Follow these step-by-step procedures to learn this skill which is presented in the *Workbook* (Job skill 10-5 and 10-8) for practice. The rationale for each step is to comply with CMS documentation guidelines.

1. Write the date of the chart entry.
2. State if it is a new prescription or a refill.
3. Insert the name of the medication.
4. Include the dosage.
5. List the amount given.
6. Write the directions.
7. Sign or initial the chart entry with your professional title.

Step-by-Step Procedures show how tasks are performed efficiently while meeting the privacy requirements of HIPAA. Each Procedure includes the performance objective, equipment and supplies needed, and the sequential steps to achieve the objective.

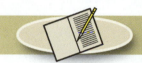

WORKBOOK ASSIGNMENT

To develop competency-based job skills, refer to the *Workbook* and complete the:

- Abbreviation and Spelling Review
- Review Questions
- Critical Thinking Exercises
- Job Skill activities which are outlined at the beginning of this chapter under "Performance Objectives in the *Workbook.*"

At the end of each chapter, the workbook assignment offers the learner the opportunity for hands-on practice to develop specific skills. Content review questions help reinforce the concepts studied in the chapter.

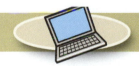

COMPUTER ASSIGNMENT

To review the concepts you have learned in this chapter, insert the *Student Practice* CD-ROM into a computer and work through the *StudyWARE* activities and games. Answer review questions in the practice mode and read the feedback, studying the questions you have missed. Take the chapter quiz until you achieve a minimum score of 90%. Successfully completing the *Critical Thinking Challenge* at the end of this course will help you think through scenarios and develop problem solving skills.

The learner is directed to the *Practice Software CD-ROM* included with the textbook. For each chapter, quizzes or games (hangman, flash cards, concentration, and the championship game) offer a wealth of content to reinforce vocabulary and understanding of concepts.

FOCUS ON CERTIFICATION*

CMA Content Summary
- Medical terminology
- Psychology
- Individual self worth, social and emotional behavior
- Maslow's hierarchy
- Hereditary, cultural, and environmental influences on behavior

RMA Content Summary
- Medical terminology
- Human/Interpersonal relations
- Age-specific responses/support
- Communication methods
- Active listening

Focus on Certification, summarizes key areas for students to study who are preparing to take certification examinations to become a CMA, RMA, or CMAS.

REVIEW **EXAM-STYLE QUESTIONS**

Exam-Style Review Questions, offer a quick review of key points in the same multiple-choice format as seen on certification examinations.

1. Basic elements in the communication cycle include:
   a. sender and receiver
   b. sender, message, and receiver
   c. sender, message, channel, receiver, feedback
   d. sender, message, channel, receiver, questions
   e. sender, message, verbal/nonverbal, receiver, feedback

   avoid something, the defense mechanism is known as:
   a. avoidance
   b. compensation
   c. displacement
   d. rationalization
   e. regression

CMS-1500 CLAIM FORM INSTRUCTIONS AND COMMERCIAL INSURANCE TEMPLATE

Appendix A provides a quick reference to completing the health insurance claim form CMS-1500 for various types of payers (third-party payers, commercial payers, Medicare, and TRICARE). These instructions and template guide learners through the completion of claim forms where accuracy is essential.

APPENDIX A

CMS-1500 (REVISED 08/05) CLAIM FORM FIELD-BY-FIELD INSTRUCTIONS AND A COMMERCIAL INSURANCE TEMPLATE

The following instructions contain information needed to complete the revised CMS-1500 claim form (08/05) using optical character recognition (OCR) guidelines for commercial payers, Medicare (Medicare/Medicaid, Medicare/Medigap, and Medicare Secondary Payer), and TRICARE programs. Information on specific coverage guidelines, program policies, and practice specialties are not included for conciseness and because guidelines for completing claim forms vary at the state and local levels. Consult your local intermediary or commercial insurance carrier for detailed instructions.

To use these instructions, follow these steps:

1. Locate the field number you need instruction for. Field numbers match those on the CMS-1500 claim form.

2. Identify the type of insurance program you are completing the claim for; titles appear in bold face, color-coded capital letters.

3. Read the instructions for specific field requirements. Guidelines for completing *Workbook* exercises are indented and appear in color when there are optional ways of completing a field.

5. Screened areas on insurance templates do not apply to the program examples illustrated and should be left blank. See Figure A-1 and Figures 16-3, 16-6, and 16-9 in Chapter 16.

When generating paper claims from a computer, some software programs insert the commercial carrier's name and address in the top right corner of the CMS-1500 claim form; however, new revised guidelines state that this area is to be left blank. When completing a claim form for the *Workbook* exercises, follow this format to indicate where the claim is to be sent.

Program icons and descriptions are as follows:

ALL THIRD-PARTY PAYERS: Guidelines cover all private insurance companies and all federal and state programs.

COMMERCIAL PAYERS: Guidelines cover all private insurance companies.

MEDICARE: Guidelines cover federal Medicare programs as well as Medicare/Medicaid, Medicare/Medigap, and Medicare Secondary Payer (MSP).

TRICARE: Guidelines cover TRICARE Standard (formerly CHAMPUS), TRICARE Prime, and TRICARE Extra programs.

KEY: **R** = Required fields that must always be completed

C = Conditional fields that may need to be completed depending on the circumstances of the insured

HOW TO USE THE PRACTICE SOFTWARE CD-ROM

STUDYWARE INTERACTIVE SOFTWARE

StudyWARE includes learning activities and quizzes to help you study key concepts from the book and test your comprehension. The activity and quiz content corresponds with each chapter in the book.

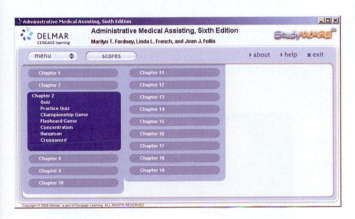

The activities for each chapter include Hangman, Flash Cards, Concentration, Crossword Puzzles, and a Championship game.

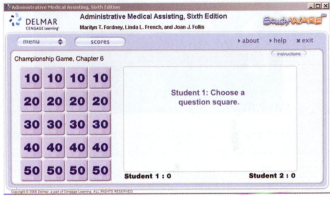

Each chapter contains a quiz made up of multiple choice and true/false questions, that can be taken in practice mode or quiz mode. Practice mode gives immediate feedback after each question and helps improve your mastery of the material. Use Quiz Mode when you are ready to test yourself and keep a record of your score.

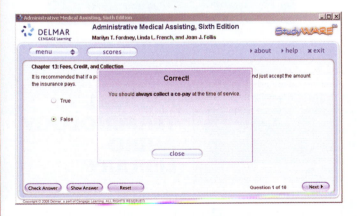

THE CRITICAL THINKING CHALLENGE

In the Critical Thinking Challenge you are on a 3-month externship in a medical office. You will be confronted with a series of situations in which you must use your critical thinking skills to choose the most appropriate action in response to the situation.

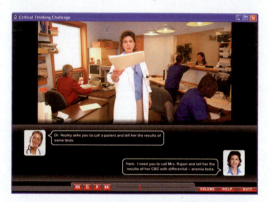

You may consult with members of the office staff and document resources to help you choose the best action, but not all of these resources will be available at all times or always office helpful advice.

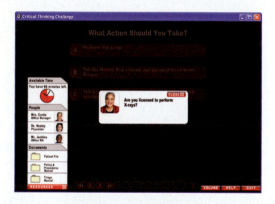

Your decisions will be evaluated in three categories: how your decisions affect the practice, the patient, and your career.

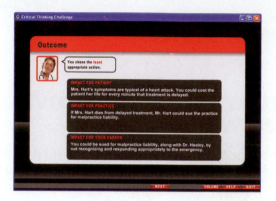

Your goal is to be hired by the medical office as a full-time medical assistant. However, if you show a lack of critical thinking skills that threatens the well-being of the practice and the patients, your externship will be terminated and you will have to start over.

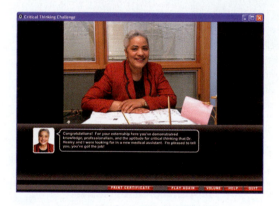

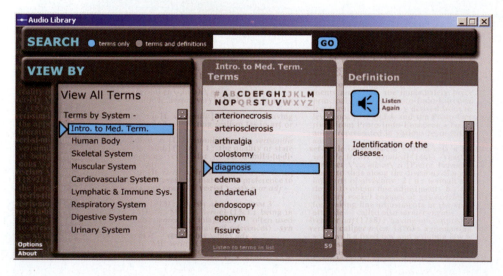

MEDICAL TERMINOLOGY AUDIO LIBRARY

Practice your pronunciation and recognition of medical terms using the Audio Library. You may search for terms by word or body system. Once you've selected a word, it is pronounced correctly and defined on the screen.

UNIT 1

Professional and Career Responsibilities

CHAPTER 1

A Career
As an Administrative
Medical Assistant

OBJECTIVES

After reading this chapter and learning step-by-step procedures to gain job skills,* you should be able to:

Learning Objectives

▌ Demonstrate how customer service skills are applied in the medical office.

▌ Describe the variety of career advantages, employment opportunities, and areas of specialization open to those trained as administrative medical assistants.

▌ Itemize 10 job responsibilities of an administrative medical assistant.

▌ List interpersonal skills needed to be an administrative medical assistant.

▌ Compare and contrast assertive and aggressive behavior.

▌ Discuss patient reactions to health problems and your role when interacting with a distressed patient or family member.

▌ Explain various patient reactions to death and name stages of dying.

▌ Define stress and identify strategies to reduce stress and burnout.

▌ State various components in professionalism.

▌ Understand the importance of and opportunities for certification or registration in your area of study.

▌ Relate how a health care professional can keep current in medical knowledge, policies, procedures, and the latest trends in the medical community.

Performance Objectives (Procedures) in This Textbook

▌ Interpret and accurately spell medical terms and abbreviations (Procedure 1-1).

---

*This textbook and the accompanying Workbook meet the educational components for entry-level administrative and general competencies outlined by CAAHEP and ABHES.

Performance Objectives (Job Skills) in the Workbook

■ Interpret and accurately spell medical terms and abbreviations (Job Skill 1-1).

■ Use the Internet to obtain information on certification and/or registration (Job Skill 1-2).

■ Use the Internet to test your knowledge of anatomy and physiology or medical terminology (Job Skill 1-3).

■ Develop a medical practice survey (Job Skill 1-4).

OUTLINE WITH LECTURE NOTES

Welcome to Administrative Medical Assisting

_____
_____
_____
_____

Customer Service–Oriented Practice

_____
_____
_____
_____

Career Advantages

_____
_____
_____
_____

Employment Opportunities
Administrative Medical Assistant

_____
_____
_____
_____

Clinical Medical Assistant

_____
_____
_____
_____

Administrative Medical Assistant Job Responsibilities

_____
_____
_____
_____

Interpersonal Skills
Listen and Observe

_____
_____
_____
_____

Interest and Concern

_____
_____
_____
_____

Sensitivity to Others

_____
_____
_____
_____

Empathetic and Positive Attitude

_____
_____
_____
_____

Job Motivation

_____
_____
_____
_____

Medical Assistant's Creed

_____
_____
_____
_____

Team Interaction

_____
_____
_____
_____

Understanding Work-Related Emotional and Psychological Problems

Aggressive versus Assertive Behavior

_____
_____
_____
_____

Grieving or Distressed Patients

_____
_____
_____
_____

Death and Dying

_____
_____
_____
_____

Stress and the Health Care Worker

_____
_____
_____
_____

Professionalism

Personal Image

_____
_____
_____
_____

Health and Physical Fitness

_____
_____
_____
_____

Licensure, Accreditation, Certification, and Registration

_____
_____
_____
_____

Keeping Current

_____
_____
_____
_____

KEY TERMS

accreditation
administrative medical assistant
aggressive

American Association of Medical
  Assistants (AAMA)
American Medical Technologists (AMT)

assertive
burnout
certification
Certified Medical Administrative Specialist
     (CMAS)
Certified Medical Assistant (CMA)*
clinical medical assistant
continuing education units (CEUs)
empathy
flextime
hospice

interpersonal skills
licensure
multiskilled health practitioner (MSHP)†
National Center for Competency Testing (NCCT)
National Certified Medical Assistant (NCMA)
National Certified Medical Office Assistant
     (NCMOA)
professionalism
Registered Medical Assistant (RMA)
stress
sympathy

HEART OF THE HEALTH CARE PROFESSIONAL

Service

Motto: "Think with empathy, act through service."

The heart of the health care professional should be directed at serving patients. Regardless of your duties, your approach should be service oriented because service is woven into all areas of medical assisting.

WELCOME TO ADMINISTRATIVE MEDICAL ASSISTING

Welcome to *Administrative Medical Assisting.* You have taken the first step into a world that will stimulate your mind, motivate your curiosity for learning, energize your work ethic, and enliven your spirit so that you will want to contribute something good to today's society.

A typical day in a medical office might include expediting an appointment so an anxious mother can bring in her ill infant, building rapport with a teenager who is afraid to tell the doctor about her promiscuous behavior, calming down a patient who is angry about a bill, reassuring a pregnant mother who is experiencing morning sickness for the first time, or offering a listening ear to a patient who has just received a problematic diagnosis. Every day is different and exciting, and each day offers challenges and opportunities for personal growth and advancement. It is an ever-changing, dynamic field, one where fascinating breakthroughs are taking place in patient care and technology and one in which the rewards always outweigh the task at hand.

Whether you are learning administrative skills to perform as an administrative medical assistant, pharmacy technician, massage therapist, or other type of health care professional, this book will help you learn step-by-step procedures needed to perform a full range of activities to master job skills that will enable you to demonstrate customer service, educate patients, and call upon your newly learned knowledge. As you become proficient in medical terminology and learn guidelines and laws, they will help you manage patient care and create a safe environment to promote healing. You will play an integral role in a medical office as you work closely with physicians or pharmacists and become a lifeline to many patients who rely upon you to educate and assist them.

CUSTOMER SERVICE–ORIENTED PRACTICE

A vibrant medical practice is a service-oriented practice where the elements of customer service are demonstrated by the physician, management team, and all employees. The key to a health care provider's success are satisfied patients, and a willingness to serve patients is an attribute that all health care professionals need—those who do not have this attitude are in the wrong career. Serving means putting someone else's needs before one's own. Patients often interrupt daily work routines, so it is imperative to continually

---

*Effective January 1, 2008, the certified title will change to "Certified Medical Assistant (AAMA)" and the certification abbreviation to "CMA (AAMA)."

†This definition was adopted by the National Multiskilled Health Practitioner Clearinghouse (NMHPC) advisory panel.

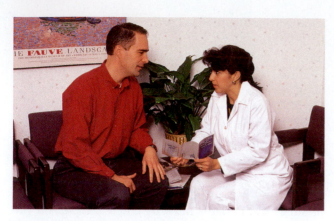

Figure 1-1. Patient education requires skill in communicating instructions to patients in language appropriate to their needs

remind oneself that serving the needs of patients is the reason for going into this profession.

Within "The Heart of the Health Care Professional," as shown at the beginning of each chapter, is a variety of ways to serve patient needs. As you work your way through this text and study the step-by-step procedures that will help you perform new job skills, you will be able to determine different ways that you can provide good customer service. Remember, each employee and patient may have a different idea about what "good" service means. All employees are customer service personnel at the same time they are performing other duties. Any time an employee has contact with a patient it has an effect. As you learn new job skills, the following questions will help you determine where customer service occurs. Always put the patient first when deciding what level of service you would like to provide in the medical practice.

* How is the task that you are performing beneficial to the patient?

* How can this task be accomplished efficiently?

* Are you observing patient interactions, and are you aware if there is patient involvement or problems?

* Has the patient been dealt with in a courteous, respectful, and caring manner?

* What is the desired outcome for the patient?

* Have the patient's expectations been met?

* Have you seized every opportunity to educate the patient?

* Has the patient's confidentiality been protected and their physical safety ensured?

CAREER ADVANTAGES

Medical assisting, both clinical and administrative, attracts individuals with an interest in people and medicine. The skills and knowledge required for this career will last a lifetime, for they are not easily lost. The training prepares the individual for a variety of employment opportunities. Work is available anywhere in the world that medicine is practiced. The training program for medical assistants may be combined with further education and can result in both certification or registration and a college degree. The work is rewarding and challenging because of its variety and everchanging nature. Part-time, **flextime**, and full-time employment are available in a variety of medical settings, as described in Chapter 2.

Flextime offers the employee a range of hours (instead of fixed hours), which may include a split-shift, coming in early, leaving late, or working different times on different days to maximize the efficient running of the office.

EMPLOYMENT OPPORTUNITIES

According to experts in career outlook, a variety of positions in the health care field are estimated to grow up to 60 percent in the next five to ten years. Among those are clerical or administrative jobs in medical assisting and specialty career options such as anesthesiologist assistant; cardiovascular technologist; cytotechnologist; dental assistant; exercise physiology assistant; kinesiology therapist assistant; medication assistant; pharmacy technician; physical

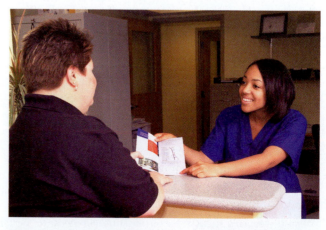

Figure 1-2. An administrative medical assistant often serves a patient by explaining office policies

therapist aid or assistant; occupational therapist assistant, ophthalmic medical technician, technologist, or assistant; orthotist or prosthetist assistant; pathologist assistant; and pediatric medical assistant; some of which offer specialized certifications. Although the terms medical assistant and administrative medical assistant are used primarily in this text, many of the job functions are similar to the clerical duties performed by other health care professionals specializing in these areas.

Administrative Medical Assistant

A career as an administrative medical assistant offers the satisfaction of helping others as well as the opportunity to serve on a health care team. As the population continues to grow, so will the need for health care and the demand for workers in this field. Employment opportunities for those with clerical skills are available in physicians' offices (both solo and group practices), clinics, hospitals, dental offices, foundations, research institutes, public school health service departments, prisons, the armed services, insurance companies, public health departments, medical departments of large companies, Medicare agencies, managed care organizations, offices of nurse practitioners, outpatient facility centers, laboratories, pharmaceutical companies, and medical instrument and supply firms; in the fields of manufacturing, publishing, and teaching; and in freelancing, for example, self-employed insurance biller or medical transcriptionist, now known as a *medical language specialist* (MLS) or *speech recognition technician* (SRT).

Clinical Medical Assistant

The **clinical medical assistant** performs back-office, or clinical duties, such as sterilizing instruments, assisting with minor surgery, giving injections, performing electrocardiograms (ECGs), obtaining vital signs, assisting during physical examinations, maintaining treatment rooms, performing phlebotomy, and doing laboratory procedures. Some states allow medical assistants to take x-rays without licensure, others require that the assistant be licensed.

Those who want active involvement and a great variety of duties can become medical assistants performing both administrative and clinical duties. (Chapter 19 has information on finding a job.)

The clinical duties mentioned however, are beyond the scope of this book.

ADMINISTRATIVE MEDICAL ASSISTANT JOB RESPONSIBILITIES

The position of **administrative medical assistant** requires medical knowledge, organizational and business skills, and the ability to meet accepted performance standards of health care workers. Managed care has had an impact on the way in which medical assistants perform their jobs, and additional paperwork must be completed for preauthorization of tests or surgeries. Patients must be greeted, either on the telephone or on their arrival at the office. Appointments must be carefully scheduled for efficient use of every working moment. Written correspondence involves composing or transcribing dictated letters, and a medical assistant should have a good command of the English language—and sometimes additional languages. Insurance forms need to be completed and submitted either electronically or manually. The mail must be screened for security, opened, sorted, and acted on. Patient's charts must be typed and notes must later be inserted to record the progress of the patient. Medical records must be filed, photocopied for recordkeeping, or faxed to other facilities. Medical and office supplies have to be ordered and an inventory kept. The medical assistant oversees the reception room, making certain that furniture and magazines are in order and plants are fed and watered.

The administrative medical assistant is also in charge of collecting fees, billing patients, maintaining records on accounts receivable, and collecting overdue accounts, so basic mathematic skills are necessary. When invoices arrive, there are checks to be written for payment and records to be maintained on accounts payable. Banking and payroll are two more of the medical assistant's functions.

Computer technology is now routinely found in the medical office, and medical assistants need to know computer programs for word processing, accounting, transmitting insurance claims electronically, obtaining information from the Internet, and communicating via electronic mail with patients and other businesses. A fluency in medical terminology is imperative so communication can take place between the medical assistant and the physician, office manager, coworkers, patients, and outside professionals. Medicolegal knowledge is vital in avoiding medical professional liability suits.

When the physician attends a convention or delivers a lecture the assistant may be responsible for preparing the manuscript and setting up travel arrangements. Hospital admissions need to be arranged as well as surgeries scheduled. Telephone calls come in from patients, laboratories, physicians, representatives of pharmaceutical companies, equipment manufacturers, and the physician's family, and all require expertise and tact. The administrative medical assistant performs a multitude of job skills and is responsible for the smooth functioning of the medical office.

In addition, within the field of administrative medical assisting, it is possible to specialize in medical transcribing, insurance billing, insurance coding, bookkeeping, or some other discipline. Figure 1-3 presents a generic job description for an entry-level administrative medical assistant. Although this is not a complete list of job responsibilities or performance standards, it provides an overview of what an individual does on the job when working in this career. It may also serve as a guideline for an employer who is developing a job description. Subsequent chapters and job skills in the *Workbook* that accompany this text will help the reader achieve the many skills outlined in this job description.

INTERPERSONAL SKILLS

Being a medical assistant is more than a job—it is a career. The career of medical assisting requires many office and **interpersonal skills**. These are exemplary personality characteristics, and include dedication, commitment, integrity, consideration and respect for others, friendliness, genuineness, openness, displaying a sense of warmth and sensitivity, having a positive attitude, and a willingness to learn and take on responsibility. However, the most important personality traits are liking people and being able to get along with other individuals.

Listen and Observe

Listening and *observing* are important tools to use when trying to understand a viewpoint or evaluating a patient's behavior. They allow one to decide what response is best.

Interest and Concern

Patients expect the assistant to act toward them with a sincere desire to help. To show *interest* and *concern* for their welfare acknowledges patients as individuals with special needs. Tone of voice can convey this concern over the telephone.

Sensitivity to Others

It is important to be *sensitive* to a patient's feelings; pretending that feelings do not exist does not serve the patient's best interest. Dealing with ill people who are often cranky, depressed, or angry at their situation makes it even more important to always be pleasant. It requires tact to know what to say in a variety of situations.

Empathetic and Positive Attitude

When an emergency arises, *the ability to follow instructions* is imperative, as is using sound judgment, maintaining a calm demeanor, and displaying **empathy**. Being able to put yourself in the patient's situation or understanding their point of view (Example 1-1) is the basis of empathy; you need not agree with their point of view. **Sympathy**, on the other hand, is displaying feelings that are so close to the person affected that you are similarly affected. This can inhibit you from helping.

A patient's mental state has a strong influence on his or her overall health. A *positive attitude* plays an important role in wellness. A medical assistant with a positive attitude may act as a role model and may help encourage patients who are naturally negative or *pessimistic*.

EXAMPLE 1-1

Empathetic Phrases

"You seem to be upset."
"That must have been painful."
"How disturbing."
"What a frustration."

Job Motivation

Initiative and high *motivation* indicate job satisfaction to the employer, who is, of course, pleased with employees who are content and productive. With effective time management an efficient medical assistant with good organizational abilities can often take over chores from the physician, freeing him or her to spend more time with patients. The medical assistant should be able to prioritize and perform multiple tasks. The ability to keep information confidential honors not only patients' rights but instills trust. Patients need to know they can count on health care workers to be discreet. Everything a medical assistant sees, hears, or reads in the office is privileged information.

ADMINISTRATIVE MEDICAL ASSISTANT JOB DESCRIPTION

Knowledge, skills, and abilities

1. Minimum education level consists of high school graduation or equivalent and (a) a certificate from a one- or two-year medical assisting program emphasizing administrative procedures, (b) an associate degree, or (c) the equivalent in work experience and continuing education.
2. Knowledge of basic medical terminology, math skills, and insurance claims completion; anatomy and physiology, diseases, surgeries, medical specialties, and various administrative procedures as required in areas of responsibility.

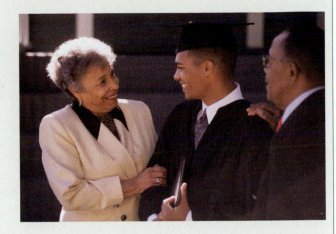

3. Ability to operate computer, scanner, photocopy, facsimile, and calculator equipment.
4. Understand commercial medical software programs, electronic medical record management, and telemedicine.
5. Written and oral communication skills, including grammar, punctuation, and style.
6. Knowledge of and the ability to use procedure and diagnostic codebooks as well as an understanding of computerized coding programs.
7. Ability to key or type a minimum of 45 wpm.
8. Ability to follow directions, participate as part of a team, as well as work independently.

Working conditions

Medical office setting. Sufficient lighting and work space, adjustable chair, and adequate office supplies.

Physical demands

Prolonged sitting, standing, and walking, using computer equipment or a typewriter. Some stooping, reaching, climbing, and bending. Occasional lifting of several pounds to a height of 5 feet. Hearing and speech capabilities necessary to communicate with patients and staff in person and on telephone. Vision capable of viewing computer monitors, calculators, charts, forms, text, and numbers for prolonged periods.

Salary

Employer would list range of remuneration for the position.

Job responsibilities	Performance standards
1. Exhibits an understanding of ethical and medicolegal responsibilities related to protecting the patient, physician, and business.	1.1 Observes policies and procedures related to confidentiality, medical records, and all professional liability matters in a physician's office practice.
	1.2 Meets standards of professional etiquette and ethical conduct.
	1.3 Recognizes and reports potential medicolegal problems to appropriate individuals.
2. Receives incoming telephone calls, places calls, and documents certain types of calls.	2.1 Screens incoming telephone calls properly.
	2.2 Logs telephone calls and documents certain types of phone calls in patient's medical records.
3. Schedules and reschedules appointments.	3.1 Maintains appointment book accurately and keeps it up to date.
	3.2 Obtains precertification, predetermination, and/or preauthorization for services and procedures when necessary.

(continues)

Figure 1-3. A generic job description for an entry-level administrative medical assistant. This is a practical, useful compilation of the basic job responsibilities. It is not a complete list of duties and responsibilities but may be used as a guideline when developing a job description.

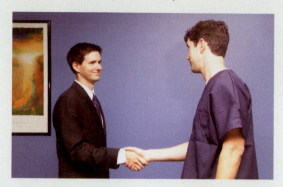

Job responsibilities	Performance standards
4. Greets and receives patients and visitors.	4.1 Receives each patient in a professional manner.
	4.2 Makes eye contact with patients to acknowledge them when otherwise occupied by various duties.
5. Registers new patients and updates existing records.	5.1 Issues proper forms to new and established patient files for good recordkeeping.
	5.2 Reviews documents for accurate and complete information.
	5.3 Collects, photocopies, and returns insurance cards to patients.
6. Screens for security, opens, sorts, and distributes mail, electronic mail, and faxed communications.	6.1 Handles daily mail using proper screening techniques, carefully sorting and distributing it.
	6.2 Faxes using legal guidelines to maintain confidentiality.
	6.3 Communicates by e-mail using proper format and etiquette.
7. Maintains reception room and business office.	7.1 Keeps reception room and business office clean and organized so it presents a professional image at all times.
8. Maintains inventory and orders supplies.	8.1 Reviews inventory and orders office and medical supplies at proper time intervals.
9. Documents prescription refills.	9.1 Logs prescription refills made via telephone, fax, or electronic mail.
10. Prepares charts.	10.1 Obtains patient information data and assembles into a chart using required labels.
11. Files and refiles patient charts and documents.	11.1 Organizes and maintains files efficiently using appropriate filing systems for ease in retrieval.
12. Operates computer and calculator equipment.	12.1 Operates equipment skillfully and efficiently.
	12.2 Evaluates condition of equipment and reports need for repair or replacement.
13. Keys or types correspondence and/or transcribes patient's chart notes.	13.1 Formats and keys correspondence and medical records according to employer's guidelines.
14. Prepares and posts transactions in computer or on daysheets.	14.1 Posts entries into computer or daysheet with appropriate bookkeeping expertise, bringing totals forward.
15. Posts transactions in computer or on ledgers (accounts).	15.1 Posts charges, payments, and adjustments in computer or by hand, calculating a running balance, to patient accounts/ledgers with appropriate accounting expertise as professional services are rendered.
16. Executes banking responsibilities.	16.1 Writes and posts checks correctly.
	16.2 Makes timely bank deposits.
	16.3 Reconciles bank statements using proper bookkeeping procedures.
	16.4 Maintains petty cash fund daily.

Figure 1-3 (*continued*). A generic job description for an entry-level administrative medical assistant

ADMINISTRATIVE MEDICAL ASSISTANT JOB DESCRIPTION
(continued)

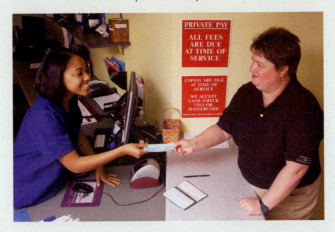

Job responsibilities

17. Collects payments from patients and/or bills patients.

18. Follows up on delinquent accounts and insurance claims.
19. Reconciles daily receipts received.

20. Processes managed-care forms and paperwork.
21. Follows employer's policies and procedures.

22. Enhances knowledge and skills to keep up-to-date.

23. Employs interpersonal expertise to provide good working relationships with patients, employer, employees, and individuals contacting the medical office.

24. Optional: Makes travel arrangements for physician's medical conferences.
25. Optional: Prepares employee payroll.

26. Optional: Completes insurance claim forms.

27. Optional: Performs library research responsibilities and types manuscripts.

Performance standards

17.1 Communicates effectively with patients to collect payments.
17.2 Sends statements at proper intervals using appropriate dun messages.

18.1 Telephones patients for payment of monies owed and and traces insurance claims in a timely manner.
19.1 Reconciles daily monies with appropriate financial expertise.

20.1 Completes appropriate managed-care paperwork with accuracy according to each plan's guidelines.
21.1 Arrives punctually for work and is dependable.
21.2 Answers routine inquiries related to the medical practice, insurance, and so forth.

22.1 Attends continuing education activities on an ongoing basis.
22.2 Obtains current knowledge applicable to all administrative medical assisting duties.

23.1 Works with employer and employees cooperatively as a team.
23.2 Communicates effectively with patients and individuals who come in contact with the medical practice.
23.3 Executes job assignments with diligence and skill.
23.4 Assists other employees when needed.

24.1 Telephones travel agent to arrange for physician's business trips in a timely manner.
25.1 Calculates payroll deductions, writes checks, and maintains financial business records accurately.
25.2 Prepares federal and state forms within time limits.

26.1 Inserts data on insurance claims accurately.
26.2 Codes procedures and diagnoses correctly.
26.3 Transmits claims electronically.

27.1 Formats and types manuscripts according to guidelines of professional association or publication.
27.2 Researches information using the library or Internet.

Figure 1-3 (*continued*). A generic job description for an entry-level administrative medical assistant

Medical Assistant's Creed

Perhaps nothing states personal qualifications better than the Medical Assistant's Creed, which was adopted in 1996 by the American Association of Medical Assistants House of Delegates. It reads:

> *"I believe in the principles and purposes of the profession of medical assisting. I endeavor to be more effective. I aspire to render greater service. I protect the confidence entrusted to me. I am dedicated to the care and well-being of all people. I am loyal to my employer. I am true to the ethics of my profession. I am strengthened by compassion, courage, and faith."*

Team Interaction

Working as a medical assistant requires a *team effort.* The assistant should view every task as important and no job as too small or insignificant to do. One should establish a good working relationship with coworkers, treating them with respect and support. It is also important to get along with supervisors, accept criticism, and show regard for their authority. Those who can join in doing their part, no matter how small, are viewed as a vital part of a team. An assistant should reinforce effective rather than ineffective behavior and, instead of complaining about problems, focus on finding solutions. More staff members lose their positions because of an inability to get along with coworkers than because of an inability to perform office duties. Positive relations are further fostered by handling the special needs of people who are disabled with kindness and courtesy and by remaining composed when dealing with people who are unruly or inconsiderate.

UNDERSTANDING WORK-RELATED EMOTIONAL AND PSYCHOLOGICAL PROBLEMS

Even though there is a spirit of interdependence and teamwork among medical office staff, some frictions and irritations may arise. The medical assistant who is aware of types of behavior and conditions that may cause negative reactions, stress, and burnout, and who understands those reactions can attempt to head off problems before they become a matter of concern and affect productivity.

Aggressive versus Assertive Behavior

Sometimes there is a fine line between being aggressive and assertive. **Aggressive** people are forward, pushy, and overbearing. They may not intend to behave this way as they try to convince or manipulate others, but they often depict a righteous attitude that can lead to confrontation. They come across as if they think they are superior and often make derogative remarks. They may have underlying resentment or anger, which leads to a defensive attitude and behavior. They are usually more concerned with their own agenda than another person's needs.

Being **assertive** reflects professional confidence. The assertive health care worker shows respect for others and does not feel threatened. To be assertive you need to trust your instincts, feelings, and opinions when you are communicating with coworkers and patients. An example of acting assertively based on your instincts (instead of being passive and doing nothing) is when you see a coworker or patient that looks fatigued, speaking up and saying something like, "You look tired. Are you getting enough rest or is something bothering you that I can help you with?" Being assertive takes practice but will help you develop leadership ability and resolve conflicts peacefully.

Grieving or Distressed Patients

Unstable health, poor diagnosis, or a terminal illness will cause a variety of emotions in patients and families, including being subdued or quiet, talkative or inquisitive, loud or volatile, and distraught. The patient may go into emotional shock from being told bad news. People in shock react differently and may cry loudly, sit quietly, or talk incessantly. They may feel like they want to leave the office abruptly or have a sense that they are outside their bodies hearing and watching all of the events. Physically, the patient may start crying uncontrollably (hysteria), have increased breathing, begin trembling, experience a change in skin color, or sit with a blank stare. These are all normal and understandable reactions to upsetting news.

When patients receive unfortunate news about themselves or loved ones it is important to offer assistance and provide follow-up support. Patients may be so upset or shocked that they are unable to remember anything said during such times. Written instructions, health care pamphlets, or other materials about the patient's particular diagnosis should be offered. These should include cause of illness, treatment options, prognosis, and contact sources where additional information may be found. Follow-up appointments should be arranged to further discuss the situation after the patient and family have time to digest the news. When dealing with a distressed patient, follow these guidelines:

1. Be open and honest by asking what they would like to know about the situation.

2. Treat every problem with concern no matter how small it may seem.

3. Offer support through words, actions, and resources.

4. Do not give false reassurances.

Death and Dying

If the patient has a terminal illness, the rights of patients and their families must be considered and honored when making decisions regarding family issues, quality of life, and quantity of life. The assistant should become familiar with *living will* and *durable power of attorney* documents and help the patient complete these, especially in regard to decisions about life support, resuscitation, and artificial feeding. These advanced directives are further discussed and shown in Chapter 3.

The way people face death may include extreme responses, and the health care worker needs to be aware of and respect each patient's reactions. Each person should be allowed the freedom and dignity to have an active part in the choices made. The dying patient should retain some control over financial decisions as well as his or her treatment.

If the survivor of the deceased comes to your office also, you may want to give him or her a list of support groups that offer grief counseling. The listing should contain both religious and secular groups. Demonstrate kindness by sending a sympathy card—your thoughtfulness will be appreciated. Reassure the survivor that he or she does not need to worry about the medical bill right now, and that the billing department will work with them.

Elisabeth Kubler-Ross introduced several stages typical of someone diagnosed with a terminal illness in her book *Death: The Final Stage of Growth.* Each stage takes varying amounts of time and may or may not occur in the order shown. The medical assistant needs to accept the various emotions expressed by patients and their families. Experiencing a loss is

painful, and each person must be allowed to grieve. There is no standard as to how long grief, the readjustment period, or the recovery time lasts. Demonstrating sincere concern with a warm smile and an expression of sympathy will provide comfort to grieving family members.

Stages of Dying

Denial—In the first stage, denial appears to be a defense mechanism and may recur at other times during the dying process. The patient refuses to believe that life is coming to an end and may continue to go about his or her daily activities as if nothing were wrong.

Anger—During the second stage, anger may be directed at anyone and everyone. A common question the patient asks him- or herself is, "Why me?" This is a difficult time for family, friends, and the health care worker.

Bargaining —While experiencing the third stage, the patient may keep information private, so others may or may not be aware of any problem. The patient pleads and tries to negotiate his or her life for a period of time. There may be an upcoming event that the patient may want to experience, expressing, "If I can only last until . . ." The bargaining may be with God, with fate, or with other people.

Depression—At the fourth stage as the illness progresses, so do the pain, weakness, and other symptoms. The patient has trouble denying what is happening. Bargaining is futile and anger begins to

PATIENT EDUCATION

An administrative assistant trained in patient education can help motivate patients and extend the physician's reach and effectiveness. The medical assistant may need to help family members of a patient who is dying by educating them about the stages Kubler-Ross describes in the dying process, that is, denial, anger, bargaining, and depression, before being able to accept the situation. Being open, answering questions, and rendering support will show care and concern. Supplying information about community services and contacting a hospice agency makes evident your regard for their situation.

give way to sorrow. The patient may slip into a depression over the impending loss and separation that are about to be experienced.

Acceptance—During the last stage one hopes the patient has had enough time and has been able to work through the other stages. Being able to *accept* what is *inevitable* will help the patient be at peace as he or she awaits what is about to happen.

Death With Dignity Act

The *Death With Dignity Act* became law in the state of Oregon in 1997. This act allows licensed Oregon physicians (MDs or DOs) to prescribe lethal medications for voluntary self-administration by residents of Oregon. The Oregon Department of Human Services collects information on patients and physicians who participate in death with dignity. A patient must meet the following criteria to be eligible:

1. Eighteen years of age or older

2. Resident of the state of Oregon

3. Able to make and communicate health care decisions for him- or herself

4. Diagnosed with a terminal illness that will lead to their demise within six months

This act does not cover *euthanasia*, in which a doctor injects a patient with a lethal dose of medication. Euthanasia is illegal in every state, including Oregon. Health care workers should take a neutral position when dealing with patients that request "death with dignity." They should respect individual patient decisions and not offer opinions or reflect personal judgment.

Hospice

The **Hospice** Foundation of American is a national program that offers medical care and support to patients and family members dealing with a terminal illness and the loss of a loved one. The hospice staff consists of an interdisciplinary team comprising physicians, nurses, social workers, home health aids, counselors, therapists, chaplains, and trained volunteers on call 24 hours a day, 7 days a week.

The earlier the hospice team enters a terminal case the more help they can provide. All members of the team are trained in dealing with the various aspects a patient and their family face during a life-threatening illness and the dying process. They provide medical equipment, medicine, and pain management, answer questions, acknowledge emotional and psychological needs, promote independence at home, assist with

PATIENT EDUCATION

"Hospice," a term used in the Middle Ages to signify a place where weary pilgrims could stop, rest, and refresh themselves before continuing on with their journey, has become a worldwide movement symbolizing a new kind of care for the terminally ill. In 1967, a British physician, Dr. Cicely Saunders, founded St. Christopher's Hospice in a London suburb and now, in the United State alone, there are over 1,500 hospice programs serving over 100,000 patients a year affiliated with the National Hospice Organization. Hospice information pamphlets are available for educational purposes and the professional staff promotes comfort, safety, meaningful living, and closure for patients and families.

funeral arrangements, and help with the transition that both patients and family members are faced with; their primary focus is on quality of life and the dignity of the dying patient.

Stress and the Health Care Worker

Stress is a condition comprising physical, psychological, and emotional reactions to time constraints and frightening, exciting, confusing, endangering, or irritating circumstances. Coping with illness, life and death issues, and emotionally upset patients on a daily basis can cause stress for the health care worker. A fast-paced office, demands of the physician, lack of private time or space, and interactions with coworkers and other professionals can all add to the pressure and tension that is felt by the medical assistant. Also, personal circumstances such as financial obligations, relationship problems, or the illness or death of a loved one contributes to the emotional overload that sometimes occurs. Even positive events such as marriage, pregnancy, moving, or a promotion can add stress to the mix.

Ongoing stress can be overwhelming and a barrier to communication. As mentioned, events and situations, both positive and negative can cause physical and psychological tension. The less control you have over the event or situation, the more stress is felt. Both physical and mental changes occur when stress levels increase and symptoms such as forgetfulness, stomach pain, shortness of breath, or a nervous tic can appear. It is considered a contributing factor to many disorders society experiences today such as depression, headaches, hormonal changes, hypertension, and lowered resistance to disease. Some emotional components are crying, shouting, drinking alcohol, taking drugs, sleeping more than necessary, and becoming angry.

Coping with Stress

Different people can cope with different amounts of stress. Certain people become motivated by stress while others shut down and cannot function. To deal with stress you first need to be aware of what causes it. The multiple duties of the health care worker and changes in your work environment or home situation are common causes. Frustration may build, anger sets in, and before you know it, you are stressed out. After you identify its root, evaluate the situation to see if you can eliminate some of the sources that are the cause. Confront the problem directly and work toward a solution so you feel as if you have some control over the situation. Cultivate healthy relationships, take regular breaks at work, and schedule fun outings to help take your mind off of the more serious side of life. Use the following guidelines to help manage stress in the workplace:

PATIENT EDUCATION

Educating patients is part of the service performed by a medical assistant. He or she is in a prime position to orient the patient to office policies so that information is gathered, schedules are kept, and treatment is uninterrupted. The medical assistant also relays information to patients about treatment and medications, test results, pre- and postoperative care, personal and physical safety, and community services. He or she may help the physician educate patients to take better care of themselves with respect to smoking cessation, eating a balanced diet, maintaining optimal weight, increasing exercise, hygiene, body mechanics, and learning methods for stress management. In some medical practices, the medical assistant may teach the patient using health-related educational materials, such as brochures, videotapes, or other visual aids (Refer back to Figure 1-1).

- Prepare to handle the responsibilities of your job by practicing skills. Accept your limitations and do not be afraid to acknowledge when you do not know how to do something. Instead, ask for help, get adequate instruction, and accept advice.

- Learn organizational skills, plan ahead, and prioritize tasks.

- Set realistic goals and remember there are always choices even when you feel otherwise.

- Practice relaxation techniques, such as deep breathing or focusing on something entirely different.

- Exercise your sense of humor; laughter is the best cure for tension.

- Do not overreact to problematic situations, instead be creative in exercising problem solving skills and talk over difficult work situations with your supervisor. Always be open to share ideas and receive suggestions.

- Create and rely on a good support system. Whether it be family, friends, or coworkers share your feelings and talk over your problems without complaining.

- Think positive and strive for a wholesome balance in your life. Monitor your own health by getting regular check ups, eating a balanced diet, resting adequately, exercising consistently, and relaxing regularly, taking quiet time to be alone, reflect, and reenergize your batteries.

- Seek help if necessary from professionals or support groups.

By recognizing stress, understanding its common causes, and learning to apply techniques to reduce it, you can learn to cope with it, reduce its effects on your life, and live a healthier, happy life. You can also help educate patients about stress management.

Burnout

Burnout is a term used to describe a condition that results from too much or too little stress. It may occur suddenly or develop slowly over months. Burnout occurs most often in the "helping" professions where there may be erratic hours and emergencies involving critically ill people and death. In attempting to cope, a person withdraws from interaction with others and experiences fear, anxiety, and depression, with resulting decreased energy and productivity.

The medical assistant who has a voice in the decision-making process in an office is less likely to experience burnout. Routines might be rearranged to relieve boredom or slowed down to limit physical and mental pressure. Assignments could be varied to ensure skillful backup when an employee is absent. Remember the preceding suggestions and follow the guidelines to help relieve stress from your life and avoid burnout.

PROFESSIONALISM

It is important for a medical assistant to develop and maintain a professional image and attitude as he or she performs the task assigned. The ability to make independent decisions, to take initiative, to respect confidentiality, and to carefully follow the physician's advice will project **professionalism** and establish the assistant as an efficient administrator. A professional demonstrates confidence because he or she is well trained and has mastered the skills of a given profession. All the personal attributes previously discussed are connected to professionalism, as is having the ability to adapt to new situations, being dependable and responsible in the workplace, and being emotionally stable. A professional aspires to be a better person, to reach a higher standard, to demonstrate personal integrity, and to behave according to the ethical standards of the profession. A professional uses diplomacy in dealing with difficult patients and situations and is honest and trustworthy—always respecting the patient's dignity. The term "professionalism" projects an image in the minds of all those who interact with the health care worker. This image includes both how the people present themselves and how they conduct themselves.

Personal Image

A well-groomed medical assistant conveys a professional image and creates the impression that the office procedures and medical care are of good quality, whereas a disheveled appearance suggests the office may be run carelessly. Basically, the image should be that of a professional business executive, conservative and stylish but not trendy. The dress code is usually set by the physician-employer. The medical assistant should observe other health care professionals at the top of their career ladders, and then upgrade his or her image to that level.

Female Grooming

The ideal standard dress for the medical assistant is to dress as the equivalent of physicians, that is, a business suit with the jacket removed and a white laboratory coat substituted.

One study found that when the physician's staff dressed professionally, like the physicians, there was less discrepancy in salaries. The same was true about how physicians and staff addressed one another. If the staff called the physician "Doctor" and the physician called the staff by first names, there was a greater discrepancy in salary. Keep this in mind when going for a job interview.

The next most professional look is a uniform, then pants and top or jacket or jumpsuit. In some office settings, it is all right to wear surgical scrub suits (scrubs). If a medical facility, such as a pediatrician's office, prefers the staff to wear colors other than white, choose jewel-tone colors or deeper muted colors (Figure 1-4).

For female medical assistants, it is equally important to wear makeup and a hairstyle that flatter the individual. The hair should be clean and neatly styled. Eye makeup should be subdued for the day. Fingernails should be carefully manicured. Do not wear long artificial nails, and do not paint on designs or have rhinestones glued to fingernails. It has been found that long nails not only interfere with various job tasks but they also become a hiding place for dangerous bacteria. Nail polish may be considered as part of a professional image if a clear or light pink polish is selected.

Jewelry also is considered part of the professional image for women, but it must be kept simple; earrings should not be the dangling type. A professional emblem, certification pin, or identification pin worn on the laboratory coat or uniform further identifies the medical assistant as a staff member. A certification pin should also be worn at professional functions. Consult the employer for office policy regarding body piercing and tattoos. Although perfume can be worn, use it in small amounts because it can be offensive and cause allergic reactions in some patients.

Male Grooming

Male medical assistants' hair should be clean, styled, and off the collar. Beards, mustaches, or sideburns should be neatly trimmed. A uniform may consist of white or colored slacks with a white or light-colored shirt worn with optional tie. Over this, a jacket, pullover top, or zippered or cardigan jacket may be worn. If preferred, a medium-length or classic-long labo-

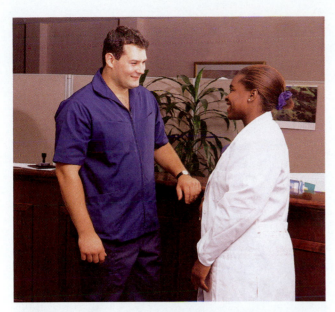

Figure 1-4. Male and female medical assistants projecting a clean, fresh, and professional image with hairstyling in good taste

ratory coat may be worn over street clothes. Shoes should be unsoiled and polished, with clean shoelaces. Limit jewelry to a ring or wedding band, professional pin, and identification badge. Personal cleanliness is of utmost importance, including daily bathing, use of deodorant, and good oral hygiene.

Health and Physical Fitness

The medical assistant should exemplify health and physical fitness. Some employers avoid hiring smokers and those who are extremely overweight because of increased health and life insurance premiums. A certain amount of physical exercise (walking, jogging, biking, swimming) is necessary to diminish stress and keep physically fit for those who have sedentary jobs. Chapter 5 discusses this subject further.

LICENSURE, ACCREDITATION, CERTIFICATION, AND REGISTRATION

Licensure is credentialing sanctioned by a state's legislature (the government), which passes laws making it illegal for an individual who is not licensed to engage in activities of a licensed occupation. For example, Registered Nurses take state boards to become licensed in the state in which they would like to prac-

tice nursing. There are no states that require a license to work as a medical assistant, although limited permits are issued in some states for invasive procedures such as injections and venipuncture or limited radiology services.

In South Dakota, a law was passed that requires that a medical assistant be a graduate from an accredited medical assisting program and register with the state board of medical and osteopathic examiners. Check with your local Department of Health or the State's Medical Examiners office to determine if there is a current law or pending legislation regarding your profession.

Accreditation can mean either meeting a state standard or being evaluated and recognized by a national organization. In Arizona, a medical assistant must have either graduated from a school accredited by the Commission of Accreditation of Allied Health Education Programs (CAAHEP) or be enrolled in an internal program at the work site that offers similar CAAHEP-accredited training. In other states, usually the minimum education requirement for the position of medical assistant is high school.

Most physicians prefer to hire a person with some education in medical terminology. Vocational and commercial schools offer 6 to 18 months of training in medical assisting. Many community colleges offer an associate-degree program that provides a broad foundation of clinical and administrative skills either separately or combined. Medical assisting courses usually cover medical terminology, medicolegal topics, medical transcription, computer training, business English, business correspondence, accounting, business math, psychology, biologic sciences, laboratory techniques, and a variety of clinical skills such as venipuncture, injections, and the autoclaving and selection of instruments using aseptic technique to assist in minor surgeries.

Certification is not controlled by the government. It implies that an individual has met either minimum competency requirements or a level of excellence in the area defined. It is based on voluntary action by a professional organization that develops a system to grant recognition to those practitioners who meet a stated level of training and experience. Once certification is attained, most organizations require recertification through a continuing education process in which the health care professional is awarded **continuing education units (CEUs)**. One hour of continuing education (1 CEU) equals one hour of activity (contact hour).

Because a medical assistant is a **multiskilled health practitioner (MSHP)** cross-trained to provide more than one function, often in more than one discipline, it is possible to gain certification in more than one area, e.g., phlebotomist, ECG technician, medical insurance billing specialist, or professional coder.

The **American Association of Medical Assistants (AAMA)** offers a national certification examination to graduates of medical assisting programs trained in both administrative and clinical areas that are accredited by CAAHEP, or Accrediting Bureau of Health Education Schools (ABHES). By passing this examination, the examinee receives the title **Certified Medical Assistant (CMA)**.*

The **National Center for Competency Testing (NCCT)** is an independent certifying agency that validates the competence of a person's knowledge in different areas of the medical profession through examination. They assess a candidate's performance against predetermined standards that are created by a job analysis survey. Medical assistants who pass the competency test receive the designation **National Certified Medical Assistant (NCMA)**. Students who focus on the administrative side of medical assisting can sit for a specialized exam, and after passing they will receive the designation **National Certified Medical Office Assistant (NCMOA)**. Following are some of the other areas of certification offered:

- National Registered Bookkeeper (NRB)
- National Certified ECG Technician (NCET)
- National Certified Pharmacy Technician (NCPhT)
- National Certified Phlebotomy Technician (NCPT)
- National Certified Insurance & Coding Specialist (NCICS)
- National Certified Patient Care Technician (NCPCT)

Registration is similar to certification and may be done on a state or national level. The **American Medical Technologists (AMT)** offers a **Registered Medical Assistant (RMA)** certification examination to any one of the following categories:

1. Students who graduate from a medical assisting program at a school accredited by

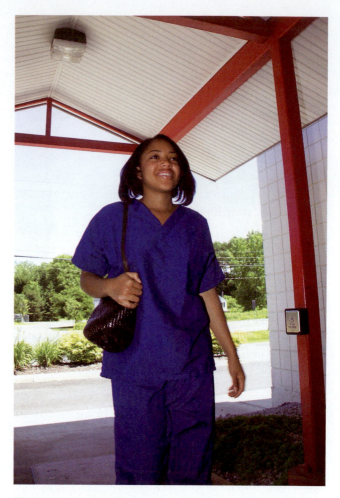

Figure 1-5. Medical assistant arriving at work

    the Accrediting Bureau of Health Education Schools (ABHES).

2. Individuals with five years of verified work experience.

3. Students who complete a medical assisting course in a school holding national accreditation recognized by the Council on Post-Secondary Accreditation (COPA) and are employed as a medical assistant for one year.

The AMT also offers a national examination for the administrative assistant who, when passing the exam, receives the credential of **Certified Medical Administrative Specialist (CMAS)**.

A number of certifications are available on a national level, depending on specialty, for example, medical transcription, diagnostic and procedural cod-

---

*Effective January 1, 2008, the certified title will change to "Certified Medical Assistant (AAMA)" and the certification abbreviation to "CMA (AAMA)."

ing, office management, and so on. Table 1-1 provides a list of certified/registered titles with abbreviations, a brief description of how to obtain the certification/registration, and the mailing address, Web site, and e-mail address to obtain more information.

Standarized testing is another way to portray a professional image. When a health care worker receives such accreditation employers and the public can be assured that an academic standard is met and that the person holds a certain body of knowledge.

Many of these organizations offer student membership and may have regional chapters.

KEEPING CURRENT

A job in a medical office is never static, always stimulating, and constantly challenging. One must be able to adapt to change. To keep up with technology and current practices, it is important for the admin-

istrative medical assistant to read professional publications, attend educational seminars, and research information on the Internet. Some publications currently of value to the administrative medical assistant are listed in Resources at the end of this chapter.

Another way to keep up-to-date in medical matters is through a membership in a professional organization, such as one of those listed in Table 1-1. State and local membership is usually automatic with national membership; there are monthly meetings, bulletins and newsletters, educational seminars and workshops, and national and state conventions.

Networking with peers at workshops and conventions is an additional way to keep in tune with the medical environment outside of your office. By building relationships with other office personnel, you can share ideas, increase your knowledge, and receive support when implementing new laws and regulations that are mandated by the government.

Table 1-1. Certification and Registration

Title and Abbreviation	Description to Obtain Certification or Registration	Professional Association Mailing Address and Telephone Number	Web Site and E-Mail Addresses
Certified Bookkeeper (CB)	Self-study program and employment experience; pass three tests	American Institute of Professional Bookkeepers 6001 Montrose Road, Ste 500 Rockville, MD 20852 (800) 622-0121	http://www.aipb.org info@aipb.org
Certified Coding: • Associate (CCA) • Specialist (CCS) • Specialist—Physician based (CCS-P)	Self-study program; pass certification examination	American Health Information Management Association 233 N. Michigan Ave, Ste. 2150, Chicago, IL 60601-5800 (800) 335-5535	http://www.ahima.org info@ahima.mhs .compuserve.com
Certified Health Care Privacy (CHP)	Self-study program; pass certification examination	American Health Information Management Association 233 N. Michigan Ave, Ste. 2150, Chicago, IL 60601-5800 (800) 335-5535	http://www.ahima.org info@ahima.mhs .compuserve.com
Certified Health Care Financial Professional (CHFP)	60 hours college/university and complete core examination and one specialty examination within 2-year period	Healthcare Financial Management Association (HFMA) 2 Westbrook Corporate Center, Ste 700 Westchester, IL 60154-5700 (800) 252-4362	http://www.hfma.org webmaster@hfma.org

(continues)

Table 1-1 (*continued*). Certification and Registration

Title and Abbreviation	Description to Obtain Certification or Registration	Professional Association Mailing Address and Telephone Number	Web Site and E-Mail Addresses
Certified Electronic Claims Professional (CECP) Certified Claims Assistant Professional (CCAP)	Self-study program; pass certification examination	Alliance of Claims Assistance Professionals 873 Brentwood Drive West Chicago, IL 60185 (877) 275-8765	http://www.claims.org askacap@charter.net
Certified Healthcare Billing and Management Executive (CHBME)	Complete comprehensive program; pass proficiency test	Healthcare Billing and Management Association 1540 South Coast Highway, Suite 203 Laguna Beach, CA 92651 (877) 640-4262	http://www.hbma.com info@hbma.com
Certified in Health Care Compliance (CHC)	Have work experience, continuing education, and pass examination	Health Care Compliance Association 6500 Barrie Rd, Ste. 250 Minneapolis, MN 55435 (888) 580-8373	www.hcca-info.org info@hcca-info.org
Certified Health Care Privacy (CHP)	Eligibility requirements and pass examination	American Health Information Management Assn. (AHIMA) 233 N. Michigan Ave #2150 Chicago, IL 60601-7349 (800) 335-5535	www.ahima.org info@ahima.mhs .compuserv.com
Certified in Health Care Privacy and Security	Pass CHP and CHS examinations	American Health Information Management Assn. (AHIMA) 233 N. Michigan Ave #2150 Chicago, IL 60601-7349 (800) 335-5535	www.ahima.org info@ahima.mhs .compuserv.com
Certified in Health Care Security (CHS)		American Health Information Management Assn. (AHIMA) 233 N. Michigan Ave #2150 Chicago, IL 60601-7349 (800) 335-5535	www.ahima.org info@ahima.mhs .compuserv.com
Certified Information Systems Security Professional (CISSP)	Pass examination and submit endorsement form	International Information Systems Security Certifications Consortium, Inc. 2494 Bayshore Blvd., Ste.201 Dunedin, FL 34698 (888) 333-4458	www.isc2.org lsc2@asestores.com
Systems Security Certified Practitioner (SSCP)		International Information Systems Security Certifi- cations Consortium, Inc. 2494 Bayshore Blvd., Ste.201 Dunedin, FL 34698 (888) 333-4458	www.isc2.org lsc2@asestores.com

Table 1-1 (*continued*). Certification and Registration

Title and Abbreviation	Description to Obtain Certification or Registration	Professional Association Mailing Address and Telephone Number	Web Site and E-Mail Addresses
Certified Medical Assistant (CMA)*	Graduate from accredited medical assisting program; apply to take national certifying examination	American Association of Medical Assistants 20 North Wacker Drive Chicago, IL 60606 (800) 228-2262	http://www.aama-ntl .org visit Web site for e-mail address
Certified Medical Biller (CMB)	Pass two-hour examination written for physician's office billers and other outpatient facilities	American Association of Medical Billers PO Box 44614 Los Angeles, CA 90044-0614	http://www.billers .com/aamb AAMB@aol.com
Certified Medical Billing Specialist (CMBS)	Pass three-hour examination		
Certified Medical Billing Specialist (CMBS)	Complete six courses and provide evaluation of billing performance by supervisor	Medical Association of Billers 2701 N. Tenaya Way Suite 190 Las Vegas, NV 89128 (702) 240-8519	http://www .physicianswebsites .com mabhelp@aol.com
Certified Medical Office Manager (CMOM)	Examination for supervisors or managers of small-group and solo practices	Professional Association of Health Care Office Managers 461 East Ten Mile Road Pensacola, FL 32534-9712 (800) 451-9311	http://www.pahcom .com pahcom@pahcom .com
Certified Medical Practice Executive (CMPE) • Nominee (1st level) • Certification (2nd level) • Fellow (3rd level) project or thesis	1st level: Eligible group managers join; membership/nominee 2nd level: Complete six- to seven-hour examination 3rd level: Mentoring	Medical Group Management Association, American College of Medical Practice Executives (affiliate) 104 Inverness Terrace East Englewood, CO 80112 (877) 275-6462	http://www.mgma .com/acmpe acmpe@mgma.com
Certified Medical Reimbursement Specialist (CMRS)	Self-study program; successfully pass 18 sections of examination	American Medical Billing Association 4297 Forrest Drive Sulphur, OK 73086 (580) 622-2624	http://www.ambanet .net/cmrs.htm larry@brightok.net
Certified Medical Transcriptionist (CMT)	Self-study program and successfully pass written and practical examinations offered by Medical Transcription Certification Commission (MTCC)	American Association for Medical Transcription 100 Sycamore Avenue Modesto, CA 95354-0550 (800) 982-2182	http://www.aamt.org aamt@amt.org

(continues)

Effective January 1, 2008, the certified title will change to "Certified Medical Assistant (AAMA)" and the certification abbreviation to "CMA (AAMA)."

Table 1-1 (continued). Certification and Registration

Title and Abbreviation	Description to Obtain Certification or Registration	Professional Association Mailing Address and Telephone Number	Web Site and E-Mail Addresses
Certified Patient Account Technician (CPAT) Certified Clinic Account Technician (CCAT) Certified Clinic Account Manager (CCAM)	Complete self-study course; pass standard examination administered twice yearly	American Association of Healthcare Administrative Management National Certification Examination Program 11240 Waples Mill Road, Suite 200 Fairfax, VA 22030 (703) 281-4043	http://www.aaham.org debra@statmarketing .com
Certified Professional Coder (CPC) Certified Professional Coder– Apprentice (CPC-A) Certified Professional Coder– Hospital (CPC-H)	Independent study program; examination approximately five hours (CPC) and eight hours (CPC-H) in length. No practical experience for CPC-A. Two years experience for CPC.	American Academy of Professional Coders 2480 South 3850 West #8 Salt Lake City, UT 84120 (800) 626-CODE	http://www.aapcnatl .org aapc@worldnet.att .net
Healthcare Reimbursement Specialist (HRS)	Successfully complete open-book examination	National Electronic Biller's Alliance 2226-A Westborough Blvd. #504 South San Francisco, CA 94080 (650) 359-4419	http://www.nebazone .com mmedical@aol.com
National Certified Insurance and Coding Specialist (NCICS)	Graduate from an insurance program; sit for certification examination given by independent testing agency at many school sites across the nation	National Center for Competency Testing 7007 College Blvd., Suite 750 Overland Park, KS 66211 (800) 875-4404	http://www.ncctinc .com staff@ncctinc.com
Registered Medical Assistant (RMA) Certified Medical Administrative Specialist (CMAS)	Sit for certification exam	America Medical Technologists (AMT) 710 Higgins Road Park Ridge, IL 60068-5765 (800) 275-1268	http://www.amt1.com amtmail@aol.com
Registered Medical Coder (RMC)	Yearly correspondence program governed by the National Coding Standards Committee and pass an examination	Medical Management Institute 11405 Old Roswell Rd Alpharetta, GA 30004-5724 (800) 334-5724	http://www .codingbooks.com dan.mistretta@archp .org
Utilization Review Accreditation Commission (URAC) Accredited Consultant	Application	Utilization Review Accreditation Commission 1220 L Street, NW, Ste 400 Washington, DC 20005 (202) 216-9010	www.urac.org ita@urac.org

PROCEDURE 1-1

STEP 1 2 3

Interpret and Accurately Spell Medical Terms and Abbreviations

Objectives: To enhance knowledge of medical terminology, interpret abbreviations, and accurately spell medical terms while reading patients' chart notes.

Equipment/Supplies: One sheet of white 8½" by 11" typing paper and pen or pencil.

Directions: Follow these step-by-step procedures, which include rationales, to learn this job skill. Job Skill 1-1 and additional exercises entitled "Abbreviation and Spelling Review" are presented at the beginning of each chapter of the *Workbook* so that you can practice this skill.

1. Read a patient's medical record.

2. Identify unfamiliar medical terms.

3. Use a medical dictionary to locate and learn the meanings of each medical term.

4. Break the term apart into word components and memorize the spelling of each medical term.

5. Find abbreviations in each chart/progress note that you do not understand or appear unfamiliar to you.

6. Decode/define each abbreviation (See Part V of the *Workbook*).

STOP AND THINK CASE SCENARIO

Listen and Observe

Scenario: A patient who is usually cheerful comes into the office and sits in the corner not talking to anyone. She is wearing a grumpy look and her posture is one of dejection.

Critical Thinking: What would you think and say to her?

_____

_____

_____

STOP AND THINK CASE SCENARIO

Positive Attitude

Scenario: A patient arrives and you ask him how he is. He responds, "Well, I won't know until I find out my test results." He also says, "The numbers probably haven't changed and I'll have to continue taking all of these pills."

Critical Thinking: Think about each statement and tell how you would respond, considering whether his statement(s) and your responses are positive, negative, or neutral.

_____

_____

_____

STOP AND THINK CASE SCENARIO

Patient Education

Scenario: Mary Lou is a three-year-old whose mother has brought her in to see the doctor for an earache. She is crying softly and wiggling around in her mother's arms. Her mother tells her to hold still and stop crying, that the doctor is going to fix her, and there is nothing to cry about.

Critical Thinking:

a. How can you tactfully educate Mary Lou's mother about her daughter's reactions?

_____

_____

b. How would you inform the mother and Mary Lou about what the physician will be doing?

_____

_____

STOP AND THINK CASE SCENARIO

Aggressive versus Assertive Response

Scenario: You have been given the assignment of directing Mrs. Hartley, a very angry and upset patient to the laboratory to have a test done and telling her that the results will not be ready until tomorrow afternoon. You feel like saying, "You need to go to ABC Laboratory to have this test done. You will not be able to find out the results until tomorrow afternoon; someone will probably call you then."

Critical Thinking: Try to reword what you would say to the patient so that it is assertive instead of aggressive.

_____

_____

_____

_____

_____

_____

FOCUS ON CERTIFICATION*

CMA Content Summary
- Medical terminology
- Understanding emotional behavior
- Professionalism
- Empathy

RMA Content Summary
- Medical terminology
- Scope of practice
- Credentialing requirements
- Ethics

*This textbook and the accompanying Workbook meet the entry-level administrative and general competencies for the CMA outlined by the AAMA Examination Content Outline and Role Delineation Study and for the RMA and CMAS outlined by the AMT Competencies and Examination Specifications (see Competency Grid in Appendix B).

- Professional development and conduct
- Interpersonal skills
- Instructing patients

CMAS Content Summary
- Medical terminology
- Professionalism
- Community referral resources

REVIEW   EXAM-STYLE QUESTIONS

1. Among a medical assistant's interpersonal skills, the most important personality trait is:

   a. dedication

   b. consideration and respect for others

   c. displaying a sense of warmth and sensitivity

   d. liking people and being able to get along with other individuals

   e. dedication to the profession of medical assisting

2. Being able to put yourself in the patient's situation is commonly referred to as:

   a. sympathy

   b. empathy

   c. having a positive attitude

   d. identification

   e. commiseration

3. The Medical Assistant's Creed was adopted in:

   a. 1954

   b. 1966

   c. 1996

   d. 1998

   e. 2000

4. Being assertive means to:

   a. respect others and reflect professional confidence

   b. be aggressive in your approach with people

   c. convince and manipulate

   d. concentrate on your own agenda

   e. confront with a righteous attitude

5. Grieving or distressed patients tend to be:

   a. subdued or quiet

   b. talkative or inquisitive

   c. loud and volatile

   d. distraught

   e. all of the above

6. Although patients do not always go through the stages of dying in the order presented, the fourth stage is usually:

   a. anger

   b. bargaining

   c. depression

   d. acceptance

   e. denial

7. The first thing you need to do in order to deal with stress is to:

   a. act out anger so it does not bottle up inside you

   b. be aware of what causes it

   c. take time off work

   d. not take your job so seriously

   e. tell the office manager so he/she can lighten your work load

8. Using diplomacy in dealing with difficult patients is a/an:

   a. sign of professionalism

   b. personal characteristic

   c. personal attribute

   d. interpersonal skill

   e. sign of having a high intellect

9. Determine the correct statement regarding the medical assistant's personal image and grooming.

    a. The dress code in a medical office is usually set by a consensus of the employees.

    b. No jewelry should be worn by men or women in the health care field.

    c. There is *no* connection between the medical assistant's personal image and the way the patient perceives how the office is run.

    d. There *is* a connection between the medical assistant's personal image and the way the patient perceives how the office is run.

    e. No beards, mustaches, or sideburns should be worn by men in the health care field.

10. Select the correct statement regarding licensure, accreditation, certification, and registration.

    a. Licensure, accreditation, certification, and registration all mean the same thing.

    b. Certification is controlled by the government.

    c. Standarized testing is a way of portraying a professional image.

    d. Licensure is required of medical assistants in all states.

    e. Certification is typically obtained on the state level.

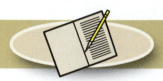

WORKBOOK ASSIGNMENT

To develop competency-based job skills, refer to the *Workbook* and complete the:

- Abbreviations and Spelling Review
- Review Questions

- Critical Thinking Exercises
- Job Skill activities, which are outlined at the beginning of this chapter under "Performance Objectives in the *Workbook*."

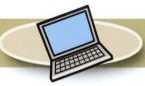

COMPUTER ASSIGNMENT

To review the concepts you have learned in this chapter, insert the *Student Practice* CD-ROM into a computer and work through the *StudyWARE* activities and games. Answer the questions in the practice mode and read the feedback, studying the questions you have missed. Take the chapter quiz until you achieve a minimum score of 90 percent. Successfully completing the *Critical Thinking Challenge* at the end of this course will help you think through scenarios and develop problem solving skills.

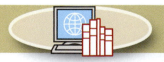

RESOURCES

To obtain answers to questions related to certification and become a member of a professional organization, refer to the data listed in Table 1-1. For additional information on health careers and job opportunities, visit the Web sites listed in Resources at the end of Chapter 19, Seeking a Position As an Administrative Medical Assistant.

Certification Review Books

American Association of Medical Assistants CMA Practice Exams:
> Anatomy and Physiology and Medical Terminology
> Web site: http://aama-ntl.org/

Appleton & Lange's Review for the Medical Assistant
> Tom Palko and Hilda Palko
> Appleton & Lange
> PO Box 120041
> Stamford, CT 06912-0041
> (800) 423-1359

The Medical Assisting Examination Guide, A Comprehensive Review for Certification
> Karen Lane
> F. A. Davis
> 1915 Arch Street
> Philadelphia, PA 19103-9954
> (800) 323-3555
> Web site: http://www.fadavis.com

Medical Assisting Review Manual
> Marcia Perkins Hemby
> Prentice Hall Publishing
> Upper Saddle River, NJ 07458
> (800) 223-1360
> Web site: http://www.pearsoned.com

Medical Assisting Review: Passing the CMA and RMA Exams, 2nd ed.
> Jahangir Moini
> McGraw Hill Company, Inc.
> 1221 Avenues of the Americas
> New York, NY 10020
> (800) 722-4726
> Web site: http://www.books.mcgraw-hill.com

Delmar Cengage Learning's Medical Assisting Exam Review: Preparation for the CMA, RMA, and CMAS Exams, 2nd ed.
> J.P. Cody and Cathy Kelly Arney
> Delmar Learning
> 5 Maxwell Drive
> Clifton Park, NY 12065-2919
> (518) 348-2300
> Web site: http://www.delmarlearning.com

MEPC: Medical Assistant, Examination Review
> LaVerne Dreizen and Thelma Audet
> McGraw Hill
> PO Box 120041
> Stamford, CT 06912-0041
> (800) 722-4726
> Web site: http://www.books. mcgraw-hill.com
> Click on "medical"

Internet

Death With Dignity Act
> Web site: http://www.oregon.gov/DHS/ph
> Search: topics—death with dignity

Newsletters

Conomikes Reports on Medical Practice Management (monthly newsletter)
> Conomikes Associates, Inc.
> 12233 W. Olympic Blvd.
> Los Angeles, CA 90064
> (800) 421-6512
> Web site: http://www.conomikes.com

The Doctor's Office (monthly newsletter)
> HC PRO
> PO Box 1168
> Marblehead, MA 01945
> (800) 650-6787
> Web site: http://www.hcpro.com

Vital Signs (quarterly)
> RMA Newsletter
> 710 Higgins Road
> Park Ridge, IL 60068
> (800) 275-1268

Professional Magazines

Advance for Health Information Professionals (biweekly)
> Merion Publications, Inc.
> 2900 Horizon Dr.
> Box 61556
> King of Prussia, PA 19406-0956
> (800) 355-1088
> Web site: http://www.advanceweb.com

CMA Today (Certified Medical Assistant) (bimonthly)
> American Association of Medical Assistants, Inc.
> 20 North Wacker Drive, Suite 1575
> Chicago, IL 60606-2903
> (800) 228-2262
> Web site: http://www.ama_ntl.org/cmatoday

Compassion and Choices
> Choice in Dying
> PO Box 101810
> Denver, CO 08250
> (800) 247-7421
> Web site: http://www.compassionandchoices.org

For the Record
    Magazine for Health Information Professionals
    Great Valley Publishing Company, Inc.
    3801 Schuylkill Rd
    Spring City, PA 19475
    (800) 278-4400
    Web site: http://www.greatvalleypublishing.com
Journal of the American Association for Medical Transcription (bimonthly)
    American Association for Medical Transcription
    PO Box 576187
    Modesto, CA 95354
    (800) 982-2182
    Web site: http://www.AAMT.org
Medical Economics (monthly magazine)
    Advanstar Publications
    131 West 1st Street
    Duluth, MN 55802
    (877) 922-2022
Perspectives on the Medical Transcription Profession (quarterly)
    Health Professions Institute
    PO Box 801
    Modesto, CA 95353
    (209) 551-2112

Professional Organizations

American Academy of Professional Coders
    309 West 700 South
    Salt Lake City, UT 84101
    (800) 626-CODE
    Web site: http://www.aapc.com
American Association of Medical Assistants, Inc.
    20 North Wacker Drive, Suite 1575
    Chicago, IL 60606
    (800) 228-2262
    Web site: http://www.aama-ntl.org

American Health Information Management Association
    233 N. Michigan Ave., Suite 2150
    Chicago, IL 60601
    (800) 335-5535
    Web site: http://www.ahima.org
Association of Healthcare Documentation Integrity (AHDI) (formerly American Association for Medical Transcription)
    4230 Kiernan Avenue, Ste. #130
    Modesto, CA 95356
    (800) 982-2182
    Web site: http://www.ahdionline.org
Medical Group Management Association affiliated with American College of Medical Practice Executives
    104 Inverness Terrace E
    Englewood, CO 80112-5304
    (877) 275-6462
    Web site: http://www.mgma.com
Professional Association of Health Care Office Managers
    461 E. Ten Mile Road
    Pensacola, FL 32534-9712
    (800) 451-9311
    Web site: http://www.pahcom.com
Registered Medical Assistant/AMT
    10700 Higgins Road
    Rosemont, IL 60018
    (847) 823-5169
    Web site: http://www.amt1.com

CHAPTER 2

The Health Care Environment: Past, Present, and Future

OBJECTIVES

After reading this chapter and learning step-by-step procedures to gain job skills,* you should be able to:

Learning Objectives

▍ Describe the past, present, and future of medical care in the United States.

▍ Understand how managed care functions; name and describe various types of managed care organizations.

▍ Analyze health care settings and compare their similarities and differences.

▍ Discuss employment opportunities in a variety of health care settings.

▍ Define different types of medical specialties.

▍ Compare the administrative medical assistant's job responsibilities among medical specialties.

▍ Learn the abbreviations for various physician specialists and health care organizations.

Performance Objectives (Procedures) in This Textbook

▍ Direct patients to specific hospital departments (Procedure 2-1).

▍ Refer patients to the correct physician specialist (Procedure 2-2).

Performance Objectives (Job Skills) in the Workbook

▍ Direct patients to specific hospital departments (Job Skill 2-1).

▍ Refer patients to the correct physician specialist (Job Skill 2-2).

▍ Define abbreviations for health care professionals (Job Skill 2-3).

▍ Determine basic skills for the administrative medical assistant (Job Skill 2-4).

*This textbook and the accompanying Workbook meet the educational components for entry-level administrative and general competencies outlined by CAAHEP and ABHES.

OUTLINE WITH LECTURE NOTES

The History of Medicine

_____
_____
_____
_____

Evolution of the Medical Assisting Career

_____
_____
_____
_____

Changes in Health Care
Current Trends

_____
_____
_____
_____

Today's Health Care Delivery System
Traditional Care

_____
_____
_____
_____

Managed Care

_____
_____
_____
_____

The Medical Practice Setting
Solo Physician Practice

_____
_____
_____
_____

Associate Practice

_____
_____
_____
_____

Group Practice

_____
_____
_____
_____

Partnership

_____
_____
_____

Professional Corporation

_____
_____
_____
_____

Urgent Care Center

_____
_____
_____
_____

Clinic

_____
_____
_____
_____

Hospital

_____
_____
_____
_____

Medical Center

_____
_____
_____

Specialized Care Center

_____
_____
_____
_____

Laboratory

_____

_____

_____

Managed Care Organization

_____

_____

Holistic Health Environment

_____

_____

_____

_____

The Physician Specialist

_____

_____

_____

_____

**Health Care Professionals'
Abbreviations**

_____

_____

_____

_____

KEY TERMS

associate practice
caduceus
capitation
clinic
exclusive provider organization (EPO)
fee-for-service (FFS)
group practice
health maintenance organization (HMO)
hospital
independent practice association (IPA)
laboratory
managed care organization (MCO)
medical assistant

medical center
MinuteClinic
multispecialty practice
partnership
point-of-service (POS) plan
preferred provider organization (PPO)
primary care physician (PCP)
professional corporation
solo physician practice
specialized care center
urgent care centers
utilization review

HISTORY OF MEDICINE

Sculptured artifacts, drawings, and hieroglyphics from prehistoric times indicate that humans have long tried to cure their illnesses. Medicine was closely connected to religion in early times, and people felt that illness was punishment indicating the gods' anger. Priests came to be the healers of illness, using magical formulas, sacrifices, and the application of herbs and other natural substances. Some of these remedies were successful and became part of folklore medicine; others have not proven so.

The first prescription (Figure 2-1) was discovered in the tomb of an Egyptian pharaoh. This first written record, from about 3000 B.C., was made by a physician, Imhotep, who attended the pharaohs and was known as the God of healing. Hippocrates, "the father of medicine," was the first to describe disease, and his descriptions were so accurate that some remain valid today. The Oath of Hippocrates is the Oath of Medicine that physicians pledge to their patients and profession on graduation from medical school (see Chapter 3).*

In Greek legend, the God of healing, Aesculapius, was represented as a serpent coiled around a staff,

_____

* *All medical schools use some form of oath, many have moved away from reciting the ancient Hippocratic oath.*

HEART OF THE HEALTH CARE PROFESSIONAL

Service

As you interact with patients, you may be responsible for guiding them through the maze of managed care. Patients can become confused with the various types of managed care organizations, authorization requirements, copayments, and so forth. By taking the time to explain plan requirements with cheerfulness and patience you will be helping the medical practice and serving patients at the same time.

which was a symbol of power. Today the **caduceus**, as this symbol is called, represents the medical profession. Its modern form is a winged staff with two snakes twined around it (Figure 2-2).

During the Middle Ages, universities in France and England began medical schools, and down through the ages, many people have developed medical instruments and techniques, conducted research resulting in remedies for disease, and contributed to medical knowledge and practice. Some of these highlights in medical history appear in Table 2-1.

EVOLUTION OF THE MEDICAL ASSISTING CAREER

In the early 1900s, the administrative side of medical practice was still relatively simple. Administrative duties could be handled by the physician or the office secretary. During World War II when office nurses were needed in hospitals, physicians began to train

their secretaries to perform this function. Since then, medical assistants have performed both administrative and clinical duties to capably manage the outpatient medical practice.

In recent years, the role of the **medical assistant** has been radically changed by an increase in the number of patients seen and a tremendous volume of paperwork and recordkeeping. Physicians now devote most of their time to taking care of patients, leaving the administrative and clinical work to one or more medical assistants. Medical assistants have greater responsibility and are given more authority than their counterparts of earlier years; therefore, they must approach this challenge with dedication and creativity. Today, the administrative assistant is an essential part of every ambulatory practice and the support functions they offer are critical, ensuring the productivity of the medical practice.

CHANGES IN HEALTH CARE

It was only a generation or two ago that country doctors traded their services for chickens, eggs, or produce. This was followed by a time when families went to physicians and opened an account, paying for services monthly or whenever they were able. As time passed, medical school costs increased, physicians' knowledge base and expertise expanded, and the cost of health care began to rise. Soon insurance companies were arriving on the scene to pick up the price tag. At this time, there were few limitations on the costs of services with minimal expense to patients while most employers paid the insurance premiums. Health care was rapidly changing from personal payments to third-party reimbursement.

As medicine advanced, so did the life expectancy of the American population. Life support measures,

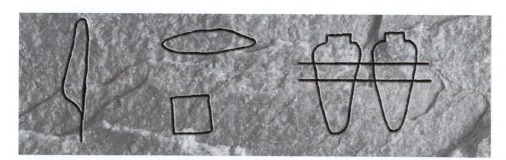

Figure 2-1. Ancient Egyptian prescription: "Six senna (pods) and fruit of colocynth are ground fine, put in honey, and eaten by the man, swallowed with sweet wine 5 ro."

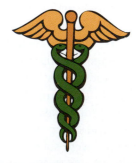

Figure 2-2. Caduceus, the symbol of the medical profession

Table 2-1. Highlights of Medical History

Medical Notable	Nationality and Accomplishment
Ambrose Pare (1510–1590)	A French surgeon, called "the father of modern surgery," who introduced advanced surgical techniques
Andraes Vesalius (1514–1564)	A Flemish anatomist, sometimes called "the father of modern anatomy," who wrote the first complete description of the human body and dissected bodies to prove his theories
William Harvey (1578–1657)	An English physician and anatomist who demonstrated the exact circulation of the blood
Anton van Leeuwenhoek (1623–1723)	A Dutch lens maker who developed the first lens strong enough to allow bacteria to be seen
John Hunter (1728–1793)	A British practitioner known as "the founder of scientific surgery"
Edward Jenner (1749–1823)	An Englishman who developed the process of vaccination and the smallpox vaccine
James Marion Sims (1813–1883)	An American gynecologist who invented the vaginal speculum and originated Sims' position
John Snow (1813–1858)	A legendary figure in the history of public health, epidemiology, and anesthesiology who determined how cholera was transmitted
Crawford Williamson Long (1815–1878)	An American physician, the first to employ ether as an anesthetic agent
Ignaz Philipp Semmelweis (1818–1865)	A Hungarian physician called "the savior of mothers," who first used antiseptic methods extensively in childbirth to prevent puerperal fever
Florence Nightingale (1820–1910)	An English hospital reformer and the founder of nursing
Clara Barton (1821–1912)	Founder of the American Red Cross
Louis Pasteur (1822–1895)	A French chemist, known as "the father of bacteriology" and "the father of preventive medicine," who developed the process called pasteurization and was involved in the prevention of anthrax (in cattle and sheep), rabies, chicken cholera, and swine erysipelas

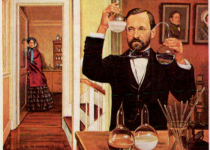

(Courtesy of Parke Davis and Company, copyright 1957)

Joseph Lister (1827–1912)	A British surgeon, known as "the father of sterile surgery," who used carbolic acid as an antiseptic in the operating room

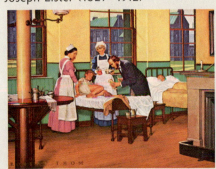

(Courtesy of Parke Davis and Company, copyright 1957)

(continues)

Table 2-1 (continued). Highlights of Medical History

Medical Notable	Nationality and Accomplishment
Robert Koch (1843–1910)	A German scientist who discovered the cause for cholera and discovered tuberculin while working with tuberculosis
Wilhelm C. Roentgen (1845–1923)	A German physicist who discovered the x-ray, which is used in diagnosing diseases and treating cancer
Walter Reed (1851–1902)	An American physician who discovered that yellow fever is caused by a virus that is carried from one person to another by a particular kind of mosquito
Paul Ehrlich (1854–1915)	A German physician known for the drug he developed to fight syphilis; also for developing chemotherapy
Pierre Curie (1859–1906) and Marie Curie (1867–1934)	French researchers known for their discovery and work with radium
Alexander Fleming (1881–1955)	An English bacteriologist who discovered penicillin, the first antibiotic drug
Frederick Banting (1891–1941)	A Canadian physician who discovered insulin
Albert Sabin (1906–1993)	An American scientist who developed an effective oral polio vaccine
Michael Ellis DeBakey (1908–)	American surgeon who contributed to techniques used to replace blood vessels including the coronary artery bypass operation; developed artificial blood vessels made of Dacron
Jonas Edward Salk (1914–1995)	An American scientist who developed an injection vaccine against poliomyelitis in 1954
Francis H. C. Crick (1916–2004) and James D. Watson (1928–)	Crick, a British biophysicist, and Watson, an American biochemist, contributed to basic understanding of the genetic code and the double-helix structure of deoxyribonucleic acid (DNA). DNA makes possible the transmission of inherited characteristics.
Christiaan Neethling Barnard (1922–2001)	A South African surgeon who performed the world's first human-heart transplant in 1967
Thomas Earl Starzl (1926–)	American surgeon who performed the first liver transplant and became known as the "Dean of Transplantation"

including quicker and better resuscitation, feeding tubes, respirators, and new drugs, helped keep individuals alive beyond normal years. More and more elderly people entered convalescent hospitals to live out the remainder of their lives when unable to care for themselves at home. Babies weighing less then two pounds made medical history when they survived the trauma of premature delivery and the complications of underdeveloped lungs. The general population began to expect the highest level of medical attention regardless of an ability to pay. Malpractice insurance soared as lawsuits increased. Physicians tried to protect themselves by ordering more, and sometimes unnecessary tests and procedures. Hospitals and outpatient centers started competing with each other by buying the largest, most advanced equipment. All these factors combined to increase health care costs.

Hospitals began investing hundreds of thousands of dollars in marketing campaigns to lure patients to their facilities, such as offering mothers-to-be bank loans and free checking accounts to be used for costs associated with the childbirth. Women especially were being targeted, after a survey showed that women make 85 percent of the medical decisions in nonemergency cases.

Current Trends

Today, with the discovery of new diseases, the increase in existing illnesses such as diabetes and obesity, and the explosion in clinical knowledge, there are increased demands on physicians' time. Reimbursement is declining for primary care services while the cost of living and operating a medical practice increases. High rents, climbing malpractice and health insurance rates, and utilization of electronic medical records and other new electronic equipment all contribute to the increase in the overhead of medical practices.

There is concern in the medical community over the effects of aging Baby Boomers who will need increased medical attention. The increase of federal regulations and the possibility of medical errors is also a primary concern. The government is proposing changes to prepare for the increase in the aging patient population and initiatives are being put in place to reduce medical mistakes. Some of the other trends in health care today include an upsurge in patient diversity, as immigration continues to increase. Consumers are more involved in health care decisions and are interested in the use of alternative medicine. The health care delivery system continues to change to try to accommodate the diverse population, comply with federal regulations, and make a profit. It is an exciting and challenging time for physicians and health care workers who must diligently work to tend to patient needs as well as focus on the future of medicine.

TODAY'S HEALTH CARE DELIVERY SYSTEM

Beginning in the mid to late 1970s, many managed care plans began to make their appearance throughout the United States. By the early 1980s health maintenance organizations (HMOs) entered the picture as a business effort to curb skyrocketing health costs. To control increased spending, a process called **utilization review** started to be used to monitor and control testing, medication, surgeries, and other areas where overuse occurred. However, this utilization process often created delays in medical care. Doctors who were once allowed to make all decisions regarding their patient's health care soon found these decisions placed in the hands of HMO personnel. Current health care delivery systems include both traditional and managed care.

Traditional Care

In traditional health care, patients may go to a physician, specialist, or facility of their choice as frequently as they desire. Physicians charge on a **fee-for-service** arrangement in which either the physician's office or the patient submits a claim to the insurance company and the full amount allowed by the insurance company is collected.

Individuals with traditional Medicare coverage may select their own **primary care physician (PCP)** who assumes the ongoing responsibility for the overall treatment of a patient, usually a general or family practitioner, internist, gynecologist, or pediatrician. They may choose to see a specialist whenever necessary, go to the hospital they prefer, and choose the facility where laboratory tests are performed. Because there is no authorization process, testing and referrals can be done immediately.

Managed Care

Managed care is a health care delivery system that strives to manage the cost, quality, and delivery of health care by emphasizing preventive medicine, utilization of services, and a network of providers. Most **managed care organizations (MCOs)** require prior approval or preauthorization for diagnostic services, hospitalization, and specialist care. Such referrals may be formal, direct, verbal, or self-directed. These are further explained in Chapter 16, Health Insurance Systems.

MCOs usually have no deductible, a small copayment at the time of each visit, and 100 percent coverage of medical expenses, including preventive services, most medications, and medical supplies. The reduced cost to patients makes MCOs a popular choice. Patients, however, have limitations in their choice of PCPs and specialty care. Often patients may have to wait for testing, some procedures, referrals to specialists, and hospitalization admissions to be approved. Many private patients and Medicare recipients who opted to go with managed care plans have seen them fail, leaving a climate of uncertainty regarding their effectiveness and benefits. They will, however, be around for a long time and are commonly referred to by their abbreviations, for example, HMOs, PPOs, and IPAs.

Types of Managed Care Organizations

Following are descriptions of some of these managed care plans.

Health Maintenance Organization (HMO)— A **health maintenance organization** is a prepaid health plan that has been in existence the longest of all managed care plans. It is a comprehensive health care financing and delivery organization offering prepaid health care for a fixed fee to subscribers in a designated geographic area. Services are rendered by a primary care physician (PCP), often considered a gatekeeper. The PCP is paid by **capitation**, a fixed fee paid monthly per enrolled patient, regardless of the number of services actually used.

Preferred Provider Organization (PPO)—A variation of the HMO, a **preferred provider organization** offers a contractual agreement between the health care providers (called preferred providers) and employers, insurance carriers, or third-party administrators to provide health care service at a discounted rate. Utilization management techniques are used and patients are given an incentive to go to a preferred provider within the network of contracted physicians and receive the benefits of lower copayments and deductibles, but may choose to go to a nonparticipating physician and pay a higher percentage of fees (Table 2-2).

Independent Practice Association (IPA)—An **independent practice association** is a group of individual health care providers that contract with HMOs and PPOs to provide care at a discounted rate. They may be paid on a fixed monthly capitation, or a fee-for-service basis. Providers are placed on the organization's approved list (physician network) and guaranteed a patient base. They remain individual practitioners and retain their own office space.

Exclusive Provider Organization (EPO)—An **exclusive provider organization**, very similar to an

PATIENT EDUCATION

Because of the change from traditional to managed care plans, the medical assistant must continually educate patients to the ever changing benefits, nonbenefits, and limitations written into their contracts that affect medical care and reimbursement. Keep abreast of plan information to be able to intelligently and accurately answer patients' questions and always follow the employer's established policies when dealing with the health care contracts.

HMO, requires members to have a designated primary care physician (PCP). It is called exclusive because it is offered to large employers who agree not to contract with any other plan. Members must choose care from providers offered within a limited physician network. State health insurance laws control such plans instead of federal and state HMO regulations.

Point-of-Service (POS) Plan—A **point-of-service plan** contracts with independent providers at a discounted rate. Members have the choice at the time services are needed (i.e., at the point-of-service)

Table 2-2. Summary of Managed Care Plan Requirements Including In- and Out-of-Network Physician Stipulations, Copayment versus Deductible Options, Payment Methods, and Authorization Requirements

Managed Care Plan	In Network	Out	Co-Pay Deductible	Payment Method	Authorization Required
HMO	X		Fixed co-pay	Capitated Some fee-for-service	Formal
PPO	X	60/40% 70/30%	Coinsurance Deductible	80/20% 90/10%	Self Verbal Direct Formal
IPA	X		Fixed co-pay	Capitated Fee-for-service	Formal Direct
EPO	X Lg employers		Fixed co-pay	Fee-for-service	Formal
POS	X	X	Fixed co-pay Deductible	Fee-for-service 80/20% 70/30%	Self Verbal Direct Formal

of receiving services from an HMO, PPO, or fee-for-service plan. A patient can self-refer himself or herself to a specialist or see a nonnetwork provider for a higher coinsurance payment.

THE MEDICAL PRACTICE SETTING

The setting in which the physician works has changed as much as the medicine he or she practices. The standard practice for many years was the single physician practice, also called the solo practice. In this chapter, a description of the different settings in which a physician practices as well as the employment opportunities for an administrative medical assistant are discussed.

Solo Physician Practice

In the **solo physician practice**, one physician works alone in a small office with a small staff. The physician is either on call 24 hours a day or shares calls with another solo practitioner. Typically, the charges are based on a fee-for-service arrangement. Although solo practices still exist in some areas, this setting is beginning to be the exception, not the rule. In many areas a solo practitioner cannot compete with large group practices and large group insurance contracts. The physician has been forced to join a group, relocate, or close the practice. Patients reap the benefits of a solo physician practice in terms of a physician and staff who know them by name, treat them like family, and offer individual attention and care. Trust and loyalty is built between the physician and the patient that is hard to obtain in any other medical setting.

Employment in a solo physician practice offers the medical assistant diverse responsibilities. In a very small practice, the medical assistant might handle both clinical and administrative duties. In an established practice, the medical assistant might be responsible for all administrative duties ranging from appointment scheduling to payroll and housekeeping. In a large solo practice, there may be two or three medical assistants sharing the administrative duties.

Associate Practice

In an **associate practice**, two or more practitioners share office expenses, employees, and the on-call schedule. They practice as solo practitioners at the same office location or at different sites billing under separate tax identification numbers and do not share the revenue. The arrangement allows a decrease in expenses and an increase in productivity.

Employment in an associate practice offers the administrative medical assistant a unique challenge. There may be two to five physicians who need to be regarded as "the boss." Duties may need to be performed for each physician in a different manner according to their specific orders, for example, keeping separate appointment schedules with varying time slots for patient treatment, lunch hours, meeting schedules, and days off. The sharing of ideas and medical decision-making can create a stimulating environment and offer patients the benefits of more sophisticated diagnosis and treatment.

Group Practice

In a **group practice**, three or more physicians agree to practice using the same office space, sharing office expenses, employees, income, and the on-call schedule. The physicians may be incorporated or in a legal partnership. A medical group is legally recognized by the American Group Practice Association. The physicians share one tax identification number and bill all claims under a group name. Three to seven physicians would be considered a small group (Figures 2-3 and 2-4). A medium group might involve eight to thirty physicians, and any group over thirty would be considered large. Most small group practices are composed of physicians of the same specialty. A variety of specialties is called a **multispecialty practice**.

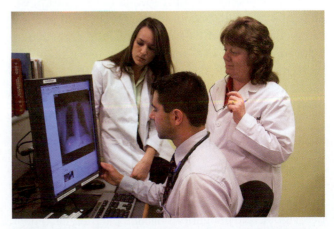

Figure 2-3. Three physicians working together in a group medical practice

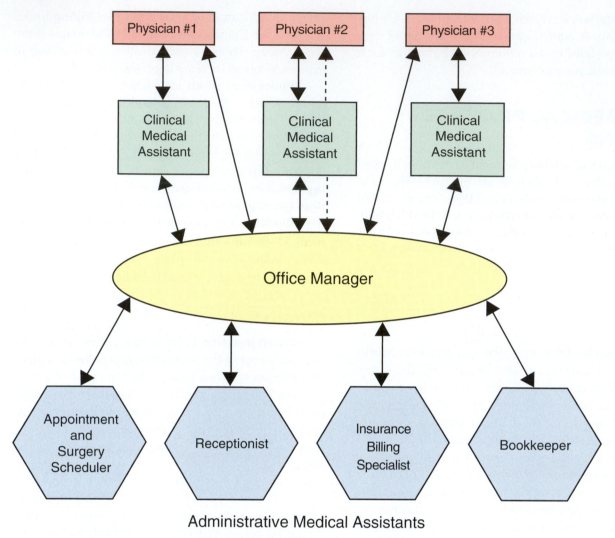

Figure 2-4. Example of physician and staff interactions in a small medical group practice

Employment in a group practice offers a variety of job duties. In a larger group, the departments become more subdivided. With more specific duties, the knowledge and job skills become more specialized, making the medical assistant a true specialist in a particular field. For example, in a large group the assistant might work in the billing department and be the Medicare specialist, while another employee might be the managed care specialist.

Partnership

In a **partnership**, two or more physicians associate in the practice of medicine under a legal partnership agreement. The agreement specifies the responsibilities, rights, and obligations of each partner. Each physician in the partnership becomes liable for the other partner's actions and conduct, making lawsuits a great disadvantage.

Employment in a partnership would be similar to working in an association or group, depending on the number of physicians.

Professional Corporation

A **professional corporation** is an entity unto itself. It has a legal and business status that is independent of its shareholders. The physician shareholders are employees in the corporation. The corporations are regulated by individual state statutes. Laws have changed making the financial advantages of a corporation less beneficial to the physician, so as a result, fewer doctors incorporate.

Employment in a corporation is similar to working in any of the previously mentioned practice settings. A solo physician, as well as a large group, can incorporate. There may be differences in the bookkeeping aspects of the corporate practice because corporations operate under a *fiscal year*, which may involve preparing budget projections and closing their books at different times during the calendar year.

Urgent Care Center

Urgent care centers, also known as freestanding emergency centers or ambulatory centers, are available in many cities throughout the country. Some centers provide extended hours to accommodate patients who have problems getting to the doctor weekdays between 8 a.m. and 5 p.m. and others are open 24 hours a day, seven days a week, including holidays. They also provide a *walk-in* capability for minor emergencies and urgent health problems. Prior to the formulation of urgent care centers, many hospital emergency rooms were overcrowded with patients requesting services for minor complaints resulting in less time to handle major emergencies. Most patients with minor complaints had insurance contracts that were paying for their emergency room services, thus contributing to the overutilization of insurance monies and increased medical costs.

An advantage of urgent care centers is the one-stop-shopping feature, because many centers have full laboratories, x-ray equipment, and physical therapy on-site.

Most urgent care centers are private, for-profit centers that employ salaried physicians who compete directly with private physician practices. After delivering primary emergency care, some centers refer patients to private physicians. Because of the competition from urgent care centers many private physicians have added walk-in hours in addition to their regularly scheduled appointment hours.

Employment with an urgent care center offers one of the most varied experiences in a health care setting because the medical assistant sees a variety of medical problems. Many centers contract with a large number of managed care plans and private insurance companies so an insurance billing specialist is needed as well as a multiskilled health practitioner. A center can be an exciting, fast-paced working environment offering many challenges. It is often the first choice of a medical assistant extern after completion of training.

Clinic

Clinics are often hard to distinguish from large group practices. Patients can be admitted for special studies and treatment by a group of health care professionals practicing medicine together. Clinics usually offer a broad range of specialties and sophisticated testing equipment. The doctors can bring a complicated case to a panel of physicians for discussion and treatment options. This approach offers patients the most advanced medical decision-making available, so patients often travel great distances to seek out clinics with prestigious reputations.

A clinic may also be a department of a hospital where patients who do not have to be admitted may be treated. Walk-in clinics, such as the urgent care centers, exist to serve patients without their having to make appointments. Satellite clinics, also known as outpatient clinics, are usually owned by a hospital, large medical group, or a managed care organization. They are located off-site from the main facility and are strategically placed to serve the needs of a different geographic area. These clinics usually employ physicians practicing a specialty so advanced care can be provided to patients who have similar physical problems. Examples of specialty clinics are abortion clinics, family planning clinics, industrial clinics, sleep diagnostic clinics, and eye clinics.

Employment in a large clinic offers a broad range of benefits to a medical assistant including job versatility and career advancement opportunities. The disadvantages of employment in such a setting are less personal contact and having to cope with bureaucratic management.

In-Store Clinic

Found in small-scale chain stores is the "**Minute-Clinic**," which offers a limited range of basic tests and treatments at a lower cost than most doctors' offices. They are operated by an outside company and generally staffed by physician assistants or nurse practitioners. They are typically patronized by people who do not have a primary care physician, do not have health insurance, and do not like waiting. They promote quick care on a walk-in basis during normal business hours.

Employment opportunities in an in-store clinic would depend on the volume of patients seen. A multiskilled assistant performing both clinical and administrative functions would be an asset to the physician assistant or nurse practitioner.

Hospital

Hospitals are facilities that provide 24-hour acute care and treatment for the sick and injured. They also provide emergency medical care. Patients are divided

HOSPITAL ADMINISTRATIVE DEPARTMENTS

Administration Department

- Oversees the management and operations of the hospital.
- The Chief Executive Officer (CEO) or President works in this department.
- The Board of Directors establishes bylaws outlining duties and responsibilities for the governing body, administrator, and all hospital committees.

Admitting Department

Handles:
- Admittance/discharge of patients
- Insurance verification
- Precertification of insurance
- Preauthorization for hospitalization and procedures

Business Department

- Provides cashiers and patient statements (bills)
- Submits insurance claims
- Collects accounts receivable

Financial Department

Oversees and controls:
- Business department
- Accounts receivable/payable
- Budgets and financial reports
- Insurance contracts
- Payroll

Human Resource Department

- Employee benefits
- Hiring
- Orientation and training
- Job evaluations

Medical Records Department

Manages:
- Coding diagnoses and procedures
- In- and outpatient medical records
- Medical transcription
- Registries

Medical Staff Department

- Processes credentialing of all allied health professionals
- Schedules and monitors department meetings

Nursing Administration Department

Supervises:
- Nursing care, staffing, and education
- Nursing care of patients in specialized medical care units
- Utilization review nurses who may report to this department

Figure 2-5A. Comprehensive listing of hospital administrative departments and their services

into units, formerly called wards, according to the type of illness or injuries incurred. In larger hospitals, these units may occupy complete floors or wings of a building. See Figures 2-5A and B for some common unit divisions and Figure 2-6 for a hospital organizational chart. By dividing the patient load in this man-ner, the nursing staff can better care for patients with similar ailments because units call for similar skills, diagnostic testing, procedures, and treatment. Larger hospitals have specialized units to serve the needs of patients who are medically unstable. See Figure 2-6 on page 43 for examples of *specialized care units*. Inten-

HOSPITAL ADJUNCT DEPARTMENTS

Dietetic/Nutrition Department

Furnishes:

- Dietitian
- Nutritional assessment
- Therapy
- Diet preparation
- Nutritional education

Emergency Department

Physician and staff on duty 24 hours a day to handle trauma and emergencies and observe and monitor patients while collecting data to make decisions regarding admissions. Sections include:

- Casting room
- Examination room
- Observation room
- Trauma room

Gastrointestinal Laboratory (GI Lab)

Performs endoscopic procedures such as:

- Colonoscopy
- Proctoscopy
- Sigmoidoscopy

Intensive Care Units

- Manage critically ill patients
- Coronary care
- Neonatal care

Laboratory Department

Offers inpatient and outpatient services such as:

- Blood bank
- Chemistry
- Cytology
- Hematology
- Histopathology
- Microbiology
- Organ bank
- Pathology
- Urinalysis

Magnetic Resonance Imaging Department (MRI)

Performs:

- MRI scans with and without contrast material

Nuclear Medicine Department

Handles radioactive materials used in tests such as:

- Bone scans
- Liver scans
- Radioimmunoassays
- Thyroid testing

One-Day Surgery Department

Takes care of patients who do not require overnight stay for procedures such as:

- Angiography
- Blood transfusion
- Heart catheterization
- Myelogram

Pharmacy Department

Supplies medication to inpatients such as:

- Injectable medications
- Intravenous solutions
- Oral medications
- Topicals, suppositories, inhalers, and so on

Physical Therapy Department

Provides:

- Inpatient physical therapy
- Outpatient physical therapy
- Occupational therapy
- Speech therapy

Physiology Department

Offers a variety of services such as:

- Cardiology (ECG, treadmill, 2-D echocardiogram)
- Electrophysiology (EMG, EEG, nerve conduction studies)
- Vascular medicine (deep vein Doppler)
- Myelogram

(continues)

Figure 2-5B. Comprehensive listing of hospital adjunct departments and their services

---

Radiology Department

Performs the following procedures:

- Barium enema
- Barium swallow
- Computed tomography
- Diagnostic x-ray

- Mammograpy
- Therapeutic radiation
- Ultrasound

Respiratory Care Department

Provides diagnostic and therapeutic services including the administration of:

- Bronchodilators
- Oxygen

Performs:

- Arterial blood gases
- Pulmonary function studies
- Spirometry

Sets up and assists with:

- Cardiopulmonary resuscitation
- Mechanical ventilators

Social Services Department

Employs medical and psychiatric social workers to work with patients and families regarding:

- Economic factors
- Emotional situations
- Social issues
- Discharge planning
- Community services
- Medical resources

Figure 2-5B (continued). Comprehensive listing of hospital adjunct departments and their services

sive care units offer 24-hour monitoring by the nursing staff for patients whose conditions are considered critical, guarded, and unstable.

It is wise for medical assistants to meet hospital personnel that they interact with by telephone. Developing a relationship with admitting clerks, billing specialists, and laboratory personnel is prudent, because establishing a relationship paves the way for good communication.

Another major function of a hospital is its surgical unit. A hospital may have several surgical suites and a delivery room in addition to an outpatient or same-day surgery unit. A major portion of the hospital's revenue and expenses is generated through its surgical cases, so a considerable amount of thought and investigation goes into the hospital's choice of staff surgeons. The prestige of the hospital and its credibility are often measured by its staff physicians. The public image of a hospital is greatly affected by having satisfied patients in the community who have had successful surgeries and hospital stays.

Hospital Categories

There are several different categories of hospitals. Hospitals can be either government-owned or non-government-owned. Government-owned hospitals

are subsidized by federal, state, county, or city government. An example of a federal hospital is a Veterans Administration hospital. The federal government also finances hospitals and health care facilities for Native Americans, Alaskans, merchant marines, and other groups. A state hospital can be a facility for chronically ill or developmentally disabled individuals, while county, district, and city hospitals are established primarily to meet the needs of a particular community.

Nongovernment-owned hospitals can be either *for-profit* or *not-for-profit*. General and community hospitals are usually nonprofit and serve a specific geographic area and need in the community. Other nonprofit hospitals include those owned by industries, unions, churches, and religious orders.

For-profit hospitals, also called private or investor-owned hospitals, are controlled by the individual, partnership, or corporation that owns them. A teaching or research hospital affiliated with a university utilizes the services of doctors who continue training after medical school.

Hospital sizes are measured by the number of beds provided with state licenses issued on that basis. Physicians apply for staff privileges at the hospitals of their choice. This involves a credentialing process with a review of the physician's curriculum vitae, practice

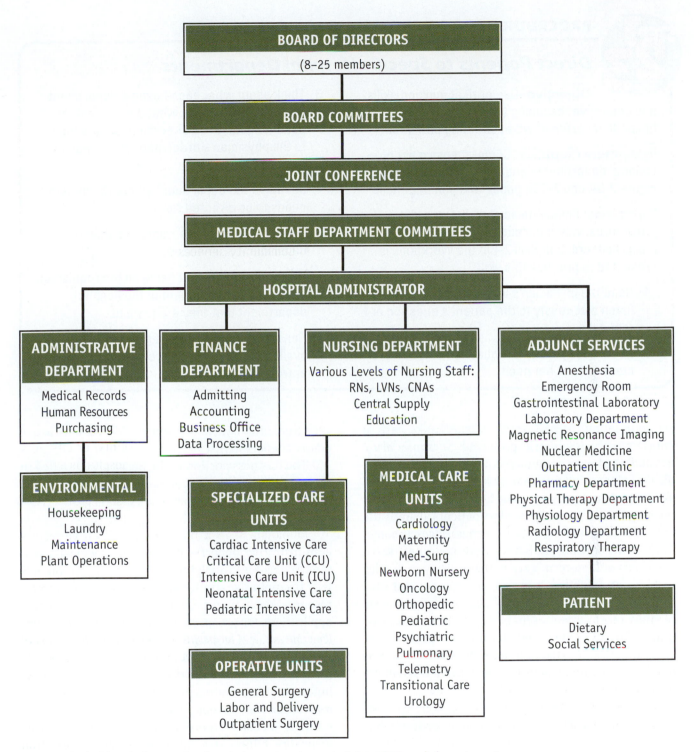

Figure 2-6. Hospital organizational chart showing administration and departments

history, hospital references, and peer references, and usually includes an oral interview. Credentials are reevaluated yearly after checking on licensure and continuing medical education via continuing education units (CEUs).

Hospital Types

Hospitals may be named for the types of patients they serve. *Acute care hospitals* treat the severely ill or injured patient. *Specialty hospitals* treat a specific type of patient such as a burn center, cancer institute, or

PROCEDURE 2-1

Direct Patients to Specific Hospital Departments

Objective: Use critical thinking skills and deductive reasoning to determine a specific hospital department when directing patients.

Equipment/Supplies: Comprehensive list of hospital departments and their services (see Figure 2-5A and 2-5B), paper, and pen or pencil.

Directions: Follow these step-by-step procedures, which include rationales, to learn this procedure. Job Skill 2-1 in the Workbook is presented to practice this skill.

1. Read the physician's instructions carefully or listen attentively to the patient's question or request.

2. Record the patient's request or question stating his or her need.

3. Think about what each hospital department offers and determine what department the patient needs to be directed to according to the physician's order, patient request, or patient question.

4. Jot down the department where the patient needs to be directed to.

5. Determine if services from more than one department are needed.

6. Write the department name on the requisition slip or inform the patient of the hospital department that they are to go to.

7. Hand the patient a map of the hospital if available, or explain where to park and which entrance to use.

---

eye foundation. *Mental health hospitals* take care of patients with psychiatric problems. *Substance abuse hospitals* deal with patients recovering from drug and alcohol abuse, and *convalescent hospitals,* for example, skilled nursing facilities, long-term-care facilities, or nursing homes, serve the needs of patients, usually the aged, who can no longer care for themselves at home. Many acute care hospitals have separate units to serve the needs of long-term-care patients. They may refer to these as extended care units or transitional care units. Convalescent hospitals also serve the needs of short-term patients rehabilitating from illness or injury. Stroke victims and hip fracture patients are two examples of patients frequently taken care of in a transitional care unit until they have recovered sufficiently to care for themselves.

Rehabilitation hospitals provide 24-hour care for patients who have been declared medically stable, but who need acute and subacute rehabilitation. Doctors on staff direct the patient's care through a multidisciplinary team of health care professionals, including physical therapists, occupational therapists, speech pathologists, recreation therapists, dietitians, nutritionists, psychologists, pulmonary specialists, and a case manager. In addition to medical care units, surgical suites, and delivery rooms, hospitals have many other units offering additional services. These services are essential to good medical care; they are referred to as adjunct services instead of ancillary or auxiliary as

they were once called. See Figure 2-5B for a listing of adjunct departments.

The business portion of the hospital is handled in many administrative departments. For a listing and explanation of these departments, see Figures 2-5A and 2-5B.

Employment in a hospital provides a variety of administrative opportunities for the medical assistant. When one is applying for a hospital position, it is wise to emphasize administrative skills. Many human resource department staff members who process applications for prospective employees do not realize that the medical assistant has been trained in most of the skills required to work in hospital administration. Hospitals often hire medical assistants for the following positions: preadmitting coordinators, admitting representatives, receptionists, unit clerks, unit secretaries, medical record technicians, clerk typists, insurance billing specialists, insurance verification coordinators, insurance coders, bed condition coordinators, cashiers, collectors, and file clerks.

Medical Center

The name **medical center** written after a hospital name usually denotes services provided at sites other than the hospital setting. Satellite clinics, rehabilitation centers, and laboratory drawing stations are additional services that may be offered at other locations.

Employment in a medical center would render the same opportunities as working in a hospital with the advantage of being able to transfer to another location when a new position at a satellite facility is available.

Specialized Care Center

Specialized care centers exist to serve the needs of a group of patients having similar medical conditions. A team of specialists with support staff treats patients in a particular area of need. Rehabilitation institutes, drug treatment centers, respiratory care centers, eye institutes, and comprehensive cancer care centers are examples of specialized care centers.

Employment in a specialized care center offers the same advantages for a medical assistant as with all its employees. It provides the opportunity to work in a specialized area, with one particular type of patient.

Laboratory

Laboratories can be independent, freestanding, or in a medical facility such as a hospital, clinic, or research center. Laboratories collect, receive, and analyze specimens. They disseminate test results via telephone, fax machine, computer transmission, and mailing of reports. Research laboratories seeking information leading to the diagnosis and cure of diseases conduct experiments on humans and animals. Laboratories are regulated by the states in which they operate and are under the direction of a licensed pathologist. Most laboratories are fully automated with high-tech computers thereby eliminating manual analysis. In many states, regulations have become so strict that doctors have closed *physician office laboratories* (POLs) and send specimens to outside laboratories.

Physicians are very dependent on laboratory results to expedite the diagnosis and treatment of their patients. The quality control standards of the laboratory, the turn-around time (speed of testing specimens and sending results to physicians), and the cost to the patient are three very important factors in choosing a dependable laboratory.

Employment in a laboratory requires precision and accuracy. Articulating and recording exact test results are skills both the clinical and administrative medical assistant should have. One transposed or misunderstood number could change the course of treatment for a patient. Other administrative skills include scheduling appointments; laboratory data entry; filing; bookkeeping; typing autopsy, forensic, coroner, and statistical reports; delivering reports; maintaining tumor and autopsy logs; labeling and filing specimens; and knowing diagnostic codes for laboratory and pathology procedures more commonly referred to as SNOMED.

Managed Care Organization

Managed care organizations operate under the concept of prepaid group health care. Managed care emphasizes preventive medicine and practices utilization review with preauthorization for services. There are many different types of prepaid health plans, but they usually fall under the headings of health maintenance organizations (HMOs), individual practice associations (IPAs), and a variation called preferred provider organizations (PPOs). See Chapter 16 for more information on this subject.

The setting of these practices usually consists of a group of doctors who act as primary care physicians (PCPs) for one or more of the previously mentioned plans. There may also be specialists at the facility. As increased efficiency and decreased costs are primary goals, the physicians may have increased patient loads resulting in less time spent with patients. The PCPs act as gatekeepers, striving to avoid unnecessary tests or referrals to specialists. The concept is to make the best utilization of time and money. Physicians are paid by capitation, which means they get a set amount per patient per month regardless of whether the patient is seen.

Employment in a managed care setting offers many of the same opportunities as a large group practice. Advocates of managed care state the advantages to employees are benefit plans, a variety of job duties, seeing health care dollars well-spent, and opportunities for advancement.

Holistic Health Environment

The holistic approach to health care evolved from the philosophy that the physical, mental, and social well-being of the "whole" person is as important as the treatment of a separate medical problem. The patient is trained to take total responsibility for his or her own or family's health from birth to death and to develop a lifestyle that produces wellness.

Complimentary and alternative medicine (CAM) physicians are used by 30 to 50 percent of the adult population according to the National Institute of Health (NIH). Although still not considered a part of conventional medical care, this group of diverse medical and health care systems, practices, and products are used in conjunction with traditional health care and include the following:

- Biofield and bioelectromagnetic-based therapies
- Chiropractic medicine and massage therapy
- Dietary supplements and herbal products
- Homeopathic, naturopathic, and traditional Chinese medicine
- Meditation, prayer, and mental healing

See "Resources" at the end of the chapter for Web site listings of licensed CAM practitioners.

Employment in a holistic health care setting would involve the medical assistant in patient education by ordering educational literature and communicating holistic principles to the patient. The medical assistant would have duties similar to other health care settings, but would need to display an optimistic attitude toward parenting, aging, and death that is characteristic of holistic thinking. The medical assistant would also be expected to encourage the patient to improve all aspects of health, including exercise, proper nutrition and diet, freedom from detrimental substance abuse such as drugs and alcohol, and a positive approach to mental health that includes freedom from stress and depression.

THE PHYSICIAN SPECIALIST

Another aspect of the medical assistant's decision about what type of practice to choose is what type of doctor to work with. There are many specialty practices available that offer a broad range of patient types and job duties. Table 2-3 contains medical specialties with a brief description and job responsibilities for each specialty.

The physician who is certified in a medical specialty must fulfill educational and internship requirements and pass an examination beyond the standard medical degree. When a physician has been certified in a field of *specialization,* he or she is known as a *diplomat.*

Many busy medical practices have found the need to free the physician's time to handle complex clinical problems. Nonphysician practitioners with advanced education and specialized clinical training that enables him or her to diagnose and treat patients with a variety of medical problems may be on the staff. These *physician extenders* might be a physician assistant (PA), *(text continues on page 51)*

PROCEDURE 2-2

Refer Patients to the Correct Physician Specialist

Objective: Use critical thinking skills and deductive reasoning to determine what physician specialist the patient needs.

Equipment/Supplies: Comprehensive list of physician specialists (see Table 2-3), paper, and pen or pencil. *Note: Most primary care physicians have a list of specialists in the community that they refer to and may collect appointment cards from those doctors so appointments may be scheduled from your office. Do not refer patients without the physician's direction.*

Directions: Follow these step-by-step procedures, which include rationales, to learn this procedure. Job Skill 2-2 in the *Workbook* is presented to practice this skill.

1. Read the physician's instructions carefully or listen attentively to the request or question from the patient, family member, or other party. Allowing the party to fully verbalize his or her request will give you

more information to determine the person's needs.

2. Record the patient's request or question stating his or her need. By writing a note you can refer back to, it will help if there is more than one request or a lengthy conversation.

3. Think about what services each type of physican specialty offers and determine if the services requested are handled by your doctor or another specialist.

4. Jot down the type of specialist the patient needs to be referred to.

5. Determine if services from more than one specialist are needed.

6. Write the physician's name and specialty on an appointment card or inform the patient of the specialist's name.

7. Offer to call and arrange the appointment and explain how to get to the office location.

Table 2-3. Medical Specialties and Administrative Medical Assisting Job Requirements

Medical Specialties	Administrative Medical Assistant Must . . .
Allergy and Immunology (All. and immun.)—Diagnosis and treatment of allergic conditions	Acknowledge and handle numerous referrals from other physicians Determine time required for tests and schedule appointments efficiently Have excellent keying/typing and transcription skills to aid in obtaining complete histories Know medical terminology, especially of respiratory system diseases and surgery
Anesthesiology (Anes.)—Administration of anesthesia for major surgery	Schedule surgery and do billing if the physician maintains an office Know types and routes of anesthesia
Bariatric Medicine Management and control of obesity	Receive referrals, obtain medical histories, schedule tests and surgery, verify insurance coverage and file insurance claims Be sensitive to the problem of obesity while referring patients for psychological evaluations Know the terminology for the various types of gastric bypass surgery Encourage and support patients
Dermatology (Derm.)—Treatment of diseases affecting the skin; proper care of the skin	Obtain accurate, detailed case histories Perform bookkeeping procedures Have excellent keying/typing skills Know medical terminology of skin diseases Be comfortable in the presence of unsightly skin disorders
Emergency medicine (Emerg. Med.)—Treatment of trauma and sudden emergent medical conditions	Handle emergent situations Be able to prioritize incoming calls and walk-in patients Calm patients and visitors Know medical terminology and billing procedures for emergencies
Family practice (FP)—Comprehensive medical care for individuals of all ages, often entire families	Manage multiple appointments and office routines Handle frequent telephone calls Complete insurance claims Perform bookkeeping procedures Enjoy people and be expert in public relations Be able to relate to children Deal well with emergencies Know medical terms for pediatrics, surgery, internal medicine, obstetrics and gynecology, and psychiatry
Gerontology (Ger or geriat)—Study of the aging process; geriatricians diagnose and treat problems and diseases of the older adult	Communicate resourcefully with patients who have hearing impairment Deal with elderly patients who have mobility problems Interact well with patients suffering visual loss or blindness Be diplomatic with elderly patients who suffer memory loss
Internal medicine (I.M.)—Consultations on and diagnosis of complex diseases, such as cardiovascular disease, endocrinology, gastroenterology, hematology, infectious disease, oncology, nephrology, pulmonary disease, rheumatology, proctology, and epidemiology	Key/type letters to referring physicians and transcribe reports Skillfully handle telephone when physician is away from office Complete insurance claims Perform bookkeeping procedures Known medical terminology Interact with elderly patients who have hearing and sight problems

(continues)

Table 2-3 (*continued*). Medical Specialties and Administrative Medical Assisting Job Requirements

Medical Specialties	Administrative Medical Assistant Must . . .
Medical Genetics Diagnosis and treatment of genetic-linked diseases	Be detail oriented and like research Process referrals and schedule tests Know biochemical terms; understand molecules, genes, and chromosomes Be sensitive to patient anxieties while undergoing testing and empathetic to those suffering from genetic abnormalities
Neonatology (Neonat.)— Dealing with disorders of the newborn, from birth to 28 days (subspecialty of pediatrics)	Understand general medical terminology Calm parents skillfully in telephone conversations Obtain from the physician detailed daily case studies Transmit records to specialists
Neurology/Neurosurgery (Neuro.)—Disorders of the nervous system that may be hereditary or caused by injuries, disease, or infection	Record physician's findings during examinations Be familiar with problems of the physically handicapped Deal with patients with emotional and abnormal behavior Know terminology of nervous system, diseases, surgeries, and anomalies
Nuclear medicine (Nuc. med.)— Diagnosis and treatment of disease by radionuclear methods	Understand radioisotopes and malignant diseases and terms relating to them
Obstetrics and gynecology (OB-GYN)—Combined specialty of the study and treatment of the female reproductive system: ob—medical care of women during pregnancy and childbirth: gyn—diagnosis and treatment of female disorders	Have a mature and dignified personality Be competent in managing appointment schedules when interruptions and delays create problems Arrange appointments with hospital for baby delivery and transmit patient records Handle postpartum referrals, detailed case records, and reports Explain patient fees and reasons for regularly scheduled visits Handle infertility patients with sensitivity Arrange for surgical scheduling of patients Interrelate well with babies in the office Know the female reproductive system, diseases, and surgical terms
Ophthalmology (Ophth.)— Treat disorders of the eye	Schedule patients to be seen when others are waiting for refraction drops to take effect Interact well with patients who are sight impaired or blind Keep diagnostic equipment in good working condition Know medical terminology of eye anatomy, diseases, surgery, and congenital anomalies
Orthopedic surgery (Orth. surg.)— Treat various parts of skeletal and muscular systems, including bones and joints	Maintain a flexible appointment schedule involving emergency appointments Schedule x-rays, MRIs, CTs, bone scans, and other various tests Schedule supplementary treatments with physical therapist Know medical terminology of skeletal, muscular, and nervous systems, diseases, surgeries, anomalies, and roentgenography Handle a large volume of industrial accident cases
Otolaryngology (ENT)— Treat disorders of the ear, nose, and throat (also called otorhinolaryngology)	Know terminology of ear, nose, and throat anatomy, diseases, surgeries, and anomalies Schedule appointments skillfully Key or type lengthy case histories, resumés, pre- and postoperative reports, and communications to referring physicians Schedule office and hospital surgery Communicate resourcefully with patients who have a hearing loss Work allergy testing and injections into daily schedule Maintain equipment in working order

Table 2-3 (continued). Medical Specialties and Administrative Medical Assisting Job Requirements

Medical Specialties	Administrative Medical Assistant Must . . .
Pathology (Path.)—Hematology, medical microbiology, neuro-pathology, and forensic medicine. Determine causes and nature of diseases and contribute to diagnosis, prognosis, and treatment	Know pathology terms Possess accurate transcription skills Telephone oral reports accurately Deliver reports File and code material

Pediatrics (Ped.) and Adolescent medicine—Medical treatment of children and adolescents
 	
  Pediatric Subspecialties
   Adolescent Medicine
   Cardiology
   Critical Care
   Development-Behavioral
   Emergency Medicine
   Endocrinology
   Gastroenterology
   Hematology-Oncology
   Infectious Disease
   Nephrology
   Neurodevelopmental
    Disabilities
   Pulmonology
   Rheumatology
   Sports Medicine
	Enjoy children and understand child psychology
	Calm upset parents skillfully on telephone and in office
	Know what information to give a parent over telephone
	Screen calls and merge emergency appointments into a full schedule
	Schedule appointments with a minimum of waiting in reception room
	Know general medical terminology
	Handle teenagers diplomatically when they have nervous or drug-related disorders

Perinatology—Specializes in maternal-fetal medicine; consultations on complications of pregnancy, genetic counseling, prematurity prevention, fetal echocardiography, and antenatal testing	Know the female reproductive system, diseases, fetal abnormalities, w surgical terms Check health insurance to verify covered and noncovered services Handle high-risk perinatal referrals from Ob-Gyn specialists Know ultrasound and amniocentesis procedures
Physiatrist Physical medicine and rehabilitation (Phys. med. rehab.)—Treatment of an ill or injured patient by massage, electrotherapy, and exercise	Know skeletal and muscular anatomy and disease and terminology Deal with patients who are in continual pain Encourage patients on long rehabilitation programs
Plastic surgery (P. surgery)—Repair or rebuild imperfect or damaged body parts	Obtain accurate, detailed case histories Have knowledge of terminology of the skeletal structure Handle emergency situations well Have knowledge of skin anatomy and medical terminology Complete insurance claims Perform bookkeeping procedures Be comfortable dealing with disfigured patients
Podiatry (DPM)—Diagnosis and treatment of conditions affecting the human foot	Be familiar with podiatric medical terminology Schedule surgery Handle elderly patients with mobility problems Manage telephone calls and appointment scheduling Take a vascular evaluation history Know diagnostic and procedure codes for podiatry

(continues)

Table 2-3 (*continued*). Medical Specialties and Administrative Medical Assisting Job Requirements

Medical Specialties	Administrative Medical Assistant Must . . .
Preventive Medicine (PM)—Protect, promote, and maintain health and well-being; prevent disease, disability, and premature death	Understand and interact with manage care plans Send recall and reminder notices to patients Schedule appointments and tests Know diagnostic and procedure codes for well check-ups, vaccinations, health history factors, and other preventive medicine procedures Understand insurance rules regarding preventive medicine
Psychiatry (Psy.) —Treatment, diagnosis, and prevention of mental disorders of a functional nature, such as stress	Deal calmly with disturbed patients Screen patients on the telephone Empathize with patients having varied mental disorders Like people Guard confidential patient records and maintain office security Transcribe and key or type lengthy case histories Know psychiatric terms and treatment, behavior, and disease terminology
Radiology (Rad.)—Diagnosis and treatment of disease using x-rays and radium	Handle referrals from physicians Know medical terminology of the anatomy and skeletal structure Know radiologic terms and general medical terminology of all body systems Telephone oral reports accurately
Surgery (Surg.)—Treatment of injuries, deformities, or disease by operation **Specific surgery disciplines:** Cardiovascular Oral Colon and rectal Orthopedic General Pediatric Hand Plastic Head and neck Thoracic Neurologic Urologic Ophthalmic Vascular	Know general medical terminology Handle patient consents for procedures Schedule in-office and hospital surgeries Schedule pre-op and post-op appointments Be able to discern and handle surgical emergencies and complications Know surgical procedure codes and billing rules File insurance claims accurately and timely
Urology (Urol.)—Disorders of the genitourinary tract: bladder, kidney, and prostate surgery	Schedule surgery with hospital personnel Know medical terminology of male and female reproductive systems, the genitourinary system, their anatomy, diseases, surgery, and congenital anomalies Have good telephone skills Perform bookkeeping procedures Complete insurance claims

nurse practitioner (NP), or a nurse midwife (NMW). Always address these individuals using their correct professional title. Be sure to correct patients who refer to a non-physician practitioner as "doctor" or to a medical assistant as "nurse." If the patient is led to believe that the medical assistant is a nurse and a lawsuit develops, the assistant may be held to standards to which nurses are held.

Health Care Professionals' Abbreviations

Table 2-4 contains a list of abbreviations of various professional positions in the field of medicine. An administrative medical assistant should be familiar with these abbreviations. The medical assistant will use them repeatedly when employed in the medical field.

Table 2-4. Abbreviations for Physician Specialists and Health Care Professionals

Physician Specialist	Abbreviation	Health Care Professional	Abbreviation
Doctor of Chiropractic	DC	Certified First Assistant (surgical)	CFA
Doctor of Dental Surgery	DDS	Certified Laboratory Assistant; certified by	CLA
Doctor of Dental Science	DD Sc	Registry of American Society of Clinical	(ASCP)
Doctor of Emergency Medicine	DEM	Pathologists	
Doctor of Hygiene	D Hy	Certified Medical Assistant	CMA
Doctor of Medical Dentistry	DMD	Certified Medical Transcriptionist	CMT
Doctor of Medicine	MD	Certified Nurse Midwife	CNM
Doctor of Optometry	OD	Certified Professional Coder	CPC
Doctor of Ophthalmology	OphD	Certified Registered Nurse Anesthetist	CRNA
Doctor of Osteopathy	DO	Certified Surgical Technician (2nd surgical asst.)	CST
Doctor of Pharmacy	Pharm D	Emergency Medical Technician	EMT
Doctor of Podiatry	DPM	Health Information Management	HIM
Doctor of Public Health	DPH	Inhalation Therapist	IT
Doctor of Tropical Medicine	DTM	Laboratory Technician Assistant	LTA
Doctor of Veterinary Medicine	DVM	Licensed Practical Nurse	LPN
Doctor of Veterinary Surgery	DVS	Licensed Vocational Nurse	LVN
Fellow of the American Academy of Pediatrics	FAAP	Master of Public Health	MPH
		Medical Technologist	MT
Fellow of the American College of Obstetricians and Gynecologists	FACOG		(ASCP)
		Physician's Assistant—Certified	PA-C
Fellow of the American College of Surgery	FACS	Public Health Nurse	PHN
Senior Fellow	SF	Registered Dietitian	RD
		Registered Nurse	RN
		Registered Nurse First Assistant (surgical)	RNFA
		Registered Nurse Practitioner	RNP
		Registered Occupational Therapist	ROT
		Registered Physical Therapist	RPT
		Registered Respiratory Therapist	RRT
		Registered Technologist (Radiology)	RT (R)
		Registered Technologist (Therapy)	RT (T)
		Visiting Nurse	VN

STOP AND THINK CASE SCENARIO

Traditional versus Managed Care

Scenario: Janet takes her two grandmothers to see the same physician who accepts Medicare and Senior Medicare. She arranges both of their appointments for Tuesday morning. Granny needs to write a check for her yearly deductible and Nana pays a $10 copayment. After they have both seen the doctor, the medical assistant appears with directions regarding their treatment plans. Granny needs to see a urologist and an appointment is made for the following day. Nana needs to have an x-ray and an authorization will be processed. The medical assistant will call when it is approved.

Critical Thinking:

1. What type of Medicare plan is Granny on?

_____

_____

2. What type of Medicare plan is Nana on?

_____

_____

3. What type of MCO does the physician belong to that enables him/her to see both of these types of patients in his/her office?

_____

_____

STOP AND THINK CASE SCENARIO

Types of Medical Practice Settings

Scenario 1: You have a desire to go to a physician who will know you by name and treat you like family.

Scenario 2: You would like to walk into a physician's office without having to make an appointment.

Scenario 3: You are looking for a job as an administrative medical assistant and benefits are more important to you than high pay.

Scenario 4: You have a friend who is a burn victim and you want to work in a setting that treats such patients.

Scenario 5: You believe that the physician should treat the body, mind, and soul, not just the physical ailment.

Critical Thinking 1: What type of practice setting will you look for?

_____

Critical Thinking 2: What type of practice setting will you look for?

_____

Critical Thinking 3: What type of practice setting will you look for?

_____

Critical Thinking 4: What type of practice setting will you look for?

_____

Critical Thinking 5: What type of practice setting will you look for?

_____

FOCUS ON CERTIFICATION*

CMA Content Summary

- Medical terminology
- Working as a team
- Patient instruction
- Appropriate referrals
- Prepaid HMO, PPO, POS

RMA Content Summary

- Medical terminology
- Patient instruction
- Insurance terminology (HMO, PPO, EPO)

CMAS Content Summary

- Medical terminology
- Prepare information for referrals

REVIEW EXAM-STYLE QUESTIONS

1. The "father of medicine" was:

   a. Imhotep

   b. Hipprocrates

   c. Pasteur

   d. Lister

   e. Salk

2. The "father of modern surgery" was:

   a. Pierre Curie

   b. Francis Crick

   c. Ambrose Pare

   d. Walter Reed

   e. William Harvey

3. The founder of the American Red Cross was:

   a. Clara Barton

   b. Florence Nightingale

   c. Ignaz P. Semmelweis

   d. John Hunter

   e. Edward Jenner

4. Managed care started the practice of "utilization review" to:

   a. review physicians' diagnostic skills

   b. review all aspects of the medical practice

   c. utilize HMO personnel more efficiently

   d. monitor and control areas in medicine where overuse occurs

   e. control doctors' decision making

5. The managed care organization that has been in existence the longest is a/an:

   a. PPO

   b. IPA

   c. HMO

   d. EPO

   e. POS

*This textbook and the accompanying Workbook meet the educational components of entry-level administrative and general competencies outlines for the CMA outlined by the AAMA Examination Content Outline and Role Delineation Study and for the RMA and CMAS outlined by the AMT Competencies and Examination Specifications (see Competency Grid in Appendix B).

6. The type of manage care organization that offers the patient flexibility when making a choice of going to a contracted or noncontracted physician at the time services are needed is a/an:

   a. POS

   b. HMO

   c. IPA

   d. EPO

   e. POS

7. A freestanding practice center that provides extended hours and walk-in appointments is a/an:

   a. medical center

   b. family practice

   c. medical clinic

   d. specialized care center

   e. urgent care center

8. A fairly new specialty that deals with the management and control of obesity is called:

   a. Weight Control Clinics

   b. Bariatric Medicine

   c. Gerontology

   d. Nuclear Medicine

   e. Medical Genetics

9. A medical specialty that determines the causes and nature of diseases and contributes to diagnosis, prognosis, and treatment is called:

   a. Gerontology

   b. Family Practice

   c. Internal Medicine

   d. Surgery

   e. Pathology

10. The abbreviation for a doctor of ophthalmology is:

   a. OD

   b. OP

   c. OphD

   d. DO

   e. MD

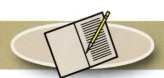

WORKBOOK ASSIGNMENT

To develop competency-based job skills, refer to the *Workbook* and complete the:

- Abbreviation and Spelling Review
- Review Questions

- Critical Thinking Exercises
- Job Skill activities, which are outlined at the beginning of this chapter under "Performance Objectives in the *Workbook*."

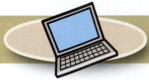

COMPUTER ASSIGNMENT

To review the concepts you have learned in this chapter, insert the *Student Practice* CD-ROM into a computer and work through the *StudyWARE* activities and games. Answer review questions in the practice mode and read the feedback, studying the questions you have missed. Take the chapter quiz until you achieve a minimum score of 90 percent. Successfully completing the *Critical Thinking Challenge* at the end of this course will help you think through scenarios and develop problem solving skills.

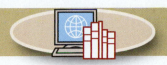

RESOURCES

Books

Health Professions Directory American Medical Association
PO Box 930876
Atlanta, GA 31193-0876
(800) 621-8335
Web site: http://www.ama-assn.org

The Managed Health Care Dictionary
Jones and Bartlett Publishers
40 Tall Pine Drive
Sudbury, MA 01776
(800) 832-0034
Web site: http://www.jbpub.com

The Managed Health Care Handbook
Jones and Bartlett
40 Tall Pine Drive
Sudbury, MA 01776
(800) 832-0034
Web site: http://www.jbpub.com

Internet

Accreditation Commission for Acupuncture and Oriental Medicine
Web site: http://www.acaom.org

American Association of Naturopathic Medical Colleges
Web site: http://www.aanmc.org

American Association of Naturopathic Physicians
Web site: http://www.naturopathic.org

American Association of Oriental Medicine
Web site: http://www.aaom.org

American Massage Therapy Association
Web site: http://www.amtamassage.org

National Center for Complimentary and Alternative Medicine
Web site: http://www.nccam.nih.gov

National Center for Homeopathy
Web site: http://www.homeopathic.org

National Certification Board for Therapeutic Massage and Bodywork
Web site: http://www.ncbtmb.com

White House Commission on Complementary and Alternative Medicine Policy
Web site: http://www.whccamp.hhs.gov/finalreport.html

United States National Library of Medicine
Web site: http://www.nlm.nih.gov

Medical Specialties

American Board of Medical Specialties
1007 Church Street, Suite 404
Evanston, IL 60201-5913
(847) 491-9091
Web site: http://www.abms.org

CHAPTER 3

Medicolegal and Ethical Responsibilities

OBJECTIVES

After reading this chapter and learning step-by-step procedures to gain job skills,* you should be able to:

Learning Objectives

▊ Define the legal terminology used in the chapter.

▊ Compare medical ethics and medical etiquette.

▊ Identify the purpose and provisions of the Health Insurance Portability and Accountability Act.

▊ State the purpose for obtaining a signed consent form.

▊ Determine reasons for disclosure that need an authorization to release medical information.

▊ State the licensing requirements for a physician.

▊ Name two types of medical professional liability insurance.

▊ List prevention measures for medicolegal claims.

▊ Distinguish three alternatives to the litigation process.

▊ Define various types of contracts.

▊ Determine instances when a minor is emancipated.

▊ Identify statutes governing subpoena of records.

▊ Describe the components of an informed consent for a procedure/service.

▊ List various types of advance directives.

▊ Name the provisions of the Uniform Anatomical Gift Act.

This textbook and the accompanying Workbook meet the educational components for entry-level administrative and general competencies outlined by CAAHEP and ABHES.

Performance Objectives (Procedures) in This Textbook

▌ Release patient information (Procedure 3-1).

▌ Accept a subpoena (Procedure 3-2).

Performance Objectives (Job Skills) in the *Workbook*

▌ Compose letter of withdrawal (Job Skill 3-1).

OUTLINE WITH LECTURE NOTES

Medical Ethics

Principles of Medical Ethics for the Physician

_____

_____

_____

_____

Principles of Medical Ethics for the Medical Assistant

_____

_____

_____

_____

Medical Etiquette

_____

_____

_____

_____

Health Insurance Portability and Accountability Act of 1996

Protected Health Information (PHI)

_____

_____

_____

_____

Compliance Plan

_____

_____

_____

_____

Security Rule

_____

_____

_____

_____

Confidentiality

Release of Medical Information

_____

_____

_____

_____

Medical Practice Acts

_____

_____

_____

_____

Medical Professional Liability

Liability Insurance

_____

_____

_____

Respondeat Superior

_____

_____

_____

Torts

_____

_____

_____

_____

Principal Defenses

_____

_____

_____

_____

Litigation Prevention

_____

_____

_____

_____

Alternatives to the Litigation Process

Screening Panel

_____

_____

_____

_____

Arbitration

_____

_____

_____

_____

No-Fault Insurance

_____

_____

_____

_____

Physician/Patient Contract

Expressed/Implied Contracts

_____

_____

_____

_____

Third-Party Contracts

_____

_____

_____

_____

Contracts and Emergency Care

_____

_____

_____

_____

Contracts with Minors

_____

_____

_____

_____

Terminating a Contract

_____

_____

_____

_____

Informed Consent

_____

_____

_____

_____

Medical Records

Subpoena

_____

_____

_____

_____

Advance Directives

Living Will

_____

_____

_____

_____

Health Care Power of Attorney

_____

_____

_____

_____

Medical Directive

_____

_____

_____

_____

Values History Form

_____

_____

_____

Health Care Proxy

_____

_____

_____

Do Not Resuscitate Form

_____

_____

_____

Uniform Anatomical Gift Act

_____

_____

_____

Advanced Directive Guidelines

_____

_____

_____

KEY TERMS

advance directive
authorization form
bioethics
bonding
civil law
complaint
compliance plan
consent form
defendant
emancipated minors
ethics
etiquette
expert testimony
grievance committee

health care power of attorney
Health Insurance Portability
    and Accountability Act
implied contract
litigation
living will
protected health information (PHI)
plaintiff
privileged information
respondeat superior
subpoena
subpoena duces tecum
tort

HEART OF THE HEALTH CARE PROFESSIONAL

Service

The health care professional has the responsibility to conduct business in a legal and ethical manner. Serving patients' needs presents the perfect opportunity to exhibit high values and principles. It is through service-oriented duties that your moral character will stand out, be noticed, and be appreciated.

MEDICAL ETHICS

Before entering the profession of administrative medical assisting, it is advisable to have some basic knowledge of ethical and legal responsibilities as they pertain to the medical profession. Professional medical **ethics** are not laws but are standards of conduct generally accepted as a moral guide for behavior. Ethical principles should be reflected in administrative procedures. For example, the principle of the patient's right to privacy is guaranteed by an administrative rule against discussing a patient's condition with others. These moral principles and related professional standards of conduct apply equally to relationships with patients, other physicians, members of allied professions, and the public.

The focus in this chapter is on professional ethics and medicolegal responsibilities with which a medical assistant needs to be concerned. For specific questions beyond the scope of this chapter, medical assistants should seek legal advice and the counsel of an attorney; each state has its own laws pertaining to medical practice. Ethical and legal considerations relating to drugs, prescriptions, and the Controlled Substances Act of 1970 are discussed in Chapter 10.

Principles of Medical Ethics for the Physician

The first standards of *medical conduct and ethics* are those set down in the Oath of Hippocrates (Figure 3-1). Included in this famous affirmation, which some doctors graduating from medical school still swear to, are many of the basics of medical ethics. This oath was updated by Dr. Louis Lasagna and appears in Figure 3-2.

In 1980, the American Medical Association (AMA) adopted a modern code of ethics called the Principles of Medical Ethics. This code benefits health professionals and meets the needs of changing times. Refer to Figure 3-3, listing these principles, which guide a physician's standards of conduct for honorable behavior in the practice of medicine.

A physician must also adhere to a body of generally accepted practice procedures, such as the following:

- A physician may ethically receive payments from patients for medical services but cannot accept a rebate of any kind from anyone.

- A physician may accept small gifts (e.g., plastic anatomic models, stethoscopes, booklets) but may not ethically accept large "gifts" from manufacturers or distributors of pharmaceuticals, remedies, or equipment. This practice could influence him or her to prescribe a particular product.

- A physician may employ a collection agency to try to collect overdue bills but may not sell his or her delinquent accounts to the agency.

OATH OF HIPPOCRATES

I swear by Apollo, the physician, and Aesculapius and health and all-heal and all the Gods and Goddesses that, according to my ability and judgment, I will keep this oath and stipulation:

TO RECKON him who taught me this art equally dear to me as my parents, to share my substance with him and relieve his necessities if required; to regard his offspring as on the same footing with my own brothers, and to teach them this art if they should wish to learn it, without fee or stipulation, and that by precept, lecture and every other mode of instruction, I will impart a knowledge of the art to my own sons and to those of my teachers, and to disciples bound by a stipulation and oath, according to the law of medicine, but to none others.

I WILL FOLLOW that method of treatment which, according to my ability and judgment, I consider for the benefit of my patients, and abstain from whatever is deleterious and mischievous. I will give no deadly medicine to anyone if asked, nor suggest any such counsel; furthermore, I will not give to a woman an instrument to produce abortion.

WITH PURITY AND WITH HOLINESS I will pass my life and practice my art. I will not cut a person who is suffering from a stone, but will leave this to be done by practitioners of this work. Into whatever houses I enter I will go into them for the benefit of the sick and will abstain from every voluntary act of mischief and corruption; and further from the seduction of females or males, bond or free.

WHATEVER, in connection with my professional practice, or not in connection with it, I may see or hear in the lives of men which ought not to be spoken abroad I will not divulge, as reckoning that all such should be kept secret.

WHILE I CONTINUE to keep this oath unviolated may it be granted to me to enjoy life and the practice of the art, respected by all men at all times but should I trespass and violate this oath, may the reverse be my lot.

Figure 3-1. Hippocrates (c. 460 B.C.–377 B.C.), a Greek physician known as the "father of medicine," developed a code, the Oath of Hippocrates, based on the golden rule that to be a good physician one must first be a good and kind person

A MODERN HIPPOCRATIC OATH

I swear to fulfill, to the best of my ability and judgment, this covenant:

I will respect the hard-won scientific gains of those physicians in whose steps I walk, and gladly share such knowledge as is mine with those who are to follow.

I will apply, for the benefit of the sick, all measures which are required, avoiding those twin traps of overtreatment and therapeutic nihilism.

I will remember that there is art to medicine as well as science, and that warmth, sympathy and understanding may outweigh the surgeon's knife or the chemist's drug.

I will not be ashamed to say, "I know not," nor will I fail to call in my colleague when the skills of another are needed for a patient's recovery.

I will respect the privacy of my patients, for their problems are not disclosed to me that the world may know. Most especially must I tread with care in matters of life and death. If it is given me to save a life, all thanks. But it may also be within my power to take a life; this awesome responsibility must be faced with great humbleness and awareness of my own frailty. Above all, I must not play God.

I will remember that I do not treat a fever chart, or a cancerous growth, but a sick human being, whose illness may affect the person's family and economic stability. My responsibility includes these related problems, if I am to care adequately for the sick.

I will prevent disease whenever I can, for prevention is preferable to cure.

I will remember that I remain a member of society, with special obligations to all my fellow human beings, those sound of mind and body, as well as the infirm.

If I do not violate this oath, may I enjoy life and art, respected while I live and remembered with affection thereafter. May I always act so as to preserve the finest traditions of my calling and may I long experience the joy of healing those who seek my help.

Figure 3-2. The Modern Hippocratic Oath. (Reprinted with permission from Dr. Louis Lasagna, Tufts University, Boston, Massachusetts.)

PRINCIPLES OF MEDICAL ETHICS FOR THE PHYSICIAN
Preamble

The medical profession has long subscribed to a body of ethical statements developed primarily for the benefit of the patient. As a member of this profession, a physician must recognize responsibility to patients first and foremost, as well as to society, to other health professionals, and to self. The following Principles adopted by the American Medical Association are not laws, but standards of conduct which define the essentials of honorable behavior for the physician.

   I. A physician shall be dedicated to providing competent medical care with compassion and respect for human dignity and rights.

  II. A physician shall uphold the standards of professionalism, be honest in all professional interactions, and strive to report physicians deficient in character of competence, or engaging in fraud or deception, to appropriate entities.

 III. A physician shall respect the law and also recognize a responsibility to seek changes in those requirements which are contrary to the best interests of the patient.

 IV. A physician shall respect the rights of patients, of colleagues, and of other health professionals, and shall safeguard patient confidences within the constraints of the law.

  V. A physician shall continue to study, apply and advance scientific knowledge, maintain a commitment to medical education, make relevant information available to patients, colleagues, and the public, obtain consultation, and use the talents of other health professionals when indicated.

 VI. A physician shall, in the provision of appropriate patient care, except in emergencies, be free to choose whom to serve, with whom to associate, and the environment in which to provide medical care.

VII. A physician shall recognize a responsibility to participate in activities contributing to an improvement of the community and the betterment of public health.

VIII. A physician shall, while caring for a patient, regard responsibility to the patient as paramount.

 IX. A physician shall support access to medical care for all people.

Figure 3-3. Principles of Medical Ethics for the Physician; revised June 17, 2001. (Reprinted with permission from the American Medical Association, Chicago, Illinois.)

PATIENT EDUCATION

Office policies should be printed in a booklet or handout so that patients will be informed about charges for missed appointments, telephone calls, insurance form completion, and so forth. The American Medical Association considers it ethical for a physician to charge a fee for such services only if the patient has been informed of the policies beforehand. Chapter 5 covers preparation of patient information booklets.

Bioethics

Because technology has brought more sophistication to the medical profession, there is increased concern about ethical and moral issues among those in the field of medicine and the lay public. The term **bioethics** emerged as a result of issues about the transplanting of organs, genetic engineering or manipulation, maintaining life with life-sustaining equipment, physician-assisted suicide, cloning, abortion, fetal tissue research, artificial insemination, in vitro fertilization, surrogate motherhood, stem cell research, and so on. Bioethics is the branch of ethics dealing with issues, questions, and problems that arise in the practice of medicine and in biomedical research. It is a very complex field that draws on medical, scientific, philosophic, sociologic, and theologic knowledge. Examples 3-1 and 3-2 describe some bioethical issues.

Principles of Medical Ethics for the Medical Assistant

To maintain a high degree of ethical conduct in relating to patients, physicians, and coworkers, a medical assistant should:

1. Remember that everything seen, heard, or read about a patient is confidential and should not leave the office (Figures 3-4 and 3-5). Before information about a patient may be released, the patient must sign an authorization form for release of information unless subpoenaed by the court. This is discussed and illustrated later in this chapter.

EXAMPLE 3-1

Quality of Life versus Length of Life

A severely deformed infant is born with many medical problems. The decision-making process may involve whether to provide or withhold treatment, what type of treatment should or should not be used, and who will bear the expense of the treatment, which may be costly.

EXAMPLE 3-2

Physician-Assisted Suicide

An elderly, terminally ill patient is requesting physician-assisted suicide because he or she is completely dependent on others for daily care, is in continual pain, and is experiencing total loss of dignity.

2. Apply discretion when using an intercom or voice pager as there may be others in the room who may hear the information being relayed. If the system permits storing the messages, the user should try to receive messages only in private areas.

3. Avoid talking about anything of a private nature when speaking to a physician via cellular or cordless telephone because it is possible for other parties to overhear conversations electronically, thus breaching a patient's confidentiality.

4. Never discuss a patient's condition within hearing distance of others.

5. Sidestep discussing a patient with acquaintances or the patient's friends.

6. Never leave a patient's records lying exposed.

7. Remain loyal to your employer; do not criticize the physician to a patient.

8. Communicate in a dignified, courteous manner with everyone in the office and those who telephone or visit; never degrade or malign a patient.

9. Notify the physician when learning that a patient is being treated by another physician

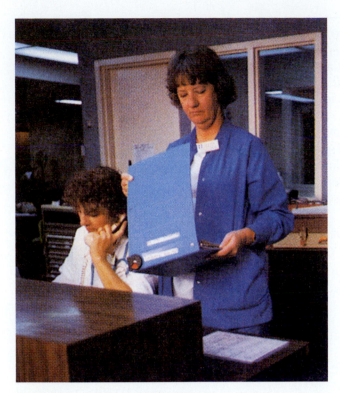

Figure 3-4. All information about patients is confidential

for the same ailment. (A consultation does not constitute treatment.)

10. Support physicians in your community. Never make critical statements about the treatment given a patient by another physician.

11. Avoid dishonest or unethical coworkers. Do not allow them to steer you into questionable practices. Keep the physician fully informed of your own work so it will be clear to everyone that any misdeeds are not yours.

The American Association of Medical Assistants (AAMA) has established a code of ethics appropriate for medical assistants whether they are members of this association or not (Figure 3-6). Other ethical issues about using computers are addressed in Chapter 9.

MEDICAL ETIQUETTE

Etiquette should not be confused with ethics. Medical **etiquette** is the customary code of conduct, courtesy, and manners in the medical profession. Courtesy in

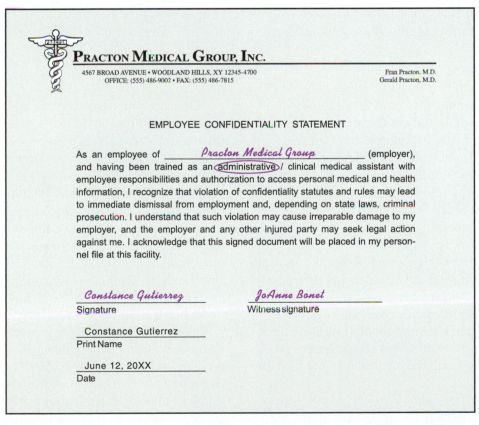

Figure 3-5. Example of an employee confidentiality agreement that may be used by an employer when hiring a new employee

---

AAMA CODE OF ETHICS

The Code of Ethics of AAMA shall set forth principles of ethical and moral conduct as they relate to the medical profession and the particular practice of medical assisting.

   Members of AAMA dedicated to the conscientious pursuit of their profession, and thus desiring to merit the high regard of the entire medical profession and the respect of the general public which they serve, do pledge themselves to strive always to:

A. render service with full respect for the dignity of humanity;
B. respect confidential information obtained through employment unless legally authorized or required by responsible performance of duty to divulge such information;
C. uphold the honor and high principles of the profession and accept its disciplines;
D. seek to continually improve the knowledge and skills of medical assistants for the benefit of patients and professional colleagues;
E. participate in additional service activities aimed toward improving the health and well-being of the community.

AAMA CREED

I believe in the principles and purposes of the profession of medical assisting.
I endeavor to be more effective.
I aspire to render greater service.
I protect the confidence entrusted to me.
I am dedicated to the care and well-being of all people.
I am loyal to my employer.
I am true to the ethics of my profession.
I am strengthened by compassion, courage and faith.

Figure 3-6. Code of medical ethics and creed for medical assistants as established by the American Association of Medical Assistants. (Reprinted with permission of the American Association of Medical Assistants, Chicago, Illinois.)

medical offices is more important than ever since customer service is emphasized and medical practices try to maximize productivity and work flow.

   The medical assistant should immediately acknowledge people when they enter the office, even if he or she is on the telephone. The assistant should look up, smile, and convey a signal that says, "I'll be with you in a moment." When other physicians visit the office to discuss a patient, it is customary to usher them into the inner office as soon as possible and not keep them waiting. Likewise, when another physician telephones, the medical assistant should connect him or her immediately without interrogation. When the physician is calling about a mutual patient, the medical assistant should take a moment to verify the patient's name, pull the medical record, and then transfer the call.

   Medical assistants should always identify themselves when answering the telephone; never leave patients on hold longer than one minute. When making a call, identify yourself and give the reason why you are telephoning.

   Etiquette among coworkers is dictated by common sense. Those in the workplace must be careful of how they act in their place of employment. It is always courteous to say, "Good morning" and "Good night" to everyone whether or not you know them personally. Use of first names is common in an informal atmosphere, but the physician should always be addressed formally (e.g., "Doctor Practon"). Respect the office's customs; for example, if everyone pitches in to handle meeting a deadline or assisting in an emergency, this might mean working late or coming in on a Saturday.

   When working as a new employee or as an extern in a medical office, never gossip and remember to use all ethical and etiquette guidelines of common courtesy presented here. (*Externship* is a training program that is part of a course of study in an educational institution. It allows the student to work alongside medical professionals in a private business and practice learned skills.)

   Etiquette is a vast subject and numerous additional instances are discussed throughout this text.

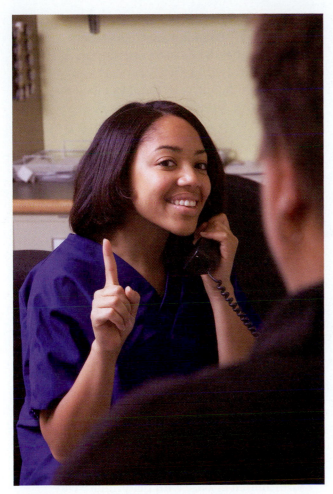

Figure 3-7. Medical assistant acknowledging a patient with a smile and gesturing that it will only be one moment before she will be able to help

Etiquette in communications is discussed in Chapter 4 (The Art of Communication). Etiquette guidelines on greeting the patient are found in Chapter 5 (The Receptionist). Additional rules of etiquette for telephone, voice mail, cell phone, and so forth are found in Chapter 6 (Telephone Procedures). When sending documents via facsimile there are both etiquette and legal confidentiality issues to be considered, which are described in Chapter 12.

HEALTH INSURANCE PORTABILITY AND ACCOUNTABILITY ACT OF 1996

The **Health Insurance Portability and Accountability Act,** commonly referred to as HIPAA (pronounced hipah), became a federal law in 1996. The purpose of HIPAA is to provide a standarized framework within which all insurance companies and providers work to:

- enhance the portability of health care coverage
- increase accuracy of data
- protect private health information and the rights of patients
- reduce fraud, abuse, and waste in the health care delivery system
- upgrade efficiency and financial management
- expedite claim processing
- lower administrative costs and simplify implementation
- promote Medical Saving Accounts
- avail better access to long-term care coverage
- improve customer satisfaction to restore trust in the health care system.

The act is divided into sections that address different issues of health care. The two main provisions are addressed in Title I and Title II; however, additional titles are listed and briefly described to provide an overview of all provisions that affect the medical office. If state laws offer protection greater than HIPAA laws, then state laws prevail. Information pertaining to HIPAA appear throughout chapters in this text where the subject matter is addressed. "Compliance" boxes are used to alert the reader to key legal issues.

- *Title I: Health Insurance Access, Portability, and Renewal*—Increases the portability of health insurance by protecting coverage when employees change jobs. It does this by prohibiting preexisting condition exclusions, disallowing discrimination of health insurance coverage based on health status, and guaranteeing renewability for certain group health plans.
- *Title II: Health Care Fraud, Abuse, Prevention, and Administrative Simplification*—Prevents fraud and abuse in health care delivery and payment for services, establishes guidelines to simplify administrative procedures, provides national standards to protect privacy, and mandates electronic transmission of certain health information.
- *Title III: Medical Savings Account (MSA) Benefits*—Addresses the MSA; increasing deductions, adding consumer protection, and addressing income tax refund payments.

- *Title IV: Group Health Plan Directives*—Details how group health plans must allow for portability, access, and renewability for members.

- *Title V: Internal Revenue Code Amendments*—Explains changes in the Internal Revenue Code of 1986 so that more revenue is generated to offset costs of implementing HIPAA.

- *Title XI: General Provisions*—Focuses on Medicare-related plans and addresses the coordination of general provisions, peer review, and administration simplification.

- *Title XXVII: Portability Assurance*—Speaks to the carry-over of health insurance plans from one plan to another.

Protected Health Information (PHI)

Protected health information (PHI),* under HIPAA is defined as information about the patient's past, present, or future health condition that contains personal identifying data. This includes patient demographics and conversations. Under the *Privacy Rule* strong federal protection is provided for the privacy of patients without interfering with the quality of health care or its access. The rule sets boundaries, defines safeguards, holds violators accountable, and gives patients more control over their health information. The use (sharing, utilizing, examining) and disclosure (releasing, transferring, or providing access) of PHI is protected under the rule.

The medical practice must have written policies and procedures that comply with HIPAA standards. This may be in the form of a Policy and Procedures Manual used both as a resource and to train employees and physicians. Revisions need to be made as necessary and documentation retained a minimum of six years.

Under HIPAA's privacy rules for PHI, patients have the right to:

1. Receive *notices* of privacy practices.
   Example: A written policy describing how the practice uses PHI and informing patients about their rights should be posted in the office and be available in a handout or booklet kept at the front desk with a signature page signed by the patient acknowledging receipt.

2. Access medical and financial records.
   Example: If a patient wants to inspect or obtain a copy of their medical record the request must be acted on within 30 days and a fee may be charged although certain information may be exempt (e.g., psychotherapy notes).

3. Ask for an amendment to the medical record.
   Example: A patient requests that changes, additions, or deletions be made to correct information. The health care provider needs to be the creator of the information and must act on the request within 60 days.

4. Receive an accounting of disclosures made. Excluded are disclosures for the purpose of treatment, receiving payment, or day-to-day operations.
   Example: A disclosure is made to the health authority reporting a communicable disease for public purposes. The log of disclosures should include the date, name of individual, purpose, and brief description of PHI disclosed.

5. Request restrictions on disclosures for certain uses (not for normal business operations, to treat the patient, or to receive reimbursement).
   Example: A patient asks her gynecologist not to share positive test results indicating a sexually transmitted disease with her primary care physician.

6. Ask that all communication be confidential.
   Example: A patient may not want to approach the front desk and talk about the reason for the visit in front of other patients, or may want to receive test results at an alternative location.

If a friend or family member is involved in a patient's care, you can disclose PHI that is relevant; however, the patient may need to agree to such a disclosure, depending on whether he or she is present and competent. The disclosure should be related only to the patient's current condition and should not include past medical history.

Compliance Plan

A **compliance plan** is a written document that includes office policies and procedures, rules to follow, and practice standards that are monitored through internal auditing. It is an ever-changing program that recognizes challenges, addresses problem areas,

---

* *The acronym PHI has been erroneously referred to as personal, privileged, or private health information.*

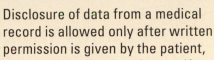

and identifies risk to the medical practice. A compliance officer, which may also be the security and privacy officer, needs to be named as the professional that conducts ongoing educational training sessions, identifies offenses, responds appropriately, and develops corrective action. Open communication is essential and guidelines need to be publicized in order to enforce disciplinary standards.

Security Rule

HIPAA's *security rule* interacts with the privacy rule as well as covering physical and technical safeguards; policies, procedures, and documentation requirements; risk analysis and risk management; and administrative safeguards to secure electronic protected health information. The rule applies to health plans, health care clearinghouses, and certain health care providers such as Medicare, Medicaid, other federal health programs and private health programs.

HIPAA violators may be subjected to fines, prison, or both. HIPAA information as it relates to insurance is further explained in Chapter 16 (Health Insurance Systems). In this chapter protected health information, confidentiality, and release of patient information are detailed.

CONFIDENTIALITY

The first policy that should be mentioned to a new employee in a medical setting is to keep information about patients confidential. Refrain from talking about patients and their problems where outsiders may overhear. A medical record contains **privileged information**; therefore, it must not be mislaid so other individuals can see it or leaf through it.

Procedures on how to retain confidentiality when using voice mail, facsimile equipment, or electronic mail are discussed in subsequent chapters.

Release of Medical Information

The medical record is the property of the physician, and he or she is legally and ethically obligated to keep it confidential unless an authorization for release of information form has been signed by the patient. With the advent of HIPAA, this has become a twofold procedure requiring a consent and/or an authorization.

Consent

HIPAA regulations state that patients have the right to know how their health information is used and may exercise control over the content of the information disclosed. Patient consent, however, is not an option; providers must obtain it. Patients can be denied treatment if they refuse to give consent. A one-time signed **consent form** is required *before* physicians use or disclose personally identifiable health information for treatment, payment, or routine health care operations, such as performance reviews, audits, training programs, and certain types of fundraising (Figure 3-8). Three basic exceptions when consent is unnecessary are:

1. When there is an emergency situation, however, providers must obtain written consent as soon as reasonably practical after the treatment.

2. When language barriers make it impossible to obtain written consent; in this case, the consent is implied.

3. When treating prison inmates.

Authorization

Under HIPAA, in addition to a signed consent form it is necessary to obtain a signed **authorization form** for use and disclosure of protected health information not included in the consent (Figure 3-9). In an

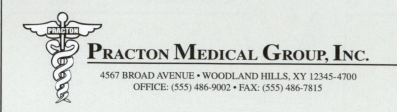

PRACTON MEDICAL GROUP, INC.

4567 BROAD AVENUE • WOODLAND HILLS, XY 12345-4700
OFFICE: (555) 486-9002 • FAX: (555) 486-7815

Fran Practon, M.D.
Gerald Practon, M.D.

CONSENT TO THE USE AND DISCLOSURE OF HEALTH INFORMATION

I understand that this organization originates and maintains health records which describe my health history, symptoms, examination, test results, diagnoses, treatment, and any plans for future care or treatment. I understand that this information is used to:

- plan my care and treatment
- communicate among health professionals who contribute to my care
- apply my diagnosis and services, procedures, and surgical information to my bill
- verify services billed by third-party payers
- assess quality of care and review the competence of health care professionals in routine health care operations

I further understand that:

- a complete description of information uses and disclosures is included in a *Notice of Information Practices* which has been provided to me
- I have a right to review the notice prior to signing this consent
- the organization reserves the right to change their notice and practices
- any revised notice will be mailed to the address I have provided prior to implementation
- I have the right to object to the use of my health information for directory purposes
- I have the right to request restrictions as to how my health information may be used or disclosed to carry out treatment, payment, or health care operations
- the organization is not required to agree to the restrictions requested
- I may revoke this consent in writing, except to the extent that the organization has already taken action in reliance thereon.

☐ I request the following restrictions to the use or disclosure of my health information.

_____

June 29, 20XX
_____
Date

Consuelo Hernandez
_____
Signature of Patient or Legal Representative

_____
Signature

_____
Date

June 29, 20XX
_____
Notice Effective Date

_____
Witness

_____
Title

_____ Accepted _____ Rejected

Figure 3-8. Example of a consent form for the use and disclosure of health information

AUTHORIZATION FOR RELEASE OF INFORMATION

Section A: Must be completed for all authorizations.

I hereby authorize the use or disclosure of my individually identifiable health information as described below.
I understand that this authorization is voluntary. I understand that if the organization authorized to receive the information is not a health plan or health care provider, the released information may no longer be protected by federal privacy regulations.

Patient name: _Hilda F. Goodman_   ID Number: _4309_

Identity of person/organization disclosing protected health information

Persons/organizations providing information:
Practon Medical Group, Inc
4567 Broad Avenue
Woodland Hills, XY 12345-4700

Persons/organizations receiving information:
Jennifer P. Lee, MD
400 North M Street
Anytown, XY 54098-1235

Identity of those authorized to use protected health information

Specific description of information [including from and to date(s)]:
Complete medical records from 4-22-XX to 9-15-XX

Specific description of information to be used or disclosed with dates

Section B: Must be completed only if a health plan or a heath care provider has requested the authorization.

Purpose for disclosure

1. The health plan or health care provider must complete the following:
   a. What is the purpose of the use or disclosure? _Patient relocating to another city_

   b. Will the health plan or health care provider requesting the authorization receive financial or in-kind compensation in exchange for using or disclosing the health information described above? Yes___ No _X_

2. The patient or the patient's representative must read and initial the following statements:
   a. I understand that my health care and the payment for my health care will not be affected if I do not sign this form.

   Initials: _hfg_

   b. I understand that I may see and copy the information described on this form if I ask for it, and that I get a copy of this form after I sign it.

   Initials: _hfg_

Section C: Must be completed for all authorizations.

The patient or the patient's representative must read and initial the following statements:

Expiration date

1. I understand that this authorization will expire on _12_ / _31_ / _20XX_ (DD/MM/YR).

   Initials: _hfg_

Individual's right to revoke this authorization in writing

2. I understand that I may revoke this authorization at any time by notifying the providing organization in writing, but if I do not it will not have any effect on any actions they took before they received the revocation.

   Initials: _hfg_

Redisclosure conditions

3. I understand that any disclosure of information carries with it the potential for an unauthorized redisclosure and the information may not be protected by federal confidentiality rules.

   Initials: _hfg_

Individual's signature

Hilda F. Goodman   _September 15, 20XX_

Signature of patient or patient's representative   **Date**
(Form MUST be completed before signing)

Date of signature

Printed name of patient's representative: _____

Relationship to the patient: _____

YOU MAY REFUSE TO SIGN THIS AUTHORIZATION
You may not use this form to release information for treatment or payment except
when the information to be released is psychotherapy notes or certain research information.

Figure 3-9. Example of an authorization form for the release of information

authorization, a minimum set of elements must be included outlining the purpose for which the health care information is to be used and disclosed. A physician is bound by the statements on the authorization and can only use or disclose the specific information listed. Requests from physicians, insurance companies, and attorneys may be honored when a patient has signed the authorization form for release of information. For cases involving continuity of patient care when requests are received to move records from hospital to hospital, physician to physician, or hospital to nursing home, if the patient has signed a consent form then it is not necessary to have the authorization form signed by the patient.

COMPLIANCE

Patients have a right to ask for an accounting of all health information disclosures (requests using the authorization form) made by a provider in the past six years. This request must be answered within 60 days. In some situations, a fee may be charged, but the majority of requests are provided at no charge.

Mandated Reporting—Although statutes may differ among states, the principal occurrences reported to the Department of Health are:

- Births, stillbirths, and deaths
- Certain communicable, infectious, or contagious diseases
- Child, spousal, or elder abuse or neglect
- Incest
- Spousal rape
- Suspicious wounds
- Injuries inflicted by oneself or by the acts of another by means of a knife, gun, pistol, or other deadly weapon
- Assaultive or abusive conduct
- Injuries inflicted in violation of any penal law
- Known or suspected drug abuse
- Epileptic seizures and related disorders

These are exceptions to the right of privacy and privileged communication that do not need an authorization form because state laws require disclosure to protect the public.

An exception also occurs in workers' compensation cases as the contract is between the physician and the insurance company. In these cases, information can be released to the insurance company without a patient's signed consent or authorization form.

Restricted Record Access—If a patient has a positive human immunodeficiency virus (HIV) test for acquired immune deficiency syndrome (AIDS), applies for life or health insurance, and signs an authorization form to release this information to the insurance company, the medical assistant should seek counsel from the proper supervisior or authorities before processing the request. Some state laws allow AIDS information to be given only to the patient's spouse. Authorization for release of information in states with restricted access about HIV test results must be carefully handled as results may appear in many sections of the health record. Use of *ICD-9-CM* codes 795.71, 042, or V08 indicates positive HIV test results, and this information must be considered confidential. The authorization form must list the specific description of particularly sensitive information to be disclosed including inclusive dates of treatment. The signed form should be retained in the health record. All information released on the request of the patient with a diagnosis of HIV infection should contain a statement prohibiting redisclosure of the information to another party without the prior authorization of the patient. The individual receiving the information should be requested to destroy the information after the stated need is fulfilled.

Patients Receiving Records—If patients request copies of their medical records, the request must be honored. However, caution should be taken because a patient may become emotionally upset due to a misunderstanding because of an inability to interpret technical or medical terms. For this reason, it is risky to release records directly to a patient or allow patients to hand-carry their records to a consultant. In an urgent situation, photocopies of the records should be sealed in an envelope or sent via facsimile using a special authorization form. The patient should sign a receipt for any radiographic films removed from the office. Consultation reports from other physicians, even if stamped "confidential," as well as accounting records may be released to a patient.

Medical Litigation—In the event of **litigation** (lawsuit), the patient waives his or her right to confidentiality and the physician's lawyer has access to the patient's medical record but must not release information to any other party unless it is subpoenaed or the patient has signed an authorization form; for example, in the case of a subpoena for a mother's obstetric records and sealed records of an adopted child, you would release only the mother's record to honor that part of the subpoena.

The patient's attorney must subpoena medical records and if he or she cannot read the physician's handwriting, the medical assistant should not try to interpret it. The assistant should make an appointment for the attorney with the physician to clarify the information.

If a photocopying service visits the office to copy a record for the attorney, the medical assistant should either number the pages released or observe the photocopying process to ensure that pages are not missing when the copying is completed. It is preferable for the physician's staff to photocopy the record and charge the attorney a fee for this service.

Medicare, Medicaid, and TRICARE Records—The Privacy Act of 1974 guarantees the right of those receiving Medicare and TRICARE, formerly known as Civilian Health and Medical Program of the Uniformed Services (CHAMPUS), benefits to have access to their records. Federal and state agencies may also have access to medical records pertaining to federal- and state-sponsored programs, such as Medicaid, but it is preferable that the patient sign an authorization form. When completing an insurance claim form for government programs the patient's signature is required in Field 12 to release medical information for claims processing.

Medicaid rules permit members of a state attorney general's staff or the department of public welfare to review Medicaid records without the patient's signed authorization form to verify billing information and determine whether the services provided were medically necessary. The information in the medical records can be used only for the audit and may not be released.

Employers Receiving Records—Special attention is required when information is to be released to an employer even with the patient's signed authorization. The exception is in worker compensation cases.

Publications Release—If a patient's medical record or photograph is requested for publication, the authorization form must contain wording that indicates the information/photograph is to be used in this manner.

Psychiatric Records—A physician caring for a patient who has had psychiatric care should always be consulted before any information is divulged, even with a signed authorization form from the patient.

Physicians can prevent psychiatric patients from gaining access to privileged information by noting on a chart that they believe knowledge of its contents would be detrimental to the patient's best interests. This entry must be entered on the chart before the patient makes the request. Usually the courts will uphold a physician's judgment in these circumstances. Many states allow for authorization for release of infor-

mation to a representative of a patient if the physician determines that the release to the patient may not be in the patient's best interests. (See Procedure 3-1.)

MEDICAL PRACTICE ACTS

By the 1800s, there was a prevalence of individuals across the United States who falsely represented having medical skills and offered cures of diseases by selling appliances and medicinal elixirs. This was known as quackery. By the early 1900s, it became necessary to protect the citizen from such unqualified medical personnel so Medical Practice Acts were passed in all states. Their purpose was for each state to establish licensure requirements for individuals to practice medicine. Each state has different requirements, but some of the basic conditions that must be met are premedical training, graduation from an approved medical school, internship approved by the State Board of Medical Examiners, and good moral character. In some states, requirements are placed on age and residency, and written and oral examinations are given by the State Board of Medical Examiners. If a physician comes from a foreign country, he or she must pass examinations and satisfy state laws before receiving permission to practice medicine in the United States.

Medical licenses are either renewed annually or every two years by payment of a licensing fee and acquiring the required continuing education units. It may be a responsibility of the administrative medical assistant to provide the medical staff office secretary at the local hospital with such information. The original license and annual renewal certificate should be displayed in the office of the medical practice. The State Board of Medical Examiners can revoke a license for conviction of a crime, unprofessional conduct, or personal or professional incapacity, such as drug addiction, alcoholism, or mental illness.

The health care professional should become familiar with the state's medical practice act to know the scope of practice for their job description and whether those duties require certificates of competency or licensure so that a *breach of duty* does not occur. A breach of duty is the failure to act as the law obligates you to act within the expected standard of care, that is, what an individual is expected to do or not to do in a given situation. The law states that you have a legal or moral obligation to act in certain circumstances on the patient's behalf.

STEP 1 2 3

PROCEDURE 3-1

Release Patient Information

Task: Determine reason for disclosure, dates of disclosure, and which disclosure form is used to legally disclose medical information.

Standards: Consent form, authorization form, pen or pencil.

Directions:

1. Determine the reason for disclosure of the personally identifiable health information and the specific dates of service being requested.

2. Verify the request.

3. Locate and retrieve the chart.

4. Identify and validate the requester.

5. Mark specific areas or pages of the document requested.

6. Select one of the following categories and continue to follow the instructions:

   a. Disclosure for treatment, payment, or routine health care operations. Prepare a consent form.

   b. Transfer of medical record to a physician for consultation. Continuity of care rules apply; no authorization needed.

   c. Transfer of medical record to a physician who will be taking over care of a specific problem. Continuity of care rules apply; no authorization needed.

   d. Transfer of medical record to an acute or convalescent hospital for inpatient treatment. Continuity of care rules apply; no authorization needed.

   e. Transfer of medical record for therapeutic purposes (e.g., to a physical therapist, occupational therapist, radiation treatment center). Continuity of care rules apply; no authorization needed.

   f. Transfer of diagnostic information from the medical record for diagnostic purposes (e.g., to a laboratory, radiology center, physiology department). Continuity of care rules apply; no authorization needed.

   g. Permanent transfer of medical record to a physician who will be taking over care (e.g., patient dissatisfied with physician's care or moving to another area). Prepare an authorization form.

   h. Transfer of sensitive information (e.g., positive HIV or AIDS test, alcohol or drug dependency, psychiatric problems). Prepare an authorization form outlining the specific information to be disclosed including dates of treatment. Note: redisclosure not allowed without patient's prior authorization.

   i. Transfer of medical record to a court of law by way of a subpoena. Refer to "Accepting a Subpoena" guidelines. Carefully read the subpoena, give it to the custodian of medical records, prepare only dates outlined in the subpoena for copy and remove to a separate record jacket, have record reviewed by the physician, and send or make appointment for copy service to copy.

   j. Transfer of medial record by court order. Certain sensitive medial records may be legally sealed for confidentiality purposes. In such cases a court order is necessary to transfer the record and identifying and nonidentifying information may be separated and treated differently. State laws vary and should be referred to regarding sealed records.

   k. Transfer of medical record requested by law enforcement official. Under HIPAA Privacy Rule, PHI may be disclosed to law enforcement officials without written authorization under the following special circumstances: (1) in response to an administrative request, (2) to comply with a court order or court-ordered warrant, or (3) for the purpose of identifying or locating a suspect, fugitive, material witness, or missing person.

   l. Transfer of medical record into patient's personal possession. Try to determine the

PROCEDURE 3-1 *continued*

reason the patient wants the records. If it is for one of the above stated reasons, offer to send the records without charge to the physician or facility in an expedient manner. If patient states he or she "just wants to have a copy," advise the physician and have the physician go over the record with the patient prior to releasing it so no misunderstandings occur due to medical terminology, abbreviations, or other language. Charge the patient according to your state's guidelines.

7. Copy only requested material.

8. Mark all transfer details in the patient's medical record and in a disclosure log.

9. File a copy of the request in the patient's medical record.

10. Select method to send or deliver documents and send/deliver.

11. Generate invoice, if billable.

12. Return chart to medical record file cabinet.

13. Receive and post payment.

Some states require medical assistants to have certificates of competency if their duties include taking x-rays, performing laboratory tests, giving injections, or performing venipunctures. In addition, as mentioned in Chapter 1, some states require that a medical assistant be a graduate from an accredited medical assisting program. Some state laws do not permit a medical assistant to perform arterial punctures, administer intravenous medication, insert urinary catheters, administer physical therapy modalities, analyze test results, advise patients about their condition, make assessments, or perform medical care decision-making.

The American Association of Medical Assistants and the American Medical Technologists have approved a document entitled Model State Legislation to Recognize and Regulate the Practice of Medical Assisting. Their hope is that this document will be adopted and used as a legislative tool to protect the medical assistant's right to practice, establish minimum qualifications to perform medical assisting duties, and disqualify or suspend individuals who are found to violate provisions of the Act or perform acts beyond the scope of training or competence.

MEDICAL PROFESSIONAL LIABILITY

Originally the term *medical malpractice*, which literally means "bad medical practice," was commonly used to indicate negligence on the part of a physician. Today the phrase in use is *medical professional liability*, which *Black's Law Dictionary* defines as "any professional misconduct, unreasonable lack of skill or fidelity in professional or fiduciary duties, evil practice, or

illegal or immoral conduct" (from *Black's Law Dictionary 8th edition*, B. A. Garner, 2004, Thomson West).

Liability Insurance

A physician may carry two types of medical professional liability insurance. The first type is called *claims incurred*, or *occurrence insurance*; in this type, the insured is covered for any claims arising from an incident that occurred or is alleged to have occurred during the policy period regardless of when the claim is made.

The second type is called *claims-made insurance*, in which the insured is covered for any claim made rather than any injury occurring while the policy is in force. Such policies offer extended discovery options that can be purchased 30 to 60 days after purchase of the policy. This "tail" coverage allows the physician to report claims for events that occurred before the policy expiration date. When a new policy is purchased, the physician may elect to obtain "nose" coverage, which gives the doctor the privilege of reporting claims for medical incidents that occurred before that policy's effective date, under certain conditions. Medical incidents reported previously are not covered, nor are incidents of which the physician is aware, should be aware, or should have been aware.

Respondeat Superior

The doctrine of **respondeat superior**, which means "Let the master answer" (also known as vicarious liability), applies to the relationship between the physician and the medical assistant. In other words, physicians are legally responsible for their own conduct and for any actions that a medical assistant might take while in their employ. This does not mean, however, that a medical assistant cannot be sued. Even if the employer's policy does extend coverage to employees, the malpractice insurer may have the right to recover from the employee any damages paid because of the employee's negligence. If the insurer is successful in its recovery attempt, the employee is in the same position as being without insurance. Thus, for their own personal protection, many medical assistants purchase medical professional liability insurance. It is the physician's responsibility to see that all staff members are included in the office policy to provide protection against a suit.

Torts

A **tort** is an action brought when one person believes that another person conducted a wrongful act and caused harm and compensation for the damage or injury is being sought by the party bringing action. The action may also be brought to discourage the wrongdoer from committing further improper acts. When a tort is being considered, an evaluation of the circumstances must be made to determine whether there is *proximate cause.* To establish proximate cause the "cause" must be considered legally sufficient to result in damage or injury. Questions to ask when trying to establish this might be:

1. Did the physician/medical assistant act in an expedient fashion?

2. Was the patient left unattended?

3. Could the damage/injury be foreseen?

4. Was there intention to hurt or injure?

The three categories of tort liability are: intentional torts, negligent torts, and liability without fault, which will not be expanded on here because it most commonly occurs in cases of manufactured products that are found to be unsafe or cause harm. Medical products, such as pacemakers or orthopedic instrumentation could fall into this last category, but litigation would most likely be directed at the manufacturer, not the physician. Most health care incidents arise in the negligent tort category.

Intentional Torts

An intentional tort is an injury or wrong intentionally committed, with or without force, to another person or to another's property. In the medical field intentional torts are rare, but they occur. Usually, standard medical malpractice insurance policies do not cover intentional torts on the grounds that the

physician could have avoided them. Policies are usually written to protect the physician from accidents and good-faith mistakes and errors of judgment. Intentional torts are:

1. *Assault and battery.* Assault is the intentional and unlawful attempt to do bodily harm to another person.
   Example: Forcing a patient to take medication when the patient has refused to take it is an assault. Battery is a deliberate physical attack on another person. Any surgical operation is technically a "battery" regardless of the result and is excusable only when express or implied consent is given by the patient.

2. *Invasion of privacy and breach of confidential communication.* The invasion of privacy is the unwarranted appropriation or exploitation of another's personality, the publicizing of another's private affairs with which the public has no legitimate concern, or the wrongful intrusion into another's private activities, in such a manner as to cause mental anguish, shame, or humiliation. Breach of confidential communication is the unauthorized release of information.
   Examples: Publicizing a patient's medical case or showing a photograph or videotape from which the identity of a patient can be determined without the knowledge and authorization of the patient.

3. *Defamation of character, libel, and slander.* This is an attack on a person's reputation or subjecting a person to ridicule. It is called libel when written and slander when spoken.
   Example: Referring to a patient as a "malingerer" (one who pretends to be ill or incapacitated) in medical records or in correspondence about the patient.

4. *False imprisonment or personal restraint of the patient.* This is the unlawful detention of a person by another, for any length of time, whereby that person is deprived of personal liberty.
   Examples: Wrongfully refusing a patient permission to leave a hospital and using physical restraint to prevent a patient's departure.

5. *Intentional infliction of emotional distress.* This is an action that is so offensive as to cause great emotional upset.

Example: Intentionally telling a patient that a terminal illness has been diagnosed even though this is not true.

6. *Fraud or deceit.* This is an intentional perversion of truth for the purpose of inducing another (in reliance on it) to part with some valuable thing belonging to that person or to surrender a legal right.

   Example: Intentionally telling a patient that the injuries are minor when they are serious.

Negligent Torts

The health care professional, whether it be a physician or medical assistant, is expected to behave in the way a prudent person who is similarly educated and trained would behave under comparable circumstances. *Negligence* is careless conduct outside the accepted standard of care and results when the above does not take place.

   Example: Overexposing a patient to x-rays or leaving a surgical instrument in a patient. The "four D's" must be present for a judgment of negligence to be obtained against the physician. They are:

- *Duty*—Duty of care is when a moral obligation to treat is owed to the patient or when a contract has been established between the patient and physician.
- *Derelict*—When the physician did not comply with the duty that was needed, according to the situation (the patient has to show proof).
- *Direct cause*—Proof that the injury that resulted from the physician's breach of duty was a direct result of the breach, and nothing else interfered that could have caused the damage.
- *Damages*—Injuries suffered by the patient; also called compensatory damages. The two types are:
  a. *General damages* provide for compensation for pain and suffering and loss of bodily members.
  b. *Special compensation* replaces loss of earnings and cost of medical care.

Negligent torts can be categorized as:

- *Malfeasance*—Unlawful or improper treatment of the patient.
- *Misfeasance*—Lawful treatment that has been done in the wrong way.
- *Nonfeasance*—Failure to act when the physician has a duty to do so.

- *Malpractice*—Carelessness or negligence of a professional person.
- *Criminal negligence*—Reckless disregard for the safety of another; being indifferent to an injury that could occur.

Liability for the acts of others can also occur, which refers to damage/injury suffered by the patient when someone other than the physician renders a medical service, for example, injection of the wrong dosage of medication by the medical assistant at the direction of the physician.

Principal Defenses

If a patient (**plaintiff**) institutes a lawsuit against a physician, three principal defenses are available. They are:

- *Contributory negligence*—The defense that applies when a patient acts in such a manner as to contribute to his or her own disability or disfigurement. If a patient does not cooperate with the physician by following all reasonable instructions and this failure contributes to his or her problem, he or she cannot collect damages. In some states, the concept of contributory negligence has been replaced with *comparative negligence,* which means in essence that even if a patient contributes to his or her own disability, the extent of his or her negligence is compared to that of the physician; instead of being prevented from collecting damages, any monetary recovery is reduced by a percentage equal to the percentage of the patient's negligence.

- *Assumption of risk*—The defense that applies when a patient understood the risks of a particular operation or other medical procedure and signed a document giving informed consent. This document is used in the physician's defense. A patient, however, never assumes the risk of negligent medical treatment. Informed consent is explained later in this chapter.

- *Statute of limitations*—The defense that applies when the time limit for legal action on medical negligence has been exceeded. This time limit varies among states. In some states, a statutory policy involved in establishing the time limit is called the rule of discovery. This means that the statutory period does not begin until the patient discovers or should discover the negligence. The discovery date is the day a reasonable person would have known of the negligence. In the case of a minor, the statute of limitations begins when the minor reaches the age of majority.

Litigation Prevention

There are a number of ways to reduce a medical practice's malpractice exposure and the medical assistant can be involved in the process. The assistant needs to be familiar with legal terms and guidelines and know how to prevent lawsuits.

The medical assistant is expected to represent and be loyal to the physician and to execute reasonable orders; nevertheless, the assistant should never support, aid, protect, or encourage the physician or any staff member in the performance of an unlawful act even if instructed to do so. A medical assistant should execute only duties and responsibilities that are within the scope of his or her training; if asked to do something he or she cannot competently perform or has no knowledge of how to handle, then he or she should inform the physician-employer.

Guidelines to Prevent Medicolegal Claims

To prevent medicolegal claims with up-to-date knowledge of federal and state statutes follow these guidelines.

1. Refrain from discussing another physician with a patient. Sometimes patients invite criticism of methods or results of former physicians by presenting only one side of the story.

2. Assist the physician in keeping up-to-date, comprehensive, and accurate medical records. This aids in the diagnosis and treatment of a patient; assists in research of disease; substantiates procedure and diagnostic codes used for submission of patients' insurance claims; defends the physician in a lawsuit; and prevents penalties should the physician's practice be audited.

3. Avoid making any statements that might be construed as an admission of fault on the part of the physician-employer. The medical assistant's position in lawsuits is to say nothing to anyone except as required by the attorney of the physician or by the court of law. However, if the

physician is doing something illegal, the medical assistant might be held responsible by being silent.

4. Inform the physician immediately on learning a new patient is still under treatment by another physician and did not convey this information to the physician during the initial interview. It is against medical ethics for two physicians to be treating a patient for the same disease or injury. If a physician feels a specialist is necessary, he or she is expected to make a referral.

5. Never compare the respective merits of various forms of treatment or discuss the patient's ailments. Patients come to talk to the physician about their symptoms and it is the physician's job to make the diagnosis and recommend a treatment plan. The medical assistant should avoid rendering an opinion as this may contradict the physician's recommendations.

6. Inform patients who call the practice when the physician is absent that a qualified substitute is available. The patient must not be abandoned.

7. Avoid referring to consent to disclose medical information forms or authorization for release of information forms as "releases." The word "release" may give the wrong impression to the patient as these forms are designed to obtain permission to disclose or transmit information and to perform a service for the patient.

8. Keep well informed and up-to-date by reading bulletins and management magazines and by attending seminars. This may prevent legal problems from developing in a medical practice; enhance the financial part of a medical practice; keep the administrative functioning of a medical practice current.

9. Watch for hazards that might cause injury to the physician, patients, or oneself, such as frayed telephone and light cords, rugs or carpets that curl at the edges, wobbly chairs, or protruding objects. Equipment should be kept in good repair, and floors should not be highly waxed or slippery. Do not try to repair office equipment but call someone with expertise so a patient or employee is not injured.

10. Make sure the patient understands which services he or she will receive and any fees for "extras." If a patient is to be hospitalized, explain

that the fee the physician charges is for his or her services only and that there will be additional charges for the operating room, laboratory tests, anesthesia, the bed charge, and so forth. Prepare the patient for the financial impact on his or her budget, which will make it easier to collect on the account.

11. Never leave drug samples out or prescription pads lying on the desk. They should be locked in a safe location. Never recommend (prescribe) a medication, even though you may have a feeling of confidence of what the physician would order. Prescribing constitutes the practice of medicine and is unlawful for nonlicensed personnel.

12. Perform only those tasks that are within your scope of knowledge and training. Leave other tasks to individuals who are certified or licensed to perform them.

13. Create a medical disclaimer and post it and all legal policies in your office or on a Web site for the medical practice. If materials on health care are handed out or posted on the Web site, make sure patients understand that the content is not intended to be used in lieu of medical advice; it is for general informational purposes and educational use only.

14. Compose a Web site privacy policy that cautions patients that whatever they post becomes public information, that the practice cannot control the privacy policies of "links" to different sites, and that files (cookies) may be automatically downloaded to the visitor's computer and used in the future to establish identification.

Bonding

Another preventive measure for the medical assistant who handles cash is to be bonded. A *fidelity bond* is insurance against embezzlement, which unfortunately, can occur in any business or medical office that handles cash. In **bonding** an employee, an insurance or bonding company guarantees payment of a specified amount to the physician in the event of financial loss caused by an employee or by some contingency over which an employee handling money has no control. Three effective bonding methods are:

1. *Position-schedule bonding*—Also known as a "name schedule" or umbrella bond, offers coverage for a specific job, such as a bookkeeper or receptionist, rather than a named individual.

If an employee in a specified category leaves, the newly employed replacement is automatically covered. This bond generally requires little, if any, person background investigation.

2. *Blanket-position bonding*—Coverage for all employees regardless of job title.

3. *Personal bonding*—Coverage for those who handle large amounts of money; a thorough background investigation is required.

Bond coverage should be reviewed periodically with the insurance agent to make sure coverage is keeping pace with expansion of the medical practice.

To further remove any temptations for embezzlement, the physician should sign checks, periodically review bills, examine records, and scan the mail to get an idea of what payments are coming in. All encounter forms should be numbered, and a copy of the deposit slip should always be retained and stapled to the day sheet so the physician can review it at frequent but irregular intervals.

Patient Care Partnership

On February 6, 1973, the House of Delegates of the American Hospital Association (AHA) approved a Patients' Bill of Rights to provide a remedy for some recurring complaints about attitudes of and treatment by physicians and administrators. It has also helped to reduce malpractice suits as these often result from misunderstandings between the patient and physician or hospital.

In 2003, the AHA's Patients' Bill of Rights was changed into a plain language brochure, *The Patient Care Partnership*. It outlines what to expect during a hospital stay, how to prepare when going home, what information will be needed from the patient, and rights and responsibilities regarding privacy, medical bills, and insurance claims. Today's physicians are challenged and urged to include patients in medical decision making and inform patients of their rights as outlined in this brochure. Refer to the Resources at the end of this chapter for a Web address to obtain this booklet.

ALTERNATIVES TO THE LITIGATION PROCESS

Litigation is *trial by jury* following a plaintiff's filing of a **complaint** or petition. Before trial, the **defendant** who is the opposing side may file a motion called a "demurrer" to have the case dismissed if there are not sufficient grounds for action. If not dismissed, the case goes to a trial judge or pretrial conference and then to a jury trial, resulting in a verdict and the possibility of an appeal.

Screening Panel

One alternative to litigation is a *screening panel,* or physician review panel, that hears cases outside the courtroom in the hope of solving them without the expense, publicity, and difficulty of court proceedings. In states where these panels have been established, review may or may not be a prerequisite for going to court. These panels issue advisory opinions but cannot legally bar litigation. Through this review process, some nuisance suits can be avoided.

Arbitration

Another method of resolving malpractice disputes is *arbitration.* This process is used when a patient and physician have agreed before treatment (*preclaim agreement*) that both will waive the right to a court trial in case of a dispute. This legal method is provided by statute in some states and helps resolve any patient-physician controversy before an impartial panel or **grievance committee**. It saves time, is less expensive, may be fairer, and allows greater privacy for the parties involved in disagreements. For such an agreement to be binding, the patient must have plain and clear notification of all terms, which must be specifically explained. Patients are free not to sign the agreement, and signing is not a requirement for being seen by a doctor or receiving continuing medical treatment.

Usually it is the medical assistant who must explain and present the arbitration agreement to patients for signature. Using tact and a willingness to answer the patient's questions are most important in making the initial request for signature. If a lawsuit is instituted against the physician, it is the medical assistant's job to notify the physician's insurance carrier promptly and include a copy of the arbitration agreement. Not invoking arbitration at the outset can result in a waiver of the arbitration agreement. Some managed care plans and some insurance programs have preclaim agreements as a requirement or option of the policy.

A second type of arbitration agreement is a *postclaim agreement* that is transacted after a dispute occurs and both sides must agree to arbitrate rather than litigate.

No-Fault Insurance

The last and most far-reaching approach to resolution of the medical malpractice problem is *no-fault insurance.* This means an injured person is compensated without regard to fault. This is under investigation and still in preliminary stages of study to determine if such insurance is fair to all parties concerned. Supporters of no-fault insurance would set up a system similar to that of workers' compensation in which an actuarial board, calculating the risks statistically, would be set up to determine the amount of payments to be made on a standard scale, taking into account the age of the injured, the injury, the occupation, and other factors.

PHYSICIAN/PATIENT CONTRACT

Usually, patients seek a physician who they may have researched and who they believe delivers a certain standard of care. Legally, this would be interpreted to mean that the physician has a certain amount of knowledge and skill comparable to other physicians who practice in the same specialty in the community. It does not necessarily mean the physician can provide a cure to an illness. A medical assistant should never encourage false expectations on the outcome of an injury or illness. When necessary, the medical assistant should help the patient understand the course of treatment and encourage willingness to comply with the treatment advised.

Expressed/Implied Contracts

A medical contract exists when a physician performs a service after a patient has requested it. This request can be *expressed,* as in a direct verbal or written statement, or it can be implied. An **implied contract** means not expressed by direct words but gathered by implication or necessary deduction from the situation, the general language, or the conduct of the patient. If the patient goes to the doctor's office and the doctor renders professional services that the patient accepts, this is an implied contract. Although a patient has medical insurance, the contract for treatment is between the physician and the patient, and the patient is thus liable for the physician's fee.

Physicians treating patients whose medical services are paid from federal or state funds (Medicare or Medicaid cases) are contractually obligated to the government and may not receive payment if they fail to follow federal or state guidelines; however, their treatment falls under a physician-patient contract.

When a physician is under contract to a managed care plan to render medical services to enrolled individuals, the contract for treatment is between the physician and patient and occurs when the patient is first seen. If the physician no longer wishes to treat an individual, termination is handled the same as with patients insured under private insurance or state or government programs.

Third-Party Contracts

There are exceptions to the physician-patient contract and instead the physician's contract is with a third party. Industrial injuries without third-party litigation are covered by a contract between the physician and the employer's industrial insurance company. Such cases do not require a signed consent or release of information form. However, when an insurance company adjuster calls for information on a workers' compensation case, verify the caller before providing medical information.

Another example would be when a worker is hurt on a job and the employer decides to pay for the medical expenses but does not report the incident as an industrial injury. Although the employer may not be complying with state law, such cases appear at physician's offices. After rendering treatment, if the employer does not pay, then the physician may find it impossible to collect the fee.

Another instance might be if a patient is brought in suffering a bite from a neighbor's dog and the neighbor says he will pay the bill. After treatment, what happens if the neighbor decides not to pay? In an implied contractural agreement, the assumption is the patient is responsible for the bill. Although this is a third-party liability case, it may be difficult to collect the fee. In such cases, always obtain a written agreement from the third party promising to pay for the services the patient receives. The agreement should be signed and witnessed. If an agreement is not obtained, there is no legal right to seek payment from the third party.

Contracts and Emergency Care

In emergency situations, when a patient may be unconscious and unable to give valid consent, the consent is implied. A medical assistant may render first aid if a physician is not present but should do no more than is absolutely essential. General procedure is to telephone 911 and try to get emergency personnel on the premises in the interim. If the state law covers the medical assistant and he or she is certified in cardiopulmonary resuscitation (CPR), it may be rendered. The staff should attempt to contact a physician immediately after emergency measures have been taken. The office procedure manual should contain information on how the physician wishes the medical assistant to act in an office emergency. Often office policies state that the office should be locked if a physician is not present, and if a patient telephones indicating an emergent situation, he or she should be directed to a hospital emergency room.

Good Samaritan Law

When rendering first aid in a life-or-death situation, the physician is governed by the Good Samaritan Law. Generally, the *Good Samaritan Law* applies to instances of emergencies outside the office, such as highway accidents. In such situations a legal patient-physician contract relationship is not created, and the physician cannot be charged with neglect or abandonment for follow-up care. However, a physician can be held liable for injuries that result if it can be shown the physician did not provide an acceptable standard of care under the circumstances in which care was given.

Contracts with Minors

Many states have different ages of majority. In some instances, it is necessary for a parent to authorize in writing surgery or treatment for a child. If the child has a guardian, this information should be recorded in the patient's medical record. A nonemancipated minor (i.e., a minor under parental control) over 14 years of age *can almost always* consent to medical and surgical treatment under the mature minor rule. Parental consent is never required in a medical emergency that is interpreted as a life-threatening situation.

If a minor has a communicable disease that by law must be reported to the Department of Health (i.e., infectious hepatitis, tuberculosis, measles, mumps, venereal disease, acquired immune deficiency syndrome [AIDS]), the physician may treat the minor without parental consent.

If an unmarried pregnant minor requires hospitalization or medical care for the pregnancy, the laws of the state determine whether parental consent is necessary. If an abortion is requested by the minor, some states will allow it without parental consent. The medical assistant should keep up to date on the changing legalities and illegalities of abortion. In some states, it would be unwise for a physician to sterilize an unmarried minor in the absence of parental consent because of the irreversible nature of the procedure.

Emancipated Minors

Children of any age who fall outside the jurisdiction and custody of their parents or guardians are called **emancipated minors.** They may personally consent to medical, surgical, or hospital treatment. Parents are not liable for the medical expenses incurred. A minor is considered emancipated when he or she is:

1. Living apart from parents or guardians and managing his or her own financial affairs

2. Married or divorced at any age

3. On active duty in the military service

4. A college student living away from home even when financially dependent on his or her parents

5. A parent (even if not married)

To avoid disagreements with parents, the patient's records should include some evidence of emancipation, such as a minor's signed statement acknowledging the fact (Figure 3-10).

In summary, when treating minors, it is advisable to:

1. Seek parental approval in cases that are not sensitive or confidential.

2. Encourage minors to involve their parents in medical decisions that are of a sensitive nature.

3. Become familiar with state laws concerning treatment of minors.

4. Obtain another medical opinion before proceeding in cases where there is any doubt about a minor's ability to consent or about the urgency or appropriateness of therapy.

5. Make sure that minors who consent to their own care are clearly aware of the nature and consequences of the procedure and obtain a signed consent form to this effect.

Terminating a Contract

If a physician wishes to terminate a contract, he or she must do so legally so as not to be accused of abandoning a case; the proper letter should be writ-

ten explaining the withdrawal to the patient and sent by registered or certified mail with return receipt requested (Figure 3-11). The American Medical Association has published a book entitled *Medicolegal Forms with Legal Analysis* that suggests the proper wording for such letters.

When terminating a contract, it is important to allow a transition period so the patient can obtain a new physician before care terminates. The letter should state the reason for termination.

Reasons for Terminating a Contract

A patient may fail to keep an appointment, fail to follow medical advice, or fail to pay the balance due on an account. If the patient continues to disregard a recommended plan or if the patient is not to be seen again, it is recommended that an appropriate letter be written to document the action (Figure 3-12). Copies of the correspondence as well as the mail receipts are placed with the patient's medical record.

Abandonment

Abandonment is when a physician terminates supervision of a patient without notifying the patient in writing. Many instances may occur when abandonment becomes an issue. The physician may move out of town, or if the physician goes on vacation and does not arrange for coverage by another physician of equal competence in the same specialty, the physician can be liable for negligence and abandonment as this becomes an issue of continuity of care. Always document in the patient's medical record any missed or failed-to-show appointments. If an established patient telephones indicating an emergency and an appointment is denied, the physician also can be charged with abandonment and neglect.

It is equally important that the physician's answering service be given accurate information as to where the physician can be reached when the office is closed. If this is not done, a physician can be sued for patient abandonment. It is the medical assistant's responsibility to always keep the answering service informed. If the practice uses an answering machine instead of a live answering service, the prerecorded message should give information to the caller about where to telephone to obtain help in the event of an emergency.

When a patient is admitted to the hospital and the physician does not see the patient within a reasonable amount of time to check on the condition and order treatment, the physician can be charged with abandoning the patient.

Documentation Of Self-Sufficient Minor Status

For the purposes of obtaining medical, dental or surgical diagnosis or treatment, pursuant to Family Code §6922, I hereby certify that the following is true:

1. I am fifteen years of age or older, having been born on *4-21-9X* , at *Woodland Hills, XY* .
    (date)(location)

2. I am living separate and apart from my parents or legal guardian.

    2011 Edgehill Drive, Woodland Hills, XY 12345   *555-476-0215*
    (Residence)   (Phone)

    _____   _____
    (Residence of parents/guardians)   (Phone)

3. I am managing my own financial affairs.

    Hi Ho Burger, 20 Main, Woodland Hills, XY
    (Name and Address of Employer)

    None
    (Other Source(s) of Income)

    College Bank, Woodland Hills, XY
    (Location of Bank Account)

4. I understand that, under the law, I will be financially responsible for my medical, dental, or surgical care and treatment.

    Brett Hayward   *July 10, 20XX*
    (Signed)(Date)

Figure 3-10. Documentation of Self-Sufficient Minor Status form, copyright California Medical Association 2006. (Published with permission of and by arrangement with the California Medical Association. Excerpted for the 2006 *California Physician's Legal Handbook.* For ordering information, call (800) 882-1262 or visit Web site: http://www.cmanet.org.)

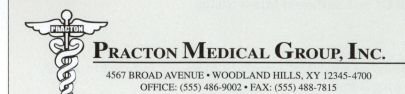

PRACTON MEDICAL GROUP, INC.

4567 BROAD AVENUE • WOODLAND HILLS, XY 12345-4700
OFFICE: (555) 486-9002 • FAX: (555) 488-7815

Fran Practon, M.D.
Gerald Practon, M.D.

LETTER OF WITHDRAWAL FROM A CASE

March 19, 20XX

Mr. David Merchant
3409 Sausalito Street
Woodland Hills, XY 12345-0433

Dear Mr. Merchant:

I find it necessary to inform you that I am withdrawing from further professional attendance upon you because you have persisted in refusing to follow my medical advice and treatment. Please find another physician as soon as possible. I will be available to attend you for a reasonable time after you have received this letter but for not more than _____ days. *(Note: time period should be designated depending on office policy.)* This will give you sufficient time to select a competent physician.

I will be glad to forward a copy of your medical history with information about the diagnosis and the treatment you received from me. Please either sign the enclosed authorization to release medical records or send a letter requesting me to do so with your signature and the address of the new physician.

Sincerely,

Gerald Practon, MD

Gerald Practon, MD

mtf

Enclosure: Authorization form

Figure 3-11. Example of letter of withdrawal from a case that is typed in modified-block style with closed punctuation. This letter should be sent certified mail with return-receipt requested.

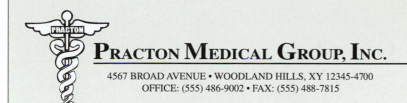

PRACTON MEDICAL GROUP, INC.

4567 BROAD AVENUE • WOODLAND HILLS, XY 12345-4700
OFFICE: (555) 486-9002 • FAX: (555) 488-7815

Fran Practon, M.D.
Gerald Practon, M.D.

LETTER TO PATIENT WHO FAILS TO KEEP APPOINTMENT

June 25, 20XX

Mr. Jonathan Reed
50 Maryland Street
Woodland Hills, XY 12345-0432

Dear Mr. Reed:

On June 24, 20XX, you failed to keep your appointment at my office.

In my opinion, your condition requires continued medical treatment. If you so desire, you may telephone me for another appointment, but if you prefer to have another physician attend you, I suggest that you arrange to do so without delay.

You may be assured that, upon your authorization, I will make available my knowledge of your case to the physician of your choice.

I trust that you will understand that my purpose in writing this letter is out of concern for your health and well-being.

Sincerely,

Gerald Practon, MD

Gerald Practon, MD

mtf

Figure 3-12. Letter on patient's failure to keep an appointment

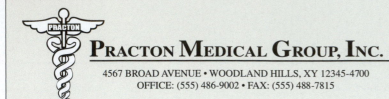

PRACTON MEDICAL GROUP, INC.

4567 BROAD AVENUE • WOODLAND HILLS, XY 12345-4700
OFFICE: (555) 486-9002 • FAX: (555) 488-7815

Fran Practon, M.D.
Gerald Practon, M.D.

LETTER TO CONFIRM DISCHARGE BY PATIENT

April 2, 20XX

Mrs. Moo McDermott
439 Nordstrom Road
Woodland Hills, XY 12345-0432

Dear Mrs. McDermott:

This will confirm our telephone conversation today during which you
discharged me from attending you as your physician in your present illness.

In my opinion, your condition requires continued medical treatment by a
physician. If you have not already obtained the services of another
physician, I suggest that you do so without delay.

You may be assured that, upon your authorization, I will furnish that
physician with information regarding the diagnosis and treatment that you
have received from me.

Sincerely,

Gerald Practon, MD

Gerald Practon, MD

mtf

Figure 3-13. Letter confirming discharge

Confirmation of Discharge

If a patient discharges a physician by telephone or discharges him- or herself from a hospital, the physician sends a letter similar to that in Figure 3-13. If there is a signed statement in the patient's hospital records in the latter case, it is not necessary for the physician to send the patient a letter.

INFORMED CONSENT

When a physician makes a diagnosis and recommends treatment, the patient then must decide whether to accept the treatment. If the patient accepts the mode of treatment, it is the obligation of the physician to inform the patient of all the risks and alternatives to the suggested procedure. The patient then decides to accept the risks and signs a consent form acknowledging the assumed risks, which include the chances of success or failure of the treatment. This is called *informed consent*. This process is important when dealing with minor or major surgical cases whether in an office or hospital setting. A patient can sue a physician if the process of informed consent has not been carried out properly and if one or more items are missing at the time the patient is informed. When a medical assistant witnesses the consent for treatment form, he or she is witnessing the signature and not the consent (Figure 3-14). For proper wording of informed consent forms, see Figure 3-15. If patients are being treated who only speak a foreign language an interpreter should be present and the forms should also be written in that foreign language.

MEDICAL RECORDS

It is essential that medical records be accurate, complete, up-to-date, and readable reflecting the history, physical examination, assessment, and treatment plan. This documentation is necessary to provide the best medical care, justify services billed to the insurance company, and defend a physician in the event of a lawsuit. Documentation of every instance of failure to

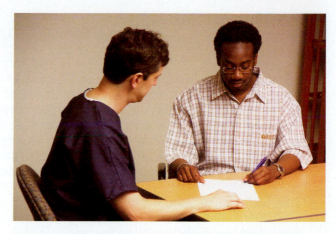

Figure 3-14. Patient signing an informed consent with a medical assistant witnessing the signature

keep an appointment or follow the physician's advice should appear in a patient's chart. Notations of prescription refills, telephone conversations, electronic mail (e-mail) messages, and faxed communications should also be documented in the patient's medical record. Because a medical record may become a legal document, it is important to use legal copy pens (permanent ink) to eliminate the possibility of alterations. Information on patients' medical records, including how to make corrections to medical documents are found in Chapter 9.

Subpoena

Subpoena literally means "under penalty," and it is an order by the court for a witness to appear at a designated place to give testimony. In medical malpractice cases, the physician may give **expert testimony** in which he or she is considered an authority on the subject matter and provides a statement that is scientific, technical, or professional in nature. A physician-employer may authorize the medical assistant to receive a subpoena in his or her name. Although a subpoena must generally be personally served to the person named in it, the medical assistant's receipt of the subpoena as the physician's representative is considered the equivalent of personal service. Neither civil nor criminal subpoenas can be served via the facsimile (fax) machine.

Civil law is a statute that enforces private rights and liabilities as differentiated from criminal law. It typically involves relations between individuals, corporations, government entities, and other organizations. Most actions encountered in the health care industry are based in civil law.

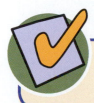

COMPLIANCE

In 35 states, minors under the age of 18 need permission for abortion procedures.

Procedure: VULVAR BIOPSY

You and your doctor are considering a biopsy of your vulva. This is a type of examination in which the doctor will take a specimen of the tissue of the vulva or private area and have it examined further. Specimens may be taken from different areas of the vulva after local anesthesia has "numbed" the area. The purpose of the test is to detect cancer or other abnormal cells. This biopsy is not treatment for any disease; it is just an examination. It is possible that an area of cancer or other abnormality may not be sampled and therefore go undected. Because of this fact, your doctor can make no guarantee as to the accuracy of the test.

This test is quite safe and complications from it are very unusual. The possibility of complications is greater in patients who have other disease or who take steroids or certain herbs or medications that effect blood clotting. Bleeding and infection are uncommon complications. In very rare cases, bleeding and infection fr om the test have resulted in the need for surgery and blood transfusions. General pain, discomfort or pain with urination, pain during sexual intercourse, and scarring may also occur. Allergic reactions to one or more of the substances used in the test are very uncommon. In very, very rare instances allergic reactions have caused death.

The vulvar biopsy is a reasonably safe and accurate method of diagnosing abnormal cells or cancer of the vulva. In those women in which the test is indicated, this procedure may provide the best chance of successful diagnosis and the lowest risk of complications.

ADDITIONAL RISKS AND ALTERNATIVES:
(To be filled here and on reverse
side by doctor as necessary)

_____

_____

_____

I CERTIFY: I have read or had read to me the contents of this form; I understand the risks and alternatives involved in this procedure; I have had the oppurtunity to ask any questions which I had and all of my questions have been answeresd.

DATE: _____ TIME: _____   SIGNED: _____
                                                                  (Signed by patient or person legally
                                                                  authorized to consent for patient)

WITNESS: _____   PHYSICIAN: _____
                                                                  (Signed by physician)

(A GENERAL CONSENT FORM MUST ALSO BE SIGNED BY THE PATIENT.)

Prepared by In-Forms No. 1494

Figure 3-15. A risk disclosure form (informed consent). Procedure: Vulvar Biopsy, prepared for the patient's signature giving permission to have the procedure performed in the physician's office. (Reprinted with permission of Phil Reeves, In-forms, P.O. Box 35194, Albuquerque, New Mexico 87176-5194, Telephone 505 255-2569, Copyright 2005. All rights reserved.)

PROCEDURE 3-2

Accept a Subpoena

Objective: Accept a subpoena for a medical record on behalf of the physician. Prepare the medical record for copying by the attorney's representative.

Equipment/Supplies: Telephone, pen or pencil.

Directions: Follow these step-by-step directions, which include rationales, to learn this procedure when a subpoena is served and the medical assistant has permission to receive it.

1. Be polite to the deputy or messenger who is serving the subpoena; ask for the fee when the subpoena is served.

2. Request to see the subpoena to decide what action to take. Determine which physician the subpoena is addressed to and ask the custodian of records for that physician to accept the subpoena.

3. If the physician is on vacation or at a medical meeting, explain to the deputy that the subpoena cannot be accepted in the physician's absence. Suggest that it be served after the physician returns or that the deputy or messenger contact the physician's attorney; then inform the attorney that this has been done. The assistant may also ask one of the other physicians in the office for advice in regard to the subpoena in question.

4. On receipt of the witness fee and subpoena, read the medical record notes for the dates of treatment requested to verify that each document is complete and that signatures and initials are identifiable. Place the patient's medical record on the physician's desk and flag the exact dates covered under the subpoena for prompt review. Willful disregard of a subpoena is punishable as a contempt of court.

5. Make an appointment within the prescribed time stated for the representative or copy service to return and copy the portion of the record named in the subpoena. It is not necessary to show the record at the time the subpoena is served unless the court order so states.

6. Verify the exact dates of treatment covered and remove those notes from the original chart and place in a copy folder. The entire medical record is not released, nor are the patient registration information sheet, encounter forms, and explanation of benefits.

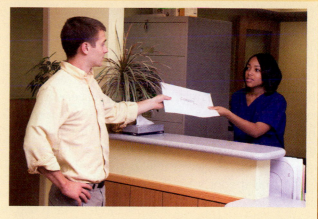

Figure 3-16. Representative of the court serving a subpoena to a medical assistant; the physician's representative

7. Refuse to give the medical record to anyone without the physician's prior permission; when a subpoena is served, a patient's signed authorization for release of information form is not required.

8. If the subpoena is for a *deposition,* verify the date and location at which the physician is to appear with an attorney.

9. If the subpoena is for a trial, verify with the court that the case is on the calendar. The physician or custodian of the record must appear in court unless permission to mail the record is granted. Failure to appear is considered a contempt of court and is subject to fine or imprisonment.

10. If the record is needed in court, make photocopies and put the record in a secure package so tampering or loss will be avoided. This will also allow detection of any altering while it is outside of custody; and if the patient is treated before the original is returned, the photocopied record will be available for reference.

11. Comply with instructions given by the court if an appearance with the record is required. In this case, do not give up possession of the medical record until requested to do so by the judge, nor allow examination of the record by anyone before identification in court. Obtain a receipt for the medical record when leaving it in the court in possession of a judge or jury.

12. Call the physician's attorney if there are additional questions or if additional information is needed.

A *subpoena duces tecum*, which literally means "under penalty you shall bring with you," is a court order for the appearance of a witness with the subpoened medical records. However, the medical record might be all that is required, as is the typical scenario experienced in most medical practices. The physician may ask the medical assistant to deliver or mail the records to the court. The subpoena service must be accompanied by a witness fee or mileage fee, and the medical assistant should request it from the deputy when the subpoena is served. Some states provide for a substitute service by mail or through newspaper publication if efforts to effect personal service have failed.

ADVANCE DIRECTIVES

Congress passed a law known as the Patient Self-Determination Act (PSDA), also known as the Danforth Bill or Medical Miranda Rights for Patients Act. It requires hospitals, hospices, physicians' offices, skilled nursing facilities, and home health providers who participate in the Medicare or Medicaid programs to ask each patient whether he or she has drawn up an **advance directive** (living will and/or health care power of attorney) and to document the response in the patient's chart. This law took effect in 1991 and requires that institutions supply patients with written information about state laws concerning advance directives and a patient's right to reject treatment. Such documents conform to state laws and detail in legal form the desires for procedures to be performed or withheld when death is imminent. Advance directives take different forms, many are simply titled "Declarations" (Figure 3-17), and several other types are mentioned here.

Living Will

Basically, a **living will** is a document stating the desires of a person should he or she become incompetent because of injury or illness and death is imminent. Living wills are not legally binding, but more than 40 states have right-to-die laws that often recognize living wills as evidence of intent. Living wills have become popular as a result of medical situations in which use of equipment assists a person to live for an undeterminable amount of time even when comatose. A living will can be revoked (usually by a simple oral statement) at any time.

Health Care Power of Attorney

Another document called a **health care power of attorney** is legally binding and is more flexible than a living will. It allows the individual to detail precise wishes about treatment. This document can be used for all medical decisions, not just those about life-prolonging treatment, and by all people, not just those who are terminally ill. Some states recognize a combination living will with a durable power of attorney for health care that allows the person to appoint another person to withhold or consent to medical care.

Medical Directive

Ezekiel and Linda Emanuel, a husband-and-wife physician team in Boston, developed a detailed document called a *medical directive.* It allows patients to specify what they would and would not want done in four specific dire situations by answering 48 questions. It can be used by itself or in conjunction with other state-authorized documents.

Values History Form

Another advance directive, a *values history form,* was developed to try to uncover a patient's value system and to guide a physician's decisions about treatment. It asks questions such as, "How important is independence and self-sufficiency in your life?" It is not a legal document, but it may be used to supplement a living will or durable power of attorney for health care.

Health Care Proxy

In Massachusetts, after many years of deliberation, legislation was enacted for a *health care proxy,* which is a type of advance directive. The patient has the responsibility to communicate his or her decisions about various forms of life support to the surrogate. If this does not occur, the surrogate is left to make decisions without direction. The responsibilities need to be explained to the patient. A physician and/or medical assistant can be valuable in aiding the patient in the choice of a surrogate.

Do Not Resuscitate Form

Some states have developed a *Do Not Resuscitate Form* for use in prehospital settings, for example, in a patient's home, in a long-term care facility, during

PENNSYLVANIA DECLARATION – PAGE 1 OF 2

INSTRUCTIONS

PRINT YOUR NAME

I, _____, being of sound mind, willfully and voluntarily make this declaration to be followed if I become incompetent. This declaration reflects my firm and settled commitment to refuse life-sustaining treatment under the circumstances indicated below.

I direct my attending physician to withhold or withdraw life-sustaining treatment that serves only to prolong the process of my dying, if I should be in a terminal condition or in a state of permanent unconsciousness.

I direct that treatment be limited to measures to keep me comfortable and to relieve pain, including any pain that might occur by withholding or withdrawing life-sustaining treatment.

In addition, if I am in the condition described above, I feel especially strongly about the following forms of treatment:

CHECK THE OPTIONS WHICH RELECT YOUR WISHES

I (   ) do (   ) do not want cardiac resuscitation.
I (   ) do (   ) do not want mechanical respiration.
I (   ) do (   ) do not want tube feeding or any other artificial or invasive form of nutrition (food) or hydration (water).
I (   ) do (   ) do not want blood or blood products.
I (   ) do (   ) do not want any form of surgery or invasive diagnostic tests.
I (   ) do (   ) do not want kidney dialysis.
I (   ) do (   ) do not want antibiotics.
I (   ) do (   ) do not want to make an anatomical gift of all or part of my body, subject to the following limitations, if any:

I made this declaration on the day of _____ (month, year).

I realize that if i do not specifically indicate my preference regarding any of the forms of treatment listed above, I may receive that form of treatment.

ADD PERSONAL INSTRUCTIONS (IF ANY)

Other instructions:

Figure 3-17. Sample declaration for making health care decisions for the state of Pennsylvania, © 2005. (Reprinted with permission of National Hospice and Palliative Care Organization, all rights reserved, Web site: http://www.caringinfo.org.)

PENNSYLVANIA DECLARATION – PAGE 2 OF 2

APPOINTING A SURROGATE	Surrogate decision-making:
	I ( ) do ( ) do not want to designate another person as my surrogate to make medical treatment decisions for me if I should be incompetent and in a terminal condition or in a state of permanent unconsciousness.
PRINT THE NAME, ADDRESS AND PHONE NUMBER OF YOUR SURROGATE	Name: _____
	Address: _____
	Phone: _____
PRINT THE NAME, ADDRESS AND PHONE NUMBER OF YOUR ALTERNATE SURROGATE	Name and address of substitute surrogate (if surrogate designated above is unable to serve):
	Name: _____
	Address: _____
	Phone: _____
PRINT THE DATE SIGN THE DOCUMENT AND PRINT YOUR ADDRESS	I made this declaration on the _____ day of _____. (day) (month, year)
	Declarant's signature: _____
	Declarant's address: _____
WITNESSING PROCEDURE	The declarant, or the person on behalf of and at the direction of the declarant, knowingly and voluntarily signed this writing by signature or mark in my presence.
YOUR TWO WITNESSES MUST SIGN AND PRINT THEIR ADDRESSES	Witness's signature: _____
	Witness's address: _____
	Witness's signature: _____
	Witness's address: _____
© 2005 National Hospice and Palliative Care Organization	*Courtesy of Caring Connections* *1700 Diagonal Road, Suite 625, Alexandria, VA 22314* *www.caringinfo.org, 800/658-8898*

Figure 3-17 (continued). Sample declaration for making health care decisions for the state of Pennsylvania, © 2005. (Reprinted with permission of National Hospice and Palliative Care Organization, all rights reserved, Web site: http://www.caringinfo.org.)

transport to or from a health care facility, and in other locations outside acute care hospitals. In some regions, emergency responders and hospitals are encouraged to honor the form when a patient is transported to an emergency room. When signed by the patient, it protects health care providers from criminal prosecution, civil liability, discipline for unprofessional conduct, administrative sanction, or any other sanction. Copies of the form are retained by the patient and physician and made part of the patient's permanent medical record. In certain regions, some ambulance companies require a copy of the form to be retained in their files. In some states, a specific organization may issue a wrist or neck medallion for identification purposes. In an emergency when a patient's heart has stopped and emergency medical services (EMS) are called, EMS providers forgo resuscitation attempts if a form is present or if the individual is wearing such a medallion. For information pertaining to laws in your region, contact the local Department of Health Services.

Uniform Anatomical Gift Act

It is the right of a competent adult to make disposition of all or part of his or her body for transplant or research purposes. The Uniform Anatomical Gift Act was approved by the National Conference of Commissioners on Uniform State Laws in July 1968. It has been adopted in all states. The act provides that a person 18 years of age or over may give all or any part of his or her body after death for research, transplant, or placement in a tissue bank.

PATIENT EDUCATION

Patients may need to be informed about the many uses of donor tissue and organs. Donor hearts or kidneys are vitally needed and many potential recipients are on waiting lists. Best results for a match occur when a donor is closely related to the recipient. Corneal transplants for individuals with scarred or opaque corneas are successful because the cornea has no blood supply and antibodies responsible for rejection of foreign tissue do not reach it. Livers, lungs, and pancreases have also been transplanted but the longevity of such transplants are not as successful.

Donor Registration

While donated organs and tissues are shared at a national level, laws that govern donations vary from state to state. A coalition on donation called Donate Life has a Web site (see Resources at the end of the chapter) that offers a state-by-state guide to donation registration. On the Web site, click on the map of the United States and select your state. Directions will appear instructing you how to sign up. At present, forty states have electronic registries. For other states you are directed to sign up by applying for a form from a state organization by downloading a donation card, or signing up at the state's Department of Motor Vehicles (see Figure 3-18). Advance directives may also have questions regarding whether you would like body parts donated.

Uniform Donor Card—Front
THIS IS A LEGALLY BINDING DOCUMENT

According to the guidelines of the Uniform Anatomical Gift Act. I choose, upon my death to:

A ___ Donate any of my organs, tissues, or parts
B ___ Donate a pacemaker (date implanted_____)
C ___ Donate parts, tissues, or organs listed _____
_____
D ___ Donate my entire body
E ___ ❏ Transplantation ❏ Medical Research ❏ Both
F ___ Not donate any organs, parts, tissues or pacemaker

SIGNATURE _____ DATE _____

WITNESS SIGNATURE _____ DATE _____
❏ Discussed with affected parties _____
DL 290 (Rev. 7/2002)   DOCTOR'S INITIALS

DMV
A Public Service Agency   ● DONOR

Uniform Donor Card—Back

IMPORTANT INSTRUCTION
If you wish to make a donation, fill out this card and put the "DONOR" dot on the front of your license or I.D. card next to the photo where indicated. Keep the card with your license or I.D. card. If you change your mind, complete a new card and remove the dot.

To refuse to donate, fill out part "F" of this card and carry it with your license or I.D. card. Do not use the dot.

NOTICE
If you are at least 18, you may choose to donate any needed organs, tissues, a pacemaker or whole body for medical transplantation or research or both, and indicate this decision on your driver license or I.D. card. According to the Uniform Anatomical Gift Act (Section 7150, Health & Safety Code), your donation will take effect on your death. (Entering the name of your next of kin below is optional)

Name _____
Address _____
Telephone No. _____
Keep this card with your driver license or I.D. card

Figure 3-18. Uniform donor card—both sides (provided by the Department of Motor Vehicles; a Public Service Agency)

Although the trend is to use online registration services because databases can be quickly accessed and donor registration confirmed, donor cards, which are legal documents, may also be distributed to patients by physicians. If cards are used, the patient and one or more witnesses must sign the card and it should be kept with the patient at all times near a driver's license or identification card. It is important for patients to inform family members of their decision to donate.

Advance Directive Guidelines

Advance directives are signed by the individual and two witnesses (preferably not relatives) and in some states must be notarized. When a patient has signed such a document, a copy of it should be filed in the patient's medical record. It is recommended that copies be given to the patient's clergy, lawyer, a close friend, relatives, and anyone to whom the patient gives the power of attorney. An advance directive should be periodically reviewed and revised. It is essential that a form be used that will be upheld by state law. Medical assistants can informally educate the patient concerning advance directives by obtaining booklets and forms and by becoming knowledgeable of the laws in the states in which they are working. Refer to the Resources at the end of this chapter to contact organizations for information on advance directive documents.

STOP AND THINK CASE SCENARIO

Ethics

Scenario: An elderly patient has severe osteoporosis and has a collapsed vertebra. She is in constant pain and only receives relief from taking a narcotic painkiller, which is addictive, four times a day.

Critical Thinking: Should the physician supply enough medication to provide relief or only enough pills for the patient to take when she is experiencing pain that she absolutely cannot bear? Think this through and formulate questions that might help you decide what stance to take.

_____

_____

_____

STOP AND THINK CASE SCENARIO

Bioethics

Scenario: You have a child who is diagnosed with cystic fibrosis and have heard that a cloning research project is progressing that holds the key to curing this disease.

Critical Thinking:
1. Would you want your child to benefit from this method of treatment if the research proves successful?

_____

_____

2. Would you advocate cloning research for other scientific breakthroughs?

_____

_____

STOP AND THINK CASE SCENARIO

Stem Cell Research

Scenario: Human embryonic stem cells are naturally created in the first days after conception. They can develop into all different types of cells, have the ability to continually renew themselves, and give rise to all organs and tissues in the human body. By fusing an embryonic stem cell to an adult human skin cell researchers report that they can create a hybrid cell that acts like an embryonic stem cell. Stem cells are also cultivated from embryos frozen in test tubes after being created by couples using in vitro fertilization and from embryos cloned from patients seeking treatment such as abortion. They hold the potential to be genetically programmed to treat various diseases by replacing diseased tissue, including:

- Brain tissue for use in patients with Parkinson's or Alzheimer's disease
- Liver tissue for use in patients with liver disease
- Nerve tissue for use in patients with spinal cord injury
- Pancreatic cells for use in diabetic patients
- Blood cells to repair ailing hearts or blocked arteries

Advocacy groups oppose the research of embryonic stem cells because human embryos are destroyed during research. Research done on a state level is also being opposed by lawyers on the grounds that it violates the state constitution because taxpayer money is being given to an organization not sufficiently controlled by the state government.

Critical Thinking: Stem cell research is fighting for its life. Think through this complex scenario. You many want to do additional research on your own or your instructor may assign this as a research/writing project. Be prepared to take a stance and debate stem cell research with your classmates. Formulate your response here.

_____

_____

_____

_____

_____

_____

_____

_____

_____

_____

_____

_____

_____

_____

_____

_____

_____

_____

_____

_____

STOP AND THINK CASE SCENARIO

Confidential Information

Scenario: Abigail Snyder hobbles into the medical office suffering from a broken right foot. The receptionist greets her and begins asking her personal questions that everyone in the waiting room can hear the answers to. Abigail tried talking softly, but the receptionist repeats her answers loudly enough so all can hear them. Abigail feels compelled to answer the questions because they pertain to her medical case.

Critical Thinking:

1. How do you think Abigail felt?

_____

2. What are the dangers of obtaining information in such a manner?

_____

_____

3. How do you think the receptionist could have handled the situation to obtain the information without jeopardizing patient confidentiality?

_____

_____

_____

FOCUS ON CERTIFICATION*

CMA Content Summary

- Medical (legal) terminology
- Performing within ethical boundaries
- Maintaining confidentiality
- Medical practice acts
- Federal compliance with right to privacy and HIPAA
- Release medical information
- Physician-patient relationships
- Office policies and procedures compliance plan

RMA Content Summary

- Medical (legal) terminology
- Medical law
- Medical ethics
- Understand and maintain patient confidentiality during check-in procedures

- Employ effective written communication skills adhering to ethics and laws of confidentiality
- Prepare and release private health information as required, adhering to state and federal guidelines

CMAS Content Summary

- Apply principles of medical law and ethics to the health care setting
- Know basic laws pertaining to medical practice
- Know and observe disclosure laws
- Know the principles of medical ethics established by the AMA
- Recognize unethical practices and identify ethical responses for situations in the medical office
- Understand and employ risk management and quality assurance concepts

*This textbook and the accompanying Workbook meet the entry-level administrative and general competencies for the CMA outlined by the AAMA Examination Content Outline and Role Delineation Study and for the RMA and CMAS outlined by the AMT Competencies and Examination Specifications (see Competency Grid in Appendix B).

REVIEW EXAM-STYLE QUESTIONS

1. Standards of conduct generally accepted as a moral guide for behavior are referred to as:

   a. laws

   b. bioethics

   c. professional medical etiquette

   d. professional medical ethics

   e. rules for medical professionals

2. The modern code of ethics adopted by the American Medical Association to guide physicians' standards of conduct is the:

   a. Oath of Hippocrates

   b. Modern Hippocratic Oath

   c. Principles of Medical Ethics for the Physician

   d. AAMA Code of Ethics

   e. AAMA Creed

3. The Health Insurance Portability and Accountability Act became federal law in:

   a. 1996

   b. 1998

   c. 1976

   d. 1956

   e. 2001

4. The correct meaning for the acronym PHI is:

   a. private health information

   b. personal health information

   c. protected health information

   d. portability of health information

   e. privileged health information

5. The "consent" form is used to disclose:

   a. sensitive information such as HIV or AIDS

   b. private information such as alcoholism or drug addiction

   c. personally identifiable health information when a patient transfers to another physician

   d. personally identifiable health information for treatment, payment, routine health care operations

   e. all of the above

6. If a patient requests copies of their medical records and signs the proper authorization, you should:

   a. honor the request

   b. seal them in an envelope before handing them to the patient

   c. take caution before complying with the request

   d. not honor the request; instead send them directly to another physician

   e. a, b, c are all correct

7. An exception to the right to privacy (privileged communication) that does not need an authorization form because it must be reported to the Department of Health is information about a:

   a. patient with multiple sclerosis

   b. patient with ALS

   c. patient experiencing epileptic seizures

   d. patient with diabetes mellitus

   e. patient with a skin rash on the genital area

8. The most common torts in health care incidents are:

   a. assault and battery torts

   b. liability without fault torts

   c. intentional torts

   d. negligent torts

   e. fraud or deceit torts

9. Unlawful treatment that has been done in the wrong way is:

   a. misfeasance

   b. malfeasance

   c. nonfeasance

   d. malpractice

   e. criminal negligence

10. Arbitration is:

    a. a physician review panel that hears cases outside the courtroom

    b. a type of no-fault insurance

    c. an alternative way of resolving malpractice disputes out of court

    d. litigation

    e. a type of lawsuit

11. When a physician recommends a surgical procedure and the patient decides to accept the risks and have the procedure, the patient must sign a/an:

    a. authorization to release medical records

    b. informed consent

    c. consent to release personally identifiable health information for treatment

    d. HIPAA consent

    e. health care power of attorney

12. With a *subpoena duces tecum*:

    a. a witness must appear

    b. a witness must appear with the medical record

    c. the physician must personally accept it

    d. the medical record may be all that is required

    e. the physician never needs to appear

13. A living will:

    a. is not legally binding

    b. is not recognized in the majority of states

    c. cannot be revoked orally

    d. can only be revoked in writing

    e. is more legally binding than a durable power of attorney for health care

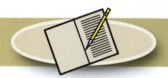

WORKBOOK ASSIGNMENT

To develop competency-based job skills, refer to the *Workbook* and complete the:

- Abbreviation and Spelling Review
- Review Questions
- Critical Thinking Exercises
- Job Skill activities, which are outlined at the beginning of this chapter under "Performance Objectives in the *Workbook*."

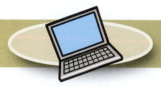

COMPUTER ASSIGNMENT

To review the concepts you have learned in this chapter, insert the *Student Practice* CD-ROM into a computer and work through the *StudyWARE* activities and games. Answer review questions in the practice mode and read the feedback, studying the questions you have missed. Take the chapter quiz until you achieve a minimum score of 90 percent. Successfully completing the *Critical Thinking Challenge* at the end of this course will help you think through scenarios and develop problem solving skills.

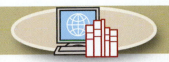

RESOURCES

Some state and local medical societies and consumer organizations can provide appropriate forms and information for advanced directives. It is important to keep well informed on legal issues affecting responsibilities of the medical assistant, and to help you there are many publications available. The following are resources to assist you.

Books

Black's Law Dictionary
Bryan A. Garner
Thomson West
610 Opperman Drive
Eagan, MN 55123-9352
(800) 328-9352
Web site: http://www.westthomson.com

Ethical Dimensions in the Health Professions
R. Purtilo
W.B. Saunders Company (Elsevier)
6277 Sea Harbor Drive
Orlando, FL 32821-9989
(800) 545-2522
Web site: http://us.elsevierhealth.com

Health Care Law and Ethics
American Association of Medical Assistants
20 North Wacker Drive, Suite 1575
Chicago, IL 60606-2903
(800) 228-2262
Web site: http://www.aama-ntl.org

Healthcare Records Management, Disclosure & Retention. The Complete Legal Guide
McGraw Hill
2 Penn Plaza
New York, New York 10121
(800) 634-3966
http://www.books.mcgraw-hill.com

Health Information Management
Edna K. Huffman
American Health Information Management Association
233 N. Michigan Ave., Suite 2150
Chicago, IL 60601-5519
(800) 335-5535
Web site: http://www.ahima.org

Insurance Handbook for the Medical Office
Marilyn T. Fordney
W.B. Saunders Company

6277 Sea Harbor Drive
Orlando, FL 32821-9989
(800) 545-2522
Web site: http://us.elsevierhealth.com

Law, Liability, and Ethics for Medical Office Professionals
Myrtle Flight
Cengage Learning
PO Box 8007
Clifton Park, NY 12065-8007
(800) 347-7707
Web site: http://www.cengagelearning.com

Medical Law, Ethics, and Bioethics in the Medical Office
M. A. Lewis and C. D. Tamparo
F. A. Davis Company
1915 Arch Street
Philadelphia, PA 19103
(800) 523-4049
Web site: http://www.fadavis.com

Medicolegal Forms with Legal Analysis
American Medical Association
515 North State Street
PO Box 10946
Chicago, IL 60610-0946
(800) 621-8335
Web site: http://www.ama-assn.org

Donor Cards

Donate Life
Online tissue donor registry service
Web site: http://donatelife.net
National Kidney Foundation
30 East 33rd Street
New York, NY 10016
(800) 622-9010
Web site: http://www.kidney.org

Internet

Compliance—Office of Inspector General (OIG)
Contains fraud and abuse settlements that can be used to identify potential problems and common risk areas in a medical practice.
Web site: http://www.hhs.gov/oig

Medical Directives

American Medical Association
    515 North State Street
    PO Box 10946
    Chicago, IL 60610-0946
    (800) 621-8335
    Web site: http://www.ama-assn.org
Caring Connections
    1700 Diogond Rd
    Suite 625
    Alexandria, VA 22344
    (800) 658-8898
    Web site: http://www.caringinfo.org
Patient Care Partnership
    American Hospital Association
    One North Franklin
    Chicago, IL 60606
    (800) 424-4301
    Web site: http://www.aha.org
Values History Form
    Center for Health Law and Ethics
    Institute of Public Law
    University of New Mexico School of Law
    1117 Stanford, N.E.
    Albuquerque, NM 87131-1431
    (505) 277-2146
    Web site: http://lawschool.unm.edu

Periodical Publications

In Confidence (bimonthly newsletter)
    American Health Information Management
    Association
    233 N. Michigan Ave., Suite 2150
    Chicago, IL 60601-5519
    (800) 335-5535
    Web site: http://www.ahima.org
Reports of the Council on Ethical and Judicial Affairs
(published annually)
    American Medical Association
    515 North State Street
    PO Box 10946
    Chicago, IL 60610-0946
    (800) 621-8335
    Web site: http://www.ama-assn.org

UNIT 2

Interpersonal Communications

CHAPTER 4

The Art of Communication

OBJECTIVES

After reading this chapter and learning step-by-step procedures to gain job skills,* you should be able to:

Learning Objectives

▊ Recognize the importance of effective communication in the medical office.

▊ List and define the basic elements of the communication cycle.

▊ Name three primary modes of communication.

▊ State and define five types of defensive mechanisms.

▊ Explain what the comfort zone is.

▊ Describe how nonverbal communication occurs.

▊ Give examples of components used in active listening.

▊ Recall three types of feedback used to evaluate whether the message sent is the message received.

▊ List things to avoid when communicating.

▊ Adapt methods of communication to meet the needs of patients in different age groups.

▊ Discuss how to handle communication problems caused by language barriers.

▊ Describe four common biases in today's society and define stereotyping, prejudice, and discrimination.

▊ Demonstrate ways to adapt communication when barriers are present such as sight-impairment, hearing-impairment, and impaired level of understanding.

▊ Discuss ways to establish positive communication with patients, coworkers, and superiors.

Performance Objectives (Procedures) in This Textbook

▊ Demonstrate active listening by following guidelines (Procedure 4-1).

*This textbook and the accompanying Workbook meet the educational components for entry-level administrative and general competencies outlined by CAAHEP and ABHES.

Performance Objectives (Job Skills) in the *Workbook*

- Demonstrate body language (Job Skill 4-1).
- Name unique qualities of other cultures (Job Skill 4-2).

OUTLINE WITH LECTURE NOTES

Essential Communications
What is Communication?

_____

_____

_____

_____

Elements and Goals of Communication

_____

_____

_____

_____

_____

Methods of Communication
Verbal Communication

_____

_____

_____

Nonverbal Communication

_____

_____

_____

_____

The Receiver

_____

_____

_____

Feedback

_____

_____

_____

Elements That Influence and Interfere with Communication
Environmental Elements

_____

_____

_____

_____

Gender

_____

_____

_____

Age

_____

_____

_____

Economic Status

_____

_____

_____

Language Barriers

_____

_____

_____

Cultural Differences

_____

_____

_____

Patients with Special Needs

_____

_____

_____

Anxious Patients

_____

_____

_____

Angry Patients

_____

_____

_____

Professional Communication

Patients and Their Friends and Family

_____

_____

_____

The Health Care Team

_____

_____

_____

_____

Office Manager

_____

_____

_____

Physician

_____

_____

_____

_____

Outside Health Care Professionals

_____

_____

_____

KEY TERMS

active listening
bias
colloquialisms
communicate
communication cycle
defensive
demeanor
discrimination
displaced anger
ethnic

enunciate
feedback
noncompliant
nonverbal communication
open-ended questions
perceptions
prejudice
reflective listening
stereotype
verbal communication

ESSENTIAL COMMUNICATION

Good interpersonal and communication skills are essential traits that should accompany the technical administrative and clinical skills each medical assistant obtains. These are referred to as *soft skills*, also called "emotional intelligence," and include such things as business etiquette, social grace, team spirit, negotiation skills, and positive behavior traits. Soft skills compliment the "hard skills" that you will learn. Of all the professionals that make up a health care team, the medical assistant will have the most interaction with the patient, therefore, the art of communication must be learned, developed, and practiced. As with other skills, it may seem easy for some and difficult for others.

HEART OF THE HEALTH CARE PROFESSIONAL

Service

Communication is the foundation of every action taken as a health care professional serves and cares for patients, regardless of the task. In good times and in times of illness you may be the lifeline that connects the patient to the physician so that they can get the help they need. Accurate communication is vital to helping maintain this connection but is often a silent component not readily seen as a way of serving patients' needs.

The health care professional who learns how to communicate effectively will be an asset to the medical practice and an important cog in the **communication cycle** (Figure 4-1). Effective communication is highly valued because it will affect office interactions, patient understanding of office policies, and various aspects of health care delivery as well as public relations.

What is Communication?

To **communicate** is to transfer information from one party to another. The information being shared is facts, feelings, ideas, opinions, and thoughts. This exchange process takes place between two individuals—a sender and a receiver. Basic elements of the communication cycle include:

- Sender—Person who has an idea or information and wants to convey it.
- Message—Content that needs to be communicated.
- Channel—Method of sending the message to the receiver.
- Receiver—Recipient getting the message and interpreting it.
- Feedback—Response from the receiver used to decide whether clarification is necessary and to determine whether the message sent is the message received.

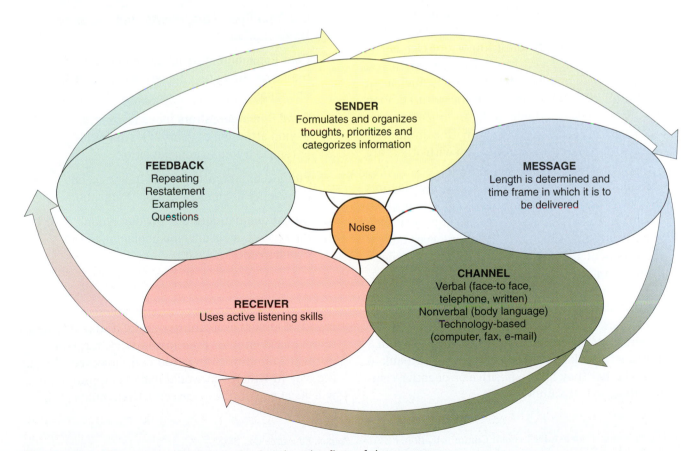

Figure 4-1. The communication cycle showing the flow of the message

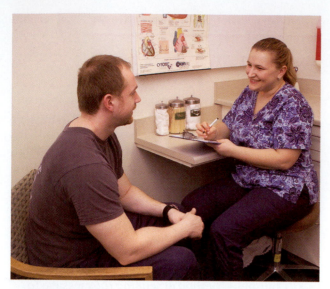

Figure 4-2. Positive communication is demonstrated by an open posture and a friendly smile

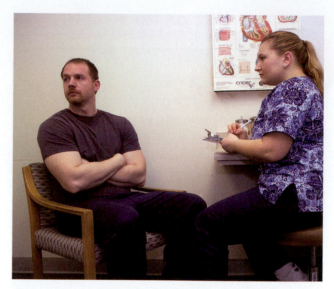

Figure 4-3. Negative communication is demonstrated by a closed posture, lack of eye contact, and a bored or disgruntled appearance

The top three ways humans communicate verbal messages are: (1) body language 55%, (2) tonality (voice tone, tempo, volume, inflection, projection) 38%, and (3) spoken word 7%.* Yes, more information is communicated by body language than words and the tone in which they are spoken. Why? One would think that words are the most important element in communication, however, this chapter will inform you of the various components involved in each element of communication and their usefulness. In addition to these elements, methods of communication, elements that influence and interfere with communication, and professional communication with others are covered.

Communication can be *positive* or *negative* (Figures 4-2 and 4-3). When you are attentive, encouraging, friendly, and show concern you are demonstrating a positive attitude. Acting bored, avoiding eye contact, being impatient, finishing another person's sentences, forgetting common courtesies, interrupting, mumbling, rushing, speaking sharply, and even doing two things at the same time when trying to communicate is received as negative communication. Observe other service industry professionals, such as a waitress in a restaurant, a clerk in a store, or a teller at the bank to assess whether they have a positive or negative communication style (Example 4-1).

EXAMPLE 4-1

Positive versus Negative Communicators

Use Your Eyes, Ears, Hearts, and Minds To Be Receptive

Poor Communicators focus on themselves—their own thoughts, feelings, experiences, and ideas.

Good Communicatiors focus on others, paying attention to everything the other person is trying to communicate.

Poor Communicators speak their part and think that the communication is finished.

Good Communicators know that what they have said is only the beginning of the communication cycle.

Take charge of your communication style, as it is a part of almost everything you do. It may be intentional, accidental, or even involuntary, but you cannot help communicating. You can, however, choose the way in which you would like to communicate, it will effect you and your career path (Example 4-2).

*The Complete Idiot's Guide to Clear Communication, *Kris Cole, Pearson Education Co., 2002*

Elements and Goals of Communication

As a health care worker, communication will take on many forms. Talking on the telephone, composing office memos or letters, and sending messages by computer or the facsimile machine are all ways of communicating. The most productive communication takes place in face-to-face conversations. For example, if you are trying to collect on an account, you can send a statement or call the patient, but if the patient comes into the office you have the best chance of collecting by having a conversation with the patient. Also, if you are trying to convey to the patient the risks of a surgical procedure you can give the patient an information pamphlet; however, if you sit down and outline the risks of the procedure and allow time for questions you will have a much better chance of being sure the patient is fully informed.

Obtaining Information

As a health care professional, much of the communication you will be involved in will be centered around gathering information. You will use informal interviewing techniques, and your goal will be to obtain accurate data that will be used by the physician and all of the professionals in your office. Asking good questions is the key to receiving accurate information. Closed-ended questions that allow the patient to answer with one word, such as "yes" or "no," should be avoided when you are trying to gather information. Such questions can be used for obtaining specific information, such as a checklist on a history form that asks whether the patient has ever had a disease (Example 4-3).

You may be communicating to schedule an appointment in the most convenient and appropriate time frame, gather insurance information to process a claim efficiently, or transfer a call to the correct staff member. Regardless of what you are communicating, first consider the area of the office in which you will be speaking to the patient, and be sure it matches the type of information you will receive. For instance, always use a private area when obtaining confidential information. Also, you will want to organize your thoughts prior to speaking. Remember to introduce yourself, wear a name badge, and let the patient know why you are trying to obtain information. You should always document the patient's responses accurately.

Building Patient Relationships

When selecting a physician, patients often ask, "Will the doctor take time with me, speak to me in a way that I can understand, and treat me with respect?" Have you ever heard someone say that they changed physicians because they could not stand the receptionist? Although patients do not often ask about the office staff, they expect the same respectful treatment from staff members as they do from the physician. Effective communication takes time and builds good relationships. Negative and poor communication damages relationships because it causes defensive reactions, misunderstandings, and a breakdown of the communication cycle. In fact, failure to communicate is the number one reason for the failure of relationships.

As a medical assistant, your goal should be to present the physician and medical practice in a positive light and to establish rapport and maintain positive relationships with patients. How you present yourself communicates a message about who you are and the medial practice in which you work. As an administrative medical assistant you can be the friendly voice, the face with the smile, or the helpful assistant to patients who are going through times of illness or distress. Each patient is unique, so treat all patients individually and with respect. When you do so, they will respond positively.

Trust begins to develop between the physician and the patient long before the patient ever meets the doctor—it begins with the relationship that is established upon first contact. This relationship between the patient and the health care professional is not equal. The power and control belongs to the person on the health care team, therefore it is important to try to equalize the relationship as much as possible. This is accomplished by showing concern and building an atmosphere of trust. Patients often open up to a medical assistant easier than with the physician. Even if a patient asks you to not tell the doctor something, you should never withhold any information that relates to health care from the physician, and patients should be reminded that all things discussed are confidential. Encourage patients to talk to the physician freely and openly.

Generally, people do not feel in control while being examined by a physician and especially when they have an illness. They often must do things they do not want to do in order to get well. It is not uncommon for patients to become inpatient, and they want the physician to help them get better immediately so they can get on with their lives with minimal interruption of their normal routine. Patients may feel guilty and think that even though the illness is out of their control, they could have done something different to avoid it. All of this may make people become anxious, and in order to cope they behave in a **defensive** manner. Defensive behavior is usually unconscious and is a response to protect oneself from a perceived threat. The threat may stem from anxiety, guilt, loss of self-esteem, or an injured ego. Understanding defense mechanisms will help you cope with patients who use them. They may become **noncompliant** and refuse to follow the doctor's treatment plan. Refer to Table 4-1

Table 4-1. Types of Defense Mechanisms

- **Apathy:** Demonstrating disinterest or indifference to what is happening. The patient may appear to have a lack of emotion or feeling and display a flippant attitude.
  Example: "Who cares what the diagnosis is, we're all going to die sometime."

- **Aggression:** Belligerent, combative attitude, such as lashing out by verbally attacking in order to avoid or diminish their role in wrong doing.
  Example: A patient arrives late for their appointment and the waiting room is full. The medical assistant calls the patient from the waiting room and says, "Would you like to come with me to the treatment room?" The patient responds, "Does the physician think we are all puppy dogs, at his beck and call?"

- **Avoidance:** Not seeing someone or not going to a place that evokes bad memories or pain.
  Example: After a physician diagnoses a patient with cancer the patient says, "I will never go to that doctor again because he gave me cancer."

- **Compensation:** Consciously or unconsciously overemphasizing something to make up for a real or imagined deficiency. This is also known as substituting a strength for a weakness and may be considered healthy in some cases.
  Example: "I know I haven't stopped smoking, Dr. Practon, but I have lost five pounds."

- **Denial:** Refusing to accept painful information or a unpleasant situation; disbelieving reality. It is often the first response after a traumatic event.
  Example: A patient is told that she has pancreatic cancer and has only three months to live. The person or a family member hears what the doctor says but goes about her business as if she was never told about the serious disease and that she is going to die. A loved-one's response may be, "My wife can't have cancer, she plays tennis three times a week, eats a healthy diet, and gets a check up every year."

Table 4-1 (*continued*). Types of Defense Mechanisms

- **Displacement:** Unconscious transfer or redirection of unacceptable emotions, feelings, or thoughts from self to someone or something else. Channeling negative feelings to an unrelated area in order to feel a sense of control in situations that are not controllable.
  Example: A patient who is upset with the doctor says a rude remark to the receptionist on the way out of the office.

- **Projection:** Taking unacceptable desires, thoughts, or impulses and falsely attributing them to others instead of admitting that they are connected to how the person feels. This defense mechanism comes out when people have feelings or urges that they do not want to admit they are experiencing. This is a sign of mental illness.
  Example: A child is fussing during an examination, and the father who has been abusing this child accuses the health care professional of being rough with the child in order to hide his feelings of wanting to hit the child.

- **Rationalization:** Making up a reason to justify unacceptable actions, behavior, or events. This is sometimes done to avoid obeying instructions or because the person knows that they are wrong and wants to avoid embarrassment or guilt. The reason used is usually a stretch of the truth; most people rationalize to some extent.
  Example: The patient tells the physician that he did not get his blood drawn as ordered because the line was too long and he did not have time to wait. Of course, he could have made an appointment and avoided the wait.

- **Regression:** Withdrawing from an unpleasant circumstance by reverting to an earlier, more secure time in life either mentally or behaviorally. Usually this is done when a person feels desperate and powerless over whatever is causing the pain.
  Example: A four-year-old reverts to baby talk after the arrival of a new baby sister.

- **Repression:** An unconscious reaction where the person seems to experience amnesia in order to block the problem from the mind. It could manifest as forgetfulness and is the mind's way of defending against mental trauma. This is not the same as outright lying. Severe cases may be associated with mental illness.
  Example: A rape victim unconsciously forgets to tell her parents that the reason she cannot go to a movie is because she was leaving a movie theater when the rapist followed her.

- **Sarcasm:** Speaking with a sharp edge; usually intended to cause pain or anger. Sometimes it is used for humor, but it is not always taken humorously.
  Example: The medical assistant comments on how good the patient looks. The patient, who is not feeling well, responds, "I guess I'll go to my grave looking great." Or children have been left in the waiting room and made a mess, and a medical assistant comments sarcastically, "I hope your children enjoyed destroying the waiting room."

- **Undoing:** Actions taken to cancel out or make up for inappropriate behavior.
  Example: Mrs. Clark brings the physician a gift, because the last time she was in the office she was very rude and spoke unkind words.

for a brief description of the various types of defense mechanisms and examples that apply to the physician's office.

Maslow's Hierarchy of Needs

An American psychologist, Abraham Maslow, studied human behavior and developed a theory that states people are motivated by needs and that their basic needs must be met before they can progress to fulfill other needs. Maslow's hierarchy pyramid (Figure 4-4) groups human needs into five levels. Basic needs are at the bottom of the pyramid, and it progresses to higher needs at each tier. The importance of understanding this concept is to be able to apply it to patients' needs. Health care professionals must realize a patient's need to fulfill his or her basic needs before expecting the patient to actually take on responsibility

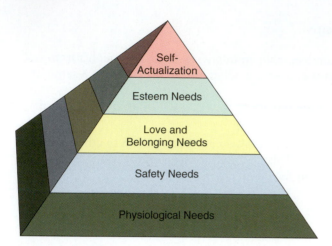

Figure 4-4. Maslow's hierarchy of needs

for their own health care. That ability is obtained only through self-actualization, the highest level of the pyramid. Following are brief descriptions of the various levels of needs.

Physiological Needs—Basic needs, or survival needs that include water, air, sleep, hygiene, and sexual activity, fall into the physiological need category and must be met before a patient can move on to consider other types of needs. Physiological needs can control thoughts and behaviors, and if not met, people can feel sick and uncomfortable. Each person has a different point of view regarding the satisfaction of these basic needs that may arise from their background or upbringing. One person may think they need three square meals per day, while another has only a cup of coffee in the morning and soup in the afternoon. These are individual perceptions and should be accepted, not judged. Once these needs are satisfied, the body recognizes a state of balance (*homeostasis*), and our minds are freed to think about other things.

Safety Needs—Once the physiological needs are met the need for safety will emerge. These needs include having a safe environment, feeling secure, and living without fear or anxiety. Patients who are injured or facing a battle with disease are often anxious and fearful. They may become preoccupied with thoughts of dying and no longer feel safe. Safety also has to do with law, order, structure, and feeling protected.

Love and Belonging Needs—After physiological and safety needs are met, social needs emerge. This involves emotionally based relationships such as feelings of belonging and being connected to our roots, friends, family, neighborhood, and so forth. To give and be shown affection and love are essential ele-

ments, and in the absence of these people feel lonely and/or depressed.

Esteem Needs—Maslow describes self-esteem as the need for respect from others (recognition, acceptance, status, appreciation), and the need for self-respect. People need to engage in activities that give a sense of contribution and self-value. The less self-assured we are, the less likely we are to place importance on our own health and elements such as inferiority complexes, inflated sense of self-importance, or snobbishness can occur.

Self-Actualization Needs—The highest level of need is that of self-actualization, or a person reaching his or her potential by making the most of unique abilities. At this level people are free to be creative, spontaneous, interested, and objective, and they have a general appreciation of life. Patients who reach this level strive to control their state of wellness and are involved in their health care decisions. All other basic needs must be satisfied before one can reach this level.

We all do not start at the bottom of the pyramid and we all do not reach the top. Sometimes circumstances cause us to go up a level but slide back down. It is important to realize where on the pyramid patients are so that you can understand how to help educate them and communicate with them effectively.

METHODS OF COMMUNICATION

In this section we look at the two parties involved in the communication cycle—the sender and the receiver. How does the sender get his message across? Does he use verbal or nonverbal communication channels? How does the recipient receive the intended information?

Verbal Communication

Verbal communication involves the use of language or spoken words to transmit messages. This is the most common form of communication, and as we talk and listen throughout the day we are sending and receiving oral messages. Select your words carefully and be aware of the power behind them. Each of us can remember a time when our feelings were hurt due to unkind words or thoughtless remarks. The meaning of some spoken words can vary depending on the settings in which they are spoken. **Perceptions**, cultural or ethic backgrounds, and a variety of other factors also impact the meanings of some words. Perceptions are based on awareness or assumptions that people make and on their point of view as they discern what is being said. Proper English, grammar, and medical terminology are necessary to communicate accurately and professionally. Speak clearly and **enunciate** (pronounce) words properly. Do not use **colloquialisms**, which are slang or informal words such as "you know" or "gonna," or phrases such as, "I'm fixin' to get your chart." To avoid misconceptions or miscommunications be sure that the words used match the voice tone and body language communicated. In other words, say what you mean clearly and use positive body language that is nonthreatening and presents a professional, compassionate tone.

Communicate according to the patient's level of education and understanding. For example, when speaking to a physician or other health care professional about a referral it would be proper to use medical terms; however, when speaking to the patient who is being referred you may need to use nontechnical language (*layman's terms*) instead.

Voice Tone

Voice tone is very important. The pitch, quality, and range within which you speak determine the overall tone. Voice tone and other nonlanguage sounds such as laughing, sobbing, sighing, and grunting often provide more information than words themselves. Remember the old saying, "it's not *what* you say but *how* you say it." The way the message is delivered affects the way it is received.

The speaker's articulation, pronunciation, and grammatical structure also offer nonlanguage clues to understanding, and can vary from region to region and can indicate the level of education and cultural background.

Nonverbal Communication

Nonverbal communication is sending a message without words. It is important that we be aware of what we communicate nonverbally. Body movements, also called nonverbal communication, accompanies oral messages and is commonly referred to as *body language*. These movements are sometimes unconscious and unintentional, or they can be natural responses to the way we feel. Body language and nonverbal communication begin in infancy, prior to speech development. We realize this when we watch how a baby communicates. Some motions and ges-

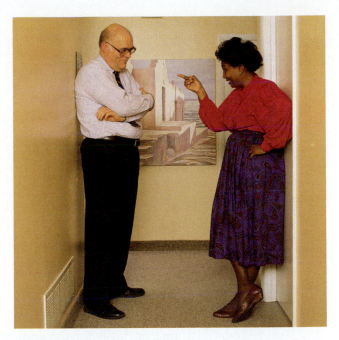

Figure 4-5. Body language can communicate more than spoken words

tures are instinctive while others may be imitated or taught. The culture in which a person is raised and the home environment greatly influence body language.

A boss's head-nod typically indicates approval. But such things as eye contact, facial movement, gestures, posture, touch, mannerisms, position, stance, gait, and attention to personal space are all nonverbal signals that can send specific messages (Figure 4-5). These expressions can be used by the medical assistant to set a professional but compassionate tone, and they can be "read" in order to better understand what patients are trying to communicate verbally. When communicating, maintain an open, relaxed body posture. See how the person is receiving the message by noticing his or her facial expressions. Following are various parts of the body and some messages that may be communicated while using them.

- *Eyes:* It is often said that the eyes are the window to a person's soul. What does that mean? The expression of anxiety, happiness, grief, joy, sorrow, and worry are reflected through the eyes. The eyes may also show interest or disinterest. Downcast eyes may indicate that you are not interested or that you are trying to avoid the person speaking; it can also be a sign of submission or avoidance. An eye-wink can communicate that you are kidding and not serious.

- *Mouth:* It can be used to offer a smile, opened wide in surprise, puckered to show dissatisfaction, or it can be set in a firm grimace to indicate impatience or anger.

- *Face:* Laugh lines around the eyes, worry lines in the forehead, or an inquisitive eyebrow all help to convey nonverbal clues. The face is the most expressive part of the body. Weathered or tanned skin indicates time spent in the sun whereas pale skin suggests time spent indoors.

- *Gait:* Walking briskly can mean the person is in a hurry or energized; it also demonstrates confidence. Walking slowly suggests fatigue or demonstrates a laid-back attitude. Problems with the gait, such as stiffness or limping can be signs of illness or injury.

- *Gestures:* Gestures are used to enhance storytelling, add drama, or clarify the size and shape of objects. Avoid informal gestures, they can be misinterpreted.

- *Hands:* Hands may be offered as a greeting, such as in a handshake. They may also be used to demonstrate size or gesture to emphasize something said. Fingers may be used to point, to indicate that all is "OK," or to snap to get someone's attention. Be aware that pointing a finger can be interpreted as very rude and "OK" signs are considered obscene in some cultures. Other mannerisms such as doodling, tapping the finger, wringing of hands, and so forth may be interpreted as indications of wandering thoughts, boredom, or anxiety. A military salute typically says "yes sir," or "you have my attention," without any spoken words.

- *Posture:* How a person holds themselves may be a sign of how a message is being received or how the person is feeling. Shoulders held back with head held high indicates confidence whereas slumped shoulders and head held down indicates tiredness or defeat. Shrugging shoulders often means, "I don't know." Arms crossed over the chest may indicate a closed demeanor.

- *Touch:* Touch is perceived in different ways among different cultures, but in America a light touch on the arm, shoulder, or back usually communicates interest or concern and can be beneficial to some patients. Like words, touch is a powerful tool and can indicate emotional support. Being touched by a stranger can have a negative affect and can make some patients uncomfortable, while hugging is usually reserved for close relationships. Reading the patient's demeanor is important when assessing a patient's response to touch. To evaluate a patient's **demeanor**, notice how they appear, what their expressions are, and try to read their body language. Learn about other cultures common to your medical practice and be sensitive to their perception of touch.

Double Messages

Patients may say one thing but show a completely different response with their body language; this is referred to as a double message. For example, a patient says, "I'd like the doctor to check my foot but it really isn't that bad," but her face is grimacing in pain with each step she takes. In this case the nonverbal clues demonstrate an inconsistent message. Patients may hide their feelings, so you need to read the nonverbal clues in addition to listening to what they tell you. As a rule, when the words spoken and the body language do not match, the body language usually depicts the true feelings of the person and their emotional state.

The Comfort Zone

The type of communication and the distance between two people communicating varies depending on how emotionally involved they are. For instance, a husband and wife communicate more intimately than two friends and would be comfortable standing or sitting very close to one another. When conversing in a health care setting the appropriate space, or "comfort zone" is usually about an arm's length, or 3 to 4 feet. This professional distance is not to be invaded and varies with individuals, circumstances, and cultures. Be aware of where patients physically place themselves in relation to others. This can be another nonverbal clue and can affect the communication process.

In a medical office it may be necessary to enter a patient's personal space, especially when delivering care. Using a professional manner, explaining what is being done, and being sensitive to patients' reactions are important when you have to work in close proximity. If you notice a patient or coworker sitting back in their chair or stepping back, you may have invaded their comfort zone. Comfort zones will vary among different people and cultures so be respectful, and ask if you are unsure. For example, "Would you like to take my arm for support while I escort you to the physician's office?" is a simple way to establish a patient's sense of personal space.

Also keep a professional distance so you can be objective. Do not become too personally involved with patients and resist the temptation to tell patients intimate information about yourself (such as financial troubles or marital problems). Do not compare or offer reassurance by telling patients about similar health care situations you or your family may have experienced. For instance, "My husband is a diabetic and is doing fine." The patient may misread your intentions and think that their diagnosis of diabetes is not very important; but to them it is.

The Receiver

When preparing to convey a message, consider the timing so that you have the best possible chance of having your message received accurately. The receiver is not always receptive and communication can be hampered if you try to send a message regardless of the receiver's mood or circumstances. For instance, if you have been wanting to talk to the doctor about a raise but there is an office emergency, it would be best to wait until another time. Or if you have been meaning to talk to your supervisor about a problem with a coworker but this is her first day back from vacation, it might not be the best time. To receive a message clearly you must be a good listener, respond to body language, and maintain eye contact.

Active Listening

Listening is not the same as hearing. In an office setting, we hear many sounds throughout the day—the copy machine running, the phone ringing, traffic outside—but we do not listen to them. We filter out these sounds and can do the same thing when someone is speaking. A wandering mind, due to anxiety or boredom, causes inattention or imprecise listening as you hear roughly what the person says but do not get the details of the message. The person who talks all the time or the one who appears to be listening but is not, does not really want to understand the message that the other person is expressing.

Active listening involves being patient while the message is spoken and giving the speaker your undivided attention. We all want to feel that we are listened to—it makes us feel understood, validated, and safe. Focus on the person with whom you are speaking and concentrate on the message being relayed. Do not think about anything else or let your mind wander. As the speaker talks, responses will come

to mind, and it may be difficult to let go of the urge to respond immediately. However, that is exactly what you should do in order to continue listening actively. This practice is an exercise that moves your mental focus from yourself to the speaker. It should be practiced over and over, otherwise you will continue to think about how you want to respond, and you will not be able to focus on what the speaker is saying. You must recognize your own attitudes and feelings so that you can put aside anything that may interfere with you concentrating on the speaker's message.

Both active and **reflective listening** help you to hear the message precisely. To listen reflectively you need to dwell on, mull over, and even study or weigh what has been said. Listen not only to the words spoken but notice the speaker's tone of voice and body language in order to receive the complete message. Be observant. When practicing active listening try to keep interruptions to a minimum. Your response to interruptions will be interpreted either positively or negatively by the other person (see Procedure 4-1).

Feedback

The oral or nonverbal response, referred to as **feedback**, is the best indicator of whether the message sent was the message received. As the speaker, the assistant should periodically verify that the person is receiving the message by being a careful observer and watching for body language as well as oral responses. Asking whether the patient understands does not always produce an honest answer. As the listener, the assistant should use feedback to verify that the message was heard correctly. Following are various techniques used to obtain feedback.

Repeating

Asking the patient to repeat back to you what was said can help verify that all the information was received. This echoing helps clarify feedback. You can prompt a patient to repeat the message by saying, "We have been talking for a while and I want to make sure you understand all of the instructions the physician has asked me to convey to you, could you please repeat them?"

Restatement or Paraphrasing

To ensure you have accurately heard what was said, you may want to restate or paraphrase the information received. Use your own words or phrases and begin with statements such as "I understood you to

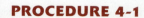

PROCEDURE 4-1

Demonstrative Active Listening by Following Guidelines

Objective: Practice active listening to develop better listening skills.

Equipment/Supplies: Two people in conversation.

Directions: Follow these guidelines when someone else is speaking to learn to listen actively and attentively.

1. Prepare yourself by leaning forward in your chair or tilting your head so that you can receive all that is said.

2. Give your full attention to the speaker. Do not pretend to listen.

3. Maintain eye contact and be sensitive to the other person's personal space.

4. Notice facial expressions, posture, and other signs of body language.

5. Remove all distractions, do not look at other things in the room, try to hear other conversations, or think about other tasks you have to accomplish.

6. Do not talk over the other person or interrupt the speaker.

7. Think before you respond and consider the other person's viewpoint.

8. Offer feedback so the sender knows you have received the message.

9. Ask questions or have the sender repeat the message if it is not understood.

---

say that . . ." or "You are saying that . . ." Paraphrasing tells the patient that you have listened and helps clarify what was said.

Requesting Examples

Requesting examples may help clarify information being communicated. For instance, if a patient is describing a rude receptionist that she encountered every time she went to a specialist's office that your physician had referred her to, ask the patient to give you an example of what happened. The patient's example should give you an insight into how the patient perceives the situation and help you better understand exactly what the patient is saying.

Questioning

When trying to encourage the patient to open up and talk, ask **open-ended questions** that allow the patient to formulate a response and elaborate if necessary. Questions that begin with *what*, *when*, or *how* or with phrases such as *tell me about*, *describe to me*, or *explain to me* are considered open-ended because they allow you to bring forth information from patients without making them feel as though they are being cross-examined. For example, "Please describe the type of pain you are having." It is a nonthreatening way to gather additional information.

Questions that begin with *why* should be avoided because they often sound judgmental or harsh and

cause people to respond defensively. The patient may feel like he or she is being accused of something, and it may incite a negative response (Example 4-4).

Summarizing

Stating a brief summary of the information you have obtained helps give the patient a chance to clarify and correct misinformation. Use this review technique when given lots of detail or a confusing message. For instance, if the patient states that he has come in to get a flu shot, but he is sick with a cold, and he then elaborates on all of his symptoms, and then says that he also has an open sore that he is worried about on his foot, review what he has said in words such as, "I understand that you wanted to get a flu shot today, but since

---

EXAMPLE 4-4

Avoid "Why" Questions

No: Why are you calling?

Yes: What may I help you with today?

No: Why are you upset?

Yes: Please describe what has upset you.

No: Why don't you call back later?

Yes: Please call back this afternoon.

you have a cold you would like to be seen for the cold, and also have the doctor take a look at the open sore on your foot." Leave time for the patient to respond and correct any misinformation. Highlight main points and use this technique to transition to a new topic.

The Silent Pause

People are often uncomfortable with periods of silence during conversation, but they can be very beneficial. Controlled silence is a well-placed pause that can be used to get someone's attention, emphasize a message, reiterate or restate thoughts, add additional information, put events in sequence, state feelings, or take the conversation in a different direction. Do not allow silent pauses to be filled with chatter or let the conversation wander. Instead, use this time wisely to gather your thoughts and formulate additional questions. Remember the power of well-placed silence–it can be an effective exclamation mark or speak louder than a raised voice.

ELEMENTS THAT INFLUENCE AND INTERFERE WITH COMMUNICATION

A number of elements can affect, interfere with, or make communication more difficult. Consider the personality type and conversational style of the person you are communicating with. Realize that a person's emotions come from within and reflect mental states such as anger, anxiety, confusion, depression, fatigue, fear, nervousness, pain, sadness, and so forth

that can interfere with communication. You may have to adapt your communication style to get your message across.

Try to stay neutral instead of agreeing or disagreeing with the patient's thoughts, ideas, or perceptions. By doing this, the patient cannot conclude that you think they are right or wrong and he or she is allowed to have personal opinions and conclusions. If you vocalize that you share the same opinion, patients may think that you agree with them, and therefore they are right. Also, if you share that you do not agree with them, they may perceive this as disapproval and then think of you as the opposition instead of someone who is trying to help them. By neither agreeing or disagreeing, you prevent displaying a moralistic attitude that implies a particular judgment upon the patient. Regardless of the communication difficulty, imagine the trip to the doctor's office through the eyes of the patient and then take the necessary steps to improve that experience. Refer to Table 4-2 for a list of things to avoid when communicating.

Environmental Elements

Outside interference can also cause difficulty in communication. Noise, visual stimuli, and touch can be distractions and can cause your concentration to wander. Distractions can come from sounds within the room, such as the conversations of others, or sounds outside the building, like the gardener operating a blowing machine. It could also be someone sighing, giggling, or coughing; someone looking at their watch, rolling their eyes, or closing their eyes; someone grabbing you, hugging you, or bumping

Table 4-2. Things to Avoid When Communicating

- Do not advise patients about their health care or other situation. This could be construed as practicing medicine without a license.
- Never belittle a patient or the feelings they have. This reflects judgment on your part and minimizes their situation or the pain they are feeling. All feelings are justified and it should never be insinuated that they are not important.
- Do not challenge patients. This makes them feel as though they have to prove what they have said is true.
- Do not change the subject if you become uncomfortable with a patient who is conveying their feelings. For instance, if a patient presents at the window and says, "I could hardly get up today I am so depressed." Do not just ask them to sign in and have a seat. Instead, address them as best you can by saying something like, "I'm sorry you are feeling so down, hopefully the doctor can help you with this."
- Do not take a defensive attitude. This may make the patient feel as though he or she must defend themselves.
- Be careful about reassuring or giving approval. When you reassure a patient they may believe that there is no need for the anxiety or pain they are feeling; instead have empathy.
- Do not jump to conclusions. This happens when you have preconceived ideas or you have your mind made up and leads to misunderstandings and miscommunication.

into you; or being uncomfortable with people who are in close proximity. Temperature deviations (being too hot or too cold) can be disturbing and affect your ability to focus. Also, being preoccupied, uncomfortable because of a poor sitting arrangement, or embarrassed because you feel half exposed in a gown can all be barriers in the communication process.

Gender

Gender is probably one of the first things that is noticed. Although generalizations about men and women should not be relied on, they should be considered. Men, for instance, often do not show their feelings and have a hard time admitting to disease and illness. Thus, they come to the physician less frequently and may not be open to admitting they have pain. Women, on the other hand, feel more free to describe their illness and are often more in tune with their bodies. When it comes to describing intimate details about their health, however, both genders feel more comfortable with a member of the same sex. These wishes should be honored if at all possible. If they cannot be honored, the issue should be discussed with the physician and the patient. Try to make the patient feel as comfortable as possible.

Each culture has its own viewpoint about gender, which includes behavioral expectations. However, in both Western and non-Western cultures, male social dominance is expected.

People declaring alternative lifestyles such as homosexuality, bisexuality, or transgender orientation should be allowed to voice their concerns with the physician and not be discriminated against. They especially need to feel safe and know that confidentiality is a mandatory requirement of all medical staff.

Age

Age is always a factor to consider when communicating. Infants, toddlers, little children, adolescents, teenagers, young adults, middle-aged persons, and older adults are all in different stages of development. Their age, life experiences, and the phase of life that they are going through affects their communication styles and abilities.

Children

When going to a doctor's office, children will often base their opinions on their past experiences and what they have been told by their parents. These

beliefs will vary greatly and affect the communication process. A parent's reaction in a health care setting is often mimicked by children. If the parent is confident and trusting the child will feel secure and open. If the parent is worried and fretful the child will feel anxious. If a child associates the visit with being sick or getting a shot they may become frightened and act out their fear in the doctor's office. Do not dismiss these emotions, instead recognize them and let them be expressed freely.

Always tailor your communication to the child's age and needs. Comprehension can vary greatly, and although a child may not understand what is said, he or she will likely respond to tone of voice, gestures, and facial expressions. Use such body language to calm the child's fears and make her feel at ease. A child needs to feel safe, so your goal should be to establish trust. Speak to the child directly and inform children of all ages, along with their parents, of what will happen during the appointment. This will help correct erroneous preexisting ideas, clarify wandering thoughts of the unknown, and establish honesty. The following guidelines will help facilitate communication with children:

1. Position yourself so that you can speak to children at eye level.

2. Speak with a soft, low-pitched voice.

3. Talk at a level they can understand and ask simple questions, rephrasing them when necessary until they are understood.

4. Allow the child to be involved—give him or her a clipboard and writing tool to use while

PATIENT EDUCATION

Parents may not realize the anxieties a child may face when he or she is ill and must continually come to the physician's office or undergo frequent tests and procedures. The parents of a seriously ill child may not know how to deal with the situation. Written pamphlets are available to help them cope with children's illnesses, understand the child's anxieties, and relate to their fears. Having pamphlets on display in the waiting room and offering them to parents helps educate them without judging their responses and actions.

the parent fills out the patient information form.

5. Offer a toy and use it or a puppet in a playful manner when asking questions. This can gain the child's attention and cooperation.

6. Recognize situations the child may be fearful of and allow each child to express fear and to cry.

7. Realize that a child may return to a lower developmental stage in order to receive comfort during an illness. For example, a child may revert to thumb sucking during a stressful event or start wetting the bed again because of fear.

Adolescence and Teenagers

Be receptive of all communication from adolescents and teenagers without being startled. If you express shock they may assume you are judging them, which can close the channel of communication. Young people may request that their parents not come into the treatment room. Teenagers may be reluctant to divulge information or ask questions if someone else is present and should be given the opportunity to speak to the physician alone. Be sensitive to such requests and inform the physician so that he or she can assess the situation and decide if the parent should be included.

Older Adults

Senior patients have special needs, and older adults do not all communicate on the same level. Mental and physical changes such as impairment in memory or judgment, may have resulted from illness, disease, or the aging process, and these changes may cause confusion or affect oral communication. Alzheimer's disease and senility are two common causes of impaired communication skills, although similar symptoms may be brought on by a head injury, depression, alcohol or drug abuse, and medication misuse. Always speak to older adults with respect, and expect them to comprehend on an adult level unless you have been advised differently. Do not speak down to them or patronize them. Generally, they will need extra patience, assistance, and instruction or explanations. When senior patients are accompanied by a spouse, relative, or friend always look directly at and speak to the patient giving them a chance to respond and speak for themselves (Figure 4-6). If they are unresponsive, forget, or you are concerned whether their recollection is accurate, ask the other adult

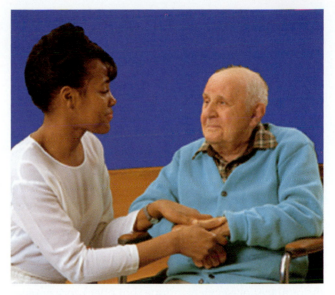

Figure 4-6. The medical assistant looks directly at the patient communicating warmth, empathy and concern

if they have anything to add. Guidelines to follow when communicating with older adults include the following.

1. Avoid misconceptions and do not prejudge.

2. Speak clearly and slowly, offering simple explanations.

3. Form short sentences and ask brief questions.

4. Rephrase statements or questions as necessary.

5. React calmly if the patient seems confused or forgetful.

6. Do not make excuses for the patient or make up explanations as to why they seem confused.

7. Tell the patient if you do not understand what they have said and ask them to repeat it.

8. Be gentle but honest and truthful in your communication so you do not mislead the patient or yourself.

9. Offer written instructions.

Economic Status

The medical assistant will interact with patients from different economic classes—both affluent and impoverished—which may lead to varied views regarding health care. In today's health care delivery system the numbers of uninsured and underinsured are increasing, and the high cost of medicines, procedures, and hospitalization causes stress and worry among patients. Many Americans struggle to pay high insurance premiums, deductibles, and copayments. People at the lowest economic levels may not be able to afford the tests, procedures, and medication that the physician recommends, which could cause them to stay away from the doctor unless absolutely necessary. Their primary concerns may be the daily issues of survival. These factors should be considered when communicating with patients and the health care professional should be aware of community assistance and government programs that they can refer patients to in such circumstances.

Wealthy patients and those in the upper middle class may not have to worry about financial problems. They are able to pay expensive premiums and use traditional fee-for-service options that offer more choices when selecting physicians and treatment alternatives. Thus, they are able to afford better insurance coverage. However, the economic status of the patient, whether they are wealthy or poor should not affect the way they are treated in the physician's office nor should it effect the way they are spoken to. All patients should be shown respect and common courtesy.

Language Barriers

As a health care professional you will likely communicate with patients who do not speak English well enough to carry on a conversation. They may, however, understand or read English. Even patients who are usually proficient in English may feel more comfortable and revert to speaking their primary language during times of stress, such as illness or injury. First determine their level of fluency and, if necessary, use a qualified health care interpreter who is professionally trained in translating medical terminology to layman's terms and who can communicate precisely in the patient's first language.

Whenever you have a non-English speaking patient, an interpreter should be scheduled when the appointment is made to ensure that the patient will receive the best medical care. Workers' compensation provides professional interpreters and physicians who treat Medicaid or State Children's Health Insurance Program (SCHIP) patients are required to create a plan for serving patients with limited English proficiency (LEP). The Department of Health and Human Services published guidelines that require physicians to consider four factors: (1) number [or proportion] of patients with limited English proficiency, (2) fre-

quency of encountering individuals with limited English proficiency, (3) importance of services provided, and (4) resources available. A staff member may be hired because they are bilingual, or telephone or video interpreting can be used, and patients may be referred to physicians with specific language capabilities. A member of the patient's family or a friend who speaks English may also be able to help; however, permission must be given by the patient, and it is important to make sure that both parties understand exactly what is being said. Some medical terms and phrases do not translate into other languages and difficulties arise when trying to communicate them accurately to a person who is not trained for this purpose.

Select an interpreter of the same sex because he or she will always be a part of personal discussions and will accompany the patient during the examination. Be aware that when discussing personal issues about the human body, interactions with members of the opposite sex may be forbidden by other cultures.

Always speak directly to the patient with the interpreter close by. Speak slowly using simple English and do not raise your voice or use slang. If the patient understands some English or if an interpreter is not available, you may have to improvise using gestures to demonstrate what you want the patient to do. Always be observant for signs that the patient understands what you are attempting to get across. You may want to learn some basic medical phrases in the patient's native language or use a dictionary or medical phrase book that has all languages that are common to the geographic region. Also, keep a note pad on hand to write down key words. Depending on the office's location, medical forms and patient information pamphlets should be made available in other languages. Bilingual classes, such as medical Spanish are offered in many areas for health care professionals.

Cultural Differences

As a medical assistant you will interact with people from varied **ethnic** (racial) backgrounds and cultural origins who bring with them beliefs and values that may differ from your own; they are not superior or inferior. Keeping an open mind and understanding those differences can aid communication and thereby improve patient care. Be sensitive to the fact that an immigrant's health care needs may differ from native citizens', as do their experiences and emotional makeup.

People move to the United States from all over the world and bring with them various cultural behaviors, traditions, and values that have been passed down through many generations. The United States was once called a melting pot because of its ethnic and cultural diversity, and the hope was that all the diverse groups would blend together as a whole. The blending does not mean ignoring heritage, and today more than ever, people are embracing their ethnic background and want to know more about where they came from. Even within the United States we have cultural differences that affect patterns of speech (accents), food preparation, beliefs, attitudes, and environments.

Variances within Cultures

The following list includes additional factors that the medical assistant should consider when shaping his or her communication with patients who have different cultural backgrounds.

- Most Americans are familiar with, and believe in, Western medicine; however, other cultures practice Eastern medicine or holistic health, which has to do with treating the body, mind, and spirit. Some cultures believe in homeopathic treatment, folk remedies, medical rituals, or healing ceremonies. Others have superstitions that affect the way they look at disease, illness, and treatment.

- Personality trends vary among cultures. In some cultures people tend to be forward or outgoing; in others they are quiet and reserved.

- The philosophy on the use of medications and other invasive tests or treatments may differ among cultures, as well as how pain is viewed and responded to.

- Nonverbal signals, such as gestures and body language, may have different meanings from yours.

- Eye contact is very important in the American culture and indicates interest and involvement. In other cultures, such as Native American, Asian, and Latin, it may be considered disrespectful to look someone straight in the eyes. Trying to maintain eye contact with someone who is uncomfortable may be perceived as aggression and create a communication barrier.

- Although Americans may feel that touch is an important way to communicate the feeling of empathy, many adults do not like to be touched by people they do not know. A handshake is a sign of respect in some cultures, whereas touching is off-limits in others. Asian children's heads, for example are considered sacred and should only be touched by a parent or elder in the family.

- Time may be viewed differently among people in general and especially among people from other cultures. For instance, in another culture, arriving 15 to 30 minutes after a scheduled appointment would be acceptable, but in the typical American medical office it would be deemed inconsiderate.

- Each person sees people and situations differently; this is referred to as perception. Do you have the ability to sense another's attitudes, moods, and feelings? Cultural background, social upbringing, and religious beliefs influence perception as well as personal values, beliefs, and convictions. Latinos, for instance, value a warm, personal relationship with their health care provider, but they often also expect an authoritative manner and professional dress from their physician. If the doctor is dressed casually, trust may be harder to establish between the patient and the physician because casualness may be viewed as being carefree.

Since it is impossible to learn of all the variances in other cultures, the medical assistant should concentrate on whatever population the medical practice serves. If the health care worker practices active listening, exhibits empathy, is genuine, and treats patients in a professional manner with equal respect, misunderstandings caused by cross-cultural differences will be minimized. Trust will be established because the patient's dignity will be preserved and their sense of self-worth maintained.

Stereotyping

Patients of different ages, cultures, genders, races, religions, lifestyles, and sexual orientation make up a medical practice, and their values may differ from yours. Judgments are often made when people are put into categories such as those mentioned above. Generalizations should not be made, and it should never be assumed that people from the same race or culture will respond in the same way. To **stereotype** is to hold an attitude that all people from the same ethnicity (or category) are the same; this should be avoided. Statements such as, "Retired people always sleep in" and "Those people are lazy and don't work for a living" are types of negative stereotyping and demonstrate **prejudice**, a judgment that is formed prior to gathering all facts. Prejudice leads to **discrimination**, which means to treat an individual or group unfairly based on the category in which they fall. All patients should be viewed individually and treated equally. When you form a **bias**, your opinion is one-sided and your judgment is influenced negatively.

Today's society holds biases that may include the belief that people who cannot afford health care should not receive the same level of care as people who can pay for full services. The prejudices of our society should not affect the communication we have with patients or the type of health care we deliver. All patients should be treated impartially and all health care services provided equally. Guard against discrimination, avoid stereotyping, and do not jump to conclusions or make determinations about patients based on the differences mentioned.

Patients with Special Needs

Many patients seeking treatment in a health care setting have special needs. Being prepared to cope with those individual needs and disabilities is very important. When a person's understanding is limited or their senses are impaired, communication can be a challenge. People with physical and other types of disabilities can fall prey to discrimination: eye contact can be avoided, staring can occur, rude remarks can be made, or an over-solicitous attitude can make the individual feel uncomfortable. Patients with disabilities prefer to be treated like other individuals. Never assume that a person with a disability needs help. Instead, ask the patient how you can be of help and

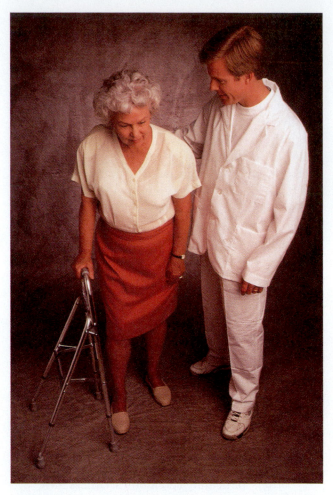

Figure 4-7. A medical assistant asking a hemiplegic patient who is using a walkcane if she needs assistance

follow his or her requests (Figure 4-7). Giving assistance without calling attention to a disability requires sensitivity and tact, and special consideration must be given in order to communicate effectively. The medical assistant can be empathetic toward a patient with special needs without offering gratuitous expressions of sympathy. The following sections offer guidance on communicating effectively with patients who have specific disabilities.

Hearing-Impaired Patients

There are many types of hearing impairments ranging from presbycusis, which is found in older patients who are hard of hearing, to congenital problems that cause complete hearing loss at an early age. Exhibit diplomacy, patience, and tact when trying to communicate with patients who cannot hear what you are saying. Guidelines to follow when communicating with hearing-impaired patients include:

1. Select a quiet place to communicate and give the patient your complete attention.

2. Eliminate distractions or background noises such as traffic, running water, or office music that may disrupt the conversation or cause confusion.

3. Choose the best seating arrangement by determining whether the patient hears out of one ear better than the other, uses a hearing aid, or reads lips. Sit on the side of the person's good ear and reduce the distance between you and the patient. A hearing aid helps but does not restore normal hearing; optimal distance for a hearing aid's effectiveness is about ten feet.

4. Face the patient in an area with good light so he or she can see your facial expressions, but do not exaggerate them while speaking. Some patients may be able to lip read so do not turn your head away from them, cover your mouth, or chew while talking. Do not sit directly in front of a brightly-lit window because your face will be shadowed.

5. Touch the patient lightly if necessary to gain his or her attention, or alert the patient by saying his or her name and then announcing the topic.

6. Speak in a natural tone, slowly, and distinctly, enunciating clearly and using a low-pitched voice; high pitched sounds are often lost with auditory nerve damage. Do not over pronounce, shout, or distort your speech.

7. Use short, simple sentences and repeat or rephrase any misunderstood statements.

8. Continue to speak directly to the patient if a sign language interpreter is present but wait for the message to be interpreted.

9. Use gestures as needed. Remember the importance of body language.

10. Write down words or phrases that you are having difficulty communicating.

11. Practice active listening techniques and get feedback by asking questions to verify understanding.

Visually Impaired Patients

When communicating with visually impaired patients, use verbal descriptions. Impaired eye sight may range from blurred vision to complete blindness and can include presbyopia, macular degeneration, cataracts, and glaucoma. If a patient looses his or her vision at an early age, other senses often take over. The patient may have more acute hearing, smell, and equilibrium, which gives them the ability to quickly recognize sounds and voices and a sense of where they are after entering a foreign space. Patients that loose their sight later in life usually have a more difficult time adjusting. When communicating with a sight-impaired patient, remember the following guidelines:

1. Approach the patient cheerfully and identify yourself by name when he or she enters the office.

2. Look directly at the patient and speak clearly in a normal tone and at a normal speed.

3. Inform the patient of others that are in the same room or area, for example, "Please have a seat in the waiting room, Mrs. Bartlett. There are a few other patients who are also waiting for Dr. Practon."

4. Let the patient know exactly what you will be doing. For example, "The medical assistant will be calling you shortly to take you to an exam room."

5. Gently take the patient's hand and allow him or her to experience different objects by touching the counter, chair, doorframe, and so forth. This will help the patient become familiar with the surroundings.

6. Ask if the patient needs your assistance with filling out paper work and comply with his or her wishes.

7. Escort the patient to the inner office or interview room by offering your arm or elbow (as directed by the patient) and helping to guide him or her. Look out for any obstacles that may be in the path. Provide verbal cues for turns, steps, and so forth, but do not steer the patient.

8. Inform the patient of the location, and tell them when you are leaving the room. Be sure to knock before reentering the room.

9. Explain the sounds of unusual noises or office machines that may be running nearby.

10. Use large-print material whenever possible or provide instructions on audiocassette.

Speech-Impaired Patients

Speech impairments can be caused by medical conditions or can result from congenital abnormalities. Stroke patients often have dysphasia or difficulty speaking. Usually they know exactly what they want to say but may be unable to form the word they are trying to speak. Be patient and allow stroke victims time to communicate without putting words in their mouths. A physical condition can leave a patient with dysphonia or voice impairment. Also a lisp, stutter, or strong accent may cause a breakdown in communication. The following guidelines are suggestions to help communicate with speech-impaired patients:

1. Look directly at the patient without making him or her feel self-conscious.

2. Allow the patient time to think through what they are going to say and give them time to speak.

3. Do not speak for them or rush the conversation; ask the person to speak slowly.

4. Do not pretend to understand. Instead, say that you are having a little difficulty understanding, and ask them to repeat the statement.

5. Do not shout; people with speech difficulty are not hard of hearing.

6. Be courteous; rudeness is never acceptable.

7. Offer a notepad if necessary.

Impaired Level of Understanding

Individuals who are developmentally disabled, emotionally disturbed, or suffering from senility or Alzheimer's disease may have below normal ability to think and reason. It is important to work closely with caregivers and to be aware of each patient's limitations. Offer assistance to each individual with dignity. Treat all such patients equally and give them the same respect and attention as other patients.

A patient's ability to communicate can be impaired by many types of mental illnesses, mental retardation, or psychiatric disorders. Common problems that occur may include patients repeating themselves, not being able to communicate at all or at the appropriate level, sitting in silence, or having outbursts or using inappropriate language. Use the following suggestions as guidelines when communicating with patients who have an impaired level of understanding.

1. Introduce yourself in a friendly manner.

2. Be professional and keep the conversation focused.

3. Speak slowly and in a calm manner.

4. Select simple words and short phrases using both verbal and nonverbal clues.

5. Use your tone of voice to express your concern; avoid letting impatience creep into your voice, as that implies the patient is slow to understand or is unintelligent. Do not raise your voice.

6. Repeat and rephrase the message you are trying to convey.

7. Use demonstration when appropriate to reinforce the message.

8. Allow more time than usual because patients with impared understanding may need more explanation than is typical.

9. Reassure the patient and do not overload him or her with information.

10. Inform the patient of what to expect prior to it happening.

11. Exhibit tolerance with patients who are withdrawn or mute; do not force answers.

12. Remind the patient why they are at the doctor's office and orient them to reality as appropriate.

13. Inform the supervisor or physician if you feel unsafe while trying to communicate.

Anxious Patients

Anxiety and anger impair communication. It is common for patients to be anxious when coming to the doctor; this reaction is called the *white-coat syndrome*. When dealing with an anxious patient realize that she may need help focusing and assume that she will not be able to remember all of the details of the conversation. Proceed at a slower pace and validate the patient's concern.

Severe anxiety may lead to an anxiety attack. Symptoms include increased heart rate (pulse rate), elevated blood pressure, diaphoresis (sweating), shaking or trembling, fast or uneven respirations, and hyperventilation. Patients may also complain of appetite changes, sleep disturbances, and being short tempered or irritable. If an anxiety attack occurs in the office notify the physician and stay with the patient until the doctor comes. Try to calm the patient by encouraging deep breaths, acknowledging that they are afraid, and getting them to talk about their fears.

Use the following guidelines when assisting an anxious patient:

1. Recognize the signs of anxiety and acknowledge them.

2. Pinpoint possible sources of anxiety, such as fear of needles.

3. Make the patient as comfortable as possible and give them ample personal space.

4. Demonstrate a warm and caring attitude.

5. Speak with confidence, calmness, and empathy, asking the patient to describe what is causing his anxiety. Allow him to describe his feelings and thoughts.

6. Listen attentively without interruption, maintain eye contact, and have an open posture.

7. Accept the patient's thoughts and feelings; do not belittle them.

8. Help the patient recognize the anxiety and cope with it by providing information and suggesting relaxation techniques such as visualization and deep breathing.

9. Inform the physician of the patient's concerns.

Angry Patients

Patients may enter the office angry or may become upset while in the office. The reason for the anger may be something completely unrelated to the office visit, this response is referred to as **displaced anger**. Or it may be caused by something that has occurred during waiting time or the visit. In either case, try to help the person identify the source and do not take it personally. Allow the patient to vent and do not let the patient's anger become contagious by responding with anger yourself. If the office has made an error, admit the mistake and apologize for it. Disarm anger by offering to help in any way you can. Do not argue—it will only add fuel to the fire—instead soften your response and avoid phrases that may ignite the situation (Example 4-5). If the person becomes loud, volatile, or threatening, take the patient aside or move to

---

EXAMPLE 4-5

Soft Responses To Help Calm Patients

Responses That May Agitate	Soft Responses
"We cannot do that!"	"That's a difficult one, Mrs. Brown. Let's see what we can do."
"I don't know!"	"That's a good question, Mr. White. Let me check that out and get back to you."
"I'll be right back."	"Can you hold Miss Gray while I check on this? It may take me a couple of minutes."
"You'll have to . . ."	"Here is how we can help you with that, Mr. Gold . . ."

---

a private office. You may have to tell that person that he or she is acting inappropriately and that shouting will not be allowed because other patients are being disturbed.

Collect information and try to pinpoint the reason for the anger. Common reasons may include feelings of resentment due to an invasion of privacy, disappointment or frustration because of a illness or circumstance beyond their control, and financial problems. If patients cannot be accommodated in the appointment schedule and cannot see their physician when they are sick and hurting, they may become frustrated. Oftentimes that frustration unravels into anger. Little things tend to agitate patients when they are feeling ill, and they may be angry about their own responses and lack of coping skills. Prolonged waiting times only aggravate these emotions. Emotional responses to physical situations are not uncommon, and an otherwise calm patient might become distressed over confusing aspects of their illness or treatment.

Guidelines to use when faced with an angry patient include the following:

1. Recognize that the patient is angry. Most of the time this emotion is obvious, but some people may disguise it by seeming disinterested,

ignoring your attempts to communicate, speaking in a monotone or unnatural voice, or avoiding eye contact.

2. Honor the patient's personal space, hold yourself with an open posture, maintain eye contact, and position yourself at the patient's eye level; do not stand over the patient.

3. Remain calm and show that you care about the patient's feelings by continuing to demonstrate genuineness and respect.

4. Focus on why the patient is there in order to uncover emotional, physical, and medical needs.

5. Listen attentively with an open mind and ask the patient to describe the cause of her anger and how it makes her feel. Let her vent openly. The patient has a right to her own feelings and perceptions; be empathetic.

6. Do not take a defensive attitude or try to talk the patient out of being angry by trying to rationalize the angry response.

7. Allow the patient time alone if he or she is so angry that it interferes with communication.

8. Determine a timeframe to get back to the patient with an answer or solution.

9. Do not stay in the room with the patient if you feel threatened or are worried about the potential for violence. Leave the room and inform the physician or another staff member.

PROFESSIONAL COMMUNICATION

As a health care professional you will communicate with patients; their families and friends; other members of the health care team; your superiors, such as the office manager and physician; and other outside professionals, such as members of the hospital staff, pharmacies, and ancillary facilities. The following section will describe techniques and guidelines that can help you communicate professionally in an efficient, constructive, and productive manner.

Patients and Their Friends and Family

In their research, psychologists have learned that the manner in which the medical staff interacts with a sick person can foster wellness or it can unintention-

ally aggravate a physical condition. They have also determined that preserving the patient's mental state is often more important than performing expert medical skills. The medical assistant should know how to create an atmosphere that will communicate a caring attitude toward the patient's feelings. To do this the medical assistant must be able to identify methods of communication. As a member of the health care team you, along with the physician, will be responsible for communicating details in order for patients to actively participate in their health care decisions. They must be informed about their diagnosis, treatment options, possibility of complications, and prognosis of their illness, injury, or disease. As an administrative medical assistant you will gather information about the patient's demographics, insurance, and medical history, as well as organize referrals and tests, procedures, and follow up examinations.

Family and friends that accompany patients to the office can provide emotional support and offer another opportunity to understand and retain detailed instructions or specific information about the patient's illness and treatment plan. Acknowledge family members and friends who accompany patients to the office and communicate with them in the same way you do with patients. Leave it up to the patient as to whether he would like to have other people in the treatment room and comply with his wishes unless the physician dictates otherwise. Be aware that in some situations patients should be seen alone, especially if the spouse or friend controls the conversation and the patient is not allowed to speak for themselves.

Follow these guidelines when communicating with patients and their families or friends.

1. Greet patients and their family members or friends with a warm smile and kind-hearted words.

2. Introduce yourself and explain what you will be doing.

3. Use a genuine, friendly approach in all interactions whether verbal or nonverbal.

4. Display a positive attitude when giving instructions or explaining such things as insurance delays, procedures, or financial statements.

5. Focus on the patient to whom you are speaking so he or she receives your undivided attention.

6. Listen carefully and allow time for questions.

7. Demonstrate confidence in the job you are doing so the patient will know you are well trained and knowledgeable.

8. Be assertive and communicate accurately, answer questions honestly, and admit when you do not know something. Tell the patient that you will find out the answers to his or her questions and follow through.

9. Keep the patient informed throughout the visit regardless of delays or interruptions.

10. Put the patient at ease by acknowledging any sources of anxiety or concern. Do not minimize their fears regardless of how trivial they may appear to you.

11. Obtain feedback to be sure the message has been received correctly.

12. Reward the patient's compliance with the doctor's treatment plan with praise. Health care professionals can offer support and guidance in things such as taking the correct medications, weight loss, smoking cessation, and so forth.

The Health Care Team

Communicating with coworkers can present some of the most difficult communication problems. Often thoughtless comments are made or a *condescending* attitude is displayed, which makes the other person feel inferior. Each person on a health care team is important and each job has value. Without all team members working together, a medical office would not run smoothly and the physician would not be able to treat all of the patients' needs successfully.

Communicate with each individual professionally and do not talk down to your peers. Regardless of the job you are doing, always show respect and be caring and thoughtful in your actions and words while displaying empathy for the other person. Even a part-time file clerk has an important job and is a vital part of the health care team. Offer words of appreciation to other members of the staff when you see that they are doing a good job.

Save lunchtime or breaks for discussion of non-work related topics. An unprofessional atmosphere is created when whispers, excessive laughter, joking, and so forth are overheard by patients. The patient in the next room may be distressed, ill, or receiving bad news from the physician, and if office staff chatter can be overheard it would appear as though the staff does not care about their patients' needs.

The following guidelines will help assure positive communication between yourself and members of your health care team:

1. Be polite and cheerful, using a friendly approach with each member of your office staff.

2. Include "please" and "thank you" in your everyday language.

3. Use correct names and titles when communicating and ask if you do not know the preference of other members of your health care team.

4. Use tact and diplomacy when attempting to resolve problems.

5. Speak calmly and respectfully and do not become angry or defensive.

6. Use proper channels of communication. Always try to work out problems on a "one to one" basis prior to going to the office manager or other supervisor.

7. Do not judge your coworkers; instead practice empathy.

8. Have a positive attitude in all your work assignments.

9. Bring issues that bother you to the forefront; do not let them fester. Be assertive about your feelings and opinions and be open to discussing them.

10. Perform all your duties and responsibilities and cheerfully bear your share of the workload.

11. Offer to help a coworker when needed and do not refuse because the task is not in your job description.

12. Avoid gossip, arguments, and uncomplimentary statements about coworkers.

13. Do not complain; instead be a problem solver.

14. Maintain your work space in an organized and orderly fashion. Respect others' work spaces and property.

15. Treat coworkers as you would like to be treated.

Office Manager

Your relationship with your supervisor differs from that of your coworkers. Your supervisor is typically your teacher, trainer, evaluator, and one who may discipline you if the need arises. A good relationship will be one with mutual respect. Always be professional when communicating with a supervisor or manager. In order to establish an open and honest relationship you will need to be able to receive critique as well as constructive criticism. Show initiative and do not fall into the habit of saying "that is not in my job description." Be willing to try new things, pitch in when necessary, and act as a team member. Be willing to share your ideas. When presented and communicated correctly, they are typically welcomed and greatly appreciated.

Keep the office manager informed of problems that occur with patients, coworkers, office equipment, and so forth. Ask if you are unsure about a request, a task, or a medical term. If you do not understand something do not try to muddle through because you are fearful of what someone will think. It is better to ask and verify the correct way to do something than go blindly along and make mistakes. If you do not find out the correct way of doing a task the first time you are asked, then in the future you will face an even bigger problem when the office manager expects you to know how to do the task but you do not.

Periodically schedule time to communicate with your supervisor in a relaxed manner, telling him or her how you are doing, sharing concerns, and offering suggestions. Before beginning such a discussion one should differentiate between an urgent and a non-urgent problem by stating, "I need to speak to you at your earliest convenience." Compare this with "I need to speak to you." Or, in order to minimize interruptions you could ask, "Do you have a minute?" "Is this a good time to talk?" or "Can I interrupt you for a moment?" If you cannot resolve a problem with a coworker or you need to report a situation that has occurred, be open, honest, and report the facts accurately. Never embellish or omit details.

Physician

Communicating with physicians in a professional manner is essential. Always address the physician as "doctor" using his or her last name unless told otherwise. Speak slowly, confidently, and use correct medical terminology. Listen carefully when given instructions to relay to a patient. The physician depends on you to communicate information to patients in a professional, accurate, and timely manner. Doctors will also rely on you to receive messages, complaints, and other data that are being relayed from patients. Do not feel intimidated if you do not understand an order. Be honest and ask for the information to be repeated or say that you do not understand and ask for an explanation. Remember that learning continues to take place in the medical office, not just in the classroom.

Outside Health Care Professionals

Whether you are making referral appointments, retrieving laboratory results, or calling the answering service for messages, you will be communicating with outside professionals who are an extension of the health care team. Use the same level of professionalism as you do with other office staff. Remember that you are representing the physician and the medical practice each time you communicate; always promote the practice through positive public relations.

When a patient is admitted to a hospital the assistant arranges for the hospital admission, schedules surgery, and advises the patient accordingly. To help the office physician, the medical assistant may act as a liaison, communicating with a variety of hospital employees in numerous departments. A successful assistant will build a rapport with hospital personnel. The medical staff coordinator notifies the physician of required staff and committee meetings, requests updated copies of credentials and licenses for hospital files, records continuing education credits, and supervises all administrative duties of the physician at the hospital. A librarian helps obtain scientific information, communicates with other health care facilities, and can do advanced computer searches to obtain the latest journal articles on diagnoses and treatment options. The nursing staff reports the changing conditions of patients to the physician and receives telephone orders. You may also work with employees in the radiology, physiology, and laboratory departments to schedule tests and receive test results. It is important to understand each of the resources that outside departments and facilities provide.

Take the time to visit the hospital departments, local pharmacies, home health care agencies, and test facilities that you deal with on a regular basis. Introducing yourself to the staff who talk with you over the telephone will go a long way toward improving communications. Always be courteous, polite, respectful, and helpful but do not be afraid to stop and clarify information if you do not understand it. For instance, if you are receiving laboratory results and the laboratory technician reads the results so fast you cannot write them down, ask for him or her to please slow down or repeat them so you can record them accurately. Likewise, if an outside physician speaks to you in a demeaning matter or too rapidly, do not be intimidated. Be courteous and ask him or her to repeat the message.

STOP AND THINK CASE SCENARIO

Feedback

Scenario: You are speaking with Mrs. Jacobson who stopped by the office and says, "I am really not feeling well, I don't know what is wrong. I wonder if the pills the doctor gave me are making me sick. I feel queasy and can't seem to keep anything down, I'm really exhausted, and sometimes I feel lightheaded like I'm going to faint. I am so tired of feeling this way! By the way, I also have a rash on my body. Do you think it's related? Could you please let the doctor know what is going on with me? I have to get home, and I'll be there if you need to get in touch with me."

Critical Thinking: Determine which kind of feedback would be most appropriate to verify that you have heard the message correctly. Formulate a written response that could be given to the physician.

_____
_____
_____
_____
_____
_____
_____

STOP AND THINK CASE SCENARIO

Communication Challenges

Scenario: You are speaking to Mrs. Stork, a long-time patient of Dr. Practon's. All of a sudden she breaks into tears and starts sobbing. You freeze and feel like walking away because you are not used to dealing with someone who is emotionally upset.

Critical Thinking: Name at least three things you would avoid doing and state the right way to help someone who breaks down.

1. _____
_____

2. _____
_____

3. _____
_____

Statement: _____
_____
_____
_____
_____

STOP AND THINK CASE SCENARIO

Socioeconomic Fairness

Scenario: Mrs. Marra drives up in a Mercedes and comes in to talk about the blood test the doctor has ordered for her. Your coworker is speaking with her and the patient demands that she call the insurance company to find out if the test is covered, what percentage they will pay, and whether any preauthorization is needed. Both you and your coworker know that it is a simple, inexpensive test and no preauthorization is required by the type of insurance plan she has. Your coworker communicates this to the patient but she insists that the insurance company needs to be called to make sure. Your coworker agrees and then leaves the front desk mumbling about how much money Mrs. Marra has, how cheap she is, how demanding she is, saying, "Just because she has money she thinks she can boss everybody around, I'm not going to waste my time calling the insurance company," even though she told Mrs. Marra she would.

Critical Thinking: How would you have handled the situation with Mrs. Marra?

_____
_____
_____
_____
_____
_____
_____
_____
_____
_____
_____
_____
_____
_____
_____
_____
_____

STOP AND THINK CASE SCENARIO

Positive versus Negative Attitude

Scenario: You arrive at the office early, in a good mood and ready to tackle the day. The lead receptionist, Sylvia, is there looking over the daily schedule and she starts complaining (like she does every day) and says, "Oh boy, Mrs. Yabarro is coming in today. What a pain she is. I hope she no-shows. And Mr. Harrington is coming back to see Dr. Practon this afternoon. I thought we got rid of him last week when he was here for three hours. What a day it's going to be! We have 30 patients scheduled and you know Dr. Practon will be late arriving from the hospital."

Critical Thinking:

1. How has the receptionist's comments affected your mood? _____

_____

2. How will you respond to the lead receptionist's comments? _____

_____

_____

3. What can you do to change this daily morning routine? _____

_____

_____

_____

FOCUS ON CERTIFICATION*

CMA Content Summary

- Medical terminology
- Psychology
- Individual self-worth, social and emotional behavior
- Maslow's hierarchy
- Hereditary, cultural, and environmental influences on behavior
- Defense mechanisms
- Adapting communication
- Verbal and nonverbal communication
- Evaluating understanding of communication

RMA Content Summary

- Medical terminology
- Human/Interpersonal relations
- Age-specific responses/support
- Communication methods
- Active listening

CMAS Content Summary

- Medical terminology
- Human relations/behaviors
- Oral communication

REVIEW EXAM-STYLE QUESTIONS

1. Basic elements in the communication cycle include:

   a. sender and receiver

   b. sender, message, and receiver

   c. sender, message, channel, receiver, feedback

   d. sender, message, channel, receiver, questions

   e. sender, message, verbal/nonverbal, receiver, feedback

2. Select the three primary ways messages are communicated in the order of importance.

   a. spoken word, body language, tonality

   b. body language, tonality, spoken word

   c. tonality, body language, spoken word

   d. spoken word, tonality, body language

   e. body language, spoken word, tonality

3. If a patient makes up a reason to justify unacceptable actions or behavior in order to avoid something, the defense mechanism is known as:

   a. avoidance

   b. compensation

   c. displacement

   d. rationalization

   e. regression

4. In a health care setting, the comfort zone is approximately:

   a. 1 to 2 feet

   b. 2 to 3 feet

   c. 3 to 4 feet

   d. 4 to 5 feet

   e. 5 to 6 feet

This textbook and the accompanying Workbook meet the entry-level administrative and general competencies for the CMA outlined by the AAMA Examination Content Outline and Role Delineation Study and for the RMA and CMAS outlined by the AMT Competencies and Examination Specifications (see Competency Grid in Appendix B).

5. When using nonverbal communication:

   a. the eyes, face, and hands can be used to communicate

   b. gestures are utilized

   c. it is referred to as body language

   d. touch can send signals

   e. all of the above are correct

6. Active listening involves:

   a. dwelling on or mulling over what the speaker has said

   b. giving the speaker your undivided attention

   c. verbal and nonverbal responses to a message

   d. focusing on yourself in addition to the speaker

   e. intuitive and immediate responses

7. Questioning, requesting examples, and paraphrasing a message are:

   a. ways to improve active listening

   b. types of nonverbal communication

   c. types of feedback

   d. not recommended when listening actively

   e. interpersonal skills

8. Which of the following is an example of negative stereotyping?

   a. All Italians are loud.

   b. I don't like Italian food.

   c. Italians should not be allowed in this medical office.

   d. I'm married to an Italian, therefore I know what they're like.

   e. I love all Italians.

9. Verbal descriptions are needed when communicating with:

   a. hearing-impaired patients

   b. patients with impaired level of understanding

   c. sight-impaired patients

   d. speech-impaired patients

   e. patients undergoing stressful situations

10. Some of the most difficult communication problems exist when communicating with a/an:

    a. physician

    b. office manager

    c. coworker

    d. patient

    e. outside health care professional

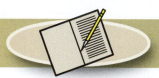

WORKBOOK ASSIGNMENT

To develop competency-based job skills, refer to the *Workbook* and complete the:

- Abbreviation and Spelling Review
- Review Questions

- Critical Thinking Exercises
- Job Skill activities, which are outlined at the beginning of this chapter under "Performance Objectives in the *Workbook*."

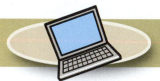

COMPUTER ASSIGNMENT

To review the concepts you have learned in this chapter, insert the *Student Practice* CD-ROM into a computer and work through the *StudyWARE* activities and games. Answer review questions in the practice mode and read the feedback, studying the questions you have missed. Take the chapter quiz until you achieve a minimum score of 90 percent. Successfully completing the *Critical Thinking Challenge* at the end of this course will help you think through scenarios and develop problem solving skills.

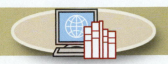

RESOURCES

Books

The Complete Idiot's Guide to Clear Communication
  Kris Cole
  Pearson Education
  PO Box 2500
  Lehanon, IN 46052
  (800) 282-0693

Multicultural Manners, Rules of Etiquette for the 21st Century
  Norine Dresser, 2005
  New York, Wiley

Racial and Ethnic Relations in America, 7ed.
  S. Dale McLemore, Harriett D. Romo
  Allyn & Bacon, 2005
  Pearson Education
  PO Box 2500
  Lebanon, IN 46052
  (800) 282-0693

Dictionary

The Nonverbal Dictionary of Gestures, Signs & Body Language Cues
  David B. Givens, Ph.D., 2005
  Spokane, Washington: Center for Nonverbal Studies Press

Internet

2004 Yearbook of Immigration Statistics
  Office of Immigration Statistics
  Homeland Security
  Web site: http://www.migrationinformation.org

Find Articles
  Use key terms to find articles (e.g., multicultural patients, language barriers)
  Web site: http://findarticles.com

Migration Policy Institute
  (202) 266-1908
  Web site: http://www.migrationinformation.org

Soft skills (Wikipedia—free encyclopedia)
  Web site: http://en.wikipedia.org
  Search: soft skills

CHAPTER 5

The Receptionist

OBJECTIVES

After reading this chapter and learning step-by-step procedures to gain job skills,* you should be able to:

Learning Objectives

▪ Open the medical office and ready it for daily activities.

▪ Welcome patients to the office in a cordial manner.

▪ Register patients by obtaining vital information.

▪ Explain the purpose of the office privacy notice to patients.

▪ Respond appropriately to patients who experience a delay in their appointment.

▪ Inspect and maintain confidentiality and orderliness in the reception area.

▪ Handle an office emergency.

▪ Perform necessary duties to close the medical office for the day.

Performance Objectives (Procedures) in This Textbook

▪ Open the medical office (Procedure 5-1).

▪ Assist patients with in-office registration procedures (Procedure 5-2).

▪ Assist patients in preparing the application form for a disabled person placard (Procedure 5-3).

▪ Develop a patient education plan for diseases/injuries related to the specialty (Procedure 5-4).

▪ Close the medical office (Procedure 5-5).

Performance Objectives (Job Skills) in the *Workbook*

▪ Prepare a patient registration form (Job Skill 5-1).

▪ Prepare an application form for a disabled person placard (Job Skill 5-2).

▪ Research materials for in-office resources and/or patient education (Job Skill 5-3).

*This textbook and the accompanying Workbook meet the educational components for entry-level administrative and general competencies outlined by CAAHEP and ABHES.

OUTLINE WITH LECTURE NOTES

Office Receptionist

First Impression

_____
_____
_____
_____

Multitasking

_____
_____
_____
_____

Opening the Medical Office

Preparing Records

_____
_____
_____

Retrieving Messages

_____
_____
_____
_____

Greeting Patients

_____
_____
_____

Patient Visit Log

_____
_____
_____

Processing Patients

Patient Registration

_____
_____
_____
_____

Medical History and Reports

_____
_____
_____
_____

Privacy Notice

_____
_____
_____
_____

Waiting in Reception Area

_____
_____
_____
_____

Escorting Patients

_____
_____
_____
_____

Instructing Patients

_____
_____
_____
_____

Reception Area

Features of the Reception Area

_____
_____
_____

Maintaining the Reception Area

_____
_____
_____
_____

Handling an Office Emergency

_____
_____
_____

Closing the Medical Office

_____
_____
_____

KEY TERMS

biohazard
face sheet
hazardous waste
infectious waste

patient instruction form
reception room
registration form
universal precautions

HEART OF THE HEALTH CARE PROFESSIONAL

Service

Old adage: "It takes months to get a new patient—and only seconds to lose one." As the first one who greets patients, the receptionist sets the tone of the office with a smile, helpful attitude, and caring approach. As the last person the patient talks to when leaving, the receptionist should seize all opportunities to leave a good impression while serving patients' needs.

OFFICE RECEPTIONIST

In past years the front office assistant was expected to welcome patients in a friendly manner, obtain demographic information, answer the telephone, make appointments, and take messages.

The emerging role of the medical receptionist includes knowing and understanding a wide variety of laws and regulations; serving as a diplomat, a negotiator, a psychologist, and a director of public relations while answering an almost constantly ringing telephone; reviewing insurance cards and determining insurance types or manage care plans; confirming the practice's participation in plans and patients' eligibility for services and copayment amounts; entering demographic data into the computer; explaining financial and medical procedures; posting a variety of transactions; and keeping up-to-date by reading monthly bulletins and newsletters. In other words, a person applying for a position as a receptionist in a medical office should be a professionally trained medical assistant who is flexible and prepared for a variety of duties.

First Impression

Since the health care worker who acts as the receptionist for a physician is usually the first person to greet a patient, by telephone or in person, and the last person the patient talks to when leaving, the assistant plays an important role in how the physician's office is perceived and remembered.

No matter how stressful the situation becomes, the receptionist must remember that first impressions always count and interruptions are a matter of daily routine. The receptionist must project a professional but empathetic and sympathetic attitude. A clean and orderly office with a friendly, well-groomed, attentive receptionist will help ease tension and make patients feel more comfortable. It is important for the assistant to be alert for cues to a patient's emotional state and to remember that most people arrive at the office ill, in pain, and anxious about their physical condition. Being attentive to the patient's needs can elicit a positive response from a patient awaiting an appointment, thereby aiding the physician at the initiation of medical treatment.

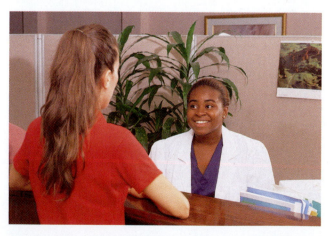

Figure 5-1. A friendly greeting with a smile from the medical assistant/receptionist sends a welcome message and is reassuring to most patients

Multitasking

Multiple tasks await the receptionist each day, and an organized approach is mandatory along with a calm demeanor. Priorities should be established, communicated, and adjusted as necessary; however, be careful about letting others change your priority list. If you are asked to do something for someone else, ask in what time-frame it needs to be completed. That will allow you to determine where on your priority list the task should fit. If you are working on a task, let your coworkers and patients know the time-frame you expect to complete it. Desk management systems can assist with multitasking and help you obtain organi-zation skills if you are not experienced in managing your time and multiple tasks. Although interruptions are constant, if patients are treated with respect, dignity, and kindness, they will in turn respect the receptionist's time and the job that he or she is doing.

OPENING THE MEDICAL OFFICE

Generally, the first and last duties of each day are to open and close the office just as you would any place of business. When arriving, disarm the security system, turn on lights and sound system, make sure the

STEP 1 2 3

PROCEDURE 5-1

Open the Medical Office

Objective: To open the office at the beginning of the day to promote efficient operation of the medical practice all through the day.

Equipment/Supplies: A simulated office setting.

Directions: Follow these step-by-step procedures and guidelines, which include rationales, and role-play the actions outlined to practice this job skill. Describe the action and rationale while performing each step. An exercise is presented in the *Workbook* acts as a stepping stone to practice this skill.

1. Unlock the outside door and disarm the security system so the alarm will not be triggered in error.
2. Turn on the office lights to ensure proper lighting throughout the day.
3. Check the room temperature for comfort and adjust thermostats if necessary.
4. Turn on office equipment; for example, computer, printer, photocopier, autoclave, diagnostic equipment, and so forth.
5. Check fax machine for documents and distribute them as needed. Important data may be communicated via facsimile while the office is closed.
6. Unlock drawers, cabinets, and files that are usually unlocked during business

hours and open those that require quick access.

7. Check answering machine and/or call the answering service for messages. Turn off answering machine during business hours. Record, relay, and/or respond to messages.
8. Check e-mail messages; deliver and/or answer as necessary.
9. Unlock door and check reception area to make sure it is neat and clean. Vacuum, dust, and water plants when necessary to ensure a pleasant environment.
10. Straighten magazines, check for condition, and date and discard if old, torn, or damaged.
11. Check for frayed electric wires, damaged furniture, or flooring that might cause a patient to fall. Report unsafe conditions to the office manager.
12. Check bathrooms to be sure they are adequately stocked and clean.
13. Restock daily office supplies (pens, pencils, note pads, paper clips).
14. Open the daysheet, and fill in the date, if a manual bookkeeping system is used.
15. Check to see that all coworkers and work before transferring telephone calls.
16. Unlock outside door to reception area when office is designed to open.

temperature is comfortable in both front and back office, or open windows for fresh air. Turn on machinery such as computers, printers, and copy machines so that they can warm up and be ready for operation. Before unlocking the outer office door each morning, the medical receptionist checks the **reception room** where patients wait until the physician is ready to see them to be sure that it is presentable. Office desks should also be checked to see that they are tidy and uncluttered and supplies are in place.

Preparing Records

Medical records for an established patient, which typically have been pulled and prepared the evening before (see Closing the Office) are retrieved from locked cabinets and put on the receptionist's desk. They were retrieved in alphabetical order but are now arranged in the order in which patients will be seen, according to the office schedule. If it is noted that consultation reports or test results are not in the chart, you now have ample time to check the incoming mail or call the appropriate facility to obtain a faxed copy prior to the patient's arrival. New patient's charts will be made up either the evening before the appointment or the morning of (see Chapter 9, Patient's Medical Records).

Retrieving Messages

Call the answering service or retrieve messages from the answering machine and note all messages on appropriate forms. Deliver urgent messages to the physician and other messages to staff members as appropriate. Return telephone calls and take action on messages that pertain to the receptionist's duties. Chapter 6 (Telephone Procedures) has information on telephone guidelines and message taking.

Greeting Patients

Before each patient arrives, the receptionist should note the name on the appointment sheet and watch for the patient's arrival in order to greet him or her by name, making sure to pronounce the name correctly. Recording the pronunciation of a particularly difficult name phonetically on the patient's chart is helpful. Customizing requests and comments by adding the patient's name will prevent you from sounding like a broken record (Example 5-1).

Using a personalized greeting, special comment, or expression with the right choice of words adds a personal touch that is cordial but not unprofessional.

EXAMPLE 5-1
Welcoming Remarks

- "Good morning, Mrs. Baker. Dr. Practon will be with you in a few minutes."

- "Hello, Mr. Cain. How is that new grandson of yours getting along?"

- "Nice to see you again, Mrs. Steinhouse."

- "How are you today, Mr. Atkins? Nancy, our clinical medical assistant will be taking you back shortly."

To accomplish this, place a self-adhesive note on the chart regarding something that is happening in the patient's life (e.g., wedding, trip, move) so the patient can be asked about it at their next visit—it is appreciated. For example, "You sure look rested. Did you have a great time in Hawaii, Mr. Warner?" A comforting touch or handshake (Figure 5-2) also conveys warmth and friendliness, as does noticing something unique about the patient and commenting on it. For example, "That's a beautiful scarf you have on Mrs. Anderson," "Is that your granddaughter Mr. Huang? She sure is adorable." By offering compliments you add sincerity to your greeting and convey interest in the patient's life.

Calling out patients' names who are seated in the reception area is not a violation of HIPAA. However,

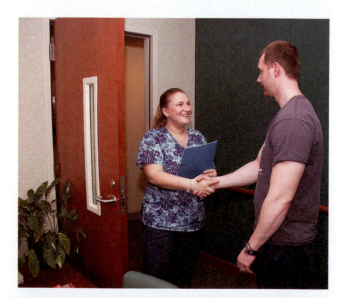

Figure 5-2. A medical assistant offering a warm greeting with a friendly handshake while making eye contact makes patients feel at ease

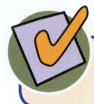

sometimes you may need to select alternatives because names alone can reveal health information in highly specialized facilities. For example, having your name associated with a fertility clinic or oncology unit can reveal protected health information (PHI). Take precautions to protect health information at all times and in special situations assign each patient a number or pager instead of using names.

Addressing Patients

It should be standard practice to get to know patients' names and to learn how they prefer to be addressed. Greet patients using a professional but friendly tone. Address them with the correct title (e.g., Mr., Mrs., Ms., Miss) and use their last names unless they indicate to you that they would like to be called by a first name or nickname. If so, indicate the name of choice on the chart so all medical personnel can use it. Children or young teenagers may be called by their given names. Do not refer to patients or staff by only their last names or by their medial conditions (e.g., "Smith is in the waiting room," "Sprained foot in Room 3," "Phone call for Practon on Line 1"). Even if only overheard by other staff members, it sounds degrading and can lead to bad habits. Never use terms that belittle the individual's dignity such as *darling, honey, sweetie,* and so forth. These terms are offensive and used in personal not professional communication.

When speaking to someone in the reception area or talking on the telephone as patients arrive, the assistant should look up, nod, and smile to acknowledge their arrival. Later a more personal welcome can be extended. Although a patient may see the physician only a few times in the course of treatment, the medical assistant who establishes positive personal relations will build trust and confidence.

Patient Visit Log

Some medical offices still use a patient visit log attached to a clipboard and have patients sign in as they arrive. This reduces the chance of a waiting patient being overlooked; however, legally a sign-in sheet is a breach of confidentiality if it prompts

patients to reveal "reason for visit." If they are there because of a sensitive medical condition it would violate privacy rules to have it written on a sign-in sheet. The open display of patient's names seen that day to all who sign in or just want to take a look is also a violation of privacy.

Secure methods to protect confidentiality while logging patients' arrival times and processing patients' information are:

1. Obtain a confidential patient sign-in log that uses layered, perforated, prenumbered tickets (forms) printed on no-carbon-required (NCR) paper (Figure 5-3A). When the patient arrives, he or she prints arrival time, name, reason for visit, and physician's name on the ticket, detaches the ticket from the log, and either places it in a box or gives it to the receptionist. The prenumbered 8 1/2″ × 11″ double sheet underneath all the tickets has a top sheet that is darkly obliterated, and when pulled apart the bottom sheet contains all the patients' data as recorded on sign-in (Figure 5-3B). This may be retained in a three-hole binder for future reference.

2. Purchase small preprinted, prenumbered adhesive labels (Figure 5-4A). As each patient arrives, he or she can write appointment time, name, arrival time, and the physician's name. The receptionist removes the label and adheres it to the Patient Visit Log, which is kept out of sight (Figure 5-4B). This may be retained in a three-hole binder for future reference.

3. Have patients check in verbally when they arrive. Either check their name off a preprinted appointment log for each physician, noting the time of their arrival, or stamp their encounter form with a date/time stamp and attach it to their chart.

4. Assign patients' numbers when they arrive and call out the number instead of their names.

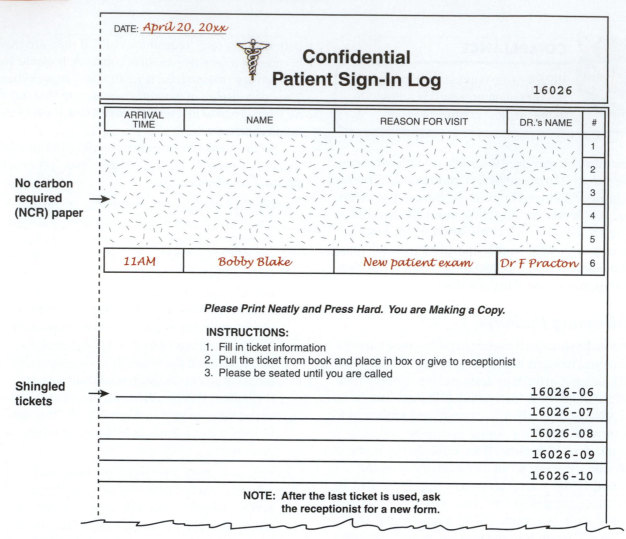

DATE: *April 20, 20xx*

Confidential
Patient Sign-In Log

16026

ARRIVAL TIME	NAME	REASON FOR VISIT	DR.'s NAME	#
				1
				2
				3
				4
				5
11AM	Bobby Blake	New patient exam	Dr F Practon	6

No carbon required (NCR) paper →

Please Print Neatly and Press Hard. You are Making a Copy.

INSTRUCTIONS:
1. Fill in ticket information
2. Pull the ticket from book and place in box or give to receptionist
3. Please be seated until you are called

Shingled tickets →

16026-06
16026-07
16026-08
16026-09
16026-10

**NOTE: After the last ticket is used, ask
the receptionist for a new form.**

Figure 5-3A. Confidential patient sign-in log with layered, perforated shingled tickets (forms) printed on no-carbon-required (NCR) paper. (Courtesy of Bibbero Systems, Inc., Petaluma, CA. Phone: 800-242-2376; Fax: 800-242-9330; Web site: http://www.bibbero.com.)

DATE: *April 20, 20xx*

Confidential
Patient Sign-In Log

16026

ARRIVAL TIME	NAME	REASON FOR VISIT	DR.'s NAME	#
10:00AM	Adrian Stewart	Annual physical exam	Dr G Practon	1
10:30AM	Jane Avery	BP Check	Dr F Practon	2
10:30AM	Joe Rangley	Dressing change	Dr G Practon	3
10:45AM	Baby O'Brian	Immunization exam	Dr F Practon	4
11AM	Kathy McCall	Ins exam	Dr G Practon	5
11AM	Bobby Blake	New patient exam	Dr F Practon	6

Log revealed under NCR paper →

Figure 5-3B. Confidential patient sign-in log revealed under NCR paper. (Courtesy of Bibbero Systems, Inc., Petaluma, CA. Phone: 800-242-2376; Fax 800-242-0330; Web site: http://www.bibbero.com.)

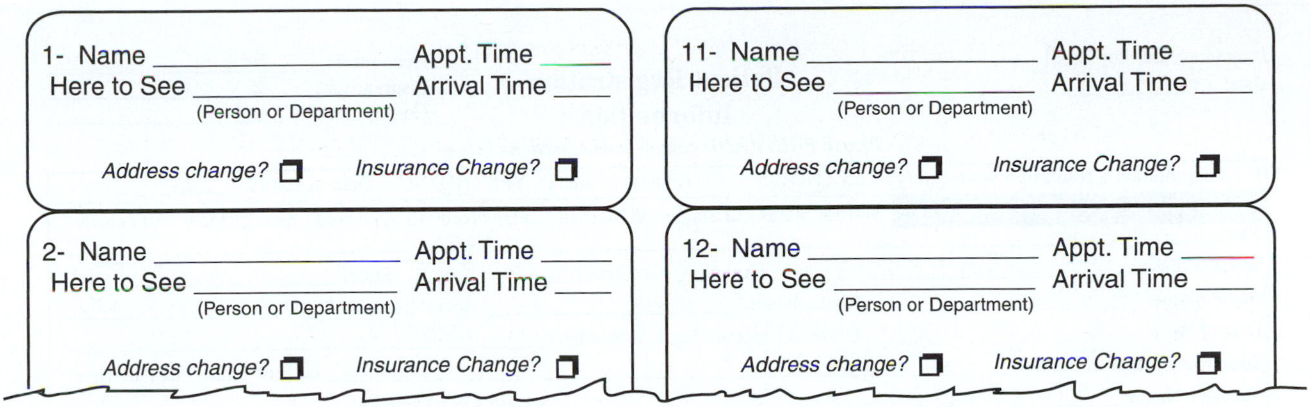

Figure 5-4A. Small, preprinted, prenumbered adhesive labels that patients complete as they arrive for an office appointment. (Courtesy of Bibbero Systems, Inc., Petaluma, CA. Phone: 800-242-2376; Fax: 800-242-9330; Web site: http://www.bibbero.com.)

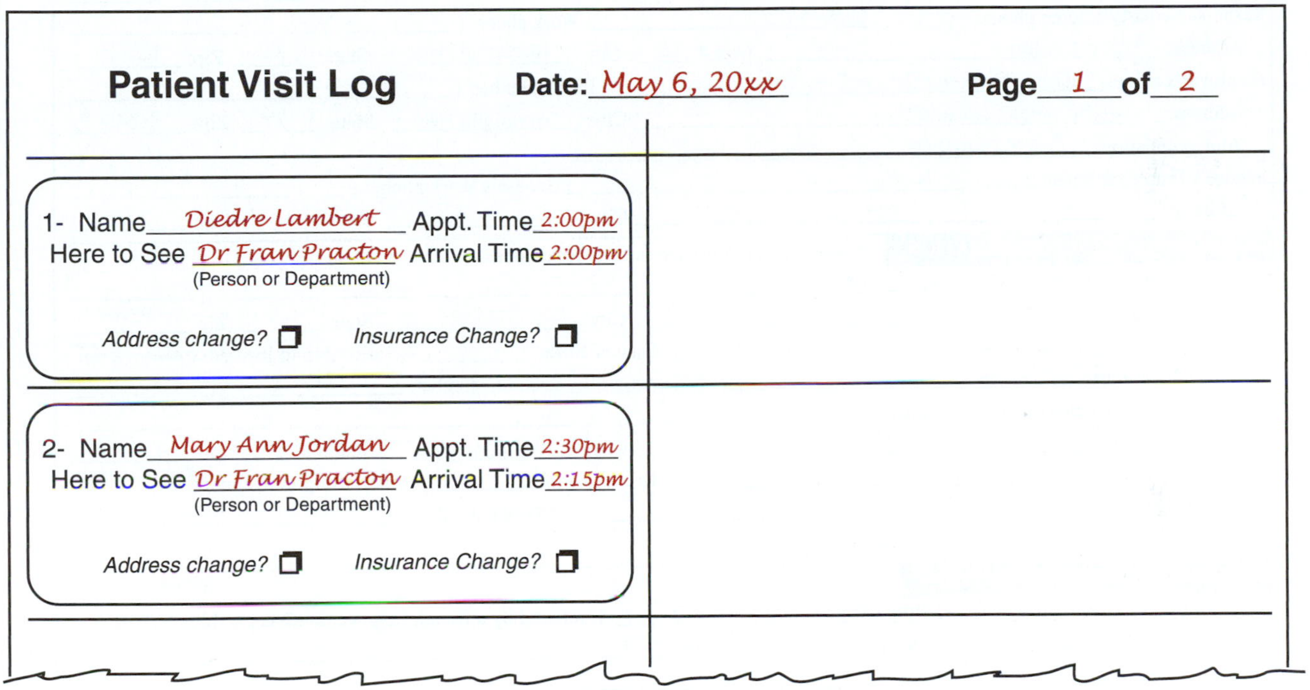

Figure 5-4B. Adhesive labels placed on patient visit log after completion by each patient. (Courtesy of Bibbero Systems, Inc., Petaluma, CA. Phone: 800-242-2376; Fax: 800-242-9330; Web site: http://www.bibbero.com.)

5. Give each patient an electronic device that vibrates or lights up when it is his or her turn to enter the back office to see the physician. Such devices are similar to ones distributed to guests waiting for tables in restaurants.

PROCESSING PATIENTS

After patients have arrived and signed in at the reception desk, it is necessary to register them or update their registration, verify that they have received a privacy notice, collect health insurance information (Chapter 16), and address all administrative issues before they are called to see the physician. After seeing the doctor, patients are given instructions pertaining to the physician's treatment plan, future appointments are made (Chapter 7), and fees are collected or their health insurance is billed (Chapters 13 and 16).

Patient Registration

At the patient's first office visit, a comprehensive but concise **registration form** (Figure 5-5) designed to record and index a patient's personal and financial data should be obtained. If the patient is to record the information at the first office visit, request that he or

Insurance cards copied ☑
Date: Feb 20, 20XX

Patient Registration Information

Please PRINT AND complete ALL sections below!

Account # : 62153
Insurance # : 572-xx-8966A
Co-Payment: $ N/A

Is your condition a result of a work injury? YES (NO)   An auto accident? YES (NO)   Date of injury: N/A

PATIENT'S PERSONAL INFORMATION   Marital Status ☐ Single ☑ Married ☐ Divorced ☐ Widowed   Sex: ☐ Male ☑ Female

Name: Peterson _____ last name _____ Mayze _____ first name _____ F. _____ initial

Street address: 851 So. Adams   12   (Apt # 12) City: Woodland Hills   State: XY   Zip: 12345

Home phone: (555) 289-4413   Work phone: (__) N/A   Social Security # 572 - xx - 8966

Date of Birth: Aug. / 07 / 1936   Driver's License: (State & Number) XY V045369X
         month   day   year

Employer / Name of School   Retired   ☐ Full Time ☐ Part Time

Spouse's Name: Peterson _____ last name _____ first name _____ initial   Spouse's Work phone: (__) _____

How do you wish to be addressed? Mrs. Peterson   Social Security # 572 - XX - 6022

PATIENT'S / RESPONSIBLE PARTY INFORMATION

Responsible party: Roy Peterson   Date of Birth: March 03, 1937

Relationship to Patient: ☐ Self ☑ Spouse ☐ Other _____   Social Security # 572 - XX - 6022

Responsible party's home phone: (555) 289-4413   Work phone: (__) N/A

Address: 851 So. Adams   (Apt # 12) City: Woodland Hills   State: XY   Zip: 12345

Employer's name: Retired Pasadena School District   Phone number: (__) N/A

Address: 44185 West Colorado Blvd.   City: Woodland Hills   State: XY   Zip: 12345

Your occupation: Retired Teacher

Spouse's Employer's name: N/A   Spouse's Work phone: (__) _____

Address: _____   City: _____   State: _____   Zip: _____

PATIENT'S INSURANCE INFORMATION   Please present insurance cards to receptionist.

PRIMARY insurance company's name: Medicare

Insurance address: P.O. Box 879   City: Los Angeles   State: CA   Zip: 12345

Name of insured: Mayze Peterson   Date of Birth: _____   Relationship to insured: ☑ Self ☐ Spouse ☐ Other ☐ Child

Insurance ID number: 572-XX-8966A   Group number: N/A

SECONDARY insurance company's name: Blue Cross

Insurance address: P.O. Box 1022   City: Woodland Hills   State: XY   Zip: 12345

Name of insured: Mayze Peterson   Date of Birth: _____   Relationship to insured: ☑ Self ☐ Spouse ☐ Other ☐ Child

Insurance ID number: 572-XX-8966   Group number: 00276A

Check if appropriate: ☑ Medigap policy ☐ Retiree coverage

PATIENT'S REFERRAL INFORMATION   (please circle one)

Referred by: Glenda Marshall (Mrs. T.K.)   If referred by a friend, may we thank her or him? (YES) NO

Name(s) of other physician(s) who care for you: Gerald King, M.D.

EMERGENCY CONTACT

Name of person not living with you: Kathryn Miller   Relationship: cousin

Address: 691 So. Brand Ave.   City: Woodland Hills   State: XY   Zip: 12345

Phone number (home): (555) 362-5711   Phone number (work): (___) _____

Assignment of Benefits • Financial Agreement

I hereby give lifetime authorization for payment of insurance benefits to be made directly to _____ Dr. G. Practon _____ , and any assisting physicians, for services rendered. I understand that I am financially responsible for all charges whether or not they are covered by insurance. In the event of default, I agree to pay all costs of collection, and reasonable attorney's fees. I hereby authorize this healthcare provider to release all information necessary to secure the payment of benefits.

I further agree that a photocopy of this agreement shall be as valid as the original.

Date: Feb. 20, 20XX   Your Signature: Mayze Peterson

Method of Payment: ☐ Cash ☑ Check ☐ Credit Card

FORM # 58-8423 • BIBBERO SYSTEMS, INC. • PETALUMA, CA. • TO ORDER CALL TOLL FREE : 800-BIBBERO (800-242-2376) • FAX (800) 242-9330   (REV. 7/94)

Figure 5-5. Patient registration information form showing completion of personal and financial data obtained from the patient prior to, or on her first visit to the office. (Courtesy of Bibbero Systems, Inc., Petaluma, CA. Phone: 800-242-2376; Fax: 800-242-9330; Web site: http://www.bibbero.com.)

she arrives at least 20 minutes early so ample time is allowed to complete the form. Preprinted registration/information forms are commercially available or can be designed by office management and supplied by a printing company in standard letter size. An extra telephone book in the reception room will save the staff interruptions and allow the patient a reference for finding addresses and telephone numbers asked for on the form.

One way to identify patients is to photocopy the driver's license picture or attach an instant photo to the registration form. It is best to verify spelling of all patient names.

Some patients may refuse to divulge certain information on the form, and in such instances it is wise to adopt a pay-at-the-time-of-service office policy. If a patient expects insurance to pay for services and has not provided information, such as insurance policy number or birth date, the insurance company will probably deny payment when processing the claim. This should be explained to the patient in a concerned manner. It may not have been something to which the patient has given much thought or consideration.

Preregistration

To ease and reduce in-office work, mail or fax the patient a registration form to complete in the comfort of his or her own home and a map giving directions so the patient can easily find the office. Ask the patient to bring the completed form in when he or she comes for the first visit.

Some offices may prefer to obtain new patient information by telephone. Be sure to verify you have the correct person, then the patient can be interviewed and data entered directly into the computer system. By calling to confirm the appointment the day before, the medical assistant can then prepare the file folder with labels and assemble a chart. The assistant needs to review the form while the patient is present to verify its accuracy and completeness. Regardless of where the form is completed, all elements need to be addressed by either completing them or referencing "not applicable" (NA) in the blank area.

Registration Member Cards

Some medical practices are starting to issue "premier member" cards to regular patients. The first time the patient is seen you collect all of the patient's information and enter it into the computer system. A plastic member card is generated with the patient's own account number or personal code, which contains all patient information. Each time the patient calls in for an appointment or is seen after that, the information is brought up on the computer screen and the patient is asked whether any changes should be made. If changes occur, new information can be downloaded to the card and if not, the card can be swiped at any affiliate location to obtain information.

Registering Patients Under Managed Care Plans

As more patients are calling or arriving at the front desk with managed care coverage, the medical assistant is faced with increased information requirements to avoid insurance and billing problems. At or prior to the initial visit, the first question the assistant should ask is: "Do you have your insurance card so that I can determine if the physician participates in the plan?" Identify the insurer's particular plan and the name of the insurer. Then photocopy both sides of the insurance card. Additional important information includes the following:

- Authorization requirements for the patient to see the physician for a visit or for elective or major surgery
- Name and phone number of referring physician
- Patient's identification numbers for the plan (policy and group)
- Copayment? (Yes/No) Amount/percentage?
- Exclusions: lab, x-ray, waiting period, other
- Preventive health visit covered/authorized? (Yes/No)
- Well-baby/child visit covered/authorized? (Yes/No)
- Allergy treatments covered/authorized? (Yes/No) What is authorized?
- Vision/hearing examinations covered/authorized? (Yes/No)
- Plan telephone number/fax number, address, city, state, and zip code

For reference, an alphabetic listing of all plans to which the physician is a participant should be handy—perhaps on a grid or in the computer system. If the office does not belong to the prospective patient's plan, explain that the physician does not participate in that plan. If the physician does belong, more screening information may be necessary prior to scheduling the office visit.

Authorization for Visits—For the primary care physician who is a participant in a managed care plan, an authorization is not required for patient visits.

STEP 1 2 3 PROCEDURE 5-2

Assist Patients with In-Office Registration Procedures

Objective: To obtain pertinent identifying information and properly register new and established patients.

Equipment/Supplies: Patient registration/information form, clipboard, pen, patient information booklet, consent form, assignment of benefits form, appointment list, and photocopy machine.

Directions: Follow these step-by-step procedures and guidelines, which include rationales, to learn this Job Skill (5-1) which is presented in the *Workbook* for practice.

1. Greet the patient and hand him or her a registration form on a clipboard with pen. Ask the patient to complete the form offering to assist as needed. Use of a clipboard allows the patient to sit comfortably and write independently on a hard surface.

2. Instruct the patient to answer all questions and complete all blank lines indicating nonapplicable (NA) for areas that do not apply. This ensures that the patient has read all areas and addressed all questions on the form.

3. Give the patient a patient information booklet outlining the policies of the medical practice unless it is office policy to mail a welcoming letter, map, booklet, and questionnaire before the first visit.

4. Ask for an insurance card and photocopy both sides.

5. Verify that the physician is covered by the health insurance contract.

6. Confirm patient eligibility and enrollment for insurance coverage or monthly capitation.

7. Ask for a prior authorization form if the patient is in a managed care plan and has been referred by another physician. An authorization to see the patient must be approved and received by the physician before the patient arrives for an appointment,

otherwise the physician would be denied payment for the service.

8. Collect and review the form for legibility, completeness, and accuracy. Ask the patient for information for any areas left blank. Correct information assists in billing and collections. The form should contain:

   a. Patient's full name (verify spelling with insurance card)

   b. Marital status

   c. Gender

   d. Home address (including street address if a post office box is listed) and e-mail address

   e. Telephone, cell phone, pager, and fax numbers—home and business (including extension number)

   f. Social Security number

   g. Birth date recorded as eight digits for computer processing (01-16-1945)

   h. Driver's license number

   i. Occupation with name and address of employer

   j. Spouse's or legal guardian's full name, work phone, and Social Security number

   k. Name and telephone number of person responsible for payment (guarantor)

   l. Insurance information; names, addresses, and telephone numbers—with policy and group numbers—of primary and secondary insurance (copy of insurance card may be placed in this area if all information is included)

   m. Name of person who referred patient and other physicians caring for patient

   n. Name of close friend or relative with daytime telephone number for emergency contact

9. Collect the copayment amount before the visit. This helps avoid sending bills for small amounts, thus reducing overhead costs.

PROCEDURE 5-2 *continued*

10. Explain the patient's financial responsibility. Collection is made easier if the patient knows his or her financial obligation before receiving service.

11. Ask if there is any changed information if the patient is an established patient. Patients may not remember to let you know about changes in personal information, for example, new insurance, new married name, and so on.

12. Ask the patient to sign the consent form, assignment of benefits form, and responsibility for the account section of the form.

13. Insert a check mark on the appointment list indicating the patient has arrived for his or her appointment. This record must be retained as documentation for financial purposes.

14. Affix the patient registration form to the front inside cover of the patient's chart.

15. Place the history form and any other forms/reports into the patient's medical record.

16. Secure a multipurpose billing form (encounter form) on the patient's chart. The multipurpose billing form is explained in detail in Chapter 13, Fees, Credit, and Collection.

17. Ask the patient to be seated and give an approximation of how long it will be before the examination. This keeps the patient informed and will reduce his or her anxiety.

18. Put the patient's medical record with multipurpose billing form in the appropriate place to indicate to the physician or clinical medical assistant that the patient is in the reception room and ready to be seen.

A great number of plans require the patient to receive an authorization from the primary care physician to see a specialist or to receive outside services. If plans require authorizations, the assistant can remind patients to bring the authorization forms at the time of their scheduled visit. If test results are to be sent or faxed to the practice, the assistant in charge of scheduling may want to put a special note in the appointment log to confirm that the results have been received—preferably one or two days before the scheduled visit. Otherwise the patient's appointment may have to be rescheduled pending necessary test results.

Registering Patients Coming from a Hospital

If you work for a surgeon, a new patient who the physician has already seen or performed emergency surgery on at the hospital may come to the office. Often the only information you get is the patient's name, diagnosis, and the procedure the surgeon performed. First, obtain the **face sheet** from the hospital admitting office or have the physician bring a copy from the patient's hospital record. If the hospital face sheet does not contain all the needed information call the hospital ward unit coordinator or the insurance verifier in the admitting office. The patient's primary care physician can also be contacted regarding basic insur-

ance information. If the doctor does not remember the patient's name, call the operating room desk at the hospital to identify the patient. Remember, HIPAA does not forbid sharing patient information for the purpose of treating the patient; however, if the hospital does not want to divulge the information the physician may need to call or take up the problem with the medical record supervisor.

Updating Information

When a patient returns, the original information is reviewed to make sure it is still accurate. This can be accomplished by printing the patient information and having the patient review it and make any changes in red ink. A patient information update form is also available for this purpose. Some offices use a confidential patient sign-in log that may be used to determine if there have been any changes (address, telephone number, insurance data) since a previous visit. Verifying patient information should be done at three-month intervals for all patients who are not being treated for ongoing problems (Figure 5-6).

Medical History and Reports

A history form can be mailed with the new patient registration form allowing the patient time to look up pertinent information and complete it accurately.

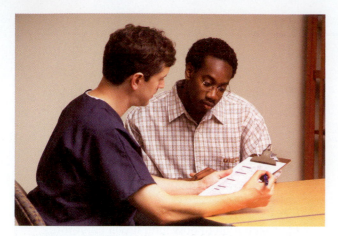

Figure 5-6. A medical assistant and patient are in a private area discussing the patient's completed registration/information form

To facilitate gathering medical information, ask new patients to request previous medical records from their former physician or to come in to sign an authorization to release information in advance of their appointment. The physician will then have time to review the past history allowing a more relaxed initial interview. If laboratory results are to be sent or faxed to the practice, the assistant in charge of scheduling may want to put a special note in the appointment log to confirm that the results have been received—preferably one or two days before the scheduled visit. Otherwise, the patient's appointment may have to be rescheduled pending necessary test results.

Privacy Notice

After the patient is registered with the medical practice, a privacy notice should be presented to the patient and signed. HIPAA's privacy rule and practices were described in Chapter 3. The privacy notice needs to be posted in the reception room and on the practice's Web site where patients can easily find it. The medical assistant must be trained in presenting this notice to the patient (Example 5-2).

A privacy officer should be available to discuss the privacy rule with the patient if there are complex questions. A common question is, "Will you release information to my family members?" The answer would be, "The privacy notice addresses to whom your health information may be released." This is a good time to find out whether the patient has a family member or friend whom he or she would like to have listed in case of an emergency or unusual situation. Some computer software allows the date the

EXAMPLE 5-2

Privacy Notice Distribution

Spoken to the patient when handing out the privacy notice: "Federal privacy law requires that we provide this notice to inform you how we will use your health information. It also outlines your rights regarding your own health information. Please sign this acknowledgement to indicate you have received a copy."

patient received the privacy notice to be noted on the patient registration screen. This will help document the distribution process. If such software is not available, an area on the patient registration form could be designed to include a receipt statement with date, or a date stamp could be made with the information.

Waiting in Reception Area

After the patient has been registered and the privacy notice obtained, insurance information must be collected (see Chapter 16), and the patient is then seated to wait for the medical assistant to escort him or her to the back office to see the physician. Waiting is expected but should be kept to a minimum. A study has shown that the average person can sit and wait for approximately 20 minutes before getting bored, fidgeting, worrying, or getting angry. Following are ways to ease the tension during long wait times.

- Post a sign in the waiting room that says, "Please approach the reception desk if you have waited more than 15 minutes."

- Keep patient expectations reasonable by including a statement in the waiting room, in the patient brochure, and on your Web site that states, "Our goal is to keep all appointments as scheduled, and we know your time is valuable. If a delay occurs we apologize and hope that you will understand that we are trying to accommodate all patients in the timeframe allowed."

- Give patients options. If a delay occurs and the 20-minute threshold is approaching, try to find out what is causing the delay and inform patients how long they can expect to wait before seeing the physician; be honest!

If the wait time is expected to run 30 or more minutes, ask the patient, "Would you like to reschedule, leave to do an errand and return in a half-hour, or continue to wait?" This common courtesy will go a long way toward smoothing patient relationships and patients will appreciate having choices and being informed.

Do not ignore patients by shutting the security window, avoiding eye contact, or acting as though you do not know how long they have waited or will have to wait—find out.

Escorting Patients

Generally, patients will arrive and approach the reception desk, check in and fill out paper work, then have a seat in the reception area. It is usually the responsibility of the clinical medical assistant to call and direct patients into the treatment area of the physician's office; however, on occasion the administrative medical assistant may need to escort or direct a patient. If you see a patient fumbling with the front door, go assist by holding the door open until he or she enters. If you are working in a large clinic, patients will need to be directed to various departments. Good communication skills should be utilized to give clear directions.

The assistant can reduce the likelihood of a patient misplacing or losing a personal article such as a sweater or purse by suggesting that patients hold their belongings or leave them in a closet with a posted sign stating "Not Responsible for Personal Items." It should be routine to hang heavy coats and rain attire on a rack outside the treatment room in inclement weather. Office insurance should cover loss of personal items as well as damage to a patient's clothing, should a mishap occur.

Not all visitors to the medical office will be patients. Family members should be escorted to the location of their relative. Other physicians should be greeted pleasantly and ushered into the back office immediately. Visits from sales representatives may be handled by the assistant, postponed, or scheduled for another time if the physician is busy.

Patients with Special Needs

Processing a patient with special needs takes skill and forethought. Patients who are *physically impaired* with deformities that alter their functions or appearance may require preliminary steps from the receptionist to ensure a pleasant atmosphere and an expedited visit. Consider the following when arranging for the arrival of elderly or physically impaired patients:

- Give consideration when setting up the appointment to allow extra time, a special treatment room, and concern for transportation; reserve time for midday appointments.
- Reserve at-the-door parking.
- Watch for the arrival of the patient and promptly escort him or her into the office after asking whether assistance is needed. By asking if assistance is needed a direct response is given, and the patient can describe how you can help; this attentiveness conveys a caring attitude.
- Become familiar with mobility devices such as a canes, crutches, walkers, or wheelchairs (Figure 5-7). It may be necessary to prepare a place for a wheelchair in the waiting room, provide a footstool for a patient who arrives on crutches, or move furniture to ease navigation.
- Speak to a disabled person at eye level, if possible, to ensure eye contact. There should be no awkwardness or hesitation when speaking to these patients.
- Verify in the patient's file that an appropriate contact is noted for emergencies.
- Enunciate clearly and speak slowly especially if the office treats patients from different ethnic

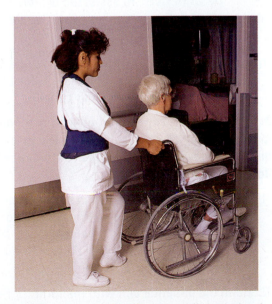

Figure 5-7. A medical assistant guiding a wheel chair–bound patient after making sure there are no obstacles

backgrounds. Concentrate on the speaker and do not interrupt.

- Avoid terms that are offensive to the disabled such as crippled, deformed, or handicapped. "Disabled" and "impaired" are more acceptable terms.

- Provide help in filling out insurance forms in a well-lighted area and become knowledgeable on supplemental insurance; provide privacy.

- Maintain a warm temperature in examination rooms.

- Keep carpet in good repair and attach handrails where needed, for example, entrance, stairs, by examination chair, and so on.

- Type information sheets in large print, (e.g., surgery aftercare).

- Print information sheets on special subjects related to geriatric infirmities, such as arthritis and osteoporosis.

- Distribute emergency stickers with the physician's name and telephone number to be attached to the patient's telephone.

- Offer to complete a Department of Motor Vehicles form, Statement of Facts, and Application for Disabled Person if the patient has a temporary or permanent disability so he or she may obtain a parking placard.

- Maintain a file with information on various senior citizen agencies that provide activities and senior daycare.

- Provide maps for directions and a list of public transportation services, with schedules. A contract with a firm to provide taxi service is cost-effective when elderly patients have transportation problems and often miss scheduled appointments.

Disabled Driver Placard or License Plate Form— A physically disabled patient who wishes to park in specially labeled spaces to reduce walking distance to a business or office may obtain a permit by getting a form provided by the state (see Figure 5-8). Most state agencies provide standardized forms to individuals with legitimate physical problems. The physician may be required to provide a complete description of the

---

PROCEDURE 5-3

STEP 1 2 3

Assist Patient in Preparing an Application Form for a Disabled Person Placard

Objective: To assist the disabled patient in completing a form for a parking placard or plate.

Equipment/Supplies: Application/Statement of Facts for Disabled Person Parking Placard or Plates form, clipboard, and pen or pencil.

Directions: Follow these step-by-step procedures and guidelines, which include rationales, to learn this Job Skill which is presented in the *Workbook* (Job Skill 5-2) for practice.

1. Obtain a form provided by the state for the physically disabled patient who wishes to park in specially labeled parking spaces. As a courtesy, many medical practices may keep the forms on hand.

2. Hand the patient a pen with the form attached to a clipboard. Use of a clipboard allows the patient to sit comfortably and write on a hard surface.

3. Direct the patient to complete the applicant's section of the form (top area) and to sign and date in the appropriate area. Offer to assist in its completion. Areas may be highlighted for patient.

4. Ask the patient to make out a check to the Department of Motor Vehicles for the necessary fee.

5. Review the filled in form for legibility, completeness, and accuracy.

6. Complete the attending physician's statement (bottom portion) and obtain the doctor's signature certifying that the patient is temporarily, moderately, or permanently disabled.

7. Make a photocopy of the form before sending it to the Department of Motor Vehicles in your state.

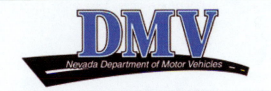

555 Wright Way
Carson City, NV 89711
Reno/Sparks/Carson City (775) 684-4DMV (4368)
Las Vegas area (702) 486-4DMV (4368)
Rural Nevada or Out of State (877) 368-7828
www.dmvnv.com

APPLICATION FOR DISABLED PERSONS LICENSE PLATES AND/OR PLACARDS
NRS 482.384

You may select either plates and one (1) placard, or two (2) placards.

☐   Disabled Plates *(permanent disability only)*   Disabled Placard(s) ☐ One ☐ Two

☐   Disabled Motorcycle Plates (permanent disability only)   Disabled Motorcycle Sticker ☐ One ☐ Other _____

First time applications for a Disabled Persons license plate or motorcycle sticker must be made in person.

In order to apply for disabled persons license plates or disabled motorcycle stickers(s) your name must appear on the vehicle registration certificate. If your vehicle is currently registered, you have the option of maintaining your current vehicle registration expiration date, or renewing for a full twelve (12) month period. Credit for any unused portion of your current registration is transferable to your disabled license plate registration. In applicable counties, if you are renewing for a full 12-month period, and your previous evidence of compliance with emissions standards was obtained more than 90 days ago, the vehicle must be re-inspected prior to registration. **You must have a permanent disability to qualify for Disabled Persons license plates** *(see description below).*

Please Print or Type

Applicants Name_____ _____/_____/_____
(Disabled Person)   First   Middle   Last   Date of Birth

Address_____
       Address   City   State   Zip Code

County of Residence _____ Nevada DL or ID No. _____ Daytime Telephone No (_____)_____

Signature of Applicant _____ Date _____

A LICENSED PHYSICIAN MUST COMPLETE THIS PORTION*

As a Physician for the above-named patient, I hereby certify that the applicant:

1. _____   Cannot walk two hundred feet without stopping to rest.

2. _____   Cannot walk without the use of a brace, cane, crutch, wheelchair, or other device or another person.

3. _____   Has a cardiac condition to the extent that functional limitations are classified as a Class III or Class IV according to standards adopted by the American Heart Association.

4. _____   Is restricted by a lung disease.

5. _____   Is severely limited in his/her ability to walk because of an arthritic, neurological, or orthopedic condition.

6. _____   Is visually handicapped.

7. _____   Uses portable oxygen.

I further certify that my patient's condition is a:

☐   **Temporary Disability** (6 months or less) Must indicate length of time not to exceed 6 months *beginning* _____
     ending _____

☐   **Moderate Disability** (reversible but disabled longer than 6 months)
     Must indicate length of time not to exceed 2 years *beginning* _____ *ending* _____

☐   **Permanent Disability** (irreversible, permanently disabled in his/her ability to walk, certification is valid indefinitely).

Please Print or Type

Physician's Name_____

Mailing Address _____
       Address   City   State   Zip Code

Physicians License Number _____ Telephone No (_____)_____

Physicians Signature _____ Date _____
    * Physicians Assistant Certified (PA-C) or Advanced Practice Nurse (APN) are not authorized to complete this document.
SP27 (Rev 4/2007)

Figure 5-8. Application/Statement of Facts for Disabled Person Parking Placard or Plates to be completed by patient and attending physician

illness or disability. City laws vary on the percentage of handicapped parking places for parking lots as this is not standardized.

Instructing Patients

At the conclusion of the patient's visit, a **patient instruction form** completed by the physician with handwritten short statements will improve compliance by the patient, legally protect the physician because items are in writing (documented), reduce telephone calls, and cement the bond between the physician and patient (Figure 5-9). The form designed by the physician can be developed in a single-page format modified for the particular practice with patients' identifying data (i.e., patient's name, date of appointment, and diagnosis), and a checklist of topics that can include:

1. Tests
2. Medications
3. Precautions
4. Expectations
5. Activities to decrease or increase
6. Miscellaneous
7. Date of next appointment

The original form with physician's signature would remain with the patient's chart in the office, and a copy would be given to the patient.

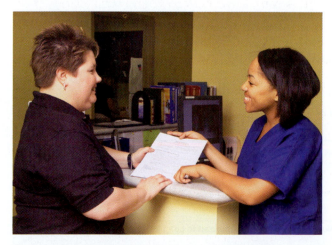

Figure 5-9. A medical assistant and patient reviewing a patient instruction form that was completed by the physician

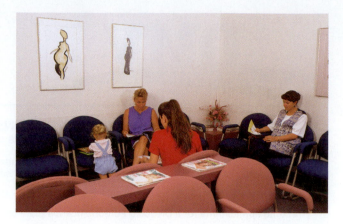

Figure 5-10. An inviting and pleasant reception area has seating arranged so that patients are comfortable sitting together or away from other patients

RECEPTION AREA

The first area that people see when they enter a physician's office is the reception room. Create a welcoming area, a place where people will want to spend time when waiting for appointments. It should be well designed, well maintained, and attractive.

Patients often spend more time in the reception room with the staff than in the examining room with the physician; for this reason a clean appearance and an atmosphere of relaxation are desirable (Figure 5-10).

A counter with a window or shoulder-high shield assists to secure privacy and security. If the reception room is separated from the office by a sliding window, a bell should be placed by it so the medical assistant knows when a patient has arrived. The medical assistant should open and close the window quietly to reduce noise. Some patients react negatively

COMPLIANCE

If the receptionist is frequently called away from his or her work station, adjust the timing of the computer screen saver to protect open documents. Most screen savers can be activated after 1 to 60 minutes of inactivity. Select a setting by right clicking the mouse while on the desktop. Select "Properties" then "Screen Saver." Choose how many minutes of time you would like to lapse before the screen saver is activated where it says "Wait _____ minutes."

to a closed window because they feel cut off from the staff—it seems to depersonalize the office.

Open reception rooms are acceptable according to HIPAA; however be sure that patients cannot view computer screens or charts. Protected health information should never be overheard, so discussions should not take place in waiting rooms or hallways. Portable room dividers may be utilized to add privacy and privacy filters for computer screens may be used to safeguard documents.

Features of the Reception Area

The reception area should include stable but comfortable chairs. Couches may be used, but they are less durable and are not as flexible for seating arrangements. The carpet should be of an industrial type that provides a cushion to walk on, reduces noise, and offers the feel of a comfortable living room. Window dressings should be simple and shades or blinds used to control lighting. The type of furniture, colors, and fabrics vary according to the taste of the physician or designer and create whatever atmosphere is desired. All items should be durable enough to handle large volumes of patient traffic and easy to maintain. A coat-rack is a functional item often placed near the outside door where patients may put coats and umbrellas during inclimate weather. Following are other features typically found in the reception area.

Business Cards

Business cards for all physicians and physician extenders (nurse practitioner/physician assistant) of the medical group should be available on the reception counter. Sometimes other office personnel (e.g., office manager, bookkeeper, medical insurance biller) also have business cards displayed for patients.

Signs

Signs in the reception area should be simple and direct. They should help people feel welcome as well as advise. A "No Smoking" sign could be displayed

COMPLIANCE

A notice should be posted in the reception area explaining the office's Health Insurance Portability and Accountability Act (HIPAA) policy on confidentiality.

in a conspicuous place and a receptacle provided outside to extinguish cigarettes before entering the office.

Air, Temperature, and Lighting

Air should circulate freely in the waiting room. A door or window left ajar, a ceiling fan moving slowly, or air circulating through the air conditioning system can help avoid a stale smell. The temperature should be adjusted so the thermostat registers 68 or 70 degrees and is comfortable to staff members. Be aware of outside temperatures and the way the office is facing (i.e., sunny exposure versus northern exposure), which can affect inside temperatures. Periodically check with patients to see that they are comfortable and be aware that elderly patients and babies may feel a draft or cold when others are comfortable. Lighting should be bright and cheerful allowing for easy reading of materials and viewing of surroundings.

Music

Music from a stereo system or CD player may help create a peaceful atmosphere but should be inoffensive, light, breezy, and quiet so as not to bother anyone; just loud enough to provide a soothing background and calm nerves. Light jazz, classical music, and soft rock are appropriate choices.

Plants and Decorative Items

Plants and terrariums can add decorative accents to the reception area and help create an inviting place for patients to wait. Be careful when adding fresh flowers; although they are beautiful, many flowers emit strong fragrances and can cause allergic reactions. Decorative items such as paintings, sculptures, mobiles, and aquariums provide a focus and add interest to the waiting area.

Reading Material

Reading material that reflects the interests of the patient population should be available in racks or on tables (Figure 5-11). Select a variety of recent issues of magazines that will appeal to both men and women, young and old, without being controversial or political in nature. Popular magazines may be brought in by staff or patients, but they should be in good condition with the address labels removed. Brochures in the reception area can supply information about the medical practice and offer suggestions and information about diseases and other topics such as

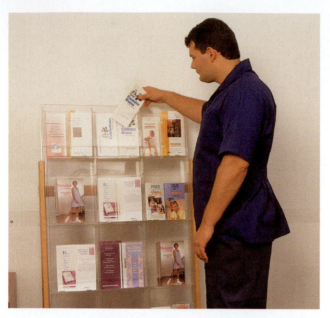

Figure 5-11. Brochures and handouts should be accessible and inviting to patients and office visitors

pregnancy, child rearing, menopause, and so forth. See Chapter 17 on designing office brochures.

Food and Drink

Food and drinks may be made available, depending on the type of practice. A water cooler is always welcome and items such as coffee, tea, or even baked

goods communicate to patients that they are welcome. Food, however, can easily soil carpet and furniture and should be discouraged in certain reception areas.

Television

Television programs playing constantly disrupt the quiet setting of the reception area and should be avoided, it sends the message that you expect patients

---

STEP 1 2 3

PROCEDURE 5-4

Develop a Patient Education Plan for Diseases/Injuries Related to the Medical Specialty

Objective: To make and carry out a plan to properly educate patients about treatment of diseases or injuries related to the specialty.

Equipment/Supplies: Patient information booklet, information pamphlets from professional medical associations, office schedule of physicians and staff, paper, pen or pencil, and bulletin board.

Directions: Follow these step-by-step procedures and guidelines, which include rationales, to learn this Job Skill.

1. Carefully assess the medical practice patients' needs for education.

2. Obtain patient educational devices, for example, information pamphlets from professional medical associations about

diseases and treatments, plastic anatomic models, and pamphlets explaining surgical procedures.

3. Devise methods to educate those patients with disabilities, for example, vision or hearing impaired, imitations of mobility, language barriers (e.g. audiotapes).

4. Read information so you can be knowledgable and answer questions.

5. Document information given to the patients in their medical record.

6. Place a suggestion box in the reception room with a short questionnaire requesting patient opinions about the quality of their care, office efficiency, and staff promptness and courtesy.

to wait. Playing educational materials is acceptable, but the sound should be turned to a low volume so as not to disturb patients who are trying to read or are not interested in listening.

Bulletin Board

A bulletin board hung in the reception room can be filled with interesting items for patients to look at; for example, color pictures of the office staff with names and brief biographies. In an obstetrician's office, color pictures of new mothers and their infants would be appropriate. A colorful wall map to guide patients to local laboratories and specialists would simplify directing patients to other sites.

In a multiphysician group, items tacked to the bulletin board might include new office schedules for physicians and staff, letters from patients, announcement cards, and newspaper clippings that have been date-stamped. It can be divided into sections for each physician so that reminders, articles, and notes for each one can be written or pinned on it. Check the bulletin board at least once a week to discard outdated material.

Toys

Toys and puzzles help entertain children and are best placed in an activity center or corner of the room so children do not disturb other patients while playing. Disinfect or sanitize toys on a regular basis and be sure to avoid easily breakable items and small toys or ones that can be pulled a part and swallowed. Cover all accessible light switch plates and place electric cords behind furniture so they are not accessible to children. Select and view all items in the reception area with safety in mind and remember, the best feature of any waiting room is an immediate acknowledgement and friendly welcome when people arrive.

Maintaining the Reception Area

If a medical office is orderly and immaculately clean, patients will associate its cleanliness with good medical practices. Many medical offices contract with private cleaning agencies or janitorial services to clean their facilities (see Chapter 17; Office Managerial Responsibilities) but regular light cleaning is usually left up to the office staff.

Divide housekeeping chores equitably among all office personnel so that no one person will feel imposed on, and the result will be an accident-free, sanitary office for both the patients and the staff.

Housekeeping Tasks

The medical assistants' housekeeping responsibilities begin where those of the cleaning service leave off. The medical assistant is assigned housekeeping duties to create a comfortable place for patients to wait, as opposed to cleaning the office. However, everything within reach should be polished and dusted by the assistants in an orderly process with items such as mirrors and medical equipment given special attention.

Avoid making patients feel as though someone is picking up after them when stepping into the reception room to straighten magazines, adjust lighting, empty wastebaskets, and arrange furniture. If the office closes for lunch, this would be a good time to freshen up the reception room.

Plants usually need to be watered weekly and fertilized occasionally. An assistant who does not have a green thumb might contact a plant service. Periodicals can be protected from theft and from becoming thumb-worn by placing them in vinyl covers or binders.

Additional housekeeping tasks might include emptying wastebaskets in the front and back office, sweeping the reception room quietly with a carpet sweeper if someone has dropped something, replenishing paper supplies, removing fingerprints from work station divider windows, and tidying restrooms.

Most housekeeping tasks assigned to the administrative medical assistant are in the outer office, where, for instance, an uncluttered secretarial work station with personal items out of sight should be the rule. To increase desktop space and secure personal items, each staff member may be assigned a drawer, locker, or cupboard that can be locked. Storing office paperwork in a desk-drawer or file upon completion is recommended.

Unsightly or dangerous conditions, such as something spilled in any part of the medical facility or debris on the floor, should be attended to immediately by the first staff member to observe it, without regard to who is responsible.

Wear gloves for protection when doing any cleaning, and remove stains when first noticed. Blot the stain, apply cleaning solution, create friction while rubbing, and use cold water instead of hot to rinse the area. If **infectious waste**, such as blood and urine (body fluids) or human waste, which can be dangerous to individuals and the environment, need to be cleaned up in the reception area, use **universal precautions** and treat all as if it were infectious. You probably will not have to worry about hazardous waste, such as needles, scalpels, or slides with cultures contaminating the reception room; however, a patient may remove a wound dressing, which would necessitate using universal precautions and following hazardous waste guidelines. Hazardous waste kits may be purchased for such situations and the waste deposited in a biohazard container.

Larger tasks such as cleaning cabinets inside and out using a bactericidal agent is done when the physician is away from the office for an extended period so cabinets can be allowed to dry thoroughly when normal office routine will not be disrupted.

Be on the lookout for frayed cords, damaged furniture, and objects on the floor that might cause accidents.

Cleaning equipment and supplies are more economically priced if purchased from a wholesaler or discount supplier.

HANDLING AN OFFICE EMERGENCY

The medical receptionist needs to maintain a flexible attitude so he or she can adjust on a moment's notice to the unexpected, for example, when a patient arrives without a scheduled appointment or calls about an accident or sudden illness (see Chapter 7). Reacting calmly in a situation that demands immediate attention includes following planned procedures and is especially important if the reception room is crowded with patients awaiting their own appointments.

The administrative medical assistant may be the staff person to orchestrate emergency efforts within an office. If an emergency arises in a treatment room, the clinical assistant would typically notify the receptionist who then calls an ambulance. This frees the clinical medical assistant to assist the physician with the patient until emergency personnel arrive. The receptionist could direct the ambulance to the back door of the office suite, lead emergency personnel to the area where the patient is, and warn or oversee anxious patients in the reception area while emergency procedures are taking place.

If a patient should stop breathing in the reception room and the physician is not immediately present, the medical assistant should be prepared to start cardiopulmonary resuscitation (CPR) until other help arrives. Classes in this technique are frequently given in most localities. First-aid training can also help the receptionist be prepared for office emergencies.

Since a medical emergency can occur at any time and when a physician or clinical assistant is not immediately present, the handling of an emergency situation should be discussed before such an eventuality.

Usually the person who has had an accident or who suddenly has become seriously will be accompanied to the office by an anxious member of the family or by a close friend. They should be immediately escorted into an inner examining room where they can be isolated from patients in the reception room. While waiting for the physician, the medical assistant must remain calm, yet show concern. Medical advice should not be given and verbal responses should be kept to a minimum with conversation conveying emotional support. Relevant medical information confided by the patient may be related to the physician in private.

For information about legal issues pertaining to emergency care of patients see Chapter 3 and for telephone calls from patients about emergencies refer to Chapter 6.

CLOSING THE MEDICAL OFFICE

In preparing to close the office all charts are pulled for patients who will be seen the following day. If time allows, a new page is date stamped and the chart is reviewed to determine if everything is in order for the patient's arrival. If a consultation has taken place or tests have been ordered, necessary reports must be filed in the chart. If results have not been received, call the appropriate facility and make arrangements to have the information faxed, either that afternoon or the following morning. If the financial information is not kept in a computer system, ledger cards should also be pulled. A schedule of all patients is either printed from the computer system or copied from the appointment book and placed on each physician's desk and made available for all personnel who will be dealing with patients.

After all patients have left, it is necessary to shut off all equipment (including unplugging the coffee pot), close and lock drawers, cabinets, and files; secure all drugs; and straighten office areas. Make sure the fax machine is stocked with paper and is in the standby mode. The answering machine should be turned on and/or the answering service called to let them know the office is closing and to verify the physician who is on-call. Turn off lights, lock all doors, and arm the security system.

STEP 1 2 3

PROCEDURE 5-5

Close the Medical Office

Objective: To close and secure the office at the end of the day in an organized manner.

Equipment/Supplies: A simulated office setting.

Directions: Follow these step-by-step procedures and guidelines, which include rationales, and role play the actions to practice this procedure. Describe the action and rationale while performing each step.

1. Straighten the reception area and your desk, if there is time.

2. Print and photocopy a list of the patients to be seen with appointment time or photocopy the appointment book page to distribute to physicians and staff the following day.

3. Put the charts in the order of scheduled appointments.

4. Date-stamp charts and review them to determine studies that were ordered; locate and file results.

5. Turn off and/or unplug all office equipment to eliminate chance of an electrical fire.

6. Put cash received in a safe, lock in a secure area, or deposit at the bank.

7. Leave fax machine on and make sure it is loaded with paper.

8. Place files in cabinets, close and lock drawers, cabinets, and files including areas where drugs are stored.

9. Turn of photocopy machine and fill with paper.

10. Turn on the answering machine and/or telephone the answering service letting them know when you will return and where and how the physician can be reached in an emergency. Notify building security if necessary.

11. Turn off lights, lock all doors, and activate the security system.

STOP AND THINK CASE SCENARIO

Privacy Protection

Scenario: You are sitting at the reception desk and there are two patients sitting in the adjoining waiting room. A new patient appears at her scheduled appointment time and begins asking you questions related to her medical condition.

Critical Thinking: Determine three possible ways you could respond to her in order to protect her privacy without seeming rude or noncaring.

1. _____

   _____

2. _____

   _____

3. _____

   _____

STOP AND THINK CASE SCENARIO

First Impression

Scenario: You are the patient and enter a medical office. You notice a faint smell of urine and approach the reception desk where the receptionist is talking on the telephone. She never looks up and you wait at the desk for a few minutes but finally give up and sit down. She keeps talking while chewing gum and you notice her blouse is low cut.

Critical Thinking:

1. What is your impression of the medical office and the receptionist?

   _____

   _____

2. How do you feel when the receptionist does not look up to acknowledge you?

   _____

3. If you were the receptionist, what would you have done in this situation?

   _____

   _____

   _____

   _____

   _____

FOCUS ON CERTIFICATION*

CMA Content Summary

- Medical terminology
- Social and environmental influences on behavior
- Professional attitude
- Confidentiality
- Promoting competent patient care
- General office policies
- Health maintenance and disease prevention instruction
- Community resources
- Professional communication/behavior
- Interviews (registration)
- Office emergencies
- Physician delays

RMA Content Summary

- Medical terminology
- Professional conduct
- Communication methods
- Patient brochures/informational materials
- Patient instruction
- Receiving and greeting patients
- Basic emergency triage
- Patient demographics
- Confidentiality
- Assisting patients

CMAS Content Summary

- Medical terminology
- Human relations

*This textbook and the accompanying Workbook meet the entry-level administrative and general competencies for the CMA outlined by the AAMA Examination Content Outline and Role Delineation Study and for the RMA and CMAS outlined by the AMT Competencies and Examination Specifications (see Competency Grid in Appendix B).

- Health histories
- Medical emergencies
- Screening visitors/vendors
- Examination room flow
- Patient information and community resources

- Confidentiality
- Biohazardous waste, hazardous chemicals, office safety
- Maintaining facility and environment

REVIEW EXAM-STYLE QUESTIONS

1. The emerging role of the administrative medical assistant serving as a receptionist includes:

   a. knowledge of operative procedures

   b. performing account collection calls at the front desk

   c. assisting the physician in the examination room

   d. serving as a diplomat, a negotiator, a psychologist, and a director of public relations

   e. managing the medical office

2. Two things that are important while multitasking are:

   a. energy and a desire to accomplish things fast

   b. organizational skills and a calm demeanor

   c. a dynamic personality and professional presentation

   d. a slow, deliberate manner with methodical tendencies

   e. the ability to always stop what you are doing and do whatever is asked of you by whoever asks it

3. After opening up the medical office, the answering machine should:

   a. be turned off during business hours after picking up messages

   b. be left on in case you get busy and cannot get to the telephone

   c. be left for the office manager to pick up all messages; they may be important

   d. be left for the physician to pick up all messages; they might be personal

   e. never be used; an answering service should be used instead

4. When greeting patients, the easiest way to customize requests or comments is to:

   a. ask the question, "How are you today?"

   b. start all conversations with, "Welcome to Dr. Practon's office."

   c. add the patient's name

   d. look straight into the patient's eyes

   e. think of a different phrase to say to each patient so you never repeat the same phrase in the same day

5. Select the correct statement regarding HIPAA's view of confidentiality in the reception area (waiting room).

   a. It would be nice if confidentiality could be kept in the reception area, but HIPAA understands that you have no control over that area in your office.

   b. HIPAA requires all offices to have a privacy screen or window separating the receptionist from patients in the waiting room.

   c. The one area HIPAA does not address is the reception area of a medical office.

   d. HIPAA forbids calling out of patients' names in the reception area.

   e. HIPAA compliance is as important in the reception area as it is anywhere in the medical practice.

6. Select the correct statement regarding HIPAA's view of Patient Visit Logs.

   a. All sign-in logs are forbidden according to HIPAA.

   b. HIPAA does not address regulations for sign-in logs in medical offices.

   c. Sign-in logs are permitted as long as patients are not prompted to reveal sensitive medical conditions by asking "reason for visit."

   d. Sign-in logs are no longer used in physicians' offices so HIPAA does not address this issue.

   e. Physicians are being forced by HIPAA to obtain expensive alternatives to sign-in logs.

7. When registering patients who have not been seen in the medical office but who have been treated by your physician at a hospital facility, first obtain:

   a. the patient registration form from the hospital

   b. the H & P from the hospital

   c. as much information as possible from all other doctors who have been treating the patient

   d. the face sheet from the hospital admitting office

   e. the face sheet from the surgical unit

8. When appointment delays have occurred and patients are waiting in the reception area:

   a. post a sign that asks them to approach the front desk

   b. give them options so they can make a decision to wait, return, or reschedule

   c. shut the security window so that you are not disturbed while conducting office business

   d. avoid eye contact because it will incite complaints

   e. both A and B are correct

9. A Patient Instruction Form will:

   a. improve patient compliance

   b. legally protect the physician

   c. reduce telephone calls

   d. cement the bond between the patient and physician

   e. all of the above

10. The best feature of any waiting room is:

    a. cheerful décor

    b. an immediate acknowledgement and friendly welcome when people arrive

    c. stable but comfortable furniture arranged for flexible seating

    d. signs that are simple but direct patients

    e. features such as music, plants, decorative items, reading material, and so forth that give it a special touch

11. Housekeeping tasks in the medical office:

    a. include keeping the reception area neat and clean throughout the day

    b. are all left up to a professional cleaning service, which is usually hired by the office manager

    c. are all performed by the medical assistant acting as receptionist

    d. always includes cleaning the office from top to bottom so that it is spotless

    e. are never done by the medical assistant

12. An office emergency:

    a. is always taken care of by the physician and should not involve the administrative medical assistant

    b. includes following planned procedures by the administrative medical assistant

    c. always dictates calling 911 for help

    d. is always handled by the clinical medical assistant

    e. should always involve evacuation of the waiting room by the receptionist

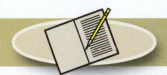

WORKBOOK ASSIGNMENT

To develop competency-based job skills, refer to the *Workbook* and complete the:

- Abbreviation and Spelling Review
- Review questions

- Critical Thinking Exercises
- Job Skill activities, which are outlined at the beginning of the chapter under "Performance Objectives in the *Workbook*."

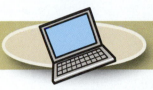

COMPUTER ASSIGNMENT

To review the concepts you have learned in this chapter, insert the *Student Practice* CD-ROM into a computer and work through the *StudyWARE* activities and games. Answer review questions in the practice mode and read the feedback, studying the questions you have missed. Take the chapter quiz until you achieve a minimum score of 90 percent. Successfully completing the *Critical Thinking Challenge* at the end of this course will help you think through scenarios and develop problem solving skills.

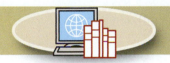

RESOURCES

Internet

Find Articles
Locate topics of interest by searching using **key terms** such as Alzheimer patients, geriatric patients, breast cancer, and so forth.
Web site: http://findarticles.com

National Organizations

Alzheimer's Association
225 North Michigan Avenue, Floor 17
Chicago, IL 60601
(800) 272-3900
Web site: http://www.alz.org

American Association of Retired Persons (AARP)
601 East Street NW
Washington, DC 20049
(888) 687-2277
Web site: http://www.aarp.org

American Cancer Society, Inc.
1599 Clifton Road NE
Atlanta, GA 30329
(404) 320-3333 (800) ACS-2345 (227-2345)
Web site: http://www.cancer.org

American Diabetes Association
1701 North Beauregard Street
Alexandria, VA 22311
(800) 342-2383
Web site: http://www.diabetes.org

American Foundation for the Blind (AFB)
11 Penn Plaza, Suite 300
New York, NY 10001
(800) 232-3044
Web site: http://www.afb.org

American Heart Association
7572 Greenville Avenue
Dallas, TX 75231
(800) 242-8721
Web site: http://www.americanheart.org

American Lung Association
61 Broadway, 6th Floor
New York, NY 10006
(800) LUNGUSA (586-4872)
Web site: http://www.lungusa.org

American Society on Aging (ASA)
833 Market Street, Suite 511
San Francisco, CA 94103-1824
(800) 537-9728
Web site: http://www.asaging.org

Arthritis Foundation Information Line
   PO Box 7669
   Atlanta, GA 30357
   (800) 568-4045
   Web site: http://www.arthritis.org
Asthma & Allergy Foundation Hotline
   1233 20th Street NW, Suite 402
   Washington, DC 20036
   (800) 7ASTHMA (727-8462)
   Web site: http://www.aafa.org
Center for Disease Control
   (800) 232-4636
   Some Topics Covered:
   AIDS
   Autism
   Birth Defects
   Cancer
   Developmental Disabilities
   Diabetes
   Fetal Alcohol Syndrome
   HIV
   Neuro Tube Defects
   Nutrition
   Sexually Transmitted Diseases
   Smoking
Meals on Wheels Association of America (MOWAA)
   Click: "Find a Local Program by City and State"
   203 South Union Street
   Alexandria, VA 22314
   (703) 548-5558
   Web site: http://www.mowaa.org
National Association of Nutrition and Aging Services
Programs (NANASP)
   Search: Nutrition provider in local area:
   (800) 677-1116
   1612 K Street NW, Suite 400
   Washington, DC 20006
   (202) 223-2099
National Center for Elder Abuse (NCEA)
   1201 15th Street, NW Suite 350
   Washington, DC 20005-2800
   (202) 898-2586
   Web site: http://www.elderabusecenter.org

National Clearinghouse on Alcohol & Drug
Information Hotline
Department of Health and Human Services
Substance Abuse and Mental Health Services
Administration (SAMHSA)
   (800) 729-6686
   Web site: http://www.health.org
National Council on the Aging
   300 D Street SW, Suite 801
   Washington, DC 20024
   (202) 479-1200
   Web site: http://www.ncoa.org
National Federation for the Blind
   1800 Johnson Street
   Baltimore, MD 21230
   (410) 659-9314
   Web site: http://www.nfb.org
National Institute on Deafness & Other
Communication Disorders
   1 Communication Avenue
   Bethesda, MD 20892-3456
   (800) 241-1044 TTY (800) 241-1055
   Web site: http://www.nidcd.nih.gov
National Kidney Foundation
   30 East 33rd Street
   New York, NY 10016
   (800) 622-9010
   Web site: http://www.kidney.org
National Mental Health Association
   2000 N Beauregard Street, 6th floor
   Alexandria, VA 22311
   (703) 684-7722
   Web site: http://www.nmha.org
National Stroke Association
   9707 East Easter Lane
   Englewood, CO 80112
   (800) STROKES (787-6537)
   Web site: http://www.stroke.org

CHAPTER 6

Telephone Procedures

OBJECTIVES

After reading this chapter and learning step-by-step procedures to gain job skills,* you should be able to:

Learning Objectives

- Communicate effectively over the telephone.
- Operate a 12-button touch-tone telephone.
- State how a cellular telephone is useful in keeping the office in contact with the physician.
- Describe different types of telephone services that can be used in a medical office.
- Place calls using proper telephone guidelines.
- Explain telephone screening and triage protocols.
- Respond appropriately to callers who have specific questions.

Performance Objectives (Procedures) in This Textbook

- Prepare and leave a voice mail message (Procedure 6-1).
- Take messages from an answering service (Procedure 6-2).
- Answer incoming telephone calls (Procedure 6-3).
- Place outgoing telephone calls (Procedure 6-4).
- Identify and manage emergency calls (Procedure 6-5).
- Handle a complaint from an angry caller (Procedure 6-6).

Performance Objectives (Job Skills) in the *Workbook*

- Screen incoming telephone calls (Job Skill 6-1).
- Prepare telephone message forms (Job Skill 6-2).
- Document telephone messages and physician responses (Job Skill 6-3).

This textbook and the accompanying Workbook meet the entry-level administrative and general competencies for the CMA outlined by CAAHEP and ABHES.

OUTLINE WITH LECTURE NOTES

Communication by Telephone

_____
_____
_____
_____

Telephone Equipment

_____
_____
_____

Touch-Tone Telephone

_____
_____
_____
_____

Cellular Telephone

_____
_____
_____
_____

Pager

_____
_____
_____
_____

Telephone Services
Speed Dialing

_____
_____
_____
_____

Redialing

_____
_____
_____
_____

Call Forwarding

_____
_____
_____
_____

Call Waiting

_____
_____
_____
_____

Caller ID

_____
_____
_____
_____

Speakerphone

_____
_____
_____
_____

Automated Attendant

_____
_____
_____
_____

Voice Mail

_____
_____
_____
_____

Answering Service

_____
_____
_____
_____

Answering Machine

_____
_____
_____
_____

Special Features

_____
_____
_____
_____

Telephone Policies and Procedures

Telephone Guidelines

_____
_____
_____
_____

Telephone Polices in Patient Information Booklet

_____
_____
_____
_____

Telephone Screening and Triage

_____
_____
_____
_____

Telephone Policies in Office Procedure Manual

_____
_____
_____
_____

Responses to Typical Telephone Calls

_____
_____
_____
_____

Waiting on Line

_____
_____
_____
_____

Callbacks

_____
_____
_____
_____

Receiving Telephone Calls and Messages

Telephone Message Slips

_____
_____
_____

_____

Telephone Logs

_____
_____
_____
_____

Computerized Telephone Messages

_____
_____
_____
_____

Special Telephone Calls

Long Distance

_____
_____
_____
_____

Toll Calls

_____
_____
_____
_____

Conference Calls

_____
_____
_____
_____

International Communications

_____
_____
_____
_____

Telephone Reference Aids

Callback List

_____
_____
_____

KEY TERMS

answering service
callbacks
cellular telephone
conference call
emergency care
pager
protocol
screening
speakerphone

telecommunication
telephone decision grid
telephone log
telephone reference aid
toll call
triage
urgent care
voice mail

HEART OF THE HEALTH CARE PROFESSIONAL

Service

The telephone becomes a lifeline to a patient calling in distress. The medical assistant who handles telephone calls can assist in calming the patient and serves as the vital link between the patient and the physician.

COMMUNICATION BY TELEPHONE

The most important public relations responsibility of the medical assistant is to place, receive, and screen telephone calls for the physician in a friendly, efficient, and courteous manner. In fact, it has been said that telephone technique can mean the success or failure of a medical practice (Figure 6-1).

Good listening habits and the ability to interact verbally are two of the most important communication skills demanded of the administrative medical assistant. They become routine only with continued practice. Two exercises that can help develop them are role-playing and tape-recording a conversation and relistening to it to evaluate voice tone, inflection, and clarity. The assistant should cultivate a cheerful and calm voice, speaking as courteously over the telephone as in face-to-face conversation. The manner in which the assistant speaks will determine the caller's response. Listen carefully and take into account patients' limitations. Use the appropriate tone of voice,

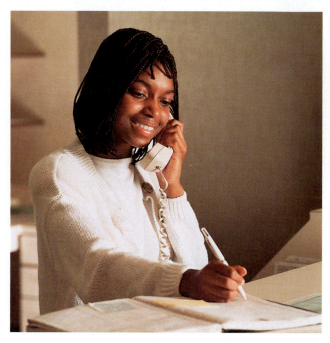

Figure 6-1. An administrative medical assistant pleasantly greeting the patient, with a smile in her voice, via the telephone

PATIENT EDUCATION

An effective medical assistant informs patients of office hours and direct extension numbers to conduct business. Patients should be encouraged to call the office during designated hours and given directions on where to call if an emergency arises.

with no inflections at the end of sentences—this will give the caller the assurance that his or her needs will be taken care of.

TELEPHONE EQUIPMENT

To telecommunicate is to transmit voice or data over a distance. The medical office assistant should periodically determine if the office is utilizing the most efficient and cost-effective **telecommunication** devices available. There is a continual need for this because telephones and services change frequently and there is a constant introduction of new equipment. Telephone companies and electronic supply businesses will demonstrate and assess the telephone demands of the office. Choice of a telephone system depends on the number of telephone calls the office makes and receives daily, and the number of physicians and staff using the equipment. A multiphysician clinic in a city would need more telephone lines than a one-doctor office in a rural location.

Touch-Tone Telephone

The standard *12-button touch-tone telephone* is arranged with 10 buttons (digits 0–9) plus 2 special buttons, a * (star) and a # (pound), that activate automatic electronic features. As each button is pressed, a tone indicates the number has been sent to the central office equipment.

This type of telephone may also accommodate multiple lines and have additional buttons that may be pressed to place a call, hold a call, transfer a call, signal, or access other office extensions (Figure 6-2). A steady button light indicates a line is in use and a flashing light indicates a line is on hold.

Wireless Headset

A telephone accessory that reduces telephone fatigue and allows you to be more productive is the wireless headset. It allows mobility so you can work, walk, and talk with both hands free. Another benefit is eliminating the need to wedge a telephone receiver between your ear and shoulder, which may result in acute neck, shoulder, upper back, and arm pain.

Cellular Telephone

A **cellular telephone** is a wireless telephone that communicates through cell sites (antenna towers). The caller and receiver are automatically transferred from cell to cell as they travel. Mountainous or airport

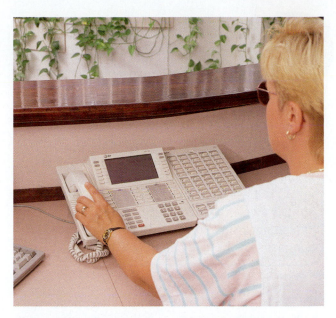

Figure 6-2. Example of a multiline telephone system

areas may cause signal interference. Cellular phone usage has become more popular and some households now have only cellular telephones and no landline phones.

A cellular phone can be purchased, leased, or rented and may or may not require installation in a vehicle depending on whether it is permanently installed or a portable unit. Hands-free operation is a must for the physician who takes calls in the car. Features can include last number redial or automatic redial, a name and telephone number directory for recalling telephone numbers, digital camera, and text messaging, as well as other options. Some cellular telephones require minutes purchased via the Internet or by purchasing a minute card. Or one can subscribe to a privately run service that has monthly fees. Their charges usually vary according to the number of incoming and outgoing calls as well as the time each call is made (on-peak or off-peak hours).

COMPLIANCE

Cellular signals are not secure, which means that other people may be able to listen to the conversations with a scanning radio. Therefore, staff and physicians should be very careful *not* to use patients' full names or reveal any confidential information when using a cellular phone.

COMPLIANCE

Health care providers are permitted to talk with others even if there is a possibility of being overheard. It is permissible to discuss a patient's condition or laboratory test results over the telephone, in a joint treatment area, or in a semi-private room with the patient, a provider, or a family member. When sharing protected health information (PHI) in these situations, use lowered voices or talk away from others. Exceptions include emergency situations, loud emergency rooms, or cases involving the hearing impaired.

Physicians have found cellular telephones to be the best tool for maintaining constant contact with their office staff and hospital personnel. The phones may be used during an emergency, to place prescription calls to a pharmacy, or to check office telephone messages without the usual office interruptions.

Pager

A **pager** is used as a means of transferring a message from one person to another using a telephone as a transmission source and a pager as the receiver. This small, handheld mobile, one-way communication device is often referred to as a "cordless personal answering machine." Pagers are used when a ringing telephone would not be appropriate and when privacy is required. The medical assistant may need to contact a physician who is on hospital rounds or who is attending a luncheon business meeting; the caller merely dials the pager number and the pager carried by the doctor beeps or vibrates. Some pagers have signal lights that flash and/or display small alphanumeric messages. The physician then uses his or her cellular telephone or preferably proceeds to a nearby telephone to return a call to the office that sent the message.

Confidentiality and privacy are better ensured when pagers are used because the physician may leave the location quietly without interruption. Then a conversation may be conducted in a private location.

TELEPHONE SERVICES

A number of telephone services are available and competition between telephone companies has increased availability of these services. Following are some of the basic services that may be encountered either in the medical office or while calling patients.

Speed Dialing

Most telephones are equipped with a *speed dialing* feature. This component electronically stores telephone numbers so that at the touch of a button or a one- or two-digit code, frequently-used numbers or pagers are directly dialed. The medical assistant, with the physician's input, may determine the most commonly dialed numbers to program them into the telephone memory. This listing can be retrieved from memory and displayed for quick access.

Redialing

An automatic *redialing* feature electronically stores the last telephone number dialed, which may be redialed by the push of a button. This redial feature may monitor a busy number for 30 minutes and alert you when the call may be put through.

Call Forwarding

A *call forwarding* feature allows all incoming calls to be automatically directed to another internal station, an outside telephone number, or to voice mail when no one is available to answer the telephone. This service may be turned on and off by dialing a sequence of numbers using activity keys.

Special call forwarding has the capacity to forward 12 preselected numbers within your service area to the telephone where you can be reached. All other calls ring as usual and may be routed to voice mail or an answering machine.

Call Waiting

Call waiting service is only for single-line telephone systems, which allows the single line to be used as a two-line phone. When using the telephone and another person calls, you hear a beep or click. By depressing the flash key (or receiver quickly), you switch to the other caller while the first caller remains on the line. You may switch back using the same method. Most medical offices do not have call waiting because their systems are multiline. A cancel call waiting feature allows you to override call waiting before you place a call so your call will not be interrupted, or before you use the Internet so you can remain connected.

Caller ID

Caller ID reveals the name and telephone number of the caller in a display panel on the telephone or separate display unit before the call is answered. If you need to return a call because you are disconnected or did not obtain the caller's number, or if an emergent patient cannot give you that information, then this feature is helpful. If your system does not have this feature, most local telephone companies provide automatic call return when you dial *69, which dials the last incoming telephone number whether it is answered or not.

Speakerphone

Most telephones have a **speakerphone.** This feature offers hands-free conversation without holding a receiver by using a built-in microphone and speaker. This feature is activated by pushing a button, then the volume may be adjusted. There are many advantages to this feature: (1) it is possible to take notes, search for a record in a file, or handle patient charts with both hands while speaking on the phone, (2) it allows you to continue working when placed on hold awaiting an answer, and (3) it allows a group of people to talk using one telephone. However, it is not good policy to initially answer calls using the speaker because it infringes on the caller's privacy, often provides a weak connection, and changes the voice quality.

COMPLIANCE

Etiquette requires that the medical assistant ask whether the caller wishes the call to be on a speakerphone. Medical ethics requires confidentiality. The caller may not want to have the conversation overheard because it may be a private matter.

Automated Attendant

Some busy medical practices choose to use an automated answering system that allows all calls to be answered immediately, without busy signals or waiting on hold. The *auto-attendant*, which is voice activated, eliminates those problems by routing calls to the appropriate person, such as the appointment scheduler, insurance biller, and so forth. Some patients have physical or sensory problems that make using auto-attendant difficult. The option of pressing "0" or saying "customer service" and reaching a live person should always be available.

An automated answering system can offer a menu in several languages. To get the most use out of an automated system, both staff and patients must accept it and use it properly. Following are suggestions for implementing such a system.

1. Advise patients in writing about the new system and how it works.

2. Instruct patients clearly on how to select options.

3. Give callers the option to select "medical emergency" right after the medical practice is identified; otherwise a medical malpractice claim could result.

4. Provide useful options such as "to schedule, change, or cancel an appointment . . . ," to speak to the billing office . . . ," to refill a prescription . . . ," and so forth.

5. Allow the option of leaving a message for the physician, but do not provide the option of speaking directly to the physician. A staff person can take messages and relay them to the doctor without messages slipping through the cracks.

6. Maintain a separate telephone line with an unlisted number for use by other physicians, the hospital staff, and physician personal calls.

Voice Mail

Voice mail is a type of answering system used to store and forward messages. It combines the technology of a telephone, a computer, and a recording device for the storage of one-way messages to be delivered immediately or at a later time. The purpose of voice mail is to leave a personal message for someone who is unavailable. Access to the system may be either an automatic connect or involves entering a code on a dial or touch-tone telephone. A recording tells the caller to dial the voice mail number of the recipient and to speak after a beep. The system converts the message into digital form. If the message cannot be delivered, it is stored in the computer's memory for later delivery. When the recipient dials into the system to receive the message, the caller's voice is reconverted into voice form and the message is relayed. When the party is not in, always ask the caller whether he or she would like to be connected to voice mail. Voice mail can be an effective way to leave detailed and more complex messages. It allows the medical assistant or other staff members to pick up messages when not busy.

Make sure the voice mail set-up has no more than four or five options for mailboxes. These options may be appointment scheduling, insurance and billing, clinical medical assistant, and prescription refills. Voice mail numbers may be printed on the monthly statement or given to frequent callers such as pharmacists, pharmaceutical representatives, relatives, or business callers. Another option might be to give frequent callers a phone number that bypasses the normal menus and puts callers speedily in contact with the mailbox they wish to reach, such as a special pharmacy line. All nonappointment callers could be encouraged to use the voice mail system after they have been advised that the special number will provide faster assistance.

To reduce telephone traffic to the receptionist, consider voice mail as a backup for receiving messages from callers. An example of a typical voice mail message, activated on the fourth ring when the assistant is away from the desk, might be: "This is Dr. Practon's office. I'm sorry we are away from the desk. Please leave a message after the beep with your name and phone number and we will return your call shortly. Thank you." When a call comes to the pharmacy line of a clinic, the message might be: "This is the pharmacy line, which will be monitored at 9 a.m., 11 a.m., 1 p.m., and 3 p.m. If your call is urgent, call 654-7150 or, if an emergency, call 911. Please leave a message with your name, telephone number, the medication you wish to fill or refill, and your choice of pharmacy. Start your message after the beep. Thank you."

Voice Mail Guidelines

If the medical office records voice mail greetings for incoming calls, instructions must be clear to be effective. Review these suggestions before recording greetings:

- Keep the recorded instruction menu short and update the greeting regularly.

- Indicate who to call in the event of an emergency.

- Make certain the calling party can select zero to quickly reach an actual person.

- Ask an employee with a pleasant voice to record the outgoing message.

- Specify in the message when calls will be received and/or returned.

- If the system has an extension directory, be certain it can be verified with the caller before forwarding the call. Example: "You have reached Dr. Practon's office, extension 567. If this selection is correct, please press star." This will prevent the caller from being connected to the wrong person.

- For after-hours medically related calls, record a special night message that goes into effect at the close of the day and tells the caller what steps to take.

Leaving a Voice Mail Message

The medical assistant should also be aware of steps to take when preparing to place a telephone message to a medical facility or patient with a voice mail or answer machine (see Example 6-1).

EXAMPLE 6-1

Answering Machine Message

"This is Jane from Dr. Practon's office and we are trying to contact Glen. Please call our office at (555) 486-9002 (repeat number twice) today if possible (give date). If Glen is unable to return the call today, please tell him that we called and would like him to return our call as soon as possible. Thank you."

Answering Service

Most physicians contract with a telephone **answering service** to personalize and handle medical calls when the office is closed. Although some medical offices use an answering service during the lunch hour, a staggered lunch hour is preferable. Unlike automatic answering, the answering service operator can execute the physician's telephone directions and be of assistance to patients. A service is usually hired to relay messages and to forward emergency calls after hours and on weekends. The selection of a competent answering service is very important because charges of negligence can be made by patients against a physician if messages are not transmitted or are incorrectly

PROCEDURE 6-1

Prepare and Leave a Voice Mail Message

Objective: To leave a voice mail message.

Equipment/Supplies: Telephone, message pad, and pen or pencil.

Directions: Follow these step-by-step directions, which include rationales, to learn this procedure. Exercises are presented throughout the *Workbook* to enhance this skill for future practice.

1. Write down and plan the message before placing the call, assuming in advance that the caller cannot be reached.

2. Give your name, the name of the medical practice, and the date and time.

3. State your telephone number *twice* (slowly) because network noise may garble one of the numbers and the person receiving the call may not be able to return the call.

4. Speak clearly and slowly, sounding conversational rather than automatic.

5. Make the message brief and simple, avoiding details and humorous remarks. Never reveal any health information when leaving a voice message.

6. Specify a time when a return call may be received.

COMPLIANCE

Telephone Voice Mail Confidentiality

The office staff should be aware of some major confidentiality concerns when using voice mail to convey messages. There are safe and unsafe ways to leave a message on a patient's home telephone. Following are some examples:

1. When leaving a message confirming an appointment with a specialist such as an oncologist or cardiologist, the identification of the type of procedure may reveal a lot about the patient and his or her medical problem. In this situation, say, "This is Erma from Dr. Practon's office. Please have Marjorie call me at (555) 486-9002."

2. When leaving a voice mail message about laboratory test results, the assistant might say, "(Patient's name) test results are in; please contact our office." This guarantees that someone other than the patient will not hear the actual test results that the patient may not want divulged.

3. Caution needs to be taken when leaving a message for a patient to call the office regarding highly confidential information. To ensure the person being spoken to is the patient, some practices assign each patient a personal identification code known only to the practice and patient. Then, to get any test results, the patient must first give his or her identification code. By following this protocol, there is a reasonable balance between the protection of confidentiality and meeting the patient's need to access personal information without having to make an office appointment.

4. Patients may be requested to sign an authorization to release the electronic transfer of information, acknowledging that the telephone might not be secure.

5. Numerous software systems have been designed to maximize the use of the office telephone. One system provides individual test results and follow-up advice recorded by the physician for 24-hour accessibility. Confidentiality is ensured because each patient is assigned a special telephone number to reach the message.

STEP 1 2 3

PROCEDURE 6-2

Take Messages from an Answering Service

Objectives: To retrieve, record, and assess the importance of messages from an answering service.

Equipment/Supplies: Telephone, message pad or telephone log, and pen or pencil.

Directions: Follow these step-by-step directions, which include rationales, to learn this procedure.

1. Call the answering service and check for messages as soon as the office opens or reopens. Callers expect responses to messages as soon as a business opens.

2. Identify yourself and the practice and say you are calling to obtain messages.

3. Record the messages in the order given.

4. Write down complete information for each message on a message pad or telephone log (name of caller, business affiliation, date, time of call, reason for the call, and home, work, and/or cellular telephone number including area code) so action can be taken and/or return calls made.

5. Confirm the correct spelling of all names and repeat any information that you are unsure of for clarification.

6. Prioritize the messages and deal with urgent calls at once and then respond or route the rest of the calls.

7. Pull medical records for clinical calls from patients and put the messages and charts in the proper location for staff or physician to respond to.

---

transmitted. To verify that the service is relaying messages and doing the job satisfactorily, a physician might periodically call his or her own office number from another telephone. The Yellow Pages of the telephone directory list the names of answering services, and recommendations from other physicians can help determine a reliable service. Since contract fees for a service are based on a predetermined number of calls per month, it is imperative that the medical assistant contact the service immediately upon arrival in the mornings to avoid additional charges.

Answering Machine

The use of a telephone *answering machine* in the medical office is not recommended because an anxious caller needs comforting through personal contact. Usually a new patient will not leave a message. However, if the office uses a machine, the caller should be asked to include not only his or her name and home, work, and/or cellular telephone number but also the date and time of the call to verify that the return call has been made within a specific period. The answering machine is a convenience that obligates a return call as soon as possible.

Special Features

Telephones are not only electronic, but now use digital technology and can be programmed to perform a variety of services such as transferring a call to another extension, placing a call at a set time, notifying the user when a previously dialed busy line is open, intercepting calls going to another extension, storing and then activating frequently called numbers, and routing long-distance calls through the most cost-efficient lines. Another service is call-block, which lets you stop 12 callers within your service area from reaching your telephone. The caller receives a recording that you are not taking calls at this time.

TELEPHONE POLICIES AND PROCEDURES

Training employees in, and advising patients of, telephone policies and procedures is part of the foundation of a medical office. Management consultants have determined that telephone calls to the medical office can be reduced by as much as 30 percent if patients understand the phone rules, particularly if the procedures have been outlined in an information booklet. In order to establish telephone policies and procedures, the following questions must be answered:

1. Who will answer telephone calls and who is the back-up person?

2. What are the designated times for patients to call the office?

3. What type of calls will the physician accept when in the office or when busy seeing patients?

4. How will calls be handled when the physician is out of the office or out of town?

5. Will patients be allowed to use the office telephone?

6. What phrase will be used when answering the telephone to identify the medical practice and person answering?

7. How soon will the telephone be answered and how will calls be placed on hold?

8. How will messages be taken?

9. When will the physician and other personnel return calls?

A number of medical practices are increasing their phone availability by answering phones one-half to one hour before the office opens, during the lunch hour, and one-half to one hour after closing time. This should be decided after analyzing patient calling patterns. Depending on the type of specialty, patients may be more likely to call early in the morning (e.g., OB-GYN, pediatrics, family practice), during the lunch hour (e.g., internal medicine) or late in the day. A telephone traffic study can be done by simply designing a sheet with spaces for 8 a.m. to 9 a.m., 9 a.m. to 10 a.m., and so forth; a separate sheet should be made for each day. Check off times when calls are received. Heavy traffic days and hours are best determined when the study is in place for at least six weeks. The practice may experience seasonal peaks and a high volume of calls after billing statements are sent out.

Telephone Guidelines

Because appointment scheduling requires asking multiple questions, many practices have found that it is best to move the phone responsibilities and/or appointment scheduling away from the reception desk. Answering the telephone and placing outgoing calls are job skills a medical assistant must master. By practicing Procedures 6-3 and 6-4 you will develop

expertise and competence in professional and efficient telephone communication.

Telephone Polices in Patient Information Booklet

The telephone section of a Patient Information Booklet outlining office policies might include:

1. Office hours

2. Telephone number patients should call when the office is closed

3. Who to call in a medical emergency

4. Designated hours during which the physician will return patient calls

5. Medical instructions and/or fee when treatment is given by telephone

6. Physician's policy on diagnosing and approving prescription refills by telephone

7. Protocol the patient should follow for laboratory test results, for example, call the office or wait to hear from the physician

8. Telephone extension to call for specific business matters, such as questions about insurance, financial accounts, or authorizations

Telephone Screening and Triage

The key to effective telephone control lies in formulating a plan for channeling and prioritizing calls, known as **screening**. Screening involves asking good questions and then following a standardized plan to route calls to the proper person. The physician usually indicates to the medical assistant his or her preference with regard to the transfer of calls. A **telephone decision grid** will guide the assistant as calls are screened and transferred (Table 6-1 on page 170). Follow the steps in the screening process to determine what action to take.

PATIENT EDUCATION

Patients should be given a booklet that outlines office telephone policies and procedures. Advise patients that telephone guidelines are included in this booklet and instruct them according to their level of understanding.

STEP 1 2 3

PROCEDURE 6-3

Answer Incoming Telephone Calls

Objectives: To answer the telephone in a physician's office in a proficient manner, take action, and accurately record messages.

Equipment/Supplies: Telephone, notepad, appointment book, and pen or pencil.

Directions: Follow these step-by-step directions, which include rationales, to learn this skill. Exercises are presented throughout the *Workbook* to enhance this skill for future practice on the job.

1. Answer an incoming telephone call before the third ring. A telephone that cannot be answered quickly may indicate inadequate staffing or a low priority toward incoming calls. The caller may hang up if the call is not answered in a reasonable amount of time.

2. Smile when answering the telephone and use a friendly, low-pitched voice with the mouthpiece held about an inch from the lips. This procedure aids the caller in clearly hearing your message.

3. Identify the office and yourself (Example 6-2). Most people do not hear the first couple of words so use a few buffer words to help avoid questions by the caller about what office they have reached. By identifying yourself, you will make the patient feel more comfortable and will inform him or her of whom to ask for in future calls.

4. Obtain the identity of the caller with his or her home, work, and/or cell number. Do not answer questions from people who cannot be identified with certainty. Try not to use one-word responses as this indicates a lack of interest.

5. Repeat the caller's name during the conversation to show attentiveness and personalize the call.

6. Stay alert to what is being said, identify emergency calls, offer assistance, transfer calls when appropriate, and take a message when necessary. Repeat the message to the caller to confirm the facts are accurate and complete. This reduces errors.

7. Be pleasant and friendly, but not too familiar. Speak in a natural, conversational tone and manner. The caller should never feel the call is an intrusion, rushed, or unimportant.

8. Pause for emphasis, avoiding monotone delivery. Speak distinctly and be expressive, pronouncing words carefully.

9. Use the words "please" and "thank you" often.

10. Be prepared to repeat or spell words when speaking to an elderly patient.

11. Use proper hold techniques if a second call should come in on another line. Politely ask the first caller to hold one moment while the other ringing line is answered. Use a notepad to jot down the name and which line the caller is on. Never put an emergency call on hold.

12. After the second caller has been identified, prioritize the two callers—an emergency

---

EXAMPLE 6-2

Answering the Telephone

Single Physician

A. "Good morning [or afternoon], Dr. Practon's office, Joan Miller speaking."

B. Good morning [or afternoon], Dr. Practon's office. This is Joan Miller, may I help you?"

Multi-Physician Office

C. "Good morning [or afternoon], doctor's office."

D. "Practon Medical Group."

PROCEDURE 6-3 *continued*

(1st), long-distance (2nd), or short-message (3rd). Never leave the caller waiting on the telephone without an explanation or without identifying the caller as it may be another physician or your employer/physician; offer to call the patient back if a delay of more than three to five minutes is anticipated.

13. Screen calls carefully, and do not be tempted to bend the truth to protect a busy schedule; just say, "The doctor is unavailable."

14. Direct any call of a clinical nature to a clinical medical assistant who can obtain pertinent facts and either relay the message or route the call to the appropriate physician.

15. Avoid comments and discussions with others while the caller is on the line; this conveys a lack of interest.

16. End the telephone call in a pleasant manner by asking if there are any other questions and thanking the caller using his or her name. By concluding the call in this manner, it conveys professionalism and gives the caller a positive image of the office. Let the caller hang up before you disconnect and replace the receiver gently.

17. Follow through on messages routing them to the proper person or department. Do not put the message on the physician's desk if it is important and needs action or if the physician will not be in the office that day. Carry through with some predetermined action or follow-up procedure.

STEP 1 2 3

PROCEDURE 6-4

Place Outgoing Telephone Calls

Objective: To place outgoing telephone calls in a physician's office in a proficient manner.

Equipment/Supplies: Telephone, notepad, reference documents (test results and/or patient's medical record), and pen or pencil.

Directions: Follow these step-by-step directions, which include rationales, to learn this skill. Exercises are presented throughout the *Workbook* to enhance this skill for future practice on the job.

1. Ask patients whether messages can be left at their residence or work and how to do so. Consider developing a form with a list of check-off possibilities, then have the patient sign it and follow his or her preferences.

2. Follow established callback routines at prescheduled times. The physician may choose certain times of the day to return calls to eliminate "telephone tag"; that is, calls being made and returned without the parties being able to reach each other. Calls to outside laboratories may be placed in the morning before the office gets busy with patients; calls regarding prescription refills or for appointment reminders may be made at slow times during the day or at the end of the day.

3. Plan the conversation and gather important papers (financial documents and/or patient's chart) for reference before placing the call.

4. Identify yourself and the office immediately when the party answers the telephone.

5. Identify party at other end.

6. Speak in a congenial but businesslike manner.

7. End each call in a friendly manner and let the other party hang up first.

Table 6-1. Telephone Decision Grid

Type of call	Refer to Physician at Once	Physician to Return Call	Refer to Clinical Personnel: RN, LPN, PA, NP, CMA, RMA	Medical Assistant Takes Action
Acute Illness				
Unconscious, in shock	X			
High fever, vomiting	X			
Severe pain	X			
Heavy bleeding	X			
Reaction to medication/injection	X			
Sudden change in patient's condition	X			
Sudden onset of critical symptoms (chest pain, acute shortness of breath)	X			
Routine				
Appointments				X
Appointment, needs physician's response		X		
New patient, ill, wants to speak to physician		X		
Patient under treatment, needs physician's response		X		
Patient's family requests information		X		
Request for consultation				X
Referral from another physician				X
Colleague wants to speak to physician	X	X		
Patient requests lab results		X	X	
Pharmacy regarding new prescription		X	X	
Patient or pharmacy regarding prescription refill		X	X	
Insurance company, attorney request for patient information				X
Hospital regarding patient (depends on which department)	X	X	X	X
Nonmedical				
Business calls for physician's attention: CPA, attorney, broker, medical society		X		
Pharmaceutical representative				X
Patient account information				X
Personal calls from physician's family members	X	X		

RN = registered nurse
LPN = licensed practical nurse
PA = physician's assistant
NP = nurse practitioner
CMA = certified medical assistant
RMA = registered medical assistant

1. Gather identifying information; identify caller (name and age), relationship to patient, and health plan information.

2. Record what the caller tells you; use quotes, for example, "I have severe stomach pain."

3. Record patient statements regarding objective measures, such as what the patient sees, hears, or records (blood pressure, temperature, and so on).

4. Record your actions and the patient's compliance with the action plan.

5. If the call is transferred to a clinician, relay basic information.

6. Sign your name with credentials.

7. Document the conversation in the patient's medical record (see Chapter 9).

The administrative medical assistant who answers the telephone may also be involved in telephone **triage**. *Triage* literally means to sort things out. Telephone triage involves conducting an oral interview to access a patient's health status and to offer treatment or referral. Establishing a good triage system will free up physicians' time and optimize constructive time spent on patient calls by determining whether patients need to be seen today, tomorrow, at a later date, or treated at home. Three levels of triage have been established to assure accurate decision making (Table 6-2). The risk factors of telephone triage should be identified, strategies need to be established, the triage levels must be understood, and telephone **protocols** (reference instructions) must be followed. All medical decisions are made by the physician and only by following a strict protocol put in place by the doctor would the medical assistant be legally able to make determinations. When performing triage, always document the patient's statement and action taken.

Telephone Policies in Office Procedure Manual

In a physician's office, the telephone policy section of an office procedure manual should summarize directives and suggest scheduling guidelines to help the assistant determine whether and when to schedule an appointment. Any protocol involving assessment of symptoms should be developed and approved by the physician. The medical assistant should be able to determine what action to take after asking three or four pertinent questions.

An alphabetic list of conditions or symptoms is another aid in eliciting the details of a patient's medical complaint. If used, the list should be included in the office procedure manual. Table 6-3 has examples of a sample triage response guide; however, the clinical medical assistant usually manages Level III of the triage process. This level requires following clinical protocols to assess medical conditions and give instructions. About two-thirds of all incoming calls deal with appointments, health insurance inquiries, financial matters, and requests for laboratory test results, most of which can be handled by the administrative medical assistant or transferred to a staff member.

Following are suggestions for the telephone section of an office procedure manual.

1. Make the manual user-friendly; arrange frequently seen medical conditions with symptoms on individual sheets in alphabetic order for quick reference.

2. Define each medical condition at the top of a sheet in a main heading.

3. Determine level of care and write separate paragraphs describing action for each condition, listing emergencies first for an EMS (911) call, followed by situations when a patient should be seen immediately, seen within four hours, seen within 24 hours, and seen within 72 hours.

4. Have physician sign each protocol.

5. Assemble pages in a three-ring notebook for easy replacement or updating; encourage assistants to suggest additions and revisions at staff meetings. Text changes may easily be updated on a computer.

Urgent and Emergent Telephone Calls

There are two types of critical situations requiring medical care that may arise, and it is important to distinguish the difference between them. The first is **urgent care**, also known as after-hours care. This involves an urgent situation requiring treatment of injuries or conditions that need prompt medical attention within 24 hours to prevent serious deterioration of a patient's health, but is not life-threatening.

Table 6-2. Telephone Triage Levels and Risk Factors

Level I:	• Patient problem documented by administrative medical assistant who is competent; competency written. • Policy in place for processing calls. • Physician makes decision based on documentation for a low-risk patient. • Physician or medical assistant calls patient. • Non-clinical staff does not make independent decisions. • No triage protocol.
Level II:	• Patient problem documented by trained clinical staff who questions patient regarding problem. • Information given to physician to review and make decision. • Physician or clinical staff calls patient. • All communication documented, including patient's understanding and willingness to comply. • No triage protocol; well defined triage policies and procedures.
Level III:	• Patient problem documented by clinical staff (a licensed practitioner may be required in some states, e.g., LVN, RN). • Communication skills and written protocol used to determine what instructions are given to patient. • All communication documented; physician to review at later time. • Well defined written triage protocols.
Responsibilities for Non-Clinical Staff— All Three Levels:	• Abide by all procedures. • Posess good communication skills. • Understand how to meet the needs of a patient with an urgent or emergent problem. • Act conservatively; error on the side of caution. • Document patient's understanding; state patient's compliance. • Assist with continuous quality improvement (CQI).
Risk Factors to Consider:	• Cannot visually see patient. • Caller does not give accurate or complete information; it may be misleading. • Caller may not be honest or who they say they are. • Communication problems may not be apparent. • Proper questions may not be asked. • Medical record not accessible to staff. • Documentation not complete. • Staff does not follow policies, procedures, and protocols or act within their scope of practice. • Physician is not consulted appropriately. • Patients get "lost" in system and/or no follow-up provided.
Patients Considered at High Risk:	• Those not seen but make repeated calls. • Those anxious about their symptoms or a child's status. • The very old and very young (elderly, infants, toddlers). • Pregnant patient with concerns. • Self-care home problems. • Those with language barriers or communication problems.

(continues)

Table 6-2 (*continued*). Telephone Triage Levels and Risk Factors

Risk Management Considerations— staff To Understand That They:	• Do not provide medical diagnosis. • Do not provide treatment advice. • Give general health information only; otherwise route to physician. • Are expected to know what to do when situation does not follow exact written protocol. • State who they are, (i.e., telephone screener, triage assistant, triage nurse). • Should not ignore or minimize routine complaints. • End all calls by advising patients to call back if symptoms worsen. • Only put patients on hold after determination is made that they do not have a medical emergency. • Understand triage categories: (1) emergent/life threatening, (2) urgent/potentially life threatening, and (3) non-urgent/non-potentially life threatening. • Document all communication including patient's understanding.

Table 6-3. Telephone Triage Response Guide

Questions to Ask Caller	**Recommendations and Instructions**	**Do Not . . .**
Fracture		
Where is it? How did it happen? When did it happen? Is there a wound? Is there any bleeding? Is there pain upon gentle pressure? Is limb cold, blue, or numb? Is limb unusable?	Carefully immobilize limb as it lays and stop bleeding (see instructions for bleeding). Use cold compresses and elevate limb. Take victim to physician's office (depending on specialty) or hospital emergency room for evaluation, or call ambulance, if multiple fractures, open fracture, or femur fracture.	Do not attempt to set or reduce fracture. Do not clean wound of an open fracture.
Hemorrhage		
Is there an injury? Where is bleeding coming from? Is bleeding profuse or scanty? Is blood bright red, pale, or brownish? Is the person vomiting blood? Is blood squirting rhythmically (as through an artery)? Is patient on blood-thinning medication?	Preferred method is to put direct pressure by hand over a dressing (sanitary napkin, paper towel, clean washcloth) for control of severe bleeding. Elevate above heart. Apply ice. If bleeding does not stop, apply second dressing over first. If bleeding does not stop, apply pressure at pressure points. Keep person lying down and quiet. Have patient taken by ambulance if necessary to hospital emergency room for immediate attention.	Do not use a tourniquet. Do not remove dressing, even if soaked.
Nosebleed		
Has bleeding been heavy? How long has it persisted? Is it associated with an accident?	Press nostrils together for five minutes with cold, damp cloth. Slowly release pressure. Apply cold compresses to forehead, back of neck, and upper lip. Keep victim quiet and sitting in upright position. Apply petroleum jelly with cotton swab to inside of nose at bedtime. Take patient to see physician if bleeding does not stop in 30 minutes.	Do not pack nostrils. Do not tilt victim's head back.
Respiratory Distress		
Is there shortness of breath, chest pain, tightness, a congestion or rash/hives?	Loosen clothing; have victim relax and sit in upright position leaning over. Make an immediate appointment with physician or take victim to hospital emergency room.	Do not give anything by mouth that contains caffeine or alcohol. Avoid smoking. Do not put patient (victim) on back. *(continues)*

Table 6-3. (continued). Telephone Triage Response Guide

Questions to Ask Caller	Recommendations and Instructions	Do Not . . .
Wounds		
Where is injury? How deep is it? How large is it? How did injury happen? What object caused injury? When was last tetanus injection?	Cleanse well with soap and running water. Stop bleeding and cover with sterile dressing. If wound is deep, long, ragged, or in facial area, it may need suturing. A puncture would should be cleansed by physician. Take victim to medical office for possible suturing of wound. If there is hemorrhage, stop bleeding and take victim to office or emergency room of hospital. Update tetanus injection if necessary.	Do not remove large foreign matter; should be done by physician. Do not clean wounds of the skull or apply pressure to skull only.

The second is **emergency care** and is a much more critical situation requiring immediate treatment to avoid putting a person's life in danger. Because time is an important element in handling any critical situation, help should be sought immediately.

It is absolutely essential that the medical assistant understand what to do should an emergency arise. In most urgent and emergent situations, the receptionist would not put the call on hold but would transfer the call to the physician, clinical assistant, registered nurse, or nurse practitioner. A note may be delivered to the physician indicating the caller's name and the nature of the emergency while remaining on the line. Or the call could be transferred immediately to a clinical triage person who could determine the seriousness of the condition and direct the patient to the office, emergency room, or advise them to call an ambulance immediately.

When the physician is not in the office, an on-call physician may handle the emergency or contact may be made to the physician's cellular phone or pager. When the physician is out of town and another doctor is covering in his or her absence, the assistant would notify the substitute physician.

It is recommended that all medical assistants attend a cardiopulmonary resuscitation (CPR) class as well as classes on emergency care offered by the American Red Cross or American Heart Association.

Certain managed care contracts require that a person certified in cardiopulmonary resuscitation (CPR) be on staff. Some medical problems that threaten life are breathing difficulty or choking, head trauma with unconsciousness, uncontrolled bleeding, severe burns, spinal injuries, shock, possible poisoning, bites, and heart attack symptoms such as chest pain. Some less severe problems that need prompt attention are minor fractures, heat exhaustion, and objects in the eye, ear, or nose.

Minor medical problems such as colds, flu, or sore throats are not legitimate medical emergencies unless the patient states that they are. The medical assistant is not the one to decide whether a case is an emergency; the patient usually makes the determination. Yet the assistant might have to stress the need for immediate medical attention in cases where the injured or sick person is unaware of the possible serious consequences. A person suffering with chest pain or having difficulty breathing should be seen immediately because of the possibility of a heart attack; some symptoms of heart attack are similar to indigestion, but this determination cannot be made by telephone. Many times these cases may be seen as hospital emergencies.

Responses to Typical Telephone Calls

The following are typical phone calls and appropriate responses.

Caller Who Fails to Identify Himself or Herself

Always screen incoming callers who request to speak to the physician. Be sure to obtain the name of the caller and the reason for the call (when appropriate). If the caller does not identify himself or herself, possible responses include those in Example 6-3.

Whether it is an incoming or outgoing call, steps should be taken to properly identify the party with

STEP 1 2 3

PROCEDURE 6-5

Identify and Manage Emergency Calls

Objectives: To determine whether a telephone call is an emergency and perform the action necessary to get help for the patient.

Equipment/Supplies: Telephone triage response guide; telephone numbers of emergency rooms, poison control centers, and ambulance services; message pad or telephone log; pen or pencil.

Directions: Follow these step-by-step directions, which include rationales, to learn this skill. Several exercises are presented in the *Workbook* for practice.

1. Allow the caller/patient time to state the problem without interruption.

2. Identify whether the call is regarding an urgent/emergent situation to determine when action should be taken.

3. Maintain a calm, even, low-pitched tone of voice and take deep breaths.

4. Use the caller/patient's name when asking specific questions about the patient. This personalizes your conversation.

5. Ask whether the patient has experienced this same problem at a prior time.

6. Ask what is being done for the patient.

7. Obtain information accurately and as quickly as possible, such as:

    a. Caller/patient's name and location of patient with telephone number (home, work, cell) and address. Obtain this first in case the patient loses consciousness or the caller gets disconnected.

    b. Caller's relationship to the patient if the patient is not calling.

    c. Patient's age.

    d. Patient's symptoms fully explained.

    e. Description of the accident or injury.

    f. Explanation of the patient's current status.

    g. Details of any treatment administered.

8. Read back the information to verify and ensure that you have written it down accurately.

9. Interrupt or transfer the call immediately to the physician, clinical assistant, registered nurse, or nurse practitioner for advice. Never diagnose. If the physician is not in the office, follow established office guidelines for handling the emergency call, which may require one or more of the following:

    a. Transfer the call to the doctor on call, clinical assistant, registered nurse, or nurse practitioner. Never put the caller on hold.

    b. Have the caller remain on the line and dial 911 to obtain an ambulance for the patient. If the patient is the caller in a true emergency, he or she may become too ill (e.g., pass out) and not be capable of following through with a telephone call. Speak to the EMS dispatcher slowly and clearly. Give the name, exact location of the sick or injured person, and the telephone number.

    c. Instruct the patient to go to the nearest emergency room.

    d. Call the poison control center while the patient remains on the line or give the caller the telephone number of the poison control center.

    e. Page the physician.

EXAMPLE 6-3

Responses to Unidentified Caller

A. "I'm sorry, but Dr. Practon has instructed me to announce his callers by name."

B. "I'm sorry, Dr. Practon is unable to take any calls at the moment. If you will leave your name, telephone number, and the reason for the call, I'll have the doctor return your call as soon as possible."

C. "I'm sorry, Dr. Practon has told me that he will be unable to return a call unless the caller has left a name and indicated the nature of the call."

EXAMPLE 6-4

Response to Insurance Questions

A. "Dr. Practon has given me the responsibility of handling health insurance claims, so I'll try to answer your questions, Mr. Acosta."

B. "Mrs. Roberts, may I transfer your call to Betty, who is our insurance billing specialist?"

whom you are speaking. Common questions include the patient's birth date or Social Security number. To ensure only authorized callers receive information, some practices assign code numbers or a password to the patient. The first or last three digits of the patient's account number could be used for this purpose. The patient is then responsible for controling the number/password and is informed that anyone calling with the number/password will be given information. In a suspicious situation where doubt occurs, ask for a call-back number and verify it with the phone number(s) on record. In rare situations you may need to ask for written authorization or ask the patient to fax the medical practice a document for a signature comparison.

Referral Inquiries

When patients call their physician for names of medical specialists, they should be given two or three names or be referred to the local county medical society for assistance. A referral list should be prepared by the physician and made available to the medical assistant for reference.

Insurance Queries

If a patient wants to talk to the physician about medical insurance, the assistant could give one of the responses in Example 6-4.

Prescription Calls

When a patient calls requesting a prescription refill, the assistant needs to know the name of the pharmacy the patient patronizes, the telephone number of the pharmacy if known, the name of the medication, dosage the patient is taking, the number of pills last prescribed, and the prescription number. Usually this information may be obtained from the patient or the chart before the message slip is handed to the physician. In the event the doctor needs to talk to the patient about the renewal or wants the patient to schedule an appointment, the patient's home, work, and/or cellular telephone number should be recorded on the message slip (Figure 6-3). Often office policy instructs the patient to call the pharmacy directly. Refer to Chapter 10 for additional information on this topic.

Caller Who Will Not Terminate Conversation

A medical assistant's office time is precious and if a call turns into a long-winded conversation, it is wise to attempt to bring the call to a close by using one of the responses listed in Example 6-5.

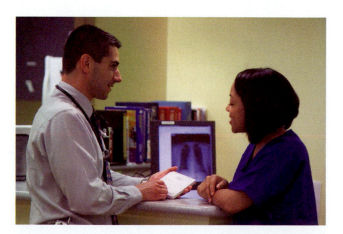

Figure 6-3. Prescription telephone messages that need immediate approval should be directed to the physician between seeing patients

---

EXAMPLE 6-5

Responses to Conclude a Call

A. "Excuse me, I must end this call to help other patients in the office. Could you please call back after 4:30 p.m. Mrs. Smith?"

B. "I'm sorry, Mr. Brown, but Dr. Practon needs me in the office now. Can I call you back?"

C. "I'm sorry, Mrs. Snyder, but I need to assist another patient now."

Angry Caller Concerned about a Bill or Delinquent Account

A call from an angry patient who is concerned about a bill or delinquent account may be avoided if billing practices have been thoroughly discussed at the time of the first office visit. The response to this call involves extreme patience and control and usually is the responsibility of the medical assistant—only in extreme situations would the physician be involved in collection matters. A suggested reply is shown in Example 6-6. See also Procedure 6-6 on page 179.

EXAMPLE 6-6

Response Regarding a Delinquent Account

"Mrs. Black, I'm sorry you are upset about the amount owed on your statement. I'll transfer your call to Roberta, who handles all bookkeeping matters and helps patients make arrangements for settling their accounts."

Inquiries from Outsiders about Patients

Do not divulge medical information about a patient without the patient's signed authorization; refer to the privacy notice. If it is a family member, the call may be transferred to the physician or you may give the response in Example 6-7.

EXAMPLE 6-7

Response to a Request to Divulge Medical Information

"I'm sorry, Mr. King, according to federal laws I'm not able to give you any information without a signed authorization for release by the patient."

When the Physician is Not in the Office

If the call is for a physician who is not in the office, refer the caller to the doctor who is on-call or ask the caller to leave a message. Some responses are listed in Example 6-8.

EXAMPLE 6-8

Response When Physician is Not in Office

A. "Dr. Practon is out of town, and I expect him to return tomorrow. If this is an emergency or urgent, Dr. Benson is on call."

B. "Dr. Practon was delayed at the hospital, but I expect him shortly."

C. "Dr. Practon is not in the office, but I do expect him to call in soon. Would you care to leave a message?"

D. "Dr. Practon is not in the office. If this is an emergency or an urgent matter, Dr. Benson is on call."

When Another Physician Calls

If the call is from another physician, try to put the call through to the doctor or ask if the physician should be interrupted. Example 6-9 shows a possible response.

When the Physician is Busy

If the call is from a patient requesting to speak to the physician and the physician is busy or behind schedule, obtain the home, work, and/or cellular telephone

EXAMPLE 6-9

Response to a Physician

"Dr. Olivas, Dr. Practon is with a patient right now. Would you like me to interrupt him or have him call you back? If you will be discussing one of the doctor's patients, I would be happy to pull the record for Dr. Practon to refer to."

number so a return call can be made later in the day. Example 6-10 shows a possible response.

EXAMPLE 6-10

Response to Patients

"Mrs. Wells, Dr. Practon is with a patient now. However, I realize your call is important so please give me your telephone number and I'll have your chart available for Dr. Practon to refer to. You can expect a return call after 4:00 p.m."

Verifying a Statement Made by the Caller

If you do not receive a clear message, always repeat or rephrase it back to the caller for verification. Use one of the suggested responses in Example 6-11.

EXAMPLE 6-11

Response to Verify a Statement

A. "Will you please repeat that?"

B. "I'm sorry, I didn't hear your name."

C. "Will you spell your name again, please?"

D. "Let me see if I understand what you are saying." Then repeat the statement or rephrase it, giving the patient an opportunity to verify it.

Obscene or Crank Call

If you receive an obscene or crank call, either hang up immediately or respond as shown in Example 6-12.

EXAMPLE 6-12

Response to an Obscene Call

"Are you there, operator? This is the call I asked you to trace—the party is on the line now."

Complaints

When handling complaints, the assistant needs to listen to the entire problem without interruption. This will allow the assistant to determine the best response, offer a solution, and then follow through on any actions promised (Example 6-13). As a general rule, the louder the caller talks, the softer the assistant should reply. A calm, quiet voice may calm the caller and make him or her listen more attentively to what is being said. If unable to meet the patient's request or needs, the assistant should explain the reason and suggest what can be done.

EXAMPLE 6-13

Response to a Complaint

"I'm sorry, no openings are available on Friday, Mr. Daventia, but I will call you if we have a cancellation."

Personal Calls

When personal calls from family or friends come in for you or a coworker, be specific and helpful, discreet, and truthful (Example 6-14). If the caller indicates it is an urgent matter and the person is busy, slip a note in front of them or interrupt politely.

EXAMPLE 6-14

Response to a Personal Call

"I'm sorry Mr. Amberly, but your wife is assisting the physician in a treatment room right now. Can I give her a message as soon as she's through?"

PROCEDURE 6-6

Handle a Complaint from an Angry Caller

Objective: To respond to a complaint from an angry caller in a professional manner while expressing empathy and taking action to resolve the problem.

Equipment/Supplies: Telephone, message pad, and pen or pencil.

Directions: Follow these step-by-step directions, which include rationales, to learn this skill.

1. Identify the person's anger and treat it seriously.

2. Slow down your rate of speech and lower your voice (pitch and volume). This practice soothes and calms the angry caller.

3. Remain calm and take time to listen carefully to the caller's complaint. This allows the caller to express the situation, release built-up feelings, and "get it off his or her chest" without forgetting something or having to repeat information.

4. Let the person have a chance to express anger without feeling rushed. Do not interrupt unless it is a medical emergency that must be taken care of immediately.

5. Do not monopolize the conversation—the angry person often can suggest the most appropriate solution to a problem if given a chance to verbalize it.

6. Change your physical position (stand up) to regain composure and take deep breaths when the irate caller is upsetting you. One cannot combat anger with anger.

7. Repeat the information to verify that you understand the problem or complaint. This procedure lets the caller know you are listening and fully understand the complaint.

8. Express your concern to help and then take action to resolve the problem or complaint.

9. Document the call and complaint on a notepad to be retained for future reference.

10. If you instruct the caller, ask him or her to repeat the instructions. People who are upset or stressed tend not to listen or comprehend parts of important conversation.

11. End the call in a cordial manner, stating what action you will take. Telephone etiquette states that the person who initiates the call should end the call.

12. Report complaint and/or angry callers to the physician or office manager. This is important in the event of litigation by a patient or if the physician wishes to follow up with a telephone call to extend more personal service.

Waiting on Line

Studies show that two-thirds of telephone callers say being put on hold makes them very angry.

A patient who has made an incoming telephone call should not be left waiting on the line. If several lines are ringing and putting someone on hold is unavoidable, identify the caller, ask the person's permission, and do not leave the caller on hold for more than 30 seconds without speaking again, even if it is just to reassure him or her that you have not forgotten the call (Example 6-15). Be appreciative when you return, and if possible, explain briefly to the caller why you must put him or her on hold. If the assistant must locate a medical chart, financial record, or other document, or the information cannot be quickly accessed on the computer, it is best to inform the patient and

---

EXAMPLE 6-15

Responding to a Waiting Caller

Ask permission:	"May I put you on hold for a moment?"
Make it short:	"Thank you for waiting, I'll be right back."
Show appreciation:	"Thank you for your patience."

EXAMPLE 6-16

Helpful Phrases:

"I apologize . . . "

"I want you to know . . . "

"I share your concern . . . "

"If I can be of further help, please let me know . . . "

"Thank you for letting me know about this . . . "

"I hope you find this helpful . . . "

"How may I help you?"

"There was no way to know this would happen."

"I can appreciate how you feel . . . "

"Is there anything you would like me to explain further?"

"I can undertand, Mrs. Arge, why you would be concerned . . . "

"So that you are never inconvenienced in this way again, may I suggest . . . "

"I'm sorry this has happened."

suggest a return call. It is acceptable for the assistant to suggest that the patient wait if it will be difficult to return his or her call and if the patient agrees. If it is foreseen that the wait may be more than five minutes, take the patient's name and number so the call may be returned.

PATIENT EDUCATION

Play educational messages while telephone callers are on hold. Messages may include: office hours, office policies, payment policies, or information on common illnesses that the medical specialist treats.

Callbacks

A designated time for routine **callbacks** that is printed in the information brochure reduces the number of incoming calls, since the patient will know when to expect a return call. Patients appreciate knowing their calls will be returned by the physician at an approximate time. Return calls might be made during the last half hour prior to lunch and at day's end when the answering service can pick up the incoming calls and transfer only the emergency calls to the doctor.

RECEIVING TELEPHONE CALLS AND MESSAGES

To receive telephone calls from patients to the physician and to chart resultant data, the proper procedure is to write messages on callback slips, repositionable adhesive notes (e.g., Post-its) or a telephone log. The message slips may be attached to the front of the patient's charts. Then during free moments or at predetermined times, perhaps before noon and at closing hours, the physician can return calls. After each telephone conversation, the physician can handwrite or dictate short notes to include in the medical record.

All patient telephone calls regarding treatment should be documented in writing and signed by the physician for transfer into the patient's chart.

In a multiphysician office where telephone lines are often busy, transferring telephone-answering responsibilities to the answering service a few minutes before the noon hour and before the end of office hours (with the understanding that all emergency messages will be put through) provides an uninterrupted time to follow through on telephone responses.

Telephone Message Slips

All incoming telephone calls should be documented by recording the date, time, caller's name, home, work, and/or cellular telephone number, reason for the call, and action to be taken. Specialized telephone record pads and booklets are designed in many formats and may be purchased at stationery stores or through medical office supply companies. Message slips with no-carbon-required (NCR) paper are available in wire-bound books. One type of repositionable adhesive message slip with a response portion can be placed on the outside of the patient's chart. After the follow-up call has been made and noted on the message slip, it may be removed from the front of the patient's folder and affixed to either the progress sheet or a telephone message carrier (Figures 6-4 and 6-5).

Telephone Logs

Use of a telephone record book provides a duplicate copy as a permanent chronologic record (**telephone log**); the original with repositionable adhesive may

MESSAGE FROM								
For Dr. *F. Practon*	Name of Caller *Carol Wise*	Rel. to Pt.	Patient *C. Wise*	Pt. Age *37*	Pt. Temp. *101*	Message Date *02.13 XX*	Message Time *3:00* AM PM	Urgent ☐ Yes ☑ No

Message: *HA over both eyes; greenish discharge from nose; cheeks hurt*   Allergies

Respond to Phone # *526-4300*	Best Time to Call *4:00* AM PM	Pharmacy Name / # *Quick Pharm. 526-1010*	Patient's Chart Attached ☑ Yes ☐ No	Patient's Chart # *0326*	Initials *T.F.*

DOCTOR - STAFF RESPONSE

Doctor's / Staff Orders / Follow-Up Action

Dr. suggested appt asap
probably sinusitis - will need Rx AB

Call Back ☑ Yes ☐ No	Chart Mess. ☐ Yes ☐ No	Follow-Up Date / /	Follow-Up Completed-Date/Time *02.13 4:30* AM PM	Response by *F.P.*

Figure 6-4. Repositionable adhesive telephone message slip designed to be shingled on a telephone message carrier sheet or affixed directly to the progress sheet. (Reprinted with permission from Bibbero Systems, Inc. Petaluma, CA. Tel. (800) 242-2376: http://www.bibbero.com.)

PATIENT'S NAME *Robert Mayhew*

ADDRESS *516 So. Palm Temecula*   INSURANCE *Medicare*

TEL. NO. *423-1127*   REFERRED BY *~*   OCCUPATION *retired*   AGE *66*   SEX *M*   S M W D

DATE	SUBSEQUENT VISITS AND FINDINGS
08/03/XX	*Office visit-Difficulty breathing + coughing, pain on*
	inhalation slight rales in LLL, Order CXR
	Advise ibuprofen 2 every 4 hours
	F. Practon, M.D.

PRIORITY ☐ | TELEPHONE RECORD ☎

PATIENT *Robert Mayhew*   AGE *66*

MESSAGE *Pt. Robt Mayhew called to report he's improving — wants results of X-ray*

CALLER *" "*

TELEPHONE *423-1127*

REFERRED TO

TEMP | ALLERGIES

CHART # *4163*

RESPONSE *X-rays negative; continue ibuprofen until pain is resolved. Call back prn.*

CHART ATTACHED ☑ YES ☐ NO

DATE *08/06/XX*   TIME   REC'D BY *W.C.*

PHY-RN INITIALS *C.K.* | DATE *08/06/XX* | TIME *4:00pm* | HANDLED BY *W.C.*

Figure 6-5. Chronologic telephone message record book slip. Duplicate copy remains in permanent record book and original with repositionable adhesive is filed in the patient's chart. (Reprinted with permission from Bibbero Systems, Inc. Petaluma, CA. Tel. (800) 242-2376; http://www.bibbero.com.)

be placed in the patient's chart either on the progress sheet or in chronologic order attached to a telephone message carrier (Figure 6-6). This is known as "shingling." Logs are important for medicolegal reasons, as a reference when patients have unlisted numbers, or when it is necessary to contact a patient on short notice. If a daily log is maintained, the procedure is similar; obtain the patient's name, reason for the call, and home, work, and/or cellular telephone number. Then pull the chart and give both the message and

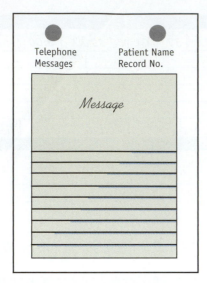
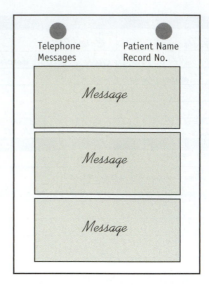

Figure 6-6. Ten telephone messages shingled on a message carrier and a full view of three messages affixed to the carrier

the chart to the physician to prepare answers to questions or requests. Calls in the log that show no action has been taken can be flagged to prevent being overlooked or forgotten.

Computerized Telephone Messages

When working with electronic medical records (EMR), messages can be taken and noted directly in the electronic medical record using word processing software. If it is a message in which action needs to be taken, a manual message can be noted, then the entire message is input and permanently recorded when the course of action has been determined.

SPECIAL TELEPHONE CALLS

The majority of telephone calls are local calls; however, depending on the type of practice and location, other types of calls may also be common. The office manager should periodically have the telephone company monitor the practice's telephone traffic to verify the volume of calls, types of calls, and busy signals received. This will aid the decision making when a telephone service plan must be contracted.

Long Distance

When placing a *long distance* call from the physician's office, the medical assistant assembles patient data before initiating the call, dials directly to save both time and money, and then keeps the conversation

brief. Directions for dialing are detailed in the telephone directory. Charges for out-of-town calls are based on distance, length of the conversation, time of day, and whether operator assistance is necessary. Rates are based on the time the call is instituted at the originating site, not on the time it is at the receiving station. The operator will give credit or solve a problem in the event of a bad connection, a number dialed incorrectly, or a disrupted call. Some offices provide telephone log slips to record long distance calls so that they may be checked against the telephone statement. Other offices block long distance calls on all telephones except those of the physician and office manager.

Toll Calls

A **toll call** is a telephone call made within a metropolitan area at widely distant locations. The call is not considered a local or a long distance call but is charged at a standard base rate taking into consideration distances between exchanges and length of time.

When placing calls within a large city or out of state, the medical assistant should make use of *toll-free numbers* whenever possible; many institutions have 800 or 888 numbers.

Conference Calls

Occasionally, the physician may seek immediate consultation with specialists concerning treatment for a patient. The **conference call,** often referred to as *teleconferencing,* is an electronic means of permitting several physicians to consult with one another at the same time from different locations. Most telephones have

Table 6-4. International Communications Telephone Aid

International Communicator's Alphabet		International Numerical Pronunciations
Alpha	**N**ovember	Zero
Bravo	**O**scar	Wun
Charlie	**P**apa	Too
Delta	**Q**uebec	Tree
Echo	**R**omeo	Foe-er
Foxtrot	**S**ierra	Fife
Golf	**T**ango	Six
Hotel	**U**niform	Seven
India	**V**ictor	Ate
Juliette	**W**hiskey	Niner
Kilo	**X**-ray	
Lima (Leema)	**Y**ankee	
Mike	**Z**ulu	

this electronic capability and one party can arrange the conference call from their site. Another method of setting up a conference call is to have the operator connect all parties with the special conference operator, who will, in turn, manually connect them with one another. This type of call is expensive because each call is charged at the operator-handled rate.

International Communications

As *international telephone communication* grows more common, the more likely it is that you may speak to someone in another country. The International Communicator's Alphabet provides clarity and ease of understanding when satellite transmission is less than perfect. For example, when saying the name "Brent" you would say, "B as in Bravo, R as in Romeo, E as in Echo, and T as in Tango." This alphabet is also standard in voice-input computer systems. Since numeric pronunciations differ internationally as well, recommended pronunciations include spelling the numbers as words. Refer to Table 6-4 to make communications clear when particular words are misunderstood.

TELEPHONE REFERENCE AIDS

There may be many frequently used telephone numbers in the medical office. To save time, place a comprehensive, alphabetized list of names and telephone numbers near the telephone for reference. Such a

telephone reference aid or list might be on a sheet of paper protected with a clear, acetate cover, laminated, or placed under the corner of a glass-covered desk, on a wall near the telephone, or on the side of a filing cabinet—wherever it is handy to see. Alternatively, the list could be in a computer file and easily viewed and updated from time to time. The list could include unlisted numbers and the numbers of hospitals, emergency services, convalescent homes, physicians, staff members, local pharmacies, business machine repair companies, and physicians designated to take over patient care when the physician is away from the office.

Callback List

Many practices are too large for the physician to have an index listing all patient telephone numbers. If the office is computerized and the physician has a computer station in his or her office, numbers can be accessed via the computerized database. A callback list consists of patients who the physician may wish to call on a regular basis—perhaps for no other reason than to give assurance. The physician who shows a personal interest by occasionally calling patients to inquire about their condition often contributes to their physical improvement. A patient might be on such a list because he or she:

1. Is trying a new medication
2. Has been unresponsive to a prescribed drug

3. Has missed an appointment, a patient usually calls when there is a good reason for missing an appointment; fear and apprehension may be involved when there is no call

4. Is depressed

5. Is experiencing a personal crisis that could affect his or her illness

6. Has seen a consulting physician

7. Has had outpatient surgery, in which case, an inquiry may be made on his or her condition and instructions about medication and diet may be reemphasized

8. Is on the physician's "worry list," that is, has a condition that the physician is concerned about and wants to monitor closely.

STOP AND THINK CASE SCENARIO

Respond to Personal Call from Friend

Scenario: Office policy states, "Do not take personal telephone calls during business hours unless it is a family emergency." A friend who telephones you continually at the medical office calls to discuss an upcoming theater date. Tickets are going fast and the play will be sold out soon.

Critical Thinking: How would you respond to him/her? Compose a personal response.

_____

_____

_____

_____

_____

STOP AND THINK CASE SCENARIO

Evaluate Telephone Equipment

Scenario: You are the receptionist answering all incoming telephone calls. The office manager informs you that she will be looking at new telephone equipment and would like your input.

Critical Thinking: What information would you gather to give to the office manager prior to purchasing new telephone equipment? Determine questions that should be answered in order to gather data.

_____

_____

_____

_____

_____

_____

_____

_____

_____

_____

STOP AND THINK CASE SCENARIO

Compose Outgoing Voice Mail Message

Scenario: You are the receptionist for Practon Medical Group and the office manager has asked you to record the voice mail message for all incoming calls.

Critical Thinking: Write a script for the message and be prepared to either read it or record it on a tape recorder to be played back to the class.

_____

_____

_____

STOP AND THINK CASE SCENARIO

Construct Questions for Telephone Triage

Scenario: Patients have called with the following problems. You interrupt the physician who is in the middle of an emergent office procedure and she asks you to get as much information as possible.

Critical Thinking: Determine questions to ask so the physician can evaluate the problems over the telephone and advise the patients whether it is necessary to come to the office and how soon, go to the emergency room, or call an ambulance. Refer to Table 6-3 (Telephone Triage Response Guide) for examples of questions.

a. Insect bite: _____

_____

_____

b. Animal bite: _____

_____

_____

c. Burn: _____

_____

_____

d. Eye injury: _____

_____

_____

e. Head injury: _____

_____

_____

f. Sunburn: _____

_____

_____

FOCUS ON CERTIFICATION*

CMA Content Summary

- Medical terminology
- Professional attitude
- Confidentiality
- Verbal communication
- Patient instruction
- Professional tact, diplomacy, courtesy
- Interview techniques
- Receive, organize, prioritize, and transmit information
- Telephone techniques
- Medical records
- Release medical information
- Telephone services and use
- Patient information booklet
- Patient education
- Personnel manual

RMA Content Summary

- Medical terminology
- Disclosure laws
- Communication methods
- Patient instruction
- Document patient encounters
- Telephone communication
- Chart information

CMAS Content Summary

- Medical terminology
- Human relation skills
- Basic charting
- Medical emergencies
- Effective oral communication
- Incoming telephone calls
- Telephone technique
- Telephone emergency protocols
- Paper charting methods
- Confidentiality

REVIEW EXAM-STYLE QUESTIONS

1. To telecommunicate is to:
   a. use a teletypewriter to communicate data
   b. use a computer to communicate data
   c. use the Internet to communicate data
   d. transmit voice or data over a distance
   e. use the telephone to communicate voice

2. Most medical offices will be using a:
   a. cellular telephone
   b. pager
   c. 12-button touch-tone telephone
   d. voice-activated telephone
   e. video phone

3. A telephone service that is a type of answering system used to store and forward messages is:
   a. voice mail
   b. automated attendant
   c. call forwarding
   d. speaker phone
   e. caller ID

This textbook and accompanying Workbook *meet the entry-level administrative and general competencies for the CMA outlined by the AAMA Examination Content Outline and Role Delineation Study and for the RMA and CMAS outlined by the AMT Competencies and Examination Specifications (see Competency Grid in Appendix B).*

4. Physicians sometimes use pagers instead of cellular telephones because:

   a. they are not as loud

   b. a ringing telephone would not be appropriate

   c. they are more reliable

   d. they are cheaper

   e. they are smaller

5. An answering service is preferable to an answering machine because:

   a. answering machines are expensive

   b. you do not have to play back messages

   c. you do not have to listen to patient complaints

   d. they will not break down

   e. they offer personalized handling of medical calls

6. How many levels of triage are there?

   a. 1

   b. 2

   c. 3

   d. 4

   e. 5

7. Which level of triage is the administrative medical assistant most likely to handle?

   a. Level I

   b. Level II

   c. Level III

   d. Level IV

   e. Level V

8. When screening a telephone call, it is important to:

   a. ask good questions

   b. gather information

   c. listen and record what the caller tells you

   d. sign your name with credentials

   e. all of the above

9. Some medical problems that threaten life are:

   a. sunburn, heat exhaustion, and exposure to cold

   b. colds, flu, or sore throats

   c. breathing difficulty, head trauma, and bites

   d. constipation, nose bleeds, and indigestion

   e. headaches, eye aches, and earaches

10. A caller who fails to identify himself but insists on speaking to the physician should be:

    a. disconnected

    b. told to call back

    c. put through to the doctor

    d. advised of office policy stating you have to announce each caller to the physician

    e. put through to the office manager

11. When you have a caller who will not terminate the call, it is proper to:

    a. allow them to continue; hanging up would be rude

    b. advise them that you must terminate the call to tend to other work

    c. listen until they stop talking

    d. hang up on them

    e. put them on hold indefinitely

12. Regarding putting patients on hold, standard practice should be to:

    a. say, "just a minute," and place them on hold

    b. say, "I'm putting you on hold"

    c. say, "I'll be right back"

    d. try not to put patients on hold but if you must, ask their permission first

    e. place them on hold as necessary

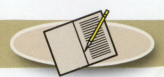

WORKBOOK ASSIGNMENT

To develop competency-based job skills, refer to the *Workbook* and complete the:

- Abbreviation and Spelling Review
- Review Questions

- Critical Thinking Exercises
- Job Skill activities, which are outlined at the beginning of this chapter under "Performance Objectives in the *Workbook*."

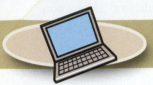

COMPUTER ASSIGNMENT

To review the concepts you have learned in this chapter, insert the *Student Practice* CD-ROM into a computer and work through the *StudyWARE* activities and games. Answer review questions in the practice mode and read the feedback, studying the questions you have missed. Take the chapter quiz until you achieve a minimum score of 90 percent. Successfully completing the *Critical Thinking Challenge* at the end of this course will help you think through scenarios and develop problem solving skills.

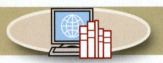

RESOURCES

Books

Documentation and Telephone Screening
Peggy M. Krueger, 2005
American Association of Medical Assistants
20 N. Wacker Drive, Suite 1575
Chicago, IL 60606

Tele-Nurse Telephone Triage Protocols
Sandi Lafferty, Marijo Baird, 2001
Delmar Cengage Learning
Cengage/PCS
Attn: Order Fulfillment
10650 Toebben Drive
Independence, KY 41051
(800) 354-9706, ext. 4
Web site: http://www.delmarhealth.com

Telephone Triage Protocols, 2 ed.
Sheila Quilter Wheeler
Delmar Cengage Learning
Cengage/PCS
Attn: Order Fulfillment
10650 Toebben Drive
Independence, KY 41051
(800) 354-9706, ext. 4
Web site: http://www.delmarhealth.com

CHAPTER 7

Appointments

OBJECTIVES

After reading this chapter and learning step-by-step procedures to gain job skills,* you should be able to:

Learning Objectives

▎ Discuss various ways an appointment template can be used.

▎ Describe how appointments are made via computer.

▎ State considerations when selecting an appointment book.

▎ Explain various flow techniques for scheduling appointments.

▎ State methods of handling various types of problem appointments diplomatically.

▎ Determine procedures for handling convalescent home and house call appointments.

▎ Identify the requirements for setting up diagnostic tests and therapeutic appointments.

▎ Choose an appointment card appropriate for the medical practice.

Performance Objectives (Procedures) in This Textbook

▎ Prepare an appointment sheet (Procedure 7-1).

▎ Schedule appointments and execute appointment procedures (Procedure 7-2).

▎ Reorganize patients in an emergency situation (Procedure 7-3).

▎ Schedule surgery, complete form, and notify the patient (Procedure 7-4).

▎ Schedule an outpatient diagnostic test (Procedure 7-5).

Performance Objectives (Job Skills) in the *Workbook*

▎ Prepare appointment sheets (Job Skill 7-1).

▎ Schedule appointments (Job Skill 7-2).

This textbook and the accompanying Workbook *meet the educational components for entry-level administrative and general competencies outlined by CAAHEP and ABHES.*

■ Prepare an appointment reference sheet (Job Skill 7-3).

■ Complete appointment cards (Job Skill 7-4).

■ Abstract information and complete a hospital/surgery scheduling form (Job Skill 7-5).

■ Transfer surgery schedule information to a letter (Job Skill 7-6).

■ Complete requisition forms for outpatient diagnostic tests (Job Skill 7-7).

OUTLINE WITH LECTURE NOTES

Appointment Schedule Template

_____

_____

_____

Scheduling Systems

_____

_____

_____

Computerized Appointments

_____

_____

_____

Appointment Book

_____

_____

_____

Patient Flow Techniques

_____

_____

_____

Scheduling Appointments
Managing Appointments

_____

_____

_____

Scheduling Tips and Types of Appointments
Follow-Up Appointments

_____

_____

Unscheduled Patient/Nonpatient Appointments

_____

_____

_____

Emergency Situations

_____

_____

_____

Referral Appointments

_____

_____

_____

Habitually Late Patients

_____

_____

_____

No-Show Patients

_____

_____

_____

Canceled Appointments

_____

_____

_____

Managed Care Appointments

_____

_____

_____

E-Mail Appointments

_____
_____
_____

Clinical Messaging Services

_____
_____
_____
_____

Telephone Appointments

_____
_____
_____
_____
_____

Scheduling Surgery

_____
_____
_____
_____

Preoperative and Postoperative Appointments

_____
_____
_____
_____

Diagnostic Testing and Therapeutic Appointments

_____
_____
_____
_____

Hospital Visits

_____
_____
_____
_____

Convalescent Hospital Visits

_____
_____
_____
_____

House Call Visits

_____
_____
_____
_____

Appointment Reminder Systems

_____
_____
_____
_____

Appointment Reference Sheet

_____
_____
_____
_____

Guidelines to Avoid Audits and Improve Scheduling

_____
_____
_____
_____

KEY TERMS

appointment abbreviations
appointment block
appointment book
appointment card
appointment schedule
clustering
established patient
fixed interval
modified wave

new patient
no-show
personal digital assistant (PDA)
program
referral
software
stream
template
true wave

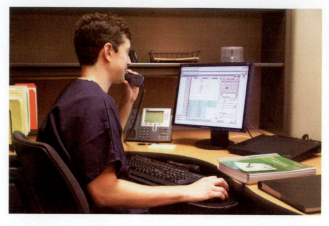

Figure 7-1. Medical assistant making an appointment for a patient using computer software

APPOINTMENT SCHEDULE TEMPLATE

In the era of two-career families, children involved in countless activities, and primary care physicians being asked to see more patients in fewer hours, a well-planned **appointment schedule** is essential.

A variety of schedule types will be introduced in this chapter, but a basic schedule consists of a list designating chronological times for patients to meet with the physician and receive medical services.

One of the most important and challenging responsibilities assigned to the medical assistant is coordinating appointments according to fixed time intervals and taking into account patient needs while maintaining a smooth schedule for patients and others who visit the physician (Figure 7-1). This task is made easier if the physician prepares a list of routine services and procedures with an estimate of the time needed for each type of visit. A **template**, which serves as a guide for scheduling various types of appointments, could be created to:

- Indicate each doctor's preferred time management schedule
- Cut down on decision making
- Allow faster access for new patients
- Meet patients' needs for urgent and emergent situations
- Decrease patient waiting times by analyzing feedback and redesigning doctors' schedules, as needed

The template is preformatted with a certain number of slots for various types of appointments per hour.

For example, one physician may choose to see established patients every 10 minutes with open periods for two new patients in the morning and three in the afternoon. An **established patient** is one who has received professional health care services within the past three years from the physician or another physician of the same specialty who belongs to the same group practice. His or her history would be somewhat familiar to the physician, thus requiring less time. A **new patient** is one who has *not* received any professional services from the physician or another physician of the same specialty who belongs to the same group practice within the past three years. Although the new patient may have been seen before by the physician and a history may be on file, if more than three years has passed, the physician will need a longer appointment to review the patient's history and get up to date on the patient's current problems.

Selected times could also be set aside for routine procedures (e.g., sigmoidoscopies on Tuesdays and Thursdays from 8:00 a.m. to 9:00 a.m.). A list of typical ailments could also be composed by the physician with time intervals needed to treat each problem. The medical assistant can then refer to this template when scheduling patient appointments.

SCHEDULING SYSTEMS

Scheduling systems can be either computerized or manual, and there are a variety of innovative scheduling techniques available. The following questions should be considered when determining what type of system will satisfy patient needs:

1. Will the system fit in with the unique demands of the specialty?

2. Will the system offer flexibility?

3. Will the system compliment the physician's style and choice of time segments for examining patients and performing procedures?

To determine a scheduling system that not only satisfies patient needs but is also flexible, the staff, including the physician, should periodically review patient flow by analyzing the schedule for a specific length of time—at least six weeks—and then adjust the times for required office procedures to better utilize the physician's time and to provide a smoother patient flow. First, the optimum number of patients that can be seen per day and half day should be determined. This decision is made by the physician. Second, determinations need to be made about how many emergencies or walk-in patients typically occur. Also consider carefully whether the practice experiences higher volumes on certain days of the week or during certain seasons (e.g., ski season for an orthopedic surgeon). Tracking the schedule for a period of 6 to 12 weeks can help determine these factors and aid in the choice of a scheduling system (Figure 7-2).

Computerized Appointments

Some offices schedule appointments using a computer software program. **Software** is defined as instruction that directs the computer or word processor to perform tasks; also referred to as a **program**. Software programs can be developed for a particular type of practice or a generic program may be purchased. The ideal appointment system will have software that performs key functions according to the unique requirements of a particular practice. The computer system supplier or vendor will assist in installation, training, and support. A good vendor will be available for questions and will assist in using the system to its full potential.

Electronic appointment scheduling is most useful in clinics or large medical facilities consisting of several doctors practicing in several locations. However, electronic appointment scheduling may be included with medical billing software and used by a single

Appointment Schedule Tracking Grid

Week	Monday	Tuesday	Wednesday	Thursday	Friday	Saturday 1/2 Day
1 (work-ins)	40 ✓✓✓✓✓✓✓	32 ✓✓✓✓✓	31 ✓✓✓	29 ✓✓✓✓	45 ✓✓✓✓✓✓	23 ✓✓✓✓✓
2 (work-ins)	36 ✓✓✓✓✓✓✓✓	31 ✓✓✓✓	37 ✓✓✓✓	32 ✓✓	39 ✓✓✓✓✓✓✓	20 ✓✓✓✓✓✓
3 (work-ins)	42 ✓✓✓✓✓✓✓	30 ✓✓✓	29 ✓✓✓✓✓	30 ✓✓✓	42 ✓✓✓✓✓✓	19 ✓✓✓✓
4 (work-ins)	38 ✓✓✓✓✓✓	29 ✓✓✓✓	30 ✓✓✓✓	27 ✓✓✓✓✓	46 ✓✓✓✓✓	25 ✓✓✓✓✓✓✓✓✓✓
5 (work-ins)	33 ✓✓✓✓	33 ✓✓✓✓✓	30 ✓✓✓✓	30 ✓✓✓✓	37 ✓✓✓✓✓	22 ✓✓✓✓✓✓✓✓
6 (work-ins)	39 ✓✓✓✓✓✓✓	35 ✓✓✓	38 ✓✓✓	30 ✓✓✓✓	35 ✓✓✓✓	24 ✓✓✓✓✓✓
Average Daily Appts.	38	31.66	32.5	29.66	40.66	23.83
Work-ins ( )	High: 8 Low: 4 Avg: 6.5	High: 5 Low: 3 Avg: 4	High: 5 Low: 3 Avg: 3.16	High: 5 Low: 2 Avg: 3.66	High: 7 Low: 4 Avg: 5.5	High: 10 Low: 4 Avg: 6.5
Walk-ins	✓✓				✓	✓✓✓
Emergencies		✓			✓✓	
Cancellations			✓	✓✓		✓
No-shows	✓✓		✓			

Figure 7-2. Appointment schedule tracking sheet for a six-week period showing number of total appointments in one day. Included in total number are number of appointments that have been worked into the schedule each day (indicated by an "✓") and number of walk-ins, emergencies, cancellations, and no-shows.

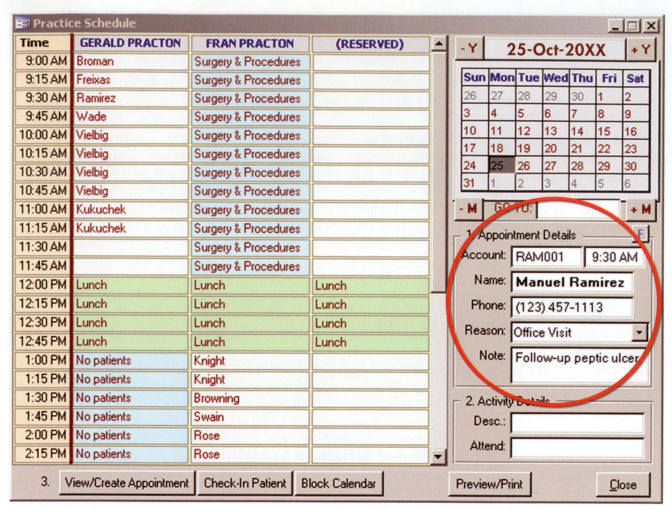

Figure 7-3. Patient appointment screen from Medical Office Simulation Software (MOSS) showing appointments for October 25, 20XX, for two providers. Note appointment details (displayed by single-clicking on a patient name) and patients with more than one (15 minute) time slot, indicating blocked time for longer appointments.

practitioner. The computer software program can be used to manage all appointments, free times, days off, and searches for available openings in the schedule. Such systems can also be used to coordinate and schedule specific treatment rooms and equipment. The system can reserve segments of time (e.g., 15 minutes, 30 minutes, 60 minutes and so forth) for specific patient types, services, or procedures. This is referred to as an **appointment block**. For example, if a consultation requires 45 minutes, the appointment scheduler would search for a 45 minute block and schedule the consult in that spot.

The appointment software can record a patient's appointment on the scheduling calendar, in the patient's computer file, and in a tickler file so the medical assistant can send a reminder notice or can telephone the patient before the appointment. If a patient calls to find out when the appointment is scheduled, the system can search by name or account number to find the time and date. From the electronic appointment schedule, a daily list of appointments can be printed for each physician (Figure 7-3).

Appointment Book

Choosing an **appointment book** consisting of lined pages used to schedule and record times set aside for patients to see health care practitioners for procedures or services involves decisions about (1) size, (2) available desktop area, (3) style requirements (taking into consideration how far in advance the appointments are to be made), (4) number of physicians in the group, and (5) medical specialty.

In a group practice, one medical assistant may schedule all the physicians' appointments on a large, multiple-column sheet, often color-coded with a dif-

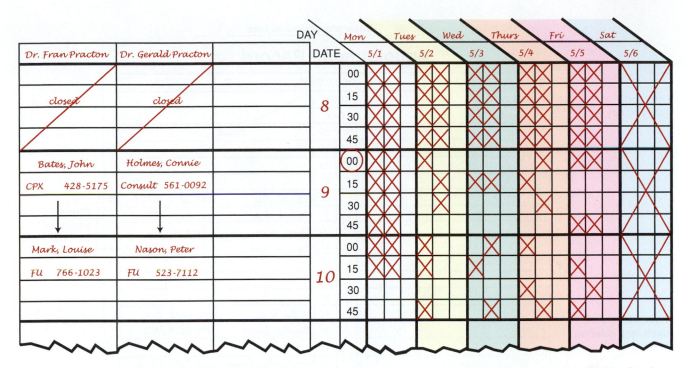

Figure 7-4. Two physician appointment sheets for one week showing part of Monday's schedule and indicating (with "X"s) appointments already blocked or booked for the rest of the week. (Courtesy of Bibbero Systems, Inc., Petaluma, CA. Phone: 800-242-2376; Fax: 800-242-9330; Web site: http://www.bibbero.com.)

ferent color for each day of the week and with a physician's name heading each column (Figure 7-4). If standardized columns contain too much or too little space devoted to particular items, self-designed, custom-made appointment sheets may be printed for a three-ring binder at reasonable cost.

Patient Flow Techniques

Because the choice of scheduling methods depends on the size and specialty of the practice, the number of physicians in the practice, and the doctors' preferences, consider these factors and the goal of maintaining smooth patient flow with a minimum of waiting time as you evaluate the following scheduling systems.

Stream

Most doctors' offices use **stream** or **fixed interval** scheduling (Figure 7-5), which gives each patient a specific appointment time. Patients seen for the first time are usually assigned 45- to 60-minute appointments, whereas follow-up examinations are scheduled every 10, 15, or 20 minutes. The time allotment will vary depending on the physicians' specialty and the circumstances.

Specialty and consulting practices also use this technique because it allows the physician time to pre-

pare for each office visit with the knowledge that the day will begin and end on schedule if patients adhere to their assigned times. The disadvantage is that there can be little deviation from the schedule for late arrivals, emergencies, walk-ins, or patients who need more or less time than scheduled.

When setting up each appointment page for a fixed schedule the assistant writes identifying information (i.e., physician's name, day, date) in ink at the top unless it is preprinted. Then as appointments are scheduled, he or she legibly enters the patient's full name (last name first) and daytime telephone number in pencil next to the time period. The reason for the appointment, known as chief complaint, is also included using standard **appointment abbreviations** (Table 7-1) so everyone can understand what is written and to save space. When training new employees, a list of acceptable abbreviations should be accessible for quick reference. For a permanent record, the patients' names may be written over in ink at the end of the day or a copy of the page may be made. The goal of the administrative medical assistant serving as a receptionist is to stay on schedule because if the appointment system fails, he or she is the one who must deal with irate patients and frustrated physicians. Refer to Procedure 7-1 (page 203) for step-by-step directions on preparing an appointment sheet and Procedure 7-2 (page 204) to schedule appointments.

(text continues on page 201)

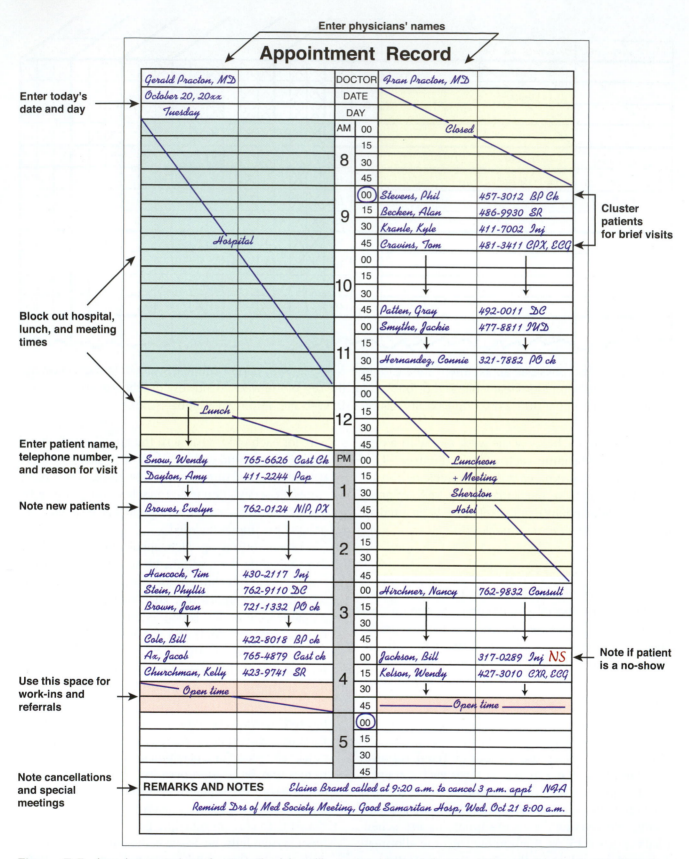

Figure 7-5. Appointment sheet for two physicians illustrating blocked time periods, appointments, no-show, canceled appointment, and special notations. (Courtesy of Bibbero Systems, Inc., Petaluma, CA. Phone: 800-242-2376; Fax: 800-242-9330; Web site: http://www.bibbero.com.)

Table 7-1. Appointment and Patient Care Abbreviations

A	allergy; abortion	C & S	culture and sensitivity
AB	antibiotic	Ca, CA	cancer, carcinoma
abd, abdom	abdominal, abdomen	canc, cncl	cancel, canceled
abt	about	cast ck	cast check
Acc, acc	accommodation	Cauc	Caucasian
accid	accident	CBC	complete blood count
adm	admit; admission; admitted	CC	chief complaint
adv	advice	CDC	calculated date of confinement
aet.	at the age of	chem	chemistry
AgNO3	silver nitrate	CHF	congestive heart failure
AIDS	acquired immune deficiency syndrome	chr	chronic
alb	albumin	ck, ✓	check
ALL	allergy	CI	color index
a.m., AM	before noon	cm	centimeter
AMA	American Medical Association	CNS	central nervous system
an ck	annual check	CO, C/O	complains of
an PX	annual physical examination	CO_2, CO2	carbon dioxide
ant	anterior	comp	comprehensive
ante	before	compl	complete
A & P	auscultation and percussion	Con, CON, Cons, Consult	consultation
AP	anterior posterior; anteroposterior; antepartum care	Cont.	continue
AP & L	anteroposterior and lateral	COPD	chronic obstructive pulmonary disease
approx	approximate	CPE, CPX	complete physical examination
apt	apartment	C section, C/S	cesarean section
ASA	acetylsalicylic acid	CT	computerized tomography
asap, ASAP	as soon as possible	CV	cardiovascular
ASCVD	arteriosclerotic cardiovascular disease	CVA	costovertebral angle; cardiovascular accident; cerebrovascular accident
ASHD	arteriosclerotic heart disease		
asst	assistant	CXR	chest x-ray
auto	automobile	Cysto, cysto	cystoscopy
Ba	barium	D & C	dilatation and curettage
Bl	biopsy	dc	discontinue
BM	bowel movement	DC	discharge, dressing change
BMR	basal metabolic rate	del	delivery
BP, B/P	blood pressure	Dg, dg, Dx, dx	diagnosis
BP ck, BP✓	blood pressure check	diag.	diagnosis, diagnostic
breast ck	breast check	diam.	diameter
Brev	Brevital	diff.	differential
BUN	blood urea nitrogen	dilat	dilate
Bx, BX	biopsy	disch.	discharged
C	cervical; centigrade; celsius		

(continues)

Table 7-1 (*continued*). Appointment and Patient Care Abbreviations

DNA	does not apply	GGE	generalized glandular enlargement
DNKA	did not keep appointment	GI	gastrointestinal
DNS	did not show	GTT	glucose tolerance test
DOB	date of birth	GU	genitourinary
dr, drsg	dressing	Gyn, GYN	gynecology
DSHA	does she have appointment	H	hospital call
DTaP*	diphtheria, tetanus, and pertussis (vaccine)	HA	headache
		HBP	high blood pressure
Dx, Dg, dx	diagnosis	HC	house call; hospital call; hospital consultation
E	emergency		
ECG	electrocardiogram; electrocardiograph	HCD	house call, day
ED	emergency department	HCl	hydrochloric acid
EDC	estimated date of confinement; due date for baby	HCN	house call, night
		hct	hematocrit
EEG	electroencephalogram; electroencephalograph	HCVD	hypertensive cardiovascular disease
		HEENT	head, eyes, ears, nose, and throat
EENT	eye, ear, nose, and throat	Hgb, Hb	hemoglobin
EKG	electrocardiogram; electrocardiograph	hist	history
EMG	electromyogram, electromyelogram	H_2O, H2O	water
epith.	epithelial	hosp	hospital
ER	emergency room	H&P	history and physical
ESR	erythrocyte sedimentation rate	HPI	history of present illness
est.	established; estimated	hr, hrs	hour, hours
etiol.	etiology	HS	hospital surgery
EU	etiology unknown	Ht, ht	height
Ex, exam.	examination	HV	hospital visit
exc.	excision	HX	history
ext	external	HX PX	history and physical examination
F	Fahrenheit; French (catheter)	I	injection
FH	family history	I&D	incision and drainage
FHS	fetal heart sounds	IC	initial consultation
flu syn	influenza syndrome	i.e.	that is
fluor	fluoroscopy	IM	intramuscualr
ft	foot; feet	imp., IMP	impression
FU, F/U	follow-up (visit)	inc	include
FUO	fever of unknown/undetermined origin	inf, INF	infection, infected
FX, Fx	fracture	inflam., INFL	inflammation
G	gravida (number of pregnancies)	init	initial
g, gm	gram	inj., INJ	injection
GA	gastric analysis	int, INT	internal
GB	gallbladder	intermed	intermediate
GC	gonorrhea	interpret	interpretation

Abbreviation approved by the Joint Commission as the preferred abbreviation.

Table 7-1 (*continued*). Appointment and Patient Care Abbreviations

IPPB	intermittent positive pressure breathing	NPN	nonprotein nitrogen
IQ	intelligence quotient	N/S, NS	no-show
IUD	intrauterine device	NTRA	no telephone requests for antibiotics
IV, I.V.	intravenous	N&V	nausea and vomiting
IVP	intravenous pyelogrm	NYD	not yet diagnosed
JVD	jugulovenous distention	O_2, O2	oxygen
K35	kollmann (dilator)	OB	obstetrical patient, obstetrics; prenatal care
KUB	kidneys, ureters, bladder	OC	office call
L	left; laboratory; living children; liter	occ	occasional
lab, LAB	laboratory	ofc	office
lac	laceration	OH	occupational history
LBP	low back pain	OP, op.	operation, operative, outpatient
L&A, l/a	light and accommodation	OPD	outpatient department
L&W	living and well	OR	operating room
lat, LAT	lateral	orig.	original
lb(s)	pound(s)	OT	occupational therapy
LLL	left lower lobe	OTC	over the counter
LLQ	left lower quadrant	OV	office visit
LMP	last menstrual period	P	pulse; preterm parity or deliveries before term
lt., LT	left	PA	posterior anterior, posteroanterior
ltd.	limited	P&A	percussion and auscultation
LUQ	left upper quadrant	PAP, Pap	Papanicolaou (test/smear)
M	medication; married	Para I	woman having borne one child (Para II, two children, and so on)
MA	mental age		
med., MED	medicine	PBI	protein-bound iodine
mg	milligram(2)	PC	present complaint; pregnancy confirmation
MH	marital history		
ml	milliliter(s)	PD	permanent disability
mm	millimeter(s)	PE	physical examination
MM	mucous membrane	perf.	performed
MMR	measles, mumps, rubella (vaccine)	PERRLA, PERLA	pupils equal, round, react to light and to accommodation
mo	month(s)	pH	hydrogen ion concentration
MRI	magnetic resonance imaging	PH	past history
N	negative	Ph ex	physical examination
NA, N/A	not applicable	phys.	physical
NaCl	sodium chloride	PI	present illness
NAD	no appreciable disease	PID	pelvic inflammatory disease
neg.	negative	p.m., PM	after noon
New OB	new obstetric patient	PMH	past medical history
NFA	no future appointment	PND	postnasal drip
NP, N/P, (N)	new patient		

(continues)

Table 7-1 (*continued*). Appointment and Patient Care Abbreviations

PO	postoperative check, phone order	SE	special examination
P Op, Post-op	postoperative check	sed rate	sedimentation rate
pos.	positive	sep.	separated
post.	posterior	SH	social history
postop	postoperative	SIG, sigmoido	sigmoidoscopy
PP	postpartum care	SLR	straight leg raising
Pre-op, preop	preoperative (office visit)	slt	slight
prep	prepare, prepared	Smr, sm.	smear
PRN, p.r.n.	as necessary	S, M, W, D	single, married, widowed, divorced
prog	prognosis	SOB	shortness of breath
procto	proctoscopic (rectal) examination	sp gr	specific gravity
		SubQ*	subcutaneous
P&S	permanet and stationary	SR	suture removal; sedimentation rate
PSP	phenolsulfonphthalein	STAT, stat.	immediately
Pt, pt	patient	STD	sexually transmitted disease
PT	physical therapy	strab	strabismus
PTR	patient to return	surg.	surgery
PX	physical examination	Sx.	symptoms
R	right; residence call; report	T	temperature; term parity or deliveries at term
RBC, rbc	red blood cell	T&A	tonsillectomy and adenoidectomy
rec	recommend	Tb, tbc, TB	tuberculosis
re ch	recheck	TD	temporary disability
re-exam, reex	reexamination	temp.	temperature
REF, ref	referral	TIA	transient ischemic attack
reg.	regular	TMs	tympanic membranes
ret, retn	return	TPR	temperature, pulse, respiration
rev	review	Tr.	treatment
Rh-	Rhesus negative (blood)	TTD	total temporary disability
RHD	rheumatic heart disease	TURB	transurethral resection of bladder
RLQ	right lower quadrant	TURP	transurethral resection of prostate
RO, R/O	rule out	TX, Tx	treatment
ROS	review of systems	U	unit
rt., R	right	Ua, U/A	urinalysis
RT	respiratory therapy	UCHD	usual childhood diseases
RTC	return to clinic	UCR	usual, customary, and reasonable
RTO	return to office	UGI	upper gastrointestinal
RUQ	right upper quadrant	UPJ	ureteropelvic junction or joint
RV	return visit	UR, ur	urine
Rx, RX, ℞	prescription; any medication or treatment ordered	URI	upper respiratory infection
		UTI	urinary tract infection
S	surgery	vac	vaccine
SD	state disability		

Abbreviation approved by the Joint Commission as the preferred abbreviation.

Table 7-1 (*continued*). Appointment and Patient Care Abbreviations

VD	venereal disease	**Symbols**	
VDRL	Venereal Disease Research Laboratory (test for syphilis)	*	birth
		c̄, /c, w/	with
W	work; white	P̄	after
WBC, wbc	white blood cell or count; well baby care	s̄, /s, w/o	without
WF	white female	c̄c, c̄/c	with correction (eyeglasses)
WI, W/I	walk-in, work-in	s̄c, s̄/c	without correction (eyeglasses)
wk	week; work	+	positive
wks	weeks	−, ō	negative
WM, W/M	white male	±	negative or positive, indefinite
WNL	within normal limits	Ⓛ	left
WR	Wassermann reaction	ⓜ	murmur
WT, Wt, wt	weight	Ⓡ	right
x, X	x-ray(s); multiplied by	♂	male
XR	x-ray(s)	♀	female
yr	year	μ	micron

Clustered Appointments

Clustering is a plan that sets aside blocks of time for similar patient problems, especially when it is known that several patients will require the same services. Physicians have determined that this system speeds up each case. Under this system, all diabetics might be scheduled in the early morning and all hypertensive patients in the afternoon. Family practice physicians may have many sports physicals or pre-school check-ups at the beginning of the school year. Arranging blocks of time to be used exclusively for similar services allows the staff to anticipate what is required to provide these services in the most efficient manner.

Single Book

Single-booking or *time-specific* is a scheduling technique used when an appointment may take a great amount of time. Specialty and consulting practices, such as psychiatry and physical or occupational therapy use this method because patients are seen for consultations, counseling, patient education, or types of therapy. Appointments may be for forty-five to fifty minutes of each hour.

Double Book

Double booking is a scheduling technique that allows two or more patients to have an appointment for a particular time, depending on the proper combina-

tion of patient complaints; for example, checking a strep throat and changing a dressing take a brief time. This system is used to work in emergencies and book in an already full schedule but involves risking the good will of the patient if he or she must always wait to see the doctor.

True Wave

True wave scheduling is a flexible appointment system that attempts to keep patient flow moving smoothly from one hour to the next. When utilizing a true wave system, all patients are told their appointments are on the hour and each is seen in the order they arrive. If one patient is late there should be another waiting to be seen. It presumes there will be some no-show patients, some walk-in patients, and some late arrivals; the expectation is that visits will average out during the hour. The number of patients to be seen in an hour depends upon the physician's specialty, which can be determined by finding the average amount of time used for each appointment and then dividing that number into one hour. In other words, if the average visit is fifteen minutes, four patients could be seen in one hour. This schedule prevents a waste of the physician's productive time. The disadvantages are that patients may wait for longer time periods and may talk to each other and discover their appointments were scheduled at the same time.

Modified Wave

In **modified wave** scheduling patients are scheduled at the first half of each hour with single ten-minute appointments; no appointments are scheduled the second half of the hour allowing for work-ins. Another example of modified wave is to schedule more than one patient at specific intervals throughout the hour, but the same number is seen during each hour. So if five patients can be seen in one hour, two are scheduled at the hour, two at twenty minutes past the hour, and one 20 minutes prior to the next hour. With staggered appointments, the patients do not have to wait unreasonable lengths of time.

This system was developed as a compromise to minimize patient waiting and to maximize use of physicians' office hours to keep the patient flow smooth. The number of patients seen is affected by the number of examination rooms available. This system works best if there is no overscheduling and if it is used consistently by both the physician and the staff. A portion of a true wave and modified wave appointment page is illustrated in Figure 7-6 A & B.

Open Access

Open access, also called *same day scheduling, same day access,* or *advanced access* allows most patients to obtain appointments the same day they call. In order

A.

Dr. Fran Practon				Wednesday, May 10, 20XX
Time	Patient	Phone	Reason for visit	Comments
9:00	Cathy Villa	488-0987	annual Px	
	Shirley Nass	985-9800	BP ✓	
	Robert Crest	480-9870	well-baby ✓	
	Mary Chin	481-9675	Pap/pelvic	
10:00	Paul Nye	988-4551	post-op visit	
	Cindy White	488-6322	cast change	
	Paul Vega	988-1200	diabetes ✓	

B.

Dr. Fran Practon				Wednesday, May 10, 20XX
Time	Patient	Phone	Reason for visit	Comments
9:00	Cathy Villa	488-0987	annual Px	
9:10	Shirley Nass	985-9800	BP ✓	
9:20	Robert Crest	480-9870	well-baby ✓	
9:30				
9:40	Mary Chin	481-9675	Pap/pelvic	
9:50				
10:00	Paul Nye	988-4551	post-op visit	
10:10	Cindy White	488-6322	cast change	
10:20	Paul Vega	988-1200	diabetes ✓	

Figure 7-6A & B. A. Example of true wave scheduling appointment page. B. Example of modified wave scheduling page.

to make this system work the back-log of current patients must be cleared. After the schedule is freed, open access will lead to a regular flow of patients and visitors who simply call and come in the same day. Many practices including large clinics such as the Mayo Clinic in Rochester, Minnesota, have adopted open access scheduling.

Open Hours

Open hours allows patients to walk in anytime within a specified time frame; they sign in with the receptionist and are seen in order of their arrival. Medical laboratories and x-ray facilities often use this scheduling procedure.

Triage

If the medical assistant is working overtime because of problems in scheduling or because many of the emergency appointments turn out to be false alarms, consideration might be given to more creative appointment scheduling and screening procedures. An example would be a system based on *triage*, as described in Chapter 6. Triage has been adapted to appointment scheduling to sort out those patients who need to be seen quickly from those who can wait. By establishing appropriate criteria, triage can be used by the staff to improve patient scheduling and to increase the certainty that real emergencies, based on the physician's determination, will receive prompt attention. Triage works well when the staff knows how to get relevant information from the patient so a real emergency can be identified and handled promptly. Emergency symptoms will, of course, vary to some extent with the type of practice or specialty. Flexible appointment systems based on triage are the *true wave*, *modified wave*, and the *clustering* or *appointment blocking* system.

SCHEDULING APPOINTMENTS

The four basic considerations that must be made when scheduling an appointment are similar to those previously discussed for determining an appointment system. They are:

1. Needs of the patient, based on the seriousness of the illness or the urgency of the medical problem

2. Convenience of the patient

PROCEDURE 7-1

Prepare an Appointment Sheet

Objective: Set up, block out, and enter information on an appointment sheet in accordance with an established format or template called a *matrix*.

Equipment/Supplies: Page from appointment book, calendar, office policy for office hours, physician's schedule, and pen or pencil.

Directions: Follow these step-by-step procedures, which include rationales, to learn this skill, which is presented in the *Workbook* (Job Skill 7-1) for practice.

1. Enter the physician's name, date, and day of the week in ink at the top of each appointment page.

2. Note the time the office opens and closes by circling the hour. (See Figures 7-4 and 7-5.)

3. Block out the hours when patients are not scheduled by inserting a diagonal line through

these time slots with a notation indicating the reason. Approximately three months of appointment sheets should be blocked out to avoid having to reschedule patients.

4. First, mark out all lunch periods and holidays.

5. Next, mark other ongoing physician responsibilities, for example, staff meetings, hospital rounds, and so on.

6. Note and block off any special luncheons, meetings, conventions, vacations, and so forth for the upcoming months.

7. Block off time to reserve space for unscheduled patients. This will allow some open time in the morning and/or afternoon for patients with urgent needs, emergencies, referred patients, walk-ins, or to let the physician and staff catch up and return calls.

PROCEDURE 7-2

Schedule Appointments and Execute Appointment Procedures

Objective: To schedule appointments, entering information in accordance with office policy for one day.

Equipment/Supplies: Page from appointment book, calendar, office policy for office hours and physician's schedule, description of patients to be scheduled, and pencil.

Directions: Follow these step-by-step directions, which include rationales to learn this skill, which is presented in the *Workbook* (Job Skill 7-2) for practice.

1. Write legibly. Erase neatly when needed. All staff who view the appointment book should be able to quickly read and locate information.

2. Determine whether the patient is new or established, which physician the patient will be seeing, and the nature of the visit when a patient requests an appointment. This information sets the stage for determining the appointment time, length, and availability. Consult office policy to determine the length of time necessary for each patient's appointment.

3. Discuss with the physician and patient any special appointment needs when making a follow-up appointment. Special needs patients may require specific appointment times as well as certain procedures and use of medical equipment.

4. Search the appointment book for a mutually agreeable date and time. Allowing for the patient's agenda is as important as considering the office schedule.

5. Write in the patient's last name, followed by the first name, telephone number (home, work, or cell), and reason for the visit (chief complaint). Listing the patient's last name first makes finding the patient's appointment

time in a busy schedule much easier. The telephone number assists in appointment confirmation, thus eliminating the need to pull charts.

6. Use abbreviations shown in Table 7-1. Standard abbreviations save space and can be understood by all staff members.

7. Indicate appointment length clearly, using vertical arrows ($\downarrow$).

8. Indicate patients requiring special preparations (preps) using a red pen or other mark (e.g., *) to ensure a call can be made to verify that correct procedures have been followed prior to arrival. For example, when a sigmoidoscopy is scheduled, check if the patient has followed the required preparatory guidelines so that visualization of the colon is maximized and the procedure does not have to be repeated.

9. Complete an appointment card to give to the patient. Medical practices that enter appointments into a computer system may print cards on card stock as the appointment is entered into the computer. This eliminates errors between the recorded appointment and what is documented on the card.

10. Reschedule all canceled appointments and indicate those not rescheduled at the bottom of the appointment sheet or on a separate list. Then record the cancellation in the patient's medical record with the current date, reason, and follow-up according to office protocol. Initial the note in the patient's medical record.

11. Indicate on the appointment sheet when the patient is a no-show by writing N/S or NS in the margin with a colored pen. Then record the no-show in the patient's medical record with the current date and your initials. Follow up according to office protocol.

3. Scheduling preferences and habits of the physician.

4. Availability of medical equipment and facilities

If the physician wishes to be reminded of his or her personal or professional appointments and to have regularly occurring events scheduled in the appointment book, time for all these should be blocked off as discussed previously.

If the physician wants personal reminders kept off the appointment schedule but wants to be reminded of such things as outside appointments, magazine renewals, and scheduled meetings, these may be noted on a separate monthly desk calendar with large squares to provide a quick reminder for the physician and all office staff members.

Managing Appointments

Physicians and their assistants often forget that a medical appointment may be just one event in a patient's, or a parent's, busy day. The available opening in the physician's schedule may conflict with school, work, or a family crisis. Therefore, the medical assistant should maintain a flexible attitude toward scheduling appointments and try to give some consideration to patients' busy schedules and personal priorities. The needs of working patients may have to be satisfied by an occasional evening, early morning, or noon appointment, or even by a Saturday morning office visit. Midday appointments may be reserved for the elderly. Toddlers and preschoolers are generally less fussy if seen early in the day. It is best to schedule after school hours for children's office visits. Late afternoon appointments may be set aside for patients who work during the day. An occasional adjustment in the schedule may have to be made for a child who must be picked up at school, a college student home for the weekend, or an office worker whose only time to visit the physician is during the lunch hour.

SCHEDULING TIPS AND TYPES OF APPOINTMENTS

To plan for unexpected patients and interruptions in scheduling, it is wise for the medical assistant to allow two 15- or 30-minute free periods during the day to fix a delayed schedule, perhaps just before the lunch hour and in midafternoon. It is also wise to schedule lightly during the first hour of the day, leaving heavier scheduling, if necessary, for hours later in the afternoon.

Bringing patients in before the actual morning start time is a good idea as long as the physician is ready to see the patient at the scheduled time. This allows time for the clinical medical assistant to take vital signs, and the patient has time to disrobe and be ready for the physician. If patients are scheduled to start at 9:00 a.m. and the first patient is in the treatment room and ready to be seen, but the physician typically arrives between 9:15 a.m. and 9:30 a.m, the schedule should be adjusted to start later. It is not good practice or realistic to process patients into multiple treatment rooms prior to the doctor's arrival; this will put the schedule immediately behind. Do not schedule according to the number of rooms available; instead schedule according to the number of health care practitioners who can see patients.

Patients who need blood work done while fasting should be scheduled early in the day. New patients, who generally require more time, might also be scheduled early in the day so they can be seen as close to their scheduled times as possible; this creates a good first impression. New patients who have not completed their paperwork should be brought in at least 30 minutes before their appointment time. Do not schedule long or time-consuming patients in the last appointment hour of the day, and speak to the physician about when he or she wants a talkative patient to be brought in. Offering patients a brief form (Figure 7-7) may help talkative patients to curtail their discussion and focus on the reason for the visit; it also helps prompt forgetful patients.

Long waiting times are equated with poor service and patient dissatisfaction. Extended waits may also leave a negative impression about the quality of health care delivered. It is noted that more patients complain about waiting times than about high fees, and according to the American Journal of Public Health, "Waiting times of 30 minutes or longer sharply reduced the likelihood that men would visit a doctor again."

In certain specialties, an early warning system might be appropriate. For example, a letter can be sent to all patients that informs them that because of the nature of the practice, appointment times are approximate and an attempt will be made to contact the patient if a delay of more than 20 minutes is expected. A sign in the office that reads, "If you have been waiting more than 20 minutes, please notify the receptionist" will call attention to a patient who may have been overlooked or failed to check in; also the waiting patient is less likely to complain to other patients about the wait. Noting each patient's arrival time and noting the time the patient is escorted to the

Patient/Physician Form

Patient Name: _____ Date: _____

To help maximize your visit, please fill out this form and present it to your physician in the treatment room. Thank you for your cooperation.

1. List the main reason for today's visit: _____
   _____
   _____

2. If you have been in an accident, please list when, where, and how it occurred. _____
   _____
   _____

3. List any other problems or concerns that you would like to speak to the physician about: _____
   _____
   _____

4. If you need any of the following, please indicate with check marks and additional details as needed.

   _____ Prescription renewal
   If "yes" please list the medication, dosage, and how you are taking it.
   _____

   _____ Forms
   List type _____

   _____ Excuse from work or school

   _____ Other
   Please explain _____
   _____

Figure 7-7. Brief memo patient fills out before seeing the physician to help outline reason for visit

treatment room helps to monitor the appointment schedule. This information may also help improve future office appointment protocol.

There are many types of appointments that a medical assistant manages during each day and these will be described subsequently.

Follow-up Appointments

Usually a patient's need for a follow-up appointment will be decided by the physician and the patient at the close of a visit. If the patient is to return, the appointment should be made at the reception desk, with the date and time made mutually clear. While the patient is determining the best time for the appointment, the assistant can guide him or her to a convenient time slot to hasten the decision. It is not advisable to schedule a patient appointment too far in advance because calendar events may not be known and the appointment may be forgotten.

The importance of writing down all appointments the moment they are made, whether by telephone or in person, cannot be overemphasized; the physician's presence in the office is often determined solely by the appointments scheduled. If an appointment is made and the assistant fails to record it, embarrassing problems can result. If possible, schedule appointments one after the other to prevent gaps in the physician's time while awaiting the next patient. When a patient is to have a series of office visits, try to schedule them at the same time and day of the week to help establish them in the patient's mind.

Unscheduled Patient/Nonpatient Appointments

Occasionally a situation may arise when a patient walks in to see the doctor without a scheduled appointment. Check office policy regarding such situations. In

STEP 1 2 3

PROCEDURE 7-3

Reorganize Patients in an Emergency Situation

Objective: To reorganize patients in an emergency situation.

Equipment/Supplies: Section of office procedure manual regarding emergencies, appointment book, telephone, and pen or pencil.

Directions: Follow these step-by-step procedures, which include rationales, to learn this skill.

1. Candidly explain to patients awaiting appointments that an emergency has interrupted the day's schedule.

2. Give patients an option to (a) reschedule their appointments, (b) run an errand and return,

(c) use the telephone if they need to alert a family member or babysitter of the delay, or (d) remain and wait.

3. If possible, notify patients by telephone about the delay, politely explaining and apologizing for the inconvenience. Give them the option of rescheduling or coming in at a later time in the day.

4. If a scheduled patient arrives before he or she can be reached, apologize and explain the situation, offering the previously mentioned options.

order for an appointment determination to be made, it is advisable to obtain the most precise assessment of the patient's medical problem and ask the physician how urgent it is to either work the patient into the day's schedule, send the patient to the emergency room or make an appointment for another day.

Unscheduled visits at peak office hours by sales representatives or drug detail people can result in wasted time for both the office staff and the sales representatives. The assistant may want to block off one or two quiet periods in the middle of the week, perhaps around the noon hour, for this type of business call. Then the salesperson will have time for a brief talk about products, and no patient care time will be lost.

Emergency Situations

When a genuine emergency situation occurs, playing havoc with a carefully planned day, the medical assistant should assess the problem and then take one or more of the following actions:

- Refer the patient to a hospital emergency facility.
- Suggest the patient come to the office immediately.
- Schedule the patient for one of the appointment periods left open for urgent or emergent problems.

- Work the patient into the schedule and enter the appointment with a colored pen or pencil.

Patients with scheduled appointments that are interrupted by an emergency should be handled in one of the ways mentioned in Procedure 7-3.

Referral Appointments

Because physicians depend upon patient **referrals** from other doctors, it is important that these patients be given appointments as soon as possible. If the referring physician calls the doctor directly regarding a referral, the appointment requirements may be assessed at that time.

Depending on the specialty, it may be appropriate to allow a block of time for referral appointments,

COMPLIANCE

Generally, it is not necessary to obtain a signed authorization for release of medical information from a patient who is being referred to another physician for the same condition. If the patient agrees to the referral, continuity of care applies and medical records regarding that specific condition may be forwarded.

which often require priority. In the managed care setting, primary care physicians refer patients to specialists when necessary.

If the physician refers many patients to other physicians, ask those physicians for their business or appointment cards. This provides the patient with the new physician's name and address and expedites the referral. Referral appointments may be flagged so the medical assistant can follow up with the referring physician to find out whether the patient kept the appointment or was a no-show.

Habitually Late Patients

When a patient is habitually late for appointments, either schedule him or her 15 minutes before the real appointment time or at the end of the day. This can prevent the patient's tardiness from disrupting the day's schedule. A coded notation could be written on the patient record as a reminder if the problem continues.

No-Show Patients

Every practice needs to establish and enforce a policy for dealing with **no-show** appointments. For example, the patient who misses a first appointment might be called at the end of the day to suggest rescheduling the visit; after a second missed appointment, an immediate call might be made to find out the reason and to remind the patient that a third no-show would result in dismissal by the physician; after a third appointment is missed, a certified letter should be sent to release the patient.

Each time an appointment is missed, the assistant should note the occurrence in the patient's medical record along with the action taken, as further explained in Chapter 8. No-shows may also be highlighted on the appointment sheet, indicated by NS or N/S with a colored pen, or noted in a computer system.

COMPLIANCE

An accurate appointment book serves as a permanent record of all appointments and can be used for documentation in medicolegal cases. Omission of information about a canceled appointment can have serious legal consequences.

Canceled Appointments

If a patient cancels an appointment and does not set up an alternative time, the name should be listed on a cancellation list for tracking purposes or remain on the appointment page with a line drawn through it and a notation in the margin to indicate a cancellation was requested by the patient. At the end of the day, the date, time, and reason for the cancellation or missed appointment is then written in the patient's medical record. If the physician thinks the missed appointment will jeopardize the patient's physical condition, the assistant should telephone the patient to suggest making another appointment.

When a patient reschedules an appointment, the medical assistant should cross out or erase the original appointment before writing in the new appointment to reduce the chance of scheduling the appointment twice. If the patient does not reschedule, the canceled appointment should be noted in the appointment book and the patient's chart. A certified letter with return-receipt requested may also be sent with a copy retained in the medical record.

Some offices charge for failure to keep an appointment. To institute this policy, the patient must be notified in advance. However, few physicians actually collect because of the poor public relations that may result.

Managed Care Appointments

One of the most important factors managed care organizations (MCOs) use as a measure of the provider's quality of care is how well appointment scheduling is organized and facilitated. This requires maximum cooperation between the front and back office staff. Services must be scheduled correctly according to a specified time frame so quality of care will not suffer. Poor appointment scheduling may provide an excuse for an MCO to closely monitor a practice's patient relations and medical outcomes. This in turn may lead to increased paperwork, reduced reimbursements, or being dropped from the MCO's network of physicians at the end of the contract period.

E-Mail Appointments

As mentioned earlier, pharmaceutical representatives may arrive unexpectedly and congest an already busy office schedule. Scheduling companies such as RepConnect and PreferredTime offer pharmaceutical companies and medical practices an Internet software tool that can be used to schedule appointments. This is a relatively new "do-it-yourself tool," so its usefulness to both the pharmaceutical industry and physician practices has yet to be determined.

Clinical Messaging Services

Patients may request appointments online and also review, reschedule, and cancel appointments using a system called *clinical messaging*. Online communication options include: completion of patient registration and medical history forms, viewing lab results, paying bills, and refilling prescriptions. Online consultations are also possible via this service, which encrypts messages and stores them in a secure Web server protected by a firewall; this offers more privacy and security than regular e-mail. Such systems decrease time spent by the physician and receptionist, save money, and offer convenience for computer-savvy patients. Refer to Resources at the end of this chapter for the names of companies that offer clinical messaging.

Telephone Appointments

In some rural areas after the initial appointment, telephone appointments can be arranged in a medical practice if no formal office visit is required. Patients are given designated times when they may call and talk to the physician. The physician must document the information in each patient's medical record. A nominal charge may be made for this service and billed to the insurance company using appropriate *Current Procedural Terminology (CPT)* codes.

Scheduling Surgery

The physician will determine the surgical procedure, specify an assistant surgeon, indicate the amount of time required, and specify the hospital preference before the assistant makes any arrangements. Then a scheduling information form or surgical flow sheet—often distinctive in color to make it stand out—may be used. This form may be designed by the staff for the physician with sections to be completed by the physician, patient, and scheduler. The form prevents scheduling problems, will help coordinate all details involving outside facilities, and will help adhere to insurance requirements. The purpose of the flow sheet is to make certain that all sequential tasks are completed. The surgical flow sheet is also helpful when the patient has managed care and prior

PATIENT EDUCATION

The physician and the medical assistant often share the responsibilities of informing the patient about a surgical procedure including what to expect before, during, and after surgery. The physician usually explains the details about the procedure, why it is needed, how it will correct the problem, how long it will take, and so forth. The medical assistant may be the one asking the patient to sign the surgical consent form, explaining when to go for preoperative testing, directing the patient to the hospital admissions office, explaining postoperative care (dietary restrictions or activity levels), and advising when a postoperative appointment should be made. The medical assistant witnesses the correct signature on the form and is not actually witnessing the consent. This is an important issue in the event the patient claims he or she did not understand or was not fully informed when verifying consent for a procedure. Special care should be taken to answer all the patient's questions and a telephone number given should additional questions arise.

authorization is required (Figure 7-8). This sheet can improve efficiency by obtaining the required information for prior authorization as part of the surgical planning process. The flow sheet has several parts:

- Patient identification and insurance information/certification
- Laboratory and other diagnostic scheduling requirements
- Clinical and preoperative results logged
- Anticipated procedures identified and scheduled
- Postoperative care plan

Referring to Figure 7-9 on page 212, Section 1 concerns the medical procedure and would be completed by the physician before surgery; Section 2 would be completed by the patient in the presence of the staff so items could be explained and insurance

XYZ SURGICAL ASSOCIATES
Surgery Flow Sheet

Date: _4/24/20XX_

Patient: _Raymond Gutierrez_   Account Number: _006492_

Telephone number: (day) _(555) 488-5323_   (evening) _(555) 487-4422_

Insurance Plan Name: _United Health Care_   Subscriber #: _209-XX-9026_

Plan Telephone Number: _1-800-XXX-1617_   Contact: _Marci_

Referring Physician: _Fran Practon, MD_   Dx: _L 4-5 herniated disc_

Authorization Requested: (date) _3/20/XX_   Received: (date) _4/15/XX_

Authorization Number: _#4062_

Lab Work:

CHEM 24 _✓_   SED rate _✓_   CBC _✓_   UA _✓_   Other _____

Laboratory: _College Hospital_   Phone: _(555) 487-6789_

Imaging:

MRI: Cervical _____   Thoracic _____   Lumbar _✓_   Other _____   W/GAD _____

Tomogram: A/P - levels _____   3 Dimensional CT Scan - levels _____

    SPECT Scan_____   Bone Scan _____   CT Scan _____

Epidural Steroid Injection - levels _L 4-5 series of two_

Myelogram: Cervical_____   Thoracic_____   Lumbar_____   Other _____

Other: _____   Facility: _____

EMG: Upper _____   Lower _✓_   Right _____   Left _____   Bilateral _✓_

Diagnostic Results (recorded in chart)   Comments:

Lab _WNL_

Imaging _Circumferential bulging of the central portion of the disc at L4–5 level_

EMG _Abn with lesion involving the right S1-S2 nerve roots_

Procedures

Cervical Arthrodesis (Fusion):

Anterior or Anterolateral	Posterior or Posterolateral	
C1-C2 (22548) _____	Occiput C2 (22590) _____	Cervical below (22600) C2 _____
Below C2 (22554)_____	Atlas-axis C1-C2 (22595)_____	

Other arthrodesis (CPT codes 22548-22830) _____   Spinal Instrumentation (22840-22855) _____

Decompressions: Cervical 1 or 2 vertebral seg. (63001) _____   3 or more (63015) _____

          Thoracic 1 or 2 (63003) _____   Thoracic 3 or more (63016)_____

          Lumbar 1 or 2 (63005) _✓_   Lumbar 3 or more (63017) _____

Discectomy: Percutaneous (62287) _____   Other (63075-63078)_____

Surgeon: Dr. X _✓_   Dr. Y _____   Dr. Z _____   Assistant: _Dr.3_

Hospital or ASC: _College Hospital_   Date: _5/26/XX_   Time: _07.30_

Post-Operative Care

Physical Therapy: _3_   X per week for _4_   weeks, starting _6/26/XX_ . P/T Facility _Sport Therapy_

Return Appointment (circle):   (1)   2   3   4   5   6   D   (W)   M   Y   PRN   Other _____

Figure 7-8. Example of a surgery flow sheet. (Reprinted with permission from Conomikes Associates, Inc., 1223 W. Olympic Boulevard, Suite 116, Los Angeles, CA 90064.)

STEP 1 2 3

PROCEDURE 7-4

Schedule Surgery, Complete Form, and Notify the Patient

Objective: To schedule surgery and complete either a hospital/surgical scheduling form or surgery flow sheet form and notify the patient.

Equipment/Supplies: Patient's chart, hospital/surgery scheduling form or surgery flow sheet form, surgical scheduling guidelines, calendar, telephone, letterhead, envelope, and pen.

Directions: Follow these step-by-step procedures, which include rationales, to learn this skill, which is presented in the *Workbook* (Job Skill 7-5) for practice.

1. Obtain detailed information from the physician and patient for Section 1 of the hospital/surgery scheduling form or the top section of the surgery flow sheet.

2. Obtain detailed information from the patient for Section 2.

3. Telephone the surgical scheduling unit at the hospital to reserve the operating room naming the surgeon, assistant surgeon, the time (hour and length), procedure, preferred date, patient's name, address, telephone number, date of birth, age, gender, and insurance/authorization information.

4. Call the hospital admissions office to give information and arrange for the patient to be admitted on the day of surgery; verify time to arrive.

5. Arrange for preadmission testing (e.g., laboratory or radiology).

6. Complete Section 3 of the hospital/surgery scheduling form or the last four sections of the surgery flow sheet.

7. Post the surgical arrangements in the appointment book blocking the appropriate time segments and indicating date, time, patient's name, procedure, name of hospital, and assistant surgeon.

8. Telephone assisting and/or referring physicians for confirmation of scheduled surgery.

9. Compose a document or letter for the patient with pertinent instructions about the scheduled surgery and send a copy to each person involved retaining a copy for the patient's medical record (Figure 7-10).

10. Schedule the preoperative and postoperative appointments.

11. Telephone one business day before surgery to remind the patient of his or her arrival time.

---

information reviewed; Section 3 would be completed by the office staff as each step is performed with dates documented and with the name of the person who did the scheduling indicated.

After the surgery has been scheduled with the supervising surgical nurse and with the hospital admissions office, the medical assistant posts the arrangements in the appointment book indicating date, time, patient's name, procedure, name of hospital, and assistant surgeon. Telephone calls are made to assisting and/or referring physicians for confirmation. After thorough verbal instructions are given, a letter or a form with pertinent information may be sent to the patient and distributed to each person involved; one copy should be filed with the patient's medical record (Figure 7-10).

The written responsibilities of the medical assistant conclude after all items on the form have been addressed. However, the assistant may want to relieve patient anxiety by telling the patient what to expect upon arrival at the hospital.

Preoperative and Postoperative Appointments

The medical assistant usually sets up the preoperative appointment the week of surgery and makes appointments for laboratory tests, and x-rays. He

HOSPITAL/SURGERY SCHEDULING FORM

Section 1   **Completed by physician**

1. ___✓___   Patient's name __*Alice Ruth Buckely*__
2. ___✓___   Procedure __*incision and drainage deep neck abscess*__
3. ___✓___   Emergency: Urgent _____   Elective ___✓___
4. ___✓___   Diagnosis: 1. __*Right neck abscess*__
                             2. _____
5. ___✓___   Hospital/Facility name __*College Hospital*__   Surgeon __*Daniel Marks, MD*__
6. ___✓___   Inpatient ___✓___   Outpatient _____   Day Surgery _____
7. ___✓___   Surgical assistant required?   Yes ___✓___   No _____
       Who preferred? ___*Ralph Curtis, MD*___
8. ___✓___   Anesthesia required?   Yes ___✓___   No _____
       Who preferred? ___*William Able, MD*___
9. ___✓___   Referring physician ___*Mary Tsongas, MD*___

Section 2   **Completed by patient**

10. ___✓___   Age of patient ___*54*___ Date of birth ___*1-15-53*___ Smoker _____ Nonsmoker ___✓___
11. ___✓___   Room accommodations: Private _____   Semi-private ___✓___
12. ___✓___   Telephone numbers: Home (*555*) __*486-1135*__   Work (____) ___*N/A*___
13. ___✓___   Insurance Company __*Acme Insurance Co.*__ Policy Number __*611-XX-9532*__
       Secondary Insurance ___*None*___   Policy Number _____
14. ___✓___   Second surgical opinion needed for insurance?   Yes ___✓___   No _____
15. ___✓___   Name of nearest relative ___*Charles Buckely*___
       Address __*49267 West Cota Drive*__   Phone number __*555-486-1135*__
16. ___✓___   Admitted to this facility previous?   Yes _____   No ___✓___
       Date _____   Type of procedure _____
17. ___✓___   Patient has had preadmission testing of CBC ___✓___ , EKG _____ , Chest x-ray _____
       within ___*1*___ weeks.
18. ___✓___   Admission and procedures reported to patient on   Date: __*October 3, 20XX*__
19. ___✓___   Preadmission and operation instructions given to me?   Yes ___✓___   No _____
20. ___✓___   Insurance and financial arrangements discussed with me?   Yes ___✓___   No _____

Section 3   **Completed by medical assistant**

21. ___✓___   Operation room reserved for surgery on this date __*Oct. 10*__ and time __*8:30 a.m.*__
       Name of hospital employee that scheduled surgery __*Betty Chapman*__
22. ___✓___   Name of surgical assistant scheduled and called __*Ralph Curtis, MD*__
23. ___✓___   Name of anesthesiologist scheduled and called __*William Able, MD*__
24. ___✓___   Reported to referring physician's office and talked to ___*Ruth Raines, RN 10/1*___
25. ___✓___   Hospital/Facility admission confirmed/preadmission test scheduled   *10/8/20XX*
26. ___✓___   Preauthorizations/second opinions obtained
       Authorization/precertification # ___*1001-62-40*___   Date provided __*10/2/20XX*__
       Who provided number? __*Acme Insurance/James Brown*__
27. ___✓___   Admitting date and surgical procedure entered in appointment book   *10/2*
28. ___✓___   Arrangements confirmed with patient   *10/2*
29. ___✓___   History and physical report ready
       Name of office employee that scheduled surgery __*Marcia Lopez, CMA*__ Date *10/2/20XX*

Figure 7-9. Example of a completed hospital surgery scheduling form

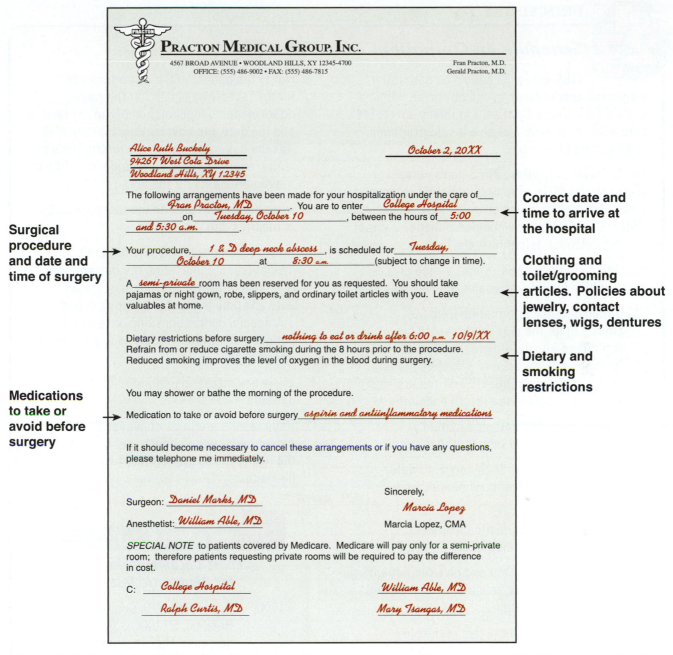

Figure 7-10. Example of a completed form letter illustrating content of important specific information related to patient's scheduled surgery

or she should exercise careful judgment in scheduling a sick person for numerous tests in sequence because too many appointments in one day may be tiring. The assistant must also have knowledge of the patient's insurance requirements that dictate in network facilities and may require preauthorization. The postoperative appointment is typically scheduled at the time surgery arrangements are made. The time interval after surgery would be specified by the surgeon and would depend on the type of procedure.

Diagnostic Testing and Therapeutic Appointments

The type of medical specialty will determine the type of diagnostic tests that are typically scheduled. Some examples are laboratory tests (blood chemistry, microbiology, pathology, cultures), radiology (x-ray, MRI, CT), physiology (ECG, treadmill, echocardiogram), and nuclear medicine (bone scan, IVP, thyroid uptake).

Examples of therapeutic appointments include physical therapy, occupational therapy, speech therapy,

STEP 1 2 3

PROCEDURE 7-5

Schedule an Outpatient Diagnostic Test

Objective: Schedule an outpatient diagnostic test ordered by the physician within a certain time frame. Confirm a mutually agreeable date with the patient and give test instructions and location of test site.

Equipment/Supplies: Physician's written or oral order for diagnostic test; patient's chart; test scheduling and preparation guidelines; name, address, and telephone number of diagnostic test facility; calendar; telephone; and pen.

Directions: Follow these step-by-step procedures, which include rationales, to learn this skill.

1. Obtain detailed information from the physician for the diagnostic test to be performed and determine the time frame for results. If it is urgent, schedule the test immediately and request STAT results, this affects the date of the return appointment.

2. Find out from the patient a mutually agreeable date and time for the test.

3. Telephone the insurance carrier to determine if preauthorization is needed and, if so, obtain it.

4. Telephone the diagnostic facility and schedule the test needed.

5. Obtain a date and time and give the patient's name, age, address, telephone number, and insurance information.

6. Notify the facility if the test results are urgently needed.

7. Obtain any special instructions for the patient, for example, dietary restrictions, fluid intake, or medications to avoid.

8. Notify the patient of the arrangements for the test giving him or her the name, address, and telephone number of the facility and the date and time to report for the test. Ask the patient to repeat the instructions to verify he or she has a clear understanding of the requirements for the test.

9. Have the patient pick up the requisition slip or mail/fax it to the patient.

10. Insert documentation in the patient's medical record indicating the current date, the name of the facility, name of the test, date and time the test is scheduled, and any special instructions. Indicate when the patient was advised about the appointment information.

11. Make a posttest appointment for the patient.

12. If the results are to be conveyed to the patient over the telephone, put a reminder in the tickler file so appropriate follow up can be made.

EXAMPLE 7-1

Chart Documentation for Diagnostic Test

5/15/XX   Scheduled MRI, College Hospital, 5/17/XX, 3:30 p.m.; no pacemaker, implants, claustrophobia. Adv. pt. via phone. Faxed requisition slip to facility. RTO 5/22/XX 10:00 a.m.

and nutritional counseling. Procedure 7-5 gives step-by-step directions for scheduling such appointments.

Hospital Visits

Postoperative visits for surgical patients and hospital visits for acutely ill patients are made by the physician at least once or twice daily. The physician may also make daily visits to patients in intensive care units, the newborn nursery, and other specialized units within the hospital. Because patient records generally do not leave the office and to facilitate recordkeeping during hospital rounds or visits the physician may choose to carry either a **personal digital assistant (PDA)**, tape recorder, small note book, 3″ by 5″ cards, or a list on which the assistant has typed the name of

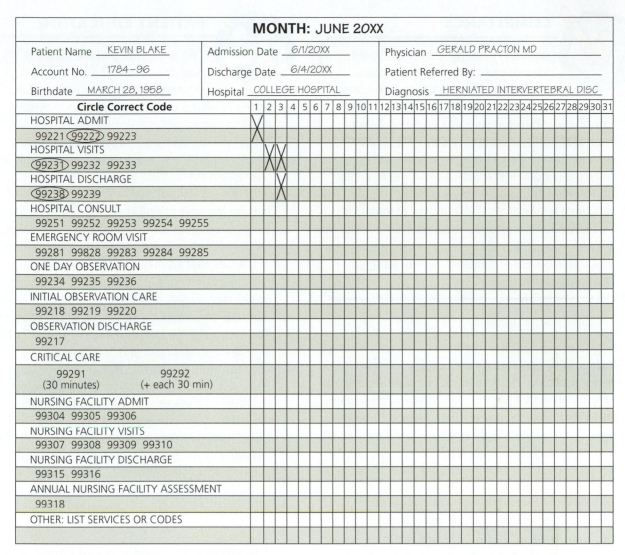

MONTH: JUNE 20XX																																	

Patient Name __KEVIN BLAKE__   Admission Date __6/1/20XX__   Physician __GERALD PRACTON MD__

Account No. __1784-96__   Discharge Date __6/4/20XX__   Patient Referred By: _____

Birthdate __MARCH 28, 1958__   Hospital __COLLEGE HOSPITAL__   Diagnosis __HERNIATED INTERVERTEBRAL DISC__

Circle Correct Code	1	2	3	4	5	6	7	8	9	10	11	12	13	14	15	16	17	18	19	20	21	22	23	24	25	26	27	28	29	30	31
HOSPITAL ADMIT	X																														
99221 (99222) 99223	X																														
HOSPITAL VISITS		X	X																												
(99231) 99232 99233		X	X																												
HOSPITAL DISCHARGE			X																												
(99238) 99239			X																												
HOSPITAL CONSULT																															
99251 99252 99253 99254 99255																															
EMERGENCY ROOM VISIT																															
99281 99828 99283 99284 99285																															
ONE DAY OBSERVATION																															
99234 99235 99236																															
INITIAL OBSERVATION CARE																															
99218 99219 99220																															
OBSERVATION DISCHARGE																															
99217																															
CRITICAL CARE																															
99291 99292 (30 minutes) (+ each 30 min)																															
NURSING FACILITY ADMIT																															
99304 99305 99306																															
NURSING FACILITY VISITS																															
99307 99308 99309 99310																															
NURSING FACILITY DISCHARGE																															
99315 99316																															
ANNUAL NURSING FACILITY ASSESSMENT																															
99318																															
OTHER: LIST SERVICES OR CODES																															

Figure 7-11. Hospital tracking form hand-carried to facility for daily record keeping. Given to medical insurance biller after patient is discharged or at end of month for posting charges.

each patient to be seen. An example of a card filled in for outside visits is shown in Figure 7-11.

A PDA is a small handheld computerized portable device that serves as an organizer, electronic book, or note taker with entries made via a key pad or by a stylus resembling a pen. It can capture, store, and manipulate a variety of information. PocketPC and Palm Pilot are two common PDAs used for simple organizational tasks, e-prescribing, ordering and checking laboratory tests, keying notes, and reading captured data. The doctor can log hospital visits and charges and this information can be transferred to the patient's financial records by the assistant later the same day by attaching the device to the desktop computer.

In a group practice, colleagues may alternate hospital rounds. One day Dr. Bernstein makes morning rounds to his own patients and those of Dr. Young. The following day Dr. Young makes rounds. The advantages of this system are that each partner gets to know the other's patients and it encourages sharing opinions on difficult medical problems.

A trend that has evolved to reduce hospital costs and shorten hospital stays is the *hospitalist*. These physicians take over when a patient is admitted to the hospital and provide inpatient care in place of primary care physicians (PCPs). They oversee tests and results, monitor changes in the patient's condition, consult with families, and discharge patients back to their regular doctor. Usually he or she is an inter-

COMPLIANCE

Any PDA used for business should have access controls and employ encryption. Passwords must be used on all PDA devices containing protected health information. PDA passwords should be different from other office computer network passwords, be a minimum of six characters, and incorporate letters and numbers. A PDA should never be left unattended and should automatically turn off following a maximum of 10 minutes of inactivity. PDAs, whether employee- or physician-owned, may be subject to audits like any other office electronic device depending on their usage for the medical practice.

PATIENT EDUCATION

The physician and the medical assistant often share the responsibilities of informing the patient about a surgical procedure including what to expect before, during, and after surgery. The physician usually explains the details about the procedure, why it is needed, how it will correct the problem, how long it will take, and so forth. The medical assistant may be the one asking the patient to sign the surgical consent form, explaining when to go for preoperative testing, directing the patient to the hospital admissions office, explaining postoperative care (dietary restrictions or activity levels), and advising when a postoperative appointment should be made. The medical assistant witnesses the correct signature on the form and is not actually witnessing the consent. This is an important issue in the event the patient claims he or she did not understand or was not fully informed when verifying consent for a procedure. Special care should be taken to answer all the patient's questions and a telephone number given should additional questions arise.

nist or family practitioner or has completed residency training. Most hospitalists are employed by managed care organizations, large clinics, or hospitals, but others are independent physicians who have agreements with PCPs and are paid for their work by insurance companies. Hospitalists do not substitute for specialists, such as surgeons or obstetricians.

Convalescent Hospital Visits

Convalescent hospital or nursing home calls are made on a monthly basis and more frequently if a patient becomes unstable. With the input of the physician, blocks of time are set aside for these outside calls, usually after hospital rounds in the morning or after office hours before the physician returns home at the end of the day.

House Call Visits

Fewer house calls are made today because most physicians do not have the time. However, they do occur on occasion especially in oncology and internal medicine. A PDA, a tape recorder, a notebook similar to those used for hospital visits, or a check-off list is prepared in advance by the medical assistant indicating the patients' name, address, and telephone number (home, work, cell). As the physician makes each call, he or she records the pertinent information about the visit. It is the medical assistant's responsibility to record financial charges for each visit to each

patient's financial account in the computer system or the patient ledger and daysheet.

APPOINTMENT REMINDER SYSTEMS

Experience has shown that custom-printed **appointment cards** simultaneously completed as the appointment is written in the appointment book or scheduled on the computer are by far the best means of avoiding misunderstandings about future office visits. Their use also reduces time-consuming telephone calls and helps prevent errors (Figure 7-12).

As mentioned earlier, some physicians trade business or appointment cards with other physicians or medical facilities so when a patient needs to seek further treatment or requires the services of a specialist, the assistant can hand one to the patient or schedule the appointment before he or she leaves the office.

Mrs. Mary Woolsey

has an appointment with

GERALD PRACTON, MD

PRACTON MEDICAL GROUP, INC.

4567 Broad Avenue
Woodland Hills, XY 12345
Tel. 555/486-9002
Fax No. 555/488-7815

for

Mon. _____ at _____

Tues. _____ at _____

Wed. *Oct. 29* _____ at *2:30 pm.*

Thurs _____ at _____

Fri. _____ at _____

Sat. _____ at _____

If unable to keep this appointment kindly give
24-hours notice.

Figure 7-12. Example of a completed appointment card

COMPLIANCE

For confidentiality purposes, a reminder card should be mailed in an envelope to established patients who have appointments scheduled periodically (Figure 7-13). Never use a postcard. Information for the reminder card may be obtained from a patient's encounter form, from dictation about the patient's visit, or retrieved from recall data entered into the computer software program. To manually keep track of periodic check-ups, the physician can clip a note to the patient's chart specifying the month the patient should be seen again. Then the assistant or the patient can address a reminder card and write the mailing date in the corner. The card is then filed alphabetically by name in a monthly tickler file and a note indicating this can be placed in the chart. At the appropriate time, the card is mailed.

facilities typically confirm only new patient, longer appointments, or appointments for in-office procedures. Also, if reminder calls (Figure 7-13) are made in advance and patients cancel their appointments, other patients who need to see the doctor may be scheduled.

APPOINTMENT REFERENCE SHEET

At the end of the previous day or before the first patients arrive each day, the medical assistant prepares a schedule of patients to be seen by the physician. It can be either a computer printout, a photocopy of the daily appointment sheet, or a typed list of names, times, and procedures (Figure 7-14).

Additional copies should be made for other office staff members. The reference sheet enables the physician to preview the day and recall established patients in order to prepare for each patient's visit. Patients' charts are pulled from the file and placed near the dated reference sheet sequenced in the order of the appointment schedule. As patients arrive, names may be checked off and/or the time of their arrival stamped or noted.

Cards introducing the referral physician with the telephone number and address may also include a place for remarks and a map to the office.

Confirmation telephone calls made by the medical assistant to patients scheduled to be seen within one or two days virtually eliminate failed appointments. Early morning or late afternoon are usually the best times to reach people at home to remind them of their appointments. Many daytime confirmation calls get "no-answers"; therefore, it might be worth having an assistant make calls in early evening hours. A flex schedule could accommodate this need and even if it requires extra pay for the work—the expense will be more than made up if only one long appointment is saved. Always indicate when the appointment is confirmed in the appointment record.

Dental offices usually confirm all appointments because many are made months in advance; medical

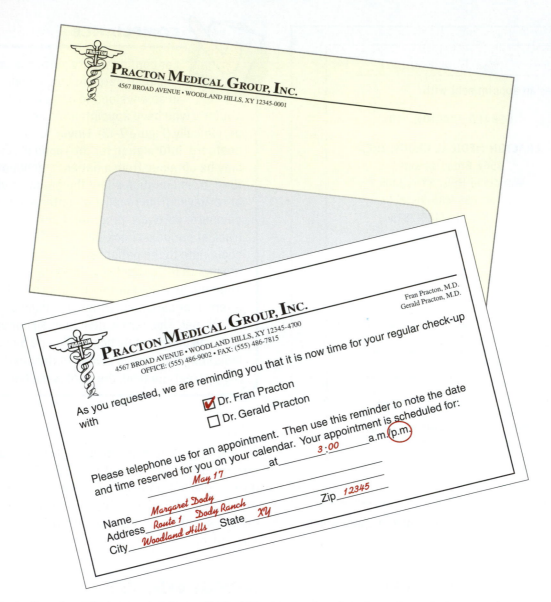

Figure 7-13. Recall reminder card to be mailed with address showing through a window envelope

APPOINTMENT SCHEDULE, FRAN PRACTON, M.D.

Tuesday, July 7, 20XX

7:30	Surgery	College Hosp.
8:15	Hospital rounds	College Hosp.
9:00	Lewis, Anthony	Annual phys.
9:45	Frame, Martha	MMR
10:00	Stewart, Adele	Heart eval.
10:30	Womochiewski, Leroy	NP; CPX
11:30	Ragland, Bill	BP check
11:45	Rowe, Ray	Chest pain

Figure 7-14. Example of a daily appointment reference sheet

GUIDELINES TO AVOID AUDITS AND IMPROVE SCHEDULING

It has been determined that appointment scheduling is the most important part of patient care. Following are a few ways to avoid an audit and improve scheduling:

- Make sure the telephone receptionist knows how much time to allow for appointments based upon the physician's determinations and guidelines.

- Block off several emergency slots during the day.

- Notify the supervisor immediately when an urgent appointment cannot be given to an established patient on the same day.

- Note the time each patient is actually seen using 15 minutes as the maximum waiting time; after a two-week check, if the waiting time is longer, bring scheduling into line with back-office reality.

- Notify patients if the physician is running 20 minutes or more behind schedule so those patients may have the option to reschedule or continue to wait.

- Utilize physician extenders to provide routine care. This gives waiting patients another immediate option.

- Limit primary-care office visits to the national average of six per hour, until it has been determined whether the work pace should be increased or decreased.

STOP AND THINK CASE SCENARIO

Handle a Patient with an Unverified Appointment

Scenario: Mr. Frederickson shows up at the office Monday morning on May 10 at 10:00 a.m. stating he has an appointment with Dr. Gerald Practon. Dr. Practon is overbooked and very busy all day. You search the appointment book and locate an appointment for the patient on the next day, Tuesday, May 11, at 10:00 a.m. When you advise Mr. Frederickson that the appointment was made for Tuesday, he becomes very agitated. He did not bring his appointment card with him but is adamant, stating, "It says Monday, May 10."

Critical Thinking: Options are: (1) Stand firm because the appointment is documented, (2) work the patient in as soon as possible, (3) work the patient in later in the morning, (4) ask the patient to come back in the afternoon and you will work him in. Decide which option you would take and elaborate on how you would word your response; give a rationale for your choice.

_____

_____

_____

_____

_____

_____

_____

_____

_____

_____

_____

_____

_____

STOP AND THINK CASE SCENARIO

Determine a Routine, Urgent, or Emergency Appointment

Scenario: Dr. Fran Practon's Friday schedule is full and Mrs. Charlene Pratt, an established patient, calls at 1:00 p.m. requesting to be seen that day for a migraine headache she has had for one week.

Critical Thinking: Below are four possible ways to respond in this situation. First, determine if this is an emergency, urgent, or routine appointment. Next, select one of the possible choices. Third, compose a response and comment on various factors used in your critical thinking and decision-making process. And last, comment on why you did not select the other choices.

a. Send her to the emergency room

_____

_____

_____

_____

_____

b. Have her see Dr. Gerald Practon, who has an opening that afternoon

_____

_____

_____

_____

_____

c. Have her come into the office and wait

_____

_____

_____

_____

_____

_____

d. Make an appointment for her first thing on Monday morning with Dr. Fran Practon

_____

_____

_____

_____

_____

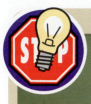

STOP AND THINK CASE SCENARIO

Explain Office Policy for Urgent and Emergent Appointments

Scenario: In Scenario #2, Mrs. Pratt indicates that she does not want to see a male doctor and decides to wait to see Dr. Fran Practon; she is worked into the schedule at 2:00 p.m. Mr. Belgum, who has an appointment at 2:00 p.m. is sitting in the waiting room and gets upset because Mrs. Pratt is taken back to see the physician before he is.

Critical Thinking: What would you say to Mr. Belgum?

_____

_____

_____

_____

_____

_____

FOCUS ON CERTIFICATION*

CMA Content Summary

- Medical abbreviations and symbols
- Disease abbreviations
- Appointment abbreviations
- Appointment office policies
- Telephone technique
- Computerized appointments
- Scheduling and monitoring appointments

RMA Content Summary

- Abbreviations and symbols
- Interpersonal skills with vendors and business associates
- Patient education
- Appointment documentation
- Medical terminology applications
- Scheduling systems

- Managing various appointments
- Telephone etiquette

CMAS Content Summary

- Medical terminology and abbreviations
- Human relation skills and professionalism
- Charting
- Medical office emergencies
- Appointment scheduling and monitoring
- Appointment cancellations, no-shows, referrals, recalls
- Hospital admissions and outside appointments
- Appointment flow
- Telephone technique
- Patient chart documentation
- Computerized appointments

---

* _This textbook and accompanying Workbook meet the entry-level administrative and general competencies for the CMA outlined by the AAMA Examination Content Outline and Role Delineation Study and for the RMA and CMAS outlined by the AMT Competencies and Examination Specifications (see Competency Grid in Appendix B)._

1. A template:

   a. serves as a guide for scheduling various types of appointments

   b. indicates each doctor's preferred time management schedule

   c. cuts down on decision making

   d. is preformatted with a certain number of slots for various types of appointments

   e. all of the above

2. A new patient is one who has:

   a. never been seen by the physician

   b. never been seen by the physician or a member of the medical practice

   c. never been seen by the physician or a member of the same specialty of the group practice

   d. not been seen by the physician or a member of the same specialty of the group practice for 3 years

   e. not been seen by the physician or a member of the same specialty of the group practice for 5 years

3. Marking the appointment book to set aside time for lunch hours, hospital rounds, regular meetings, and so forth is referred to as a:

   a. block

   b. hold

   c. reservation

   d. close

   e. flag

4. To evaluate a scheduling system, periodically review patient flow by analyzing the schedule for a minimum of:

   a. 2 weeks

   b. 4 weeks

   c. 6 weeks

   d. 8 weeks

   e. 10 weeks

5. Scheduling patients in the first half of each hour with single ten-minute appointments and no scheduled appointments the second half of the hour is called:

   a. true wave scheduling

   b. modified wave scheduling

   c. stream scheduling

   d. clustered appointments

   e. open access

6. Open access is also called:

   a. single booking

   b. double booking

   c. same day scheduling

   d. open hours

   e. triage

7. A tickler file may be used:

   a. as a template for appointment scheduling

   b. to file incoming test results

   c. to file incoming documents

   d. to place reminder cards

   e. to look up telephone numbers

8. Select what action to take when a genuine emergency situation occurs.

   a. refer the patient to a hospital emergency room

   b. suggest the patient come to the office immediately

   c. schedule the patient for one of the appointment slots left open for such problems

   d. work the patient into the schedule

   e. all the above

9. All referral appointments should be:

   a. referred to the physician

   b. referred to the doctor on call

   c. scheduled as soon as possible

   d. treated as typical new patient or established appointments

   e. handled by the office manager

10. An appointment reference sheet:

    a. can be used by all staff members

    b. is for the physician only

    c. is made for the receptionist

    d. should be kept as a permanent record

    e. is not used in computerized offices

11. A "PDA" device is a:

    a. physician's desk advisor used for scheduling appointments

    b. physician digital access component that can be connected to a computer

    c. small laptop computer

    d. personal doctor's analogue

    e. handheld computer that can be used for data transfer

12. A patient who is in a convalescent or nursing home is visited by the physician:

    a. every time the patient requests

    b. each week

    c. each month

    d. every time the nursing staff calls to report on the patient's condition

    e. as needed

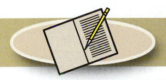

WORKBOOK ASSIGNMENT

To develop competency-based job skills, refer to the *Workbook* and complete the:

- Abbreviation and Spelling Review
- Review Questions

- Critical Thinking Exercises
- Job Skill Activities, which are outlined at the beginning of this chapter under "Performance Objectives in the *Workbook*."

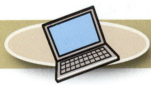

COMPUTER ASSIGNMENT

To review the concepts you have learned in this chapter, insert the *Student Practice* CD-ROM into a computer and work through the *StudyWARE* activities and games. Answer review questions in the practice mode and read the feedback, studying the questions you have missed. Take the chapter quiz until you achieve a minimum score of 90 percent. Successfully completing the *Critical Thinking Challenge* at the end of this course will help you think through scenarios and develop problem solving skills.

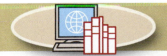

RESOURCES

Appointment Scheduling

View software selections and Internet services for appointment scheduling

Use one of the search engines, e.g., www.google.com.
Google

Lycos
Web Crawler
Yahoo
Search key phrase: physician appointment scheduling

Booklets

How to Cut Patient Wait Times

Practice Support Resources
4230 Phelps Road, Suite E
Independence, MO 64055
(800) 967-7790
Search key phrase: cut patient wait time
Web site: http://www.practicesupport.com

Office Productivity & Efficient Patient Scheduling

Practice Support Resources
4230 Phelps Road, Suite E
Independence, MO 64055
(800) 967-7790
Search key number and phrase: #157 (efficient scheduling)
Web site: http://www.practicesupport.com

Clinical Messaging

Sample companies that offer clinical messaging:
Medfusion
Web site: http://www.medfusion.net
RelayHealth
Web site: http://www.relayhealth.com

Internet

American Academy of Family Physicians

Search key term: open access scheduling
Web site: http://aafp.org/fpm/

UNIT 3

Records Management

CHAPTER 8

Filing Procedures

OBJECTIVES

After reading this chapter and learning step-by-step procedures to gain job skills,* you should be able to:

Learning Objectives

State the differences between alphabetic, subject, indirect, chronologic, electronic, and tickler filing systems.

Memorize and apply ARMA filing rules.

Select equipment and supplies to set up a filing system.

Develop a charge-out system and conduct a search for a lost record.

Prepare and sort documents for filing.

Determine the retention period for temporary and permanent records.

Understand various reprographic methods used in record storage.

Determine methods to transfer and dispose of records including confidential materials.

Performance Objectives (Procedures) in This Textbook

File using a subject filing system (Procedure 8-1).

File using a numeric filing system (Procedure 8-2).

Set up an e-mail filing system (Procedure 8-3).

Organize a tickler file (Procedure 8-4).

Determine filing units and indexing order to alphabetically file a patient's medical record (Procedure 8-5).

Label and color-code patient charts (Procedure 8-6).

This textbook and the accompanying Workbook meet the educational components for entry-level administrative and general competencies outlined by CAAHEP and ABHES.

- Prepare, sort, and file documents in patient records (Procedure 8-7).
- Locate a misfiled medical-record file folder (Procedure 8-8).

Performance Objectives (Job Skills) in the *Workbook*

- Determine filing units (Job Skill 8-1).
- Index and file names alphabetically (Job Skill 8-2).
- File patient and business names alphabetically (Job Skill 8-3).
- Index names on file folder labels and arrange file cards in alphabetic order (Job Skill 8-4).
- Color-code file cards (Job Skill 8-5).

OUTLINE   WITH LECTURE NOTES

Commercial Filing Systems
Alphabetic Filing System

_____

_____

_____

_____

Subject Filing System

_____

_____

_____

Indirect Filing System

_____

_____

_____

_____

Electronic Filing System

_____

_____

_____

_____

Tickler Filing System

_____

_____

_____

_____

Alphabetic Filing Rules
General Guidelines

_____

_____

_____

_____

Filing Equipment
Lateral Files

_____

_____

_____

_____

Full-Suspension Drawer Files

_____

_____

_____

Automated Files

_____

_____

_____

_____

Filing Supplies and Their Uses

_____

_____

_____

_____

Guides

_____

_____

_____

_____

Folders

_____

_____

_____

_____

Color-Coding File Folders

_____

_____

_____

_____

Tabs

_____

_____

_____

_____

Labels

_____

_____

_____

_____

Charge-Out and Control Systems
Outguide

_____

_____

_____

_____

Outfolder

_____

_____

_____

_____

Filing Documents in Patient Records

_____

_____

_____

_____

Misfiling

_____

_____

_____

_____

Misplaced or Lost Records

_____

_____

_____

_____

Record Retention and Storage

_____

_____

_____

_____

Financial and Legal Records

_____

_____

_____

_____

Active and Inactive Patient Files

_____

_____

_____

_____

Electronic Storage

_____

_____

_____

_____

Destroying Documents
Purging Computer Files

_____

_____

_____

_____

Recycling

_____

_____

_____

_____

KEY TERMS

alphabetic filing
Association of Records Managers and
    Administrators (ARMA International)
automated files
backup
binder file folder
caption
charge-out system
coding
commercial filing system
cut
databases
diagnostic file
download
downtime
electronic files
encryption
folder

given name
guide
indexing unit
label
lateral file
master patient index (MPI)
numeric filing
open-shelf files
outguide
password
purge
recycle
scores
subject filing
surname
tab
tickler file
virus

HEART OF THE HEALTH CARE PROFESSIONAL

Service

Patients appreciate a medical assistant who can expedite their care by performing behind-the-scenes tasks. Having information at your fingertips and being able to locate documents quickly are a great service to patients.

COMMERCIAL FILING SYSTEMS

There is an abundant variety of recorded information in physician practices, and the administrative medical assistant needs to protect and file it in an accurate and expedient manner. The information can be paper documents such as progress notes, hard-copy reports, hand-written memos, or messages, or electronic documents such as medical records, databases, or e-mail, or graphic images such as x-rays. Because medical records constitute the collective memory of a physician's practice, good judgment should be exercised in choosing a filing system that not only is easy to understand but also meets the office needs for security, expansion, and retrieval. No single filing system is "best," because every practice is unique. The office staff may choose to adopt its own filing system and rules to fit the office needs; however, general rules should be written so all staff members follow the same guidelines. Compliance by all employees is mandatory or the system will not work.

Office management considerations when determining a filing system are (1) amount of active records, (2) amount of inactive records, (3) frequency of record retrieval, (4) amount of filing space, (5) convenience of file locations, and (6) cost of the system. After the medical assistant has determined office needs, the names of dealers and manufacturers can be found in the Yellow Pages of the telephone directory or over the Internet. Medical offices often purchase some form of patented **commercial filing system** (alphabetic and/or numeric), which uses folders and guides manufactured for professional office use. Medical and financial records are filed separately.

Alphabetic Filing System

The simplest and most popular filing method is by alphabetic name sequence, because it is easy to understand and does not require a cross-reference index.

Also, if an alphabetic entry is especially confusing, the telephone book, which is a classic example of alphabetic name filing, provides an excellent reference.

Alphabetic Color-Coding

Management consultants recommend color-coded alphabetic filing that consists of colored tabs for each letter of the alphabet. Depending on the size of the practice, tabs are selected for the first, second, and third letters in the patient's last name and secured to the edge of the file folder for easy reference.

Alphabetic color-coding of medical file folders has the advantage of reducing misfiles, speeding retrieval, and making office filing more efficient. The labels are readable from front and back for open-shelf file cabinets.

In alphabetic color-coding, all letters of the alphabet are assigned specific colors. Typically the first two letters of the patient's last name would be identified on the folder tab with different colors. Any misfiled record would break the color pattern and stand out, for example, when filing the name "Franklin," the letter F could be red and the r would be color-coded green. You would quickly locate the "Fr" section in the file cabinet and file the chart using the remaining letters of the patient's surname alphabetically. An example of an open-shelf file folder using this type of color coding is shown in Figure 8-1.

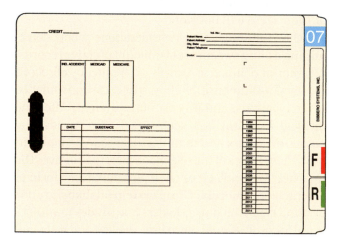

Figure 8-1. Preprinted lateral file folder with color-coded alphabetic designation for first two letters of the last name and year tab. (Courtesy of Bibbero Systems, Inc., Petaluma, CA. Telephone: (800) 242-2376; Fax (800) 242-9330; Web site: http://www.bibbero.com.)

Subject Filing System

Subject filing is an alphabetic arrangement of records filed by topic or grouped under a main theme. These themes are assigned titles that become signposts to direct you to the right file.

Business papers, other than those dealing with patients, are usually stored in a separate cabinet or desk drawer and filed in alphabetic order by subject. Miscellaneous communication dealing with matters other than patient treatment may be filed under "Correspondence."

If the physician does research, lectures, or writes for periodicals, the assistant may be in charge of organizing materials in a **diagnostic file** so the physician can easily and quickly locate current information. The main heading in this type of subject file might be the name of the disease. Then after the main heading, patient cards can be alphabetized with name, diagnosis, treatment, prognosis, and additional information outlined. A diagnostic file can be easily adapted to the office computer.

Since no two subject files are the same, the medical assistant handling the business matters of the practice usually determines the captions for the guides and folders. Examples of documents include: employee information, financial documents, insurance policies, and taxes. Then subcategories are created under each category, e.g., taxes (federal and state).

In Office Reference Files

If the physician keeps medical articles for future reference, the medical assistant should maintain a subject filing system for storing and retrieving articles and other information. Processing articles for such a system can be accomplished in the following ways:

1. The physician can write a heading on each informative article printed from the Internet or taken from newspapers, brochures, and journals. The articles may then be. filed by subject or assigned a number and cross-referenced in a subject card file. Both main subject and secondary subject headings may be referenced (see Example 8-1). If the article is on an obscure topic, it is helpful to give it a fairly general heading.

2. The physician may highlight the title of an article that is of special interest in the table of contents. The assistant will then remove the article and assign a main heading and

> ## EXAMPLE 8-1
>
> ### Subject Headings for Medical Articles
>
> A. Article title: "Advance Clues to Heart Attacks"
>   Main subject heading: "Heart Attacks"
>   Secondary subject heading: "Advance Clues"
>
> B. Article title: "Living with Multiple Sclerosis"
>   Main subject heading: "Multiple Sclerosis"
>   Secondary subject heading: "Activities of Daily Living (MS)"
>
> C. Article title: "The Menopausal Woman and Breast Cancer"
>   Main subject heading: "Breast Cancer"
>   Secondary subject heading: "Menopause"

secondary heading for a subject file. If two articles share a common page (front and back sides), one side would be photocopied for the first page of the second article.

3. The assistant can make a photocopy of the tables of contents of all journals to be kept in a loose-leaf notebook. The journals are stored elsewhere. After the physician has decided which material to retain, the remaining journals can be discarded or given away. Outdated medical magazines can be sent to medical missionaries in third-world countries, or more recent issues could be donated to a hospital library, medical school, or allied health program.

4. Articles can be accessed via computer, thus eliminating the storage of journals.

Physicians can also insert current articles directly into the patients chart so a discussion of the latest treatment option can be held when the patient returns. Maintaining a patient database by disease, symptom, medication, or device (e.g., pacemaker) will make locating patients for this purpose easier.

Software which simplifies locating and organizing bibliographic information can also be obtained.

Indirect Filing System

If privacy and convenience of expansion are important considerations, an indirect filing system may be preferable. An indirect filing system, also referred to as **numeric filing** or *unit numbering*, is used primar-

---

PROCEDURE 8-1

File Using a Subject Filing System

Objective: To demonstrate filing of documents using a subject filing system.

Equipment/Supplies: Documents to be filed by subject, subject index list, highlighter pen, and pencil.

Directions: Follow these step-by-step procedures, which include rationales, to learn this skill.

1. Read the document to find the main subject.

2. Highlight or underline the key-word that best describes the subject of the document.

3. Write the subject header in the upper right corner if it does not appear in the document.

4. Search the subject index list to match the subject of the item with an appropriate category.

5. Copy the document if it will be filed in two locations.

6. Make a cross-reference if the document contains information that may pertain to more than one topic by inserting a keyword for the second subject in the upper right corner of the document.

7. Periodically remove any outdated information.

ily to handle rapidly growing files in hospitals, clinics, and large medical practices. An indirect system might be more appropriate than an alphabetic system if the patient load exceeds 10,000. It is termed an "indirect" system because an auxiliary cross-reference index is used to determine a patient's assigned number before locating the file. A *numeric file register*, or accession file with consecutive numbers, is usually maintained to determine the last assigned number. After a number has been assigned, it is either keyed into a computer filing program or typed with the patient's name on a small index card and filed alphabetically by last name in a vertical file container or visible file such as a rotary rack, wheel, or loose-leaf binder. A cross-reference file provides rapid access to patient numbers and may also be used to record addresses, telephone numbers, and brief diagnostic notes. A disadvantage of numeric filing is the time the extra step (i.e., locating the number to find the file) takes when an assistant needs to pull a patient's chart quickly in response to a telephone inquiry.

The following methods of filing by consecutive numeric sequence result in more even distribution of active and inactive records in large medical institutions maintaining 10,000 to 100,000 records. The *middle-digit numbering sequence* arranges records by six-digit numbers. The *terminal-digit* and *triple-digit* systems use numbers to designate shelves or drawers to find charts, and all digits are color-coded. Hospital record numbers, x-ray numbers, and telephone numbers are often used as a basis for arranging records by the last digits (Example 8-2).

EXAMPLE 8-2

Indirect Numeric Filing (Terminal Digit)

A. To retrieve Mrs. Doe's case, number 294597, begin with the last number sequence and locate 97, then look for the middle number sequence 45, and finally look for the first number sequence 29.

$$294597 = 97\ 45\ 29$$

B. To obtain Mr. Benton Thomas's patient record number 516204, begin with the last number by going to Section 4, which appears as 000004 (sections 0 to 9), then the next two digits—Row 20 appears as 000204 (rows 00 to 99), then the next two digits—Shelf 16 appears as 016204 (order 00 to 99), and finally to the chart 516204 (order 0 to 9).

Record No. 516204 = 5 (chart)
16 (shelf) 20 (row) 4 (section)

Color-coding of individual digits is often used with these systems to prevent misfiling and to make it easier to find a misplaced file.

Serial numbering is used by hospitals and large facilities when file expansion is not necessary. A patient receives a new number and folder at each visit. The disadvantage is that continuity of care may

---

PROCEDURE 8-2

STEP 1 2 3

File Using a Numeric Filing System

Objective: To demonstrate filing of documents using a numeric filing system.

Equipment/Supplies: Documents to be filed by number, three- by five-inch cards, and an alphabetic card cross-reference file box.

Directions: Follow these step-by-step procedures, which include rationales, to learn this skill.

1. Inspect the file folder and assign a serial number.

2. Obtain a file card to use as the alphabetic card cross-reference.

3. Write the assigned number in the upper right corner.

4. Data such as patient's name, address, telephone numbers, and diagnoses may be indicated.

5. Place the document numerically in the file cabinet with guides for every 25 or more items.

6. Store cards alphabetically by name or subject in a card file kept near the cabinet.

be disrupted because retrieval of previous records is time-consuming.

Numeric Color-Coding

Numeric color-coding of file folder tabs assigns ten colors to represent the numbers zero through nine. An office that uses consecutive numeric color-coding will decide the number of digits to color-code—all or only one of the numbers may be color-coded depending on the size of the practice. Color-coding only the primary digits is known as two-band color-coding; four bands use primary and secondary digits, six bands color-code all numbers. In middle-digit and terminal-digit filing, two blocks of color or bars appear in each position, indicating first, second, and third units.

Master Patient Index

Large health maintenance facilities and hospitals may choose to set up **master patient index (MPI)** files that identify all patients who have ever been admitted or treated in the health care facility. The filing system is usually computerized; however, if a manual system is used and a chart needs to be retrieved, the assistant first consults the MPI card file to find the number assigned to the patient and then goes to the storage area to retrieve the file. This system is *indirect* because before the patient's data is retrieved, a numeric file must be consulted to obtain the reference number.

Chronological Files

In a *chronological* filing system, numbers are used based on dates. Files, or sections within a file are listed by year, month, and day having the most recent files in the front of the file drawer or the most recent documents in the front of the folder. In a physician's office, chronological filing is one method used to file documents within a chart so that the latest visit, laboratory text, x-ray, hospitalization, and so forth are at the beginning of each section of the file (see Chapter 9 for more information).

Electronic Filing System

With computer hard drives increasing in size and printers rapidly outputting information, different methods of media storage and retrieval have been developed. Information systems of the millennium and beyond will require much more refined and efficient techniques. Electronic filing systems offer such capabilities.

A computer can organize information and allow for easy retrieval and storage. A limited amount of information about a patient may be stored using an electronic record management system. Records may be retrieved for an individual patient or by using search parameters, such as all women between the ages of 35 and 50 with diabetes or all patients last seen 36 months prior. Patient and insurance requests for documents become simplified by automatic printouts.

With a computer it is possible to link up to a local community hospital's health information management (medical record) department using a modem. This may allow physicians to have access to their patients' hospital history and physical reports; patient chart notes; operative reports; discharge summaries; and x-ray, pathology, and laboratory reports. The physician can dictate, edit, and electronically sign all reports from the office, eliminating a trip to the hospital and expediting the completion of medical records.

Bar Codes

Some medical practices use pressure-sensitive barcode labels on patients' file folders, record boxes, or other document containers. The bar code number is scanned into the computer software. A wand may be attached to the computer for scanning purposes, making computer-based file management and tracking of the file immediately possible (Figure 8-2). A chart with a bar code can simply be swiped like a credit card as the chart passes from one area of the office to another, thus tracking the chart becomes easy. Some software systems allow on-demand printing of bar codes and folder labels, which may be color-coded for rapid visual identification.

Scanners

Some medical practices use a scanning machine to scan and index outside documents, such as explanation of benefit (EOB) reports that are received with insurance checks. Document management software digitizes the information and stores it on the hard drive of the practice's computer. Checks may be categorized by number for future reference. At the end of each month, the data may be downloaded on two CDs—one kept in the office for reference and one stored off-site for backup safety. This makes it easy to look up documents, answer patients' questions about bills, or solve payment problems with an insurer. Original EOBs may be shredded so little office space is needed for storage.

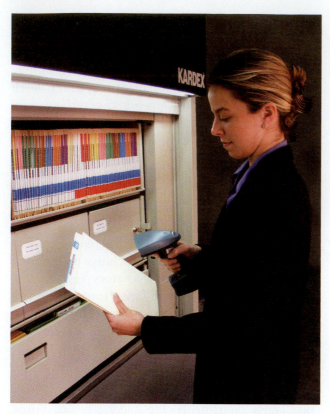

Figure 8-2. The medical assistant scanning a bar code to track where charts are located in the office. (Courtesy of Kardex.)

Databases

Various **electronic files** or **databases** are used in medical practices to store a collection of information electronically. These may consist of files pertaining to patients, drugs, diagnoses, procedures, diseases, surgeries, or other categories used to monitor information. First, the data are entered. Searches can be performed and reports printed according to patients' names, patient numbers, procedure codes, birth dates, insurance company names, or any other common factors. If a physician is doing research and wants to search for the names of all patients with a certain disease, the database can be quickly accessed and the information easily retrieved.

Other data can consist of stored form letters that can be retrieved and printed when necessary. This eliminates having to either compose original letters or order and store preprinted letters.

Financial records also are kept in electronic files.

Electronic Security

Because a patient's medical information must always be kept confidential, it is important to maintain security of the computer system. This becomes the respon-

COMPLIANCE

There are several options for controlling access to data. Those most frequently used are identification (ID) numbers and electronic passwords, also called *security codes*. A **password** can be a word or phrase, but it should contain a sequence of letters and numbers so it remains private and cannot be guessed by others to gain access. Badges, cards, and keys may also be used to access individual terminals. Biometric access controls unique to each individual may consist of fingerprints, eye patterns, or voice prints. As mentioned and shown in Chapter 3, there are statements that clearly outline the consequences of violating confidentiality rules and regulations.

sibility of every employee. Access to the systems can become threatened if medical assistants are not aware of basic security measures.

When an individual leaves a place of employment, his or her password or means of access needs to be changed. To guard against theft and embezzlement, an employer should consider whether employees need simple inquiry functions versus data entry and update functions. Only responsible employees should be given the task of deleting and updating information. Accounting procedures should be monitored frequently, and an "exceptions report" (printing write-offs or adjustments), which identifies the employee who posts the transactions, should be available only to the office manager and physician. A secure form of retaining confidentiality is a software program that stores files in coded form. This process is known as **encryption**, which makes the data look like gibberish to unauthorized users. Many computer programs are designed to record the dates and times files are altered. With a log-on feature, any employee who alters a file can be identified.

Maintaining Computer Files

Computer files can grow tremendously and then become unmanageable when the medical assistant tries to find a letter or report. Similar word documents should be placed in computerized file folders clearly labeled and sorted for easy retrieval. Computerized file management systems are also available to assist in arranging files. Using such a system not only helps

PROCEDURE 8-3

Set Up an E-Mail Filing System

Objective: To prepare an e-mail file designed for filing e-mail messages.

Equipment/Supplies: Computer, Internet access, and e-mail account.

Directions: Follow these step-by-step procedures, which include rationales, to learn this skill.

1. Separate and delete junk mail immediately upon receiving it. If you want to keep mail temporarily, it may be left after reading it; most e-mail systems will automatically delete read mail in 7 to 14 days.

2. Sort through business-related e-mail to determine which ones need to be printed for action, filed in office files (e.g., patient charts), and stored electronically.

3. Create a filing system for important e-mail items. Determine e-mail folder names that will allow you to find them easily and quickly when you need them. For example, folders could be named, "Contracts," "Supply Companies," "Maintenance," and so forth.

4. Save e-mails to appropriate folders.

5. Purge mail in folders periodically to eliminate old information.

---

with quick retrieval but also saves space on the computer hard drive.

Maintaining E-Mail Files—The medical office may get electronic mail from vendors, patients, government agencies, and other outside sources. E-mail files need to be managed the same way paper files are managed so that information can be easily retrieved. It is important to sort e-mail regularly so you can determine what is important, label it, and file it so it is easily found. Procedure 8-3 lists steps for setting up an e-mail filing system.

Backing up Computer Files

Files should be backed up periodically and always at the end of the day. A full **backup** is an exact copy of the entire hard drive that is stored on a Digital Versatile (Video) Disc (DVD), Compact Disc Read-Only Memory (CD-Rom), Zip disk, flash drive, or an external hard drive. Frequency of backups will depend on the amount of information input. If a lot, then it is wise to back up (save data) often during data entry.

It is possible to establish automated backup, where the computer itself regularly initiates the process. Good financial software programs have a screen prompt asking for backup before quitting the program. Information may be lost because of a power spike, computer breakdown, or a **virus**. To prevent a virus from infecting the computer, use a firewall or router to prevent outsiders from viewing computer data. Software can also be installed to display a mes-

sage when an infected disk is inserted. Occasionally update the antiviral program and annually purchase the latest version. When the computer is not functioning properly, this is referred to as **downtime**. A power *surge suppressor*, preferably with backup capability, will prevent computer and data file damage. Always retain the three most recent backups, recycling the older to be used for the newer.

About once a week have the computer compare the original records with the copies. This verification can take 20 percent to 30 percent longer than ordinary backup, but if a comparison is not made, there is no way to ensure it has been backed up properly. Another good insurance is to select one backup per month to keep indefinitely. Then if something should happen to the computer, it is then possible to return the data to an earlier condition and update from that point. It is important to store backup copies of computer data away from the office because of fire, flood, and theft.

Electronic Confidentiality Guidelines

Follow these guidelines for proper compliance of confidentiality when using a computer and for avoiding problems with computer files.

1. Never leave disks or tapes unguarded on desks or anywhere else in sight.

2. Always log off your computer terminal before you leave your workstation, especially if working in a local area network (LAN) environment.

3. Never write down log-on sequences, passwords, or any other codes that regulate personal access to a system; change your password periodically. If you must write down your password, hide the paper and scramble what is written; for example, New York could be written as KEWYORN, EWYOR, or YORKNEW. Each will jog your memory, but none is immediately useful to the casual observer. Do not use an obvious choice for a password. A password that includes numbers, such as BOOK91END, 22MODEM88, or PHONE64 is significantly harder to break than one composed of letters alone.

4. Never **download** (transfer data) public domain software, files from electronic bulletin boards, or other communications systems, because a virus can get into the office system.

5. Never bring in disks from outside your office.

6. Always back up files regularly to save data that might get lost through a breach of security.

7. Respect other employees' computer files the same way you do those kept in a desk file drawer. If you use another employee's computer, do not move or alter files or change the screen format.

Tickler Filing System

A **tickler file**, also called a *suspense* or *follow-up* file, is used in medical offices so the staff can remind patients of preset appointments, follow up on patients who have missed or canceled appointments, and note tests patients may need scheduled in the future (see Figures 8-3, 8-4, 8-5, and 8-6). Tickler files can be set up in computer systems to prompt the medical assis-

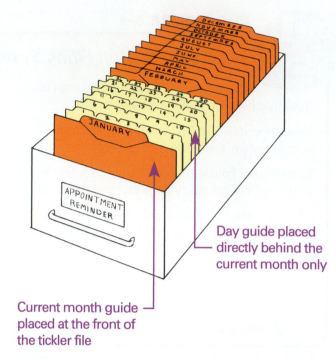

Day guide placed directly behind the current month only

Current month guide placed at the front of the tickler file

Figure 8-3. Tickler card file used as an appointment reminder system

tant to take action at specific times, such as check on an expected referral letter or laboratory report due by a specified date, order a depleted inventory item, or follow up on an unpaid insurance claim. These files may also be used to remind the physician of personal appointments, subscription renewal dates, income tax payments, and meeting dates.

Short-Notice Reminder File

In a short-notice reminder system, a file is divided into time categories appropriate to the practice, such as *urgent*, *anytime*, *a.m.*, and *p.m.* When making appointments, patients are asked if they are interested in coming on short notice or anytime there is

PATIENT EDUCATION

Offer to notify a patient prior to a future appointment. For example, if a patient has an appointment in April, he or she can address a preprinted reminder notice or card (Figure 8-4) when in the office for a visit. The assistant places the card in the tickler file (Figure 8-3) after the April guide, ready to be placed in an envelope and mailed a few weeks before the scheduled appointment. At the conclusion of the April appointment, the patient completes another card for the next appointment, which is again placed behind the appropriate monthly guide.

PRACTON MEDICAL GROUP, INC.
4567 Broad Avenue
Woodland Hills, XY 12345
Tel. 555/486-9002

As you requested, we are reminding you that it is time for your six-month checkup with *Dr. Fran Practon*

Please phone today for an appointment. Then use the space below to note the date and time reserved for you.

DAY   DATE   TIME

Figure 8-4. Preprinted tickler card used as appointment reminder

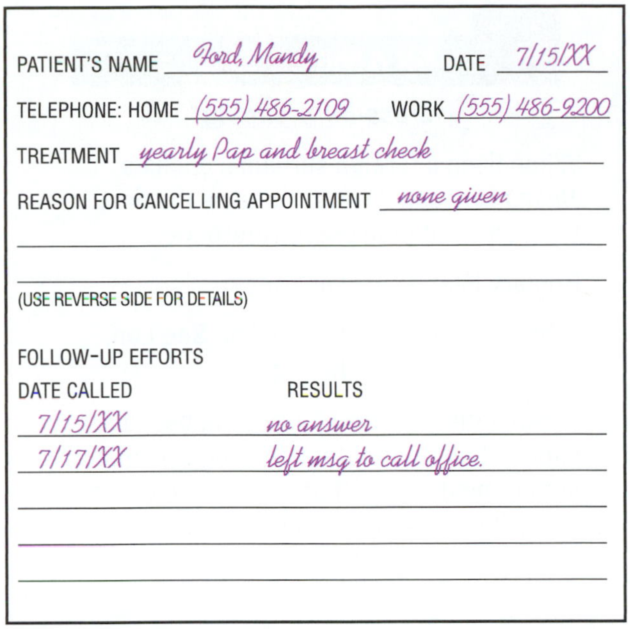

PATIENT'S NAME _Ford, Mandy_   DATE _7/15/XX_

TELEPHONE: HOME _(555) 486-2109_   WORK _(555) 486-9200_

TREATMENT _yearly Pap and breast check_

REASON FOR CANCELLING APPOINTMENT _none given_

_____

(USE REVERSE SIDE FOR DETAILS)

FOLLOW-UP EFFORTS

DATE CALLED   RESULTS

_7/15/XX_   _no answer_

_7/17/XX_   _left msg to call office._

Figure 8-5. Follow-up card documenting data on patients who have missed or canceled appointments

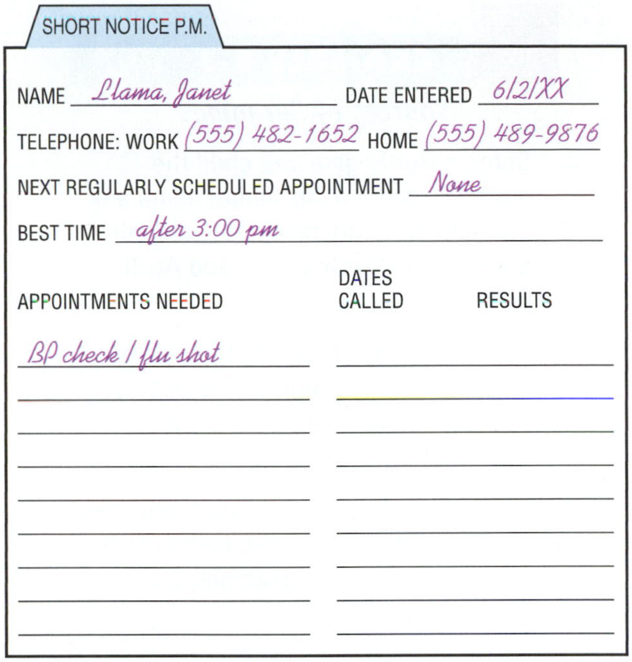

SHORT NOTICE P.M.

NAME _Llama, Janet_   DATE ENTERED _6/2/XX_

TELEPHONE: WORK _(555) 482-1652_ HOME _(555) 489-9876_

NEXT REGULARLY SCHEDULED APPOINTMENT _None_

BEST TIME _after 3:00 pm_

APPOINTMENTS NEEDED	DATES CALLED	RESULTS
BP check / flu shot		

Figure 8-6. Tickler card used as a reference to call patients on short notice for fill-in appointments

an opening. This information is placed on an appointment card and filed in the appropriate category (Figure 8-6). Then when there is a cancellation, the assistant can refer to the short-notice reminder file to select one of these people as a substitute.

Temporary Reminder File

Occasionally, a *temporary* file can be set up for items that need action but need not be kept permanently. The items can be coded with a "T" and destroyed when action has been completed.

ALPHABETIC FILING RULES

In 1986 the **Association of Records Managers and Administrators (ARMA International)** developed rules for alphabetizing that are the basis for most **alphabetic filing** systems in use today. As patterns for naming offspring are changing, moving away from the traditional use of the male surname, rules must be adopted to reflect these trends. Example 8-3 (page 238) shows alternative sources of surnames.

PROCEDURE 8-4

STEP 1 2 3

Organize a Tickler File

Objective: To prepare a tickler file designed for recalling patients by mail for future appointments.

Equipment/Supplies: Small index card storage box, three-by-five-inch index cards, 12 monthly dividers, and pen.

Directions: Follow these step-by-step procedures, which include rationales, to learn this skill.

1. Type or write the names and addresses of patients on cards. These will be mailed to patients as reminders of needed appointments.

2. Insert the month and year of the recall appointment on each card.

3. File each card behind the month preceding the patient's recall appointment. Allow enough time for mailing and response.

4. Check the tickler file at least once or twice a month to send out recall notices. This should be done enough in advance so patients can call and reserve times during the appropriate month for their future appointments.

EXAMPLE 8-3

Sources of Surnames

A. Some parents give one child the mother's maiden (surname) name and the next child the father's name, for example, Jerry Dearfield and April Lange

B. Others choose to give their children a hyphenated version of the last two names, for example, Jerry Dearfield-Lange

C. Others develop a hybrid surname linking parts of the parents' two names to form a new surname, for example, Jerry DeLange

---

EXAMPLE 8-4

Cross-Referencing

When filing a foreign surname, such as *Huang Lon*, use the last name as the first filing unit and then cross-reference.

Primary File: Lon, Huang

X-Reference File: Huang, Lon **See** Lon, Huang

When patients have identical names, alert each patient to that fact and suggest that both remind the staff at each office visit to prevent confusion about records.

To standardize filing procedures and ensure consistency, the simplified general rules considered appropriate for the medical office will be summarized with examples from the current edition of *Alphabetic Filing Rules* published by the AMRA International Standards Program. The creative medical assistant can design a specific filing system with rules for the office as long as each person handling the files knows exactly which rules to follow.

Before preparing any file-folder labels, a medical assistant needs to master either the filing rules developed by the office staff or adopt the simplified standard rules developed by AMRA International*, that follow.

General Guidelines

Names are divided into sections called *units* (last name, first name, middle name). The alphabetical process starts by comparing the first unit (last name), letter by letter. If only a last name is known, this single unit is filed before a last name with a first initial. A last name with only an initial is filed before a last name with a first name beginning with the same initial; this rule is often stated as "file nothing before something." Punctuation marks are generally disregarded, and the use of periods after abbreviations is optional. Example 8-4 shows how to cross-reference.

Rule 1: Individual Names

Names of patients are assigned **indexing units** and alphabetized by comparing the first unit in each name, letter by letter, in this order: **surname** (last name), first indexing unit; **given name** (first name), second indexing unit; and middle name (if any), third indexing unit (see Example 8-5). Second units are considered only when the first units are the same, third units are considered only when the first and second units are the same, and so on. Additional subsequent names or initials are filed as successive units. If only initials are listed, for example, E. J. Hoover, the first initial is considered a complete unit and filed before names with additional letters.

Rule 2: Prefixes

Last names with prefixes are called *surname particles* (e.g., "D," "de," "Del," "Des," "Mac," "Mc," "Saint," "St.," "Van") and are filed like other surnames as one indexing unit whether the prefix is followed by a space or not (see Example 8-6). The prefix is considered part of the surname. When filing "Saint" and "St.," they either may be filed exactly as spelled or "St." may be spelled out, depending on the wishes of the office.

Rule 3: Hyphenated Names

All hyphenated names—whether first names, middle names, or surnames—are considered to be one indexing unit. For example, when a husband and

---

* AMRA International, 13725 West 109th Street, Suite 101, Lenexa, KS 66215 Telephone: (913) 341-3808 or (800) 422-2762

wife combine their surnames with a hyphen, ignore the hyphen and file the two names as one unit. Surnames on folder labels may be typed without a hyphen, a space, or any punctuation mark such as apostrophes and periods. Hyphenated words in a business name, however, are indexed as separate units. Example 8-7 shows how to file hyphenated names.

EXAMPLE 8-5

Filing Individual Names

Name	Unit 1	Unit 2	Unit 3	Names as Typed and Filed in Drawer
Thomas Andrew Johnson	Johnson	Thomas	Andrew	JONG, NEUYEN
T. K. Johnson	Johnson	T	K	JOHNSTONE, THOMAS
Thomas Johnstone	Johnstone	Thomas		JOHNSON, THOMAS ANDREW
Neuyen Jong	Jong	Neuyen		JOHNSON, T.K.

EXAMPLE 8-6

Filing Names with Prefixes

Name	Unit 1	Unit 2	Unit 3	Names as Typed and Filed in Drawer
Marilyn McFadden	McFadden	Marilyn		vonDYKE, ROBERT
John MacArthur	MacArthur	John		ST. JAMES, MARCIA
Harvey Schmidt	Schmidt	Harvey		SCHMIDT, HARVEY
Robert vonDyke	vonDyke	Robert		McFADDEN, MARILYN
Marcia St. James	St. James	Marcia		MacARTHUR, JOHN

EXAMPLE 8-7

Filing Hyphenated Names

Name	Unit 1	Unit 2	Unit 3	Names as Typed and Filed in Drawer
Leslie Newton-Ross	NewtonRoss	Leslie		NEWTONSDAVIS, ANNAMARIE
Loretta Jane Newtonberg	Newtonberg	Loretta	Jane	NEWTONROSS, LESLIE
Anna Marie Newtons-Davis	NewtonsDavis	AnnaMarie		NEWTONJOHN, ARTHUR
Arthur Newton-John	NewtonJohn	Arthur		NEWTONBERG, LORETTA JANE
Business Names				
Smyth-Barnes Cosmetics	Smyth-	Barnes	Cosmetics	SMYTH-BARNES COSMETICS
Churchill-Clayton Pharmacy	Churchill-	Clayton	Pharmacy	CHURCHILL-CLAYTON PHARMACY

Rule 4: Abbreviated Names and Nicknames

Abbreviations of personal names (i.e., first names) are indexed as they are written (see Example 8-8). Shortened names or nicknames, such as Al or Kate, are used if they are true names or if the true names are not known.

Rule 5: Titles and Degrees

Titles, degrees, and seniority terms following the name are not units and are disregarded in the indexing unless they are needed to distinguish identical names. Arabic numbers (1, 2, 3) precede Roman numerals (I, II, III). Numeric suffixes, such as "II" and "III," and abbreviations such as "Jr." are filed before alphabetic suffixes such as "Prof.," "Dr.," or "PhD."

A man with a name identical to his father's is called "Jr." as long as his father is alive; when his father is dead, he may drop the "Jr." A male is a "III" when his father is a "Jr." A male named after his grandfather, uncle, or cousin is a "II."

These terms may be enclosed in parentheses and placed at the end of the name on file folder labels. Exception: when a name consists of a title and one name, such as Reverend Brown, the name is not transposed and the title is the first indexing unit. Example 8-9 shows how to file names with titles and degrees.

Rule 6: Married Women

Legally, the surname is the only part of her husband's name a woman assumes when she marries. Her legal name could be (1) her own first and middle names together with her husband's surname, (2) her own first name and maiden surname together with her husband's surname, or (3) her given name and her own (maiden) surname. On file folders, "Mrs." may be considered part of the third unit and placed in parentheses with the husband's first and middle names or initials and typed to the side or below the woman's legal name (see Example 8-10).

Rule 7: Hospitals, Medical Facilities, and Businesses

The names of hospitals, pharmacies, and other business facilities are indexed in the same order as written on the letterhead unless the firm name includes the complete name of a person, in which case the surname would be followed by the given name or initials. However, some offices follow an *optional* rule that does not transpose the full name in a business. Thus, in Example 8-11, Wm. Ingram's Pharmacy would be the last name in the group. Numbers are indexed as though written out and are filed as one unit. Compass directional terms are usually considered separate units. Prepositions, conjunctions, and articles are not

---

EXAMPLE 8-8

Filing Abbreviated Names

Name	Unit 1	Unit 2	Unit 3	Names as Typed and Filed in Drawer
Virgil Robt. DeKalb	DeKalb	Virgil	Robt (Robert)	DeKALB, VIRGIL ROBT
Jas. Charles Baker	Baker	Jas (James)	Charles	BAKER, JAS CHARLES
Charles L. Baker	Baker	Charles	L	BAKER, CHARLES L

EXAMPLE 8-9

Filing Names with Titles and Degrees

Name	Unit 1	Unit 2	Unit 3	Unit 4	Names as Typed and Filed in Drawer
Dr. Robt. Crespi, Jr.	Crespi	Robt.	(Jr)	(Dr)	ESPINOZA, ROBT. A (PROF.)
Congressperson Blake	Congressperson	Blake			CRESPI, ROBERT (JR) (DR)
Prof. Robert A. Espinoza	Espinoza	Robert	A	(Prof.)	CONGRESSPERSON BLAKE
Samuel T. Blake, III	Blake	Samuel	T	(III)	BLAKE, SAMUEL T (III)

units except when "a," "an," "and," "the" are the first words, in which case they are the last filing unit.

Rule 8: Addresses When Names Are Identical

If two names are identical and the physician or hospital sees patients from more than one city or state, the address may be used to make the filing decision. Index by name first, then state, city, street, and finally by number from the lowest to the highest number (see Example 8-12). Geographic names such as Las Vegas are treated as two separate indexing units.

EXAMPLE 8-10

Filing Names of Married Women

Name	Unit 1	Unit 2	Unit 3	Names as Typed and Filed in Drawer
Mrs. Nola Walker (Karl W.)	Walker	Nola	(Mrs.)	WALKER, NOLA (MRS. KARL W.)
Mrs. M. K. Bates	Bates	M	K (Mrs.)	HENSON, HILDA (MRS.)
Mrs. Arnold S. Battie (Mildred Ax)	Battie	Mildred	Ax	BATTIE, MILDRED AX (MRS. ARNOLD S.)
Mrs. Hilda Henson	Henson	Hilda	(Mrs.)	BATES, M K (MRS.)

EXAMPLE 8-11

Filing Names of Hospitals, Medical Facilities, and Businesses

Name	Unit 1	Unit 2	Unit 3	Unit 4	Names as Typed and Filed in Drawer
The Good Samaritan Hospital	Good	Samaritan	Hospital	The	WM INGRAM'S PHARMACY
Wm. Ingram's Pharmacy	Ingram's	Wm	Pharmacy		TWENTYFIFTH ST AMBULANCE
25th St. Ambulance	Twenty-fifth	St	Ambulance		GOOD SAMARITAN HOSPITAL THE

EXAMPLE 8-12

Filing Addresses When Names Are Identical

Name	Unit 1	Unit 2	Unit 3	Unit 4	Unit 5	Unit 6
John Almonzo, Rye, New Hampshire, 120 Adams	Almonzo	John	New	Hampshire	Rye	120 Adams
John Almonzo, Portage, New York	Almonzo	John	New	York	Portage	
John Almonzo, Rye, New Hampshire, 450 Adams	Almonzo	John	New	Hampshire	Rye	450 Adams

Names as Typed and Filed in Drawe

ALMONZO, JOHN NEW YORK PORTAGE

ALMONZO, JOHN NEW HAMPSHIRE RYE 450 ADAMS

ALMONZO, JOHN NEW HAMPSHIRE RYE 120 ADAMS

PROCEDURE 8-5

Determine Filing Units and Indexing Order to Alphabetically File a Patient's Medical Record

Objective: To determine each filing unit given a surname, given name, and middle name to alphabetically file patients' medical records.

Equipment/Supplies: Patients' medical records with names on labels and pen or pencil.

Directions: Follow these step-by-step procedures, which include rationales, to learn this skill, which is presented in the *Workbook* (Job Skill 8-1 and 8-2) for practice.

1. Obtain the patient's surname (last name), considered unit 1. Filing records in alphabetic order creates efficiency in filing and retrieving files. Look carefully at each letter of the name when placing it in the file.

2. Study each filing rule to see which one applies to the surname you are trying to file.

3. Consider the second unit, the first name, only when the first unit is the same as the other names in the file.

4. Study, letter by letter, the patient's given name (first name), which becomes unit 2.

5. Consider the third unit, the middle name or middle initial, only when the first and second units are the same.

6. Study, letter by letter, the middle name or middle initial (if any); this is unit 3 in the sequence of filing. Remember "file nothing before something," so an alike name without middle initials or names would be filed first.

7. Find the proper location on the shelf or in the file drawer.

8. Use your hand to make space between the existing records and place the file in the proper location.

9. If refiling a file folder where an outguide exists, pull the outguide halfway out, insert the file folder in front of the outguide, and remove the outguide. Outguides must be removed each time you refile a record that has been borrowed.

FILING EQUIPMENT

Filing equipment consists of the storage units used to keep files. Size (floor space used), accessibility (ease of use), durability, security, and appearance are all considered when selecting filing equipment.

Lateral Files

The most popular file cabinets used for storing patient medical records are the upright shelf files referred to as **lateral files**. They typically have sliding doors that open upward and recede into the top of the shelf, which resembles a bookcase (Figure 8-7). An **open-shelf file** unit with seven 36-inch shelves will hold approximately 1,000 records. File cabinets are available in colors to harmonize with office décor.

Open-shelf or lateral files are popular in medical offices because they require less floor space than conventional steel drawer cabinets. There is no drawer opening and closing to cause cabinets to tilt, and record access is quicker, thus reducing labor costs. Misfiles are reduced, especially if folders are color-coded. Doors that can be pulled out and down can provide security with locks.

Lateral shelves can be located on a wall or double as a room divider near the medical assistant's desk, and they can be found in modular-stationary or roll-out models. It is important to secure these types of files to the walls to prevent tipping during any earth

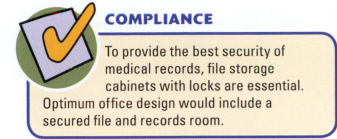

movements. File dividers keep materials upright, and visible file folders are stored perpendicularly with tabs and color-coded labels extending beyond the side of each folder to clearly show the patient's name.

Full-Suspension Drawer Files

The traditional upright steel cabinet with three to five drawers is still popular for the storage of business records in a medical office (e.g., payroll records, insurance explanation of benefit documents).

A five-drawer vertical cabinet will hold about 720 records. Desirable features in cabinets with drawers are ball-bearing drawer rollers, telescoping movable slides, steel movable blocks (compressors) that allow for expansion and contraction of files within the drawers, rods at the top or bottom of the drawers to anchor guides, and a fire insulated frame that is rigidly braced. If office files are not bolted securely

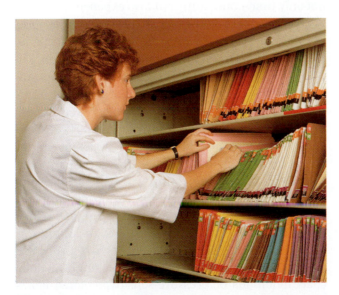

Figure 8-7. Administrative medical assistant filing at an open-shelf lateral file cabinet

to the wall or floor, the cabinet may tip forward when the two top drawers are pulled out simultaneously. It may be necessary to open a lower drawer to prevent this; however, try to keep lower drawers closed so they do not block the traffic path and cause an accident. To avoid overcrowding, leave three or four inches of extra space in each drawer.

Automated Files

An automated storage and retrieval system is practical for offices with 10,000 or more records. The records are stored in a unit with a stacker, which moves along the row until it finds the record requested by the computer. The stacker retrieves the record and delivers it to the person requesting it at the workstation. This kind of system saves space and time, reduces errors, and increases the productivity of employees.

Automated files are usually found in large clinics and hospital facilities. This type of file system is initially expensive, but it can store many records, which may be located quickly.

FILING SUPPLIES AND THEIR USES

It is important to find a reliable office supply company with a knowledgeable sales person who provides up-to-date information and supplies at reasonable costs. Companies that specialize in medical supplies will have items specific to a medical practice's needs and will incorporate new items when government mandates become law (e.g., HIPAA regulated consent forms, new CMS-1500 claim form). Following are general supply items found in a medical practice.

Guides

Guides are pressboard, manila, metal, or plastic dividers that sit slightly higher than the file folders in order to be more visible on the shelf or in the drawer. They provide support for folders and serve as signposts to direct the eyes to labeled sections. Along the top of the best quality guides is a reinforced metal tab in which labels may be inserted so the guides can be reused. Less sturdy guides with plastic-coated tabs are also available. The number of guides per shelf or drawer depends on the number of records to be stored and the filing system. Usually one divider for 25 folders

EXAMPLE 8-13

Two-Letter Secondary Guides

Primary Guide

■ B

Secondary Guides

■■ Be

■■ Bi

■■ Bo

■■ Br

CREDIT _____ Vol. No _____
Patient Name: _____
Patient Address: _____
City, State: _____
Patient Telephone: _____

DOCTOR: _____

Patient classification

| xxx Account | Medicaid | Medicare |

ALLERGIC REACTIONS

Date	Substance	Effect

CEPEDA, Joe

1991
1992
1993
1994
1995
1996
1997
1998
1999
2000
2001
2002
2003
2004
2005
2006

Figure 8-9. Preprinted lateral chart cover—outside view

is adequate. Allow four to six inches of empty space for working. In an alphabetic lateral filing system, guide labels can be placed in the extreme left position or staggered throughout the files. As the number of folders increases, two-letter (color-coded) secondary guides may be added to serve as additional signposts (Example 8-13).

Guides for shelf files are side-tabbed and as a rule are not staggered (Figure 8-8). A sturdy metal hook projects from the back of each guide to keep it attached to the cabinet so it will not work forward. Guides for file drawers have tabs on the top and are equipped with a projection at the bottom center with a metal-reinforced hole in the middle. A metal guide rod attached horizontally to the bottom of a file drawer is placed through these holes to secure the guides in place within each drawer.

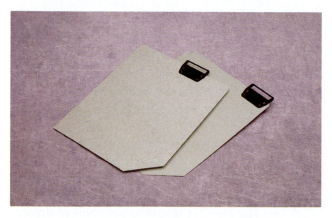

Figure 8-8. Guides separating file folders into subsections. Captions such as A, B, C (single captions) or Ab-Be, Co-Dy (double captions) are placed on the guide tabs to identify the sections.

Folders

Folders in letter size, 8½ by 11 inches, are designed to hold information to be stored in open-shelf cabinets or file drawers. Some physicians (e.g., ophthalmologists and dermatologists) may prefer smaller sizes for their charts. For these, documents may need to be folded, creating thicker file folders. Ordinary kraft or manila folders in 11-point stock are suitable for average medical practices. The choice of weight ranges from 8-point, which is very light, to 24-point, which is extra heavy, and will depend on the extent of handling. If folders are to be handled often, sturdier file folders should be purchased because redoing folders is not only time-consuming but also expensive.

The assistant can be creative in designing pre-printed chart covers so important information can be recorded on both the inside and outside (Figures 8-9 and 8-10). Commercially printed folders are economically sensible when a practice initiates a great number of new patient records a day or per week. If too much time is spent flipping through charts searching for specific information, the assistant might choose to place data in code on the cover as shown by the colored dots indicating type of insurance coverage in Figure 8-13, page 248. Information available on the outside of chart covers might include the patient's allergies, drug reactions, nicknames or titles, for example, a Ph.D. who prefers to be addressed as "Dr." The inside of the chart cover might include coded notations or pressure-sensitive colored labels alerting the staff of a patient's failure to pay a bill, legal problems, or specific medical problems such as Rh negative, diabetic, hypertension, a patient on Coumadin, and so on.

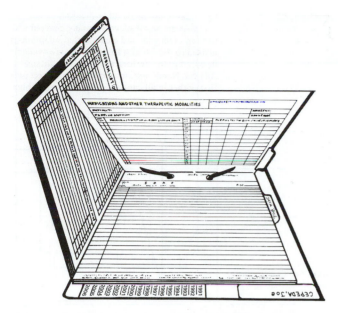

Figure 8-10. Inside view of file folder with fastener. (Courtesy of Bibbero Systems, Inc., Petaluma, CA. Telephone: (800) 242-2376; Fax (800) 242-9330; Web site: http://www.bibbero.com.)

The back half of a standard folder extends about one-half inch beyond the front to form a protruding tab. Creases at the bottom of folders, called **scores**, permit expansion of file folders (by bending the folders on the scores) to hold 100 sheets without causing records to stand unevenly on their edges. However, it is best not to overload file folders.

An 8- by 10-inch envelope folder may be used within a file folder to hold small items, such as photographs. The closed sides protect supplemental information inside from being lost when records are carried away from the files.

Binder File Folders

Binder file folders are designed with clamps or file fasteners to secure items inside, preventing lost items. Disadvantages of binder folders include the tendency of the files to bulge where the clamps are located and the time it takes to insert documents in the folder and remove them for photocopying or when filing new paperwork.

Information is placed in folders with correspondence headings visible and with most recently dated papers at the front (Figure 8-11). Special medical reports may be filed according to type of report; that is, all ECG results together, all urinalysis reports together, and so forth. It is best for a medical assistant to set aside a specific time each day to transfer and file patient data, ideally when there will be no interruptions by patients.

Stapled and Shingled Documents

Because paper clips slip off or attach to neighboring papers, stapling continuation sheets or related items diagonally in the upper left corner is preferable.

A telephone message or small laboratory-test report may be stapled, taped, or glued to a standard-size sheet of paper so that it will not be misplaced or overlooked. It may also be *shingled* as described in Chapter 6 (Figure 6-6). This method is not preferred, because data is covered and it is time-consuming to take documents apart before photocopying a medical record.

Before leaving the office at night or on arrival in the morning, the medical assistant organizes the patient file folders for the physician in the sequence of the day's appointments. The assistant also prepares labeled folders for new patients before their arrival.

When it is time to dispose of the contents of a folder, the assistant should remove labels and save the folder for reuse by placing a new label directly on top of the old one or by replacing a removable label. Some folders can be turned inside out to provide a clean folder and a clean tab. Old folders may be used for inactive storage because they will not be reviewed often.

Color-Coding File Folders

When several physicians are associated but maintain separate practices, patient folders may be color-coded to distinguish each physician. An inexpensive way to convert ordinary manila folders to color is to purchase colored tape or preglued colored tabs to affix directly to the folder tabs.

Colored dots can be used on ledger cards and patient records to distinguish at a glance the documents belonging to a particular physician.

Miscellaneous Colored Labels

Other kinds of labels are also useful. A small wraparound self-stick label printed with the last digit of each year can be attached to the edge of the folder to indicate the most recent year of service. This can be covered with a new sticker each year after the patient has seen the physician. Folders with old dates that need to be purged from the active files can be seen easily.

A fluorescent sticker placed on the left front of the chart alerts the physician to a patient's drug allergies. Dots indicating type of insurance coverage assists the physician when prescribing medication according to specific insurance formularies, sending patients to

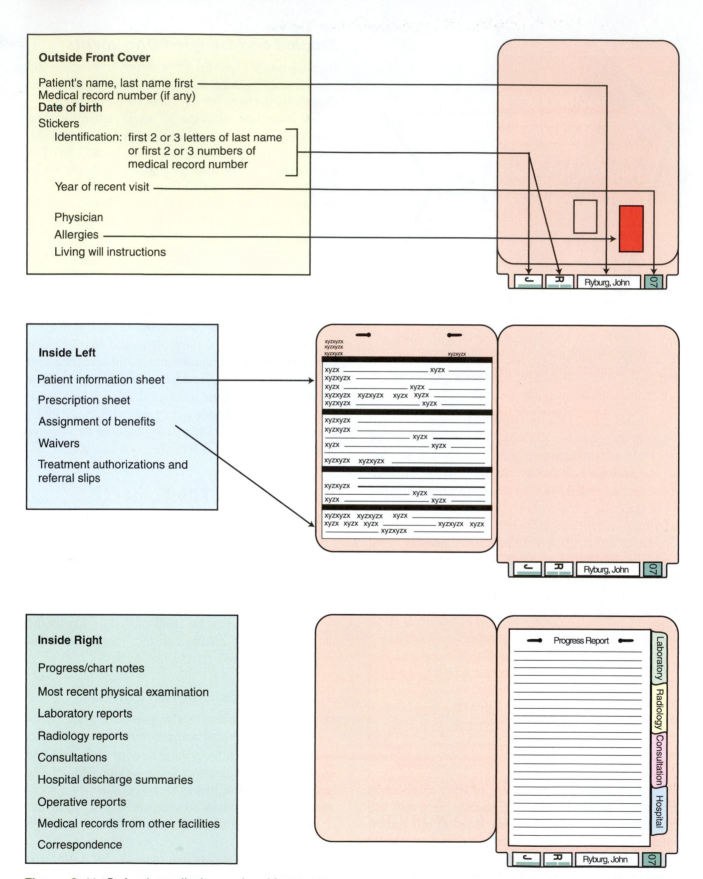

Outside Front Cover

Patient's name, last name first
Medical record number (if any)
Date of birth
Stickers
    Identification: first 2 or 3 letters of last name
                     or first 2 or 3 numbers of
                     medical record number

    Year of recent visit

    Physician

    Allergies

    Living will instructions

Inside Left

Patient information sheet

Prescription sheet

Assignment of benefits

Waivers

Treatment authorizations and
referral slips

Inside Right

Progress/chart notes

Most recent physical examination

Laboratory reports

Radiology reports

Consultations

Hospital discharge summaries

Operative reports

Medical records from other facilities

Correspondence

Figure 8-11. Patient's medical record and its contents

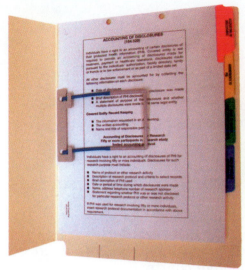

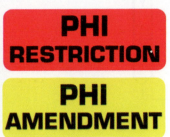

Figure 8-12. HIPAA divider sets are used in patient files to quickly identify records with protected health information (PHI); fluorescent labels are placed on the cover of the folder to alert office staff of PHI. (Reprinted with permission of Ames Color File Products and Services, Somerville, MA. Telephone: 800-343-2040; Web site: http://www.amespage.com.)

in-network facilities, and speeds the completion of insurance claims (Figure 8-13). For example, all Medicare folders are put in one pile and completed at one time.

Another brightly colored warning label can signal chronic or serious ailments, information valuable to a physician who is treating patients with similar medical problems or doing research in a specific area of medicine. For very heavy usage, file labels can be covered with Mylar overlays.

Tabs

Tabs are staggered projections in varying widths above or on the sides of the body of a file folder or guide, also used as sign posts to direct the eye to a specific label. The width of the tab, called the **cut,** is usually expressed as a fraction. *One-half cut* means that the tab takes up one-half of the back flat of the folder, while a *one-third cut*, which is the most popular, allows for three tabs of equal length to fit across the top of a standard folder. *A full tab*, often with a reinforced edge, extends the length of the back of the folder and may be used to attach color-coded labels. Straight-cut folder tabs with rounded corners stay in the best condition (Figure 8-14). To be visible, tabs of folders used in open-shelf files extend beyond the right side of the back leaf. Names arranged vertically on these side tabs are not as easily read as numbers.

Labels

Labels are small stickers usually covered with acetate or a protective overlay to keep them from wearing. After a **caption** has been typed on a label, it is affixed

COMPLIANCE

To comply with Health Insurance Portability and Accountability Act (HIPAA) regulations, fluorescent labels may be placed on the cover of the patient's folder and divider sets used for patient files (Figure 8-12). These allow quick identification of records with protected health information (PHI).

to the tab of a folder. Leave a small space between the top of the label and the top of the folder so the label will not peel off. Labels are available in various styles and colors; in continuous, perforated rolls for typewriter use; in adhesive strips; in pressure-sensitive stickers that are easily removed; and aligned on pages for a computer printer. Name captions are typed in correct indexing arrangement (last name first) either in all capital letters or in a combination of uppercase and lowercase letters, as shown in Figure 8-15. The patient's name is typed two or three spaces from the left edge of the label on the second line space from the top edge, and placement should be consistent on all labels. When children's names are different than their parents', the parents' name (guarantor—individual responsible for the bill) should be cross-referenced on the chart, as this will help locate the account or ledger for billing.

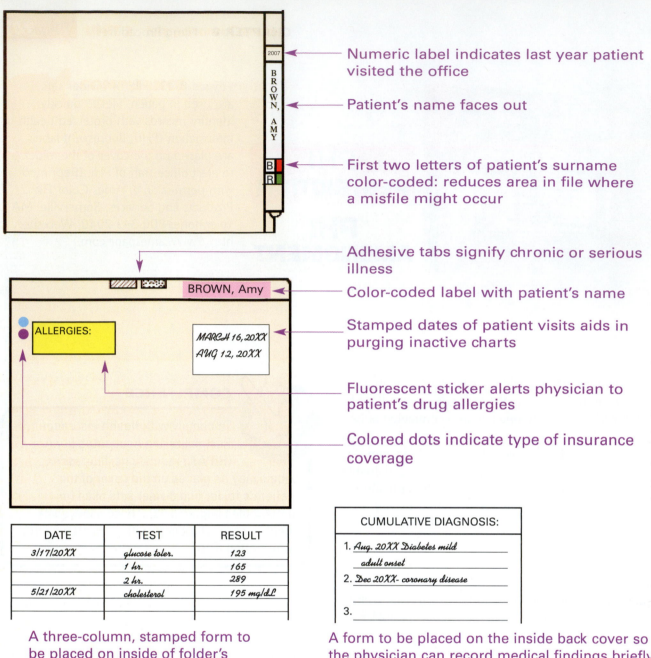

Numeric label indicates last year patient visited the office

Patient's name faces out

First two letters of patient's surname color-coded: reduces area in file where a misfile might occur

Adhesive tabs signify chronic or serious illness

Color-coded label with patient's name

Stamped dates of patient visits aids in purging inactive charts

Fluorescent sticker alerts physician to patient's drug allergies

Colored dots indicate type of insurance coverage

ALLERGIES:

MARCH 16, 20XX
AUG 12, 20XX

DATE	TEST	RESULT
3/17/20XX	glucose toler.	123
	1 hr.	165
	2 hr.	289
5/21/20XX	cholesterol	195 mg/dL

A three-column, stamped form to be placed on inside of folder's front cover to identify lab work

CUMULATIVE DIAGNOSIS:

1. Aug. 20XX Diabetes mild adult onset
2. Dec 20XX- coronary disease
3.

A form to be placed on the inside back cover so the physician can record medical findings briefly in the order in which they occur; saves time by not having to go through patient's records

Figure 8-13. Colored labels and stickers placed on the front and inside covers of chart

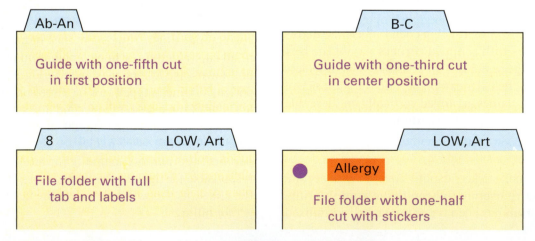

Ab-An
Guide with one-fifth cut in first position

B-C
Guide with one-third cut in center position

8   LOW, Art
File folder with full tab and labels

LOW, Art
● Allergy
File folder with one-half cut with stickers

Figure 8-14. Guides and file folders with tabs in different cuts and positions

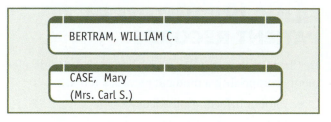

Figure 8-15. Typed file folder labels

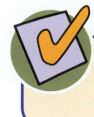

CHARGE-OUT AND CONTROL SYSTEMS

If the medical staff has trouble locating charts after they have been removed from the files, a **charge-out system** is needed to indicate when and by whom a record has been removed; one person should supervise the system and maintain control. All members of the staff who remove records, charts, or folders should be admonished to return them promptly to the files to avoid misplacement. A team effort should be made to return borrowed patient charts promptly to the files. Patients have the right to expect that their medical records will be safeguarded from unauthorized use or disclosure and that the filing system adopted by the office will assure accurate retrieval.

Outguide

An **outguide**, or substitution card, is required if control of patient records is to be maintained. It is usually made of heavy pressboard with a tab labeled "OUT."

An outguide replaces a folder that has been removed until it has been returned. Some are designed with lines to record the patient's name, date, who removed the record, and why the record was removed. Others are designed with pockets in which a written requisition form can be inserted. The form is made out by the borrower and would include the name of the patient, record number, date taken out and returned, and the location where the record has been taken. Requisition forms may consist of an original and a copy. One can be filed in the outguide folder and one attached to the medical record. When any medical record is removed from a file cabinet, it is important that the entire requisition form be filled out so there is no chance of record misplacement or loss. It cannot be overemphasized that once an outguide system is put into place, every staff member must abide by performing these procedures or it will not work.

As an alternative to outguides that indicate pulled charts, colored card stock can be cut slightly larger than the file folders and placed where sheets or whole folders have been removed. Different colors can be

---

STEP 1 2 3   **PROCEDURE 8-6**

Label and Color-Code Patient Charts

Objective: To label and color-code patient charts using a specified color-coding system to quickly file and locate charts.

Equipment/Supplies: Patient charts, color-coding system guidelines, file folders, and colored name labels.

Directions: Follow these step-by-step procedures, which include rationales, to learn this skill which is presented in the *Workbook* (Job Skill 8-6) for practice.

1. Assemble patient charts.

2. Arrange each name in indexing order so charts can be color-coded in sequence.

3. Begin with the first patient and note the first and second letters of the patient's surname (last name) and select alphabetic labels of the correct color.

4. Type in indexing order the patient's last name, first name, and middle initial and adhere the label to the file folder tab.

5. Repeat steps 3 and 4 until all charts are labeled and color-coded.

6. Look through the group of file folders to be sure the order and color of the file folders are correct and that all charts are of the same color within each letter of the alphabet grouped together.

used to identify which staff member or office location has removed the file. A red sheet might signify that it is in the billing department, a blue one might indicate the physician has removed the chart, and so forth.

If a file needs to be kept out of the cabinet for a long period of time, it may be necessary to photocopy instead of remove needed items for office use; never remove original information from a file folder. This practice should be avoided unless it is essential, and all materials should be returned as soon as possible.

Outfolder

An *outfolder* serves the same purpose as an outguide except that it provides a place to store incoming items (e.g., laboratory reports) until the regular folder is returned. Charge-out information may be written on the front of the folder, which is often printed with ruled lines.

FILING DOCUMENTS IN PATIENT RECORDS

In Chapter 9 you will learn about the various elements comprising a medical record, such as:

- Patient information sheet
- Medical history questionnaire
- Progress and chart notes
- Electrocardiogram reports
- Laboratory (log) reports
- Radiological reports
- Prescription log
- Medical reports (history and physical, consultation, operative reports, discharge summaries)

Each of these documents must be placed within every patient's file folder in an organized manner so that data can be accessed quickly. Procedure 8-7 will take you through the steps of getting documents ready for filing in a patient's medical record.

STEP 1 2 3

PROCEDURE 8-7

Prepare, Sort, and File Documents in Patient Records

Objective: To prepare, sort, and file documents in patient records.

Equipment/Supplies: Documents (letters, medical reports, diagnostic test reports), file sorter, tape, stapler, and pen or pencil.

Directions: Follow these procedures, which include rationales, to learn the skill of filing documents.

1. Examine papers that are to be filed, making sure they have been date stamped and initialed by the physician. All documents must be viewed by the physician and released before filing.

2. Separate and group documents to be filed in patient medical records, financial records, business files, and so forth.

3. Index and code documents to be filed by subject. *Indexing* is deciding on the caption; **coding** is marking the caption on the material to be filed, usually by underlining or by writing a word in the upper right corner. Both steps can be performed simultaneously. Captions

chosen and marked might be letterhead name, signature name, reference name, or the name of the person or institution to whom the letter is addressed. Coding may be unnecessary when files are supervised by one person who will be familiar with correspondents and able to quickly scan for the caption.

4. Photocopy and cross-reference data when it applies to more than one patient or subject.

5. Sort documents in filing sequence; documents are arranged in either alphabetic or numeric order. A desk sorter with a series of dividers using alphabetic or numeric classifications facilitates this step before the documents are placed in file folders. It is efficient to file in order since one patient may have several reports to be filed (Figure 8-16).

6. File documents. Items are placed in the appropriate file folder and under the appropriate file division (e.g., laboratory) face up, top edge to the left, with the most recent item placed to the front.

PROCEDURE 8-8

Locate a Misfiled Patient Medical-Record File Folder

Objective: To search for a misfiled patient medical record.

Equipment/Supplies: File cabinet (shelves or drawers).

Directions: Follow these step-by-step procedures, which include rationales to learn this skill.

1. Check in the spaces in front of and behind where the patient's file folder should be located.

2. Check above and below the shelves where the record should be kept, or in the bottom of the drawer.

3. Look for the first two colors of the patient's last name among other records if using a color-coded system. The color, if misfiled, should stand out.

4. Look under the patient's first name, instead of the last; sometimes it is difficult to distinguish between first and last names or the file folder could be set up incorrectly.

5. Search through the entire section of the first letter of the patient's last name.

6. Determine other ways the patient's name could have been spelled, as well as misspelled, transposed, and so forth.

7. Look for similar names; names that sound the same but are spelled with a different vowel.

8. Explore different areas of the office; that is, look in desk trays or in-baskets, on top of and beneath folders, and among the charts of other patients seen the same day; a variety of employees may need to use the file.

9. As a last resort if the record remains missing after a thorough search, set up another file folder or sheet, flag it with red tape for identification, and label it with the word "Duplicate" and the patient's name.

Misfiling

In order to avoid the misfiling of information, study the following guidelines and common causes of misfiles.

- Keep headings simple. Complex headings cause confusion.

- Type patient names legibly using a standardized form. Changes in the typed format of headings can be misread.

- Include adequate guides for the number of files stored. Too many or too few guides make filing difficult.

- Leave three to four inches of extra working space per shelf or drawer. Overcrowding causes misfiles, damages records, and makes filing difficult.

- Rid file folders of unnecessary items. Overloaded folders cause papers to push up and conceal file tabs.

- Staple papers when necessary. Avoid paper clips because they can cling to other papers in the file.

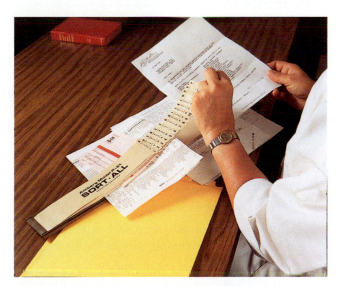

Figure 8-16. Medical assistant using a desk sorter to alphabetize reports to make filing easier

- File carefully. Hurrying causes carelessness and folders get filed in the wrong place.

- Select proper titles for subject files. Failing to properly designate the subject or name results in lost files.

Misplaced or Lost Records

Misplaced or lost records can disrupt the routine of the day, creating delays and problems for the entire staff. When a record cannot be found, the assistant conducts an organized search.

RECORD RETENTION AND STORAGE

The length of time records must be retained after a patient is discharged from care varies from state to state, but all records should be retained for at least the number of years included in the statute of limitations. Both federal and state governments have requirements for keeping business records. Sometimes a law specifies a retention period, and in other cases a law cannot be found for the retention of a particular type of record. If federal laws and state laws do not agree on the length of time a record should be kept, always keep the record for the longer period stated. Most states have statutes requiring medical or hospital records to be kept anywhere from 7 to 25 years. Because records chiefly contain information on patient care, the records may be of value to patients in later years or even to their offspring. It is, therefore, the policy of most physicians to retain medical records indefinitely.

Setting up a records retention schedule will assure that records are kept according to law and not retained unnecessarily. A retention schedule is a list of record types and the length of time each record should be kept. Steps to take when preparing a policy for retention are:

1. Sort records according to type (e.g., patient inactive records, payroll records, appointment sheets).

2. Prepare an inventory of all records to be stored.

3. Refer to the schedule for retention.

4. Determine how long to keep each type of record according to the schedule.

5. Obtain the physician's approval.

6. Implement the schedule by moving records from active to inactive files, packing storage boxes to move off site, or processing for destruction.

7. Conduct random inspections to ensure compliance with the schedule.

If storage of records involves moving boxes to another facility away from the office, follow these guidelines:

- Use 15- by 12- by 10-inch storage boxes, which will hold both letter and legal papers and are easier to lift than larger cartons.

- Leave records in standardized manila folders; if binders or hanging files are used, remove items before sending them to storage.

- Place all similar records in one container with the same destruction date.

- Clearly label the storage box with the type of records and the "from" and "to" dates of the materials enclosed or the last date (by year) the patient was seen.

- Compile an inventory list of contents for future reference (e.g., payroll 20XX).

- Destroy records according to the retention policy unless there is ongoing or pending litigation, an audit, or other inquiry.

Financial and Legal Records

Vital papers are considered permanent records and are kept indefinitely in a secure file. They include inventory reports, major contracts, deeds, income tax records, CPA audits, titles to ownership of property, and legal papers. Financial statements, active correspondence, equipment inventory, and payroll records are kept for *seven years*. Applications for employment, expired or canceled insurance policies, petty cash vouchers, purchase orders, general correspondence, and miscellaneous office reports are usually kept for *three to four years*. A loose-leaf notebook can hold a record of the physician's personal inventory, including his or her assets and savings accounts, Social Security information, military records, and educational documents; changes and additions may be made simply by adding and deleting pages.

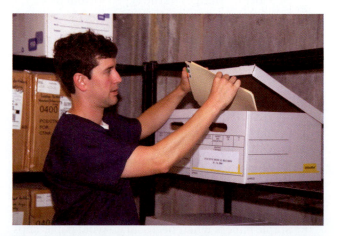

Figure 8-17. Medical assistant placing a chart in a storage box to retain off site

Active and Inactive Patient Files

Medical charts should be purged (removed) at predetermined intervals to increase shelf space and eliminate looking through inactive records when trying to file. It is often difficult for the medical assistant to determine when to transfer patient files from active to inactive status without having to read all the details on each chart. This problem can be solved by date-stamping visits or treatments on the front of each folder or by attaching colored tabs to indicate the last year of treatment (as shown in Figure 8-12). The color-coded year tabs make it easy to purge files because you can quickly see which charts have a particular year's color and remove them. The physician should have the final say on the length of time that files should be kept active, depending on the type of medical specialty.

It is basic medical office policy to purge the files from active to inactive every three to five years. The assistant should, in any case, review all files at least once a year to remove useless data, making it easier to find things and reducing bulk. This task may be worked into the regular filing routine.

Typically, the charts of a surgeon would be kept in the active file a shorter period of time than those of a pediatrician or family practitioner, whose patient care is more likely to continue over years. Physicians located near military bases or resort areas see many transient patients, whose records would be purged frequently.

COMPLIANCE

The medical assistant should retain requests made by patients to transfer or release medical information to other parties (e.g., other physicians, insurance companies). These documents become part of the permanent medical record.

Proof materials, such as x-rays, laboratory reports, and pathology specimens, should be kept indefinitely. If a patient is a minor, records should be retained until the patient reaches the age of majority, that is, 18 to 21 years, plus the time allowed in that state for a lawsuit to be instituted for injuries the patient sustained as a minor. In most states, that period is one to four years beyond the age of majority. Everything pertaining to a patient who has had a negative attitude toward his or her care should be retained.

Calendars, appointment books, and telephone logs should also be filed and stored. Cases involving radiologic injury, such as leukemia, may be considered under the statute after the injury is discovered, and this can occur 20 to 30 years after radiation exposure. Before purging records, the medical assistant should check the current statute of limitations in the state because state laws vary, or refer to the record-retention schedule in Table 8-1, keeping in mind these are only suggested guidelines.

Electronic Storage

The advantage of computerized medical records is that they can be downloaded from the computer to other media (e.g., flash drive, external hard drive, DVD) for storage. The transfer of such records is accomplished quickly and the media can be stored in a fireproof safe or off site for safe keeping.

Document Imaging

Paper-based medical and financial records can be converted into electronic documents using imaging technology. Records are scanned into the computer system, digitized, and transferred to one of the above mentioned media for storage. Archived electronic documents may then be retrieved using electronic search capabilities, saving time and space. The type of scanning equipment would determine how fast this process could be done but the money saved on medical record storage might be worth the effort and expense.

Document management software can digitize scanned information and store it on the hard drive of a computer system. Advanced programs have the capability of sorting similar documents and organizing them by check number, date, and so forth. A medical office could use such software for scanning explanation of benefits (EOBs) on a daily basis and have it available for storage purposes.

The storage of documents reduced on film using micrograph technology is still used in some hospitals, clinics, and insurance companies.

Microfilming involves a photographic process that develops medical records in miniature on film. Information is stored on cards holding single film frames or in reels or strips for projection on compact electric viewers placed at convenient office locations.

Microfiche (pronounced mi-kro-feesh) technology is similar. It is a miniature photographic system that stores rows of images in reduced size on cards with clear plastic sleeves rather than on film strips. Information can be handled manually, examined on a

Table 8-1. Records Retention Schedule

Temporary Record	Recommended Retention Period (Years)	Temporary Record	Recommended Retention Period (Years)
Accounts receivable ledger cards (patients)	7	Duplicate bank deposit slips	1
Appointment sheets	3	Employee time cards/sheets and schedules	5
Balance sheets	5	Employment applications	4
Bank deposits and statements, reconciliations	2	Expense reports	7
Cash receipt records	6	Inventory records	3
Contracts and leases (expired)	7	Invoice and billing records	6
Contracts with employees	6	Medicare financial records	7
Copies of estimated tax forms	6	Payroll records	7
Correspondence, general	5	Petty cash vouchers	3
Deceased patients' medical records	5	Postal and meter records	1
Depreciation schedules	3		

Permanent Record (Retained Indefinitely)	
Accounts payable ledgers	Equipment records
Balance sheets	Inactive patient medical records purged from active files
Bills of sale for important purchases	Income tax returns and documents
Canceled checks and check registers	Insurance policies and records
Capital asset records	Journals
Cashbooks	Magnetic tapes and disks
Certified financial statements	Patients' medical records including x-ray films
Charts of accounts	Professional liability insurance policies
Correspondence, legal	Property appraisals
Credit history	Telephone records
Deeds, mortgages, contracts, leases, and property records	

viewer (which enlarges the record), or reproduced as hard copy by high-speed photocopiers.

DESTROYING DOCUMENTS

Some large medical facilities may contract with outside vendors to destroy medical documents. Some use small paper shredders that attach to waste baskets and shred 2 to 5 sheets at a time. Stand-alone machines can shred up to 27 sheets at a time. Items of a confidential nature that might need to be shredded are meeting notes, unneeded or "bad" photocopies, computer printouts, correspondence, old employment applications, personnel documents, payroll and salary data, and obsolete reports.

Purging Computer Files

More records are being stored electronically, that is, on computer hard drives, flash drives, microfilm, optical disks, and various types of backup disks. Disposal methods may include degaussing (wiping out information using a magnet) and zeroization (which involves writing binary code zeros over the data). Refer to Table 8-2 for methods of recycling and destroying various types of media.

Table 8-2. Methods of Recycling and Disposing Protected Health Information

Type of Media	Method of Recycling and Destruction
Audiotape	Record over original tape to recycle Shred tape or crush cassette to destroy
Computer disk	Overwrite all data to recycle Crush disk or magnetically erase and incinerate to destroy
Labels for PHI created on media devices	Remove and shred or incinerate to destroy
Laser disk	Overwrite rewriteable disks to recycle Crush rewriteable and write-it-once disks to destroy
Magnetic media	Reformat and overwrite tape to recycle Magnetically erase, shred, and incinerate to destroy
Microfilm/Microfiche	Crush or shred to destroy
Videotape	Record over original content to recycle Crush or shred tape and cassette to destroy

COMPLIANCE

Deleting confidential files may not be sufficient to prevent unauthorized disclosure of information. The impression that the information, once deleted, has been removed from the system and is inaccessible to others may not always be true. Measures to prevent unauthorized disclosure of information are:

1. Encrypt confidential files.

2. Use utility software to specifically overwrite files that have been deleted.

3. Physically destroy disks that are being discarded.

4. Monitor the printer while printing, and destroy "bad" copies of confidential printouts.

5. Carefully control, or do not permit utility software designed to read and restore deleted files.

Word processor operators need to **purge** (remove or delete) stored data frequently. Dated documents hamper retrieval, increase supply costs, and use up valuable storage space. Because various types of storage media is reusable, keeping them clear will reduce supply costs. The office manager should have document originators authorize deletion dates for their documents so a procedure for regularly clear-

COMPLIANCE

Any document that identifies a patient by name should be considered confidential and disposed of in a way that ensures privacy. Obtain a written agreement with an outside company to ensure that all documents containing PHI will be handled securely.

ing unnecessary documents can be established. One way to assist purging of electronically stored files is to print a form listing the documents indicating retention time, which might be any length of time (e.g., 3 days, 6 months, 1 year). But if no retention time is set, the document may be automatically deleted after a given length of time. Any one of the following files can be an unnecessary file to be targeted for deletion:

1. A file that has been superseded by another file.

2. A backup or temporary file created by an application program. This is only a data entry, update, query, or report program that processed data for the user. In contrast, a system software program controls the internal operations of a computer system, such as operating systems, mathematical routines, graphics support programs, and so forth.

3. An older version of a software program if the newer version is on the hard drive.

4. An infrequently used file that should have been transferred to another media.

Whatever the method, it is essential that all information be completely eradicated.

Recycling

Medical assistants can show concern for the environment by supervising a waste paper **recycle** plan that is neat and orderly, with paper waste separated and placed in a container centrally located. Corrugated boxes of uniform size that provide protection from inclement weather can then be stored outside when full. A small box placed near the photocopy machine will provide storage for unclear photocopies that can be used for scrap paper as long as they are not of a confidential nature (e.g., medical records).

Most breaches of confidentiality related to paper recycling occur before the paper ever leaves the medi-

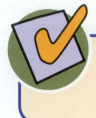

COMPLIANCE

A paper shredder should always be used to ensure confidentiality of medical records that are being discarded.

cal office. Use of closed containers with slots with one person assigned to empty them can solve the problem. Usually, white bond paper and high grades of computer paper command higher recycle prices than colored paper, business forms, newspapers, magazines, and index cards. Under most recycling programs, carbon paper, used envelopes, gummed labels, rubber bands, cellophane, plastic report covers, and photographic paper are not recyclable.

STOP AND THINK CASE SCENARIO

Locate a Missing Record

Scenario: Kathryn Holcomb's medical record cannot be located in the file cabinet and the patient is coming in this afternoon for a postoperative recheck with Dr. Fran Practon.

Critical Thinking: You have methodically checked the file cabinet. What staff members might have the file and for what purpose?

a. _____

b. _____

c. _____

d. _____

e. _____

f. _____

g. _____

What procedures can be used to prevent missing records?

_____

_____

_____

_____

_____

_____

_____

Determine Document Types and Filing Systems

Scenario: Dr. Fran Practon arrived at the office this morning and handed you the following documents to be filed: (a) list of e-mail addresses, (b) last month's bank statement, (c) recipe for apple crisp, (d) list of personal books for reading, (e) laboratory test results on patient Mary Higgins, (f) MRI results on patient Clark Brenneman, (g) phone message on patient Linda Downey, and (h) recall notice for patient Sandra Inez.

Critical Thinking: Decide (1) what type of documents these are (electronic, financial, medical, or personal), (2) how these documents should be filed (alphabetic, chronological, by subject), and (3) where these documents should be filed (medical record, personal file, tickler file). Suggest and note file names.

Example: Transcribed chart note for patient Cindy Hopkins
1. patient's medical record
2. file chronologically
3. in progress notes

a. E-mail addresses
1. _____
2. _____
3. _____

b. Bank statement
1. _____
2. _____
3. _____

c. Recipes
1. _____
2. _____
3. _____

d. Books (personal)
1. _____
2. _____
3. _____

e. Laboratory report
1. _____
2. _____
3. _____

f. MRI report
1. _____
2. _____
3. _____

g. Telephone message
1. _____
2. _____
3. _____

h. Recall notice
1. _____
2. _____
3. _____

FOCUS ON CERTIFICATION*

CMA Content Summary

- Medical terminology and abbreviations
- Release of patient information
- Priority of incoming and outgoing data
- Medical records and personal records
- Release of medical information
- Computerized storage devices
- Computer security and passwords
- File maintenance
- Needs, purposes, and terminology of filing systems
- Process for filing documents
- Patient record organization
- Filing guidelines
- Retaining and purging medical records

RMA Content Summary

- Filing terminology
- Receive, process, and document results received from outside providers
- Manage patient medical record system
- Record diagnostic test results in patient charts

- File patient and physician communication in charts
- File material according to proper systems
- Protect, store, and retain medical records according to proper conventions and HIPAA privacy regulations
- Prepare and release private health information

CMAS Content Summary

- Manage medical record systems
- Manage and file paper and electronic documents
- File records alphabetically, numerically, by subject, and by color
- Employ indexing rules
- Arrange contents of patient's charts and employ chart management
- Store, protect, retain, and destroy records appropriately
- Observe and maintain confidentiality of records, charts, test results, and protected health information

REVIEW EXAM-STYLE QUESTIONS

1. Information to be filed may be in the form of:
   a. paper documents
   b. electronic documents
   c. graphic images
   d. manila file folders
   e. a, b, and c are all correct

2. When selecting a filing system, determine two things to consider.
   a. should be difficult to understand so files cannot be tampered with
   b. security and expansion
   c. appearance and mobility
   d. lightweight and attractive
   e. sturdy and long lasting

---

* This textbook and accompanying Workbook *meet the entry-level administrative and general competencies for the CMA outlined by the* AAMA Examination Content Outline and Role Delineation Study *and for the RMA and CMAS outlined by the AMT Competencies and Examination Specifications (see Competency Grid in Appendix B).*

3. For patient medical records, the most common filing system is:

   a. indirect

   b. numeric

   c. alphabetic

   d. subject

   e. tickler

4. A subject filing system is usually used for:

   a. patient medical records

   b. hospitals, large medical practices, and clinics

   c. reminder notices

   d. business records

   e. electronic records

5. In an indirect filing system, you begin to look for a file by:

   a. going to the cross-reference index

   b. looking for the number 0

   c. looking for the patient's last name in the file cabinet

   d. looking at the middle digit

   e. looking at the terminal digit

6. A chronologic filing system:

   a. is out of date and not frequently used

   b. uses numbers to identify and locate patient records

   c. is frequently used in doctors' offices to file documents within a chart

   d. is based on the alphabet

   e. is only used for business files

7. An electronic database may consist of files pertaining to:

   a. patients

   b. drugs

   c. procedures

   d. diagnoses

   e. all of the above

8. A tickler file system is also called a/an:

   a. alphabetic filing system

   b. chronological filing system

   c. suspense file

   d. inactive filing system

   e. short-notice reminder file

9. What organization developed the rules for alphabetic filing that are still used today?

   a. AHIMA

   b. ARMA

   c. HIPAA

   d. AAMA

   e. AMA

10. The most popular file cabinets used for storing patient medical records are:

    a. lateral or open shelf files

    b. drawer files

    c. vertical files

    d. automated files

    e. telescoping files

11. The "cut" of a file folder describes the:

    a. thickness of the folder

    b. type of edge the folder has (rough, smooth)

    c. number and position of tabs

    d. number of folders in a box

    e. manufacturer

12. A record retention schedule is a:

    a. list of active records

    b. list of inactive records

    c. list of active and inactive records

    d. list of record types and the length of time each should be kept

    e. list of destruction methods used for old records

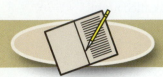

WORKBOOK ASSIGNMENT

To develop competency-based job skills, refer to the *Workbook* and complete the:

- Abbreviation and Spelling Review
- Review Questions

- Critical Thinking Exercises
- Job Skill activities, which are outlined at the beginning of this chapter under "Performance Objectives in the *Workbook*."

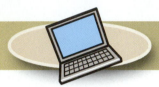

COMPUTER ASSIGNMENT

To review the concepts you have learned in this chapter, insert the *Student Practice* CD-ROM into a computer and work through the *StudyWARE* activities and games. Answer review questions in the practice mode and read the feedback, studying the questions you have missed. Take the chapter quiz until you achieve a minimum score of 90 percent. Successfully completing the *Critical Thinking Challenge* at the end of this course will help you think through scenarios and develop problem solving skills.

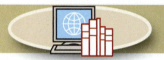

RESOURCES

Internet

American Health Information Management
    Association
    Articles, career, federal regulations
    Web site: http://www.ahima.org
Association of Records Managers and
    Administrators (AMRA International)
    Archives, compliance, federal rules,
    management and organization of records
    Web site: http://www.arma.org
Bibbero Systems, Inc.
    Filing equipment and products
    Web site:http://www.bibbero.com

Medical Records Institute
    Electronic medical record trends
    Web site: http://www.medrecinst.com

Keywords for Internet Searches

Filing rules
Filing systems
Health record systems
Medical record filing
Medical record storage
Tickler files

CHAPTER 9

Medical Records

OBJECTIVES

After reading this chapter and learning step-by-step procedures to gain job skills,* you should be able to:

Learning Objectives

▌ List reasons for maintaining medical records.

▌ Name three basic types of medical record organization systems.

▌ State the functions of a flowchart.

▌ Describe the operation of an electronic medical record system.

▌ Name various titles the physician may have in the treatment of patients.

▌ List contents of a patient's medical record file.

▌ State the differences between a manual, an electronic, and a digital signature.

▌ Describe two types of documentation formats.

▌ Distinguish subjective from objective information.

▌ Understand the contents of a history and physical examination report.

Performance Objectives (Procedures) in This Textbook

▌ Prepare and compile a medical record for a new patient (Procedure 9-1).

▌ Correct a medical record (Procedure 9-2).

▌ Abstract data from a medical record (Procedure 9-3).

Performance Objectives (Job Skills) in the *Workbook*

▌ Prepare a patient record and insert progress notes (Job Skill 9-1).

▌ Prepare a patient record and format chart notes (Job Skill 9-2).

This textbook and the accompanying Workbook meet the educational components for entry-level administrative and general competencies outlined by CAAHEP and ABHES.

■ Correct a patient record (Job Skill 9-3).

■ Abstract from a medical record (Job Skill 9-4)

■ Prepare a history and physical report (Job Skill 9-5).

OUTLINE WITH LECTURE NOTES

Patients' Medical Records

_____

_____

_____

_____

_____

Medical Record Systems

Paper-Based Medical Record System

_____

_____

_____

_____

Electonic Medical Record System

_____

_____

_____

_____

Medical Record Organization Systems

_____

_____

_____

_____

_____

Recordkeeping

Recordkeepers

_____

_____

_____

_____

Documenters

_____

_____

_____

_____

Authentication of Documents

_____

_____

_____

_____

_____

Documentation Format

_____

_____

_____

Documentaiton Guidelines

_____

_____

_____

_____

Documentation Terminology

_____

_____

_____

_____

Correcting a Medical Record

_____

_____

_____

_____

Elements of a Medical Record

Patient Information Form

_____

_____

_____

_____

Patient Medical History

_____

_____

_____

Physical Examination

_____

_____

_____

Complexity of Medical Decision Making

_____

_____

_____

Progress or Chart Notes

_____

_____

_____

Medical Reports

_____

_____

_____

Laboratory Reports

_____

_____

_____

Laboratory Log

_____

_____

_____

Radiographs (X-Ray Films)

_____

_____

_____

Electrocardiograms

_____

_____

_____

Abstracting from Medical Records

_____

_____

_____

Audit of Medical Records
Internal Review

_____

_____

_____

External Audit

_____

_____

_____

KEY TERMS

abstract
attending physician
audit
case history
CHEDDAR
consulting physician
diagnosis
electronic health record (EHR)
flow sheet

health information management (HIM)
laboratory report
medical record
medical report
objective
ordering physician
POMR
prognosis
progress report

(continues)

referring physician
sign
SOAP
subjective

symptom
treating or performing physician
x-ray report

HEART OF THE HEALTH CARE PROFESSIONAL

Service

Consider the medical record as a diary put in your care, and have a high regard for it. By respecting patients' privacy and keeping personal information confidential you will be serving all patients.

PATIENTS' MEDICAL RECORDS

A patient's **medical record** is a handwritten or type-written recording of information that documents facts and events during the administration of patient care. The legal task force of The American Health Information Management Association (AHIMA) defines the legal health record (LHR) as "the documentation of healthcare services provided to an individual, in any aspect of healthcare delivery by a healthcare provider organization." The principal reasons for maintaining medical records are:

1. To aid in the diagnosis and treatment of a patient

2. To provide written documentation of directed patient care

3. To verify that services were medically necessary

4. To assist in the research of disease and injuries so other patients may benefit from previous patient care

5. To substantiate procedure and diagnostic code selections for appropriate reimbursement

6. To comply with federal and state laws

7. To defend the physician in the event of a lawsuit

Patient records are also used in completing various reports required by law, such as reports on communicable diseases, child abuse, gunshot wounds, stabbings from criminal actions, diseases and illnesses of newborns and infants, and injury or illness that occurs in the workplace. In addition, they are used to assist in the preparation of insurance claims for private, federal, and state programs.

A medical record must be prepared for all new patients who will be seen in the medical practice. File folders and labels are used to set up the chart, as mentioned in Chapter 8.

MEDICAL RECORD SYSTEMS

With the onset of documentation guidelines and the increase of internal and external audits, it is important that a proper medical record system be used. A good medical record system is a key to quality care. It assists with accessing patients' conditions, provides others with critical information, furnishes statistical information, and protects against liability suits. The day has arrived when medical record information is available through data retrieval systems that provide computer readouts so that traditional patient charts can be updated constantly.

Paper-Based Medical Record System

Paper-based medical records are used by the majority of medical practices; however, they are costly to manage, move, and store. Many people feel secure with a hard copy of information in hand, but paper records are more vulnerable to a variety of security threats such as tampering, theft, and loss. There is

COMPLIANCE

One provision in Title II of the Health Insurance Portability and Accountability Act (HIPAA) of 1996 directs federal government programs to adopt national electronic standards for automated transfer of certain health care data among health care payers, plans, and providers. This eliminates nonstandard formats and encourages offices to convert to an electronic recordkeeping system.

STEP 1 2 3

PROCEDURE 9-1

Prepare and Compile a Medical Record for a New Patient

Objective: To prepare and compile a medical record for a new patient.

Equipment/Supplies: File folder, patient information form, file folder label, labels for special information (current year, allergies, insurance information), computer or typewriter, forms (flow sheet, progress notes, laboratory reports, and so forth), two-hole punch, and pen.

Directions: Follow these step-by-step procedures, which include rationales, to learn this skill, which is presented in the *Workbook* (Job Skills 9-1 and 9-2) for practice.

1. Select a file folder; either lateral or vertical.

2. Key or type a label for the patient's file folder with the last name followed by the first name and middle initial. Charts are filed by last name; however, if the office uses a numeric filing system, insert a number on the label.

3. Adhere the label to the tabbed edge of the file folder, which may be located at the right, left, or middle top portion of the folder or on the side.

4. Select colored letter-tabs for the first two letters of the patient's last name if a color-coded filing system is used. In larger offices additional labeling may be required. This label must be visible when the patient's record is in the filing cabinet or drawer. Colored labels aid in filing and locating lost charts because if misfiled, the color stands out from neighboring file folders.

5. Add a current year label either to the end or top tab of the file folder for a new patient. To update an established patient's record, add a year label the first time the patient comes in for an appointment for the current year. This helps when purging inactive files. (See Chapter 8.)

6. Adhere an allergy label and indicate all allergies or if there are no known allergies, write NKA. Allergy labels alert all staff members and help avoid adverse reactions.

7. Adhere an insurance label indicating the type of plan. Labels identify patients who are in specific insurance plans or categories (e.g., Medicare, HMO).

8. Insert blank forms used by the medical practice into the patient's file folder. Label each sheet with the patient's name or record number. This helps identify each page of the record.

9. Punch holes in the sheets if necessary and affix them to the folder. This will secure pages and help position information that may otherwise fall out.

---

also no easy way to search for clinical data in a paper-based system. With government mandates requiring increased security for health information and increased competition with electronic medical record software development, more physician practices will be motivated to use electronic record systems.

Converting Paper Records to Electronic Records

To digitize medical records is to convert paper documents to electronic images using a scanner. Some health care enterprises process more than 2,500 different types of documents, the most common are patient history and physical evaluations, consultations, prescriptions, reports (laboratory, EKGs, radiology), insurance claims, and billing statements. Advanced scanners can handle taped strips from fetal monitors or electrocardiography machines, envelopes, self-adhesive notes, and other odd-sized items without misfeeding or errors while reading the material.

If you are responsible for managing the conversion to an **electronic health record (EHR)** or *electronic medical record (EMR)*, it is important to consult with a **health information management (HIM)** professional to develop a plan, write a proposal, and select a vendor. Goals should be clarified and the physician needs to lead the effort. Visit other offices, network with managers who have gone through the conversion process, and attend vendor demonstrations. Verify the references of all potential vendors prior to making a selection, obtaining a commitment, and negotiating a contract.

Electronic Medical Record System

The use of legal, financial, clinical, and other business data has generated an ever-expanding volume of required forms, documentation, and reporting procedures. These data take more office time to document and require more storage space when a paper chart system is used.

New technology and cost reductions in equipment and software offer the ability to have electronic medical records (EMR) in physician offices. EMR offers fast, secure, and centralized access to health care data that can be viewed from home, satellite offices, and hospital sites (such as the emergency room or intensive care unit). One database collects medical histories, x-rays, laboratory results, and a multitude of other data that is accessible to both physicians and patients. Benefits of an EMR system include the ability to:

- Track patient histories, prescription drugs, consultations, and a variety of data
- Detect inconsistencies in diagnoses
- Monitor quality assurance standards
- Deliver prompt reports
- Achieve timely billing and reimbursement
- Decrease errors and miscommunications
- Reduce handwritten notes
- Make information more accessible
- Eliminate searching charts for clinical data

In an EMR system, a template on the computer screen is brought up and the medical assistant enters the reason for the patient's visit (see Example 9-1). A series of questions designed to find more information about the patient's complaint are then answered.

One screen may contain ongoing data about a patient, including allergies and past history of complaints. There may be a history and physical screen with two different templates. For example, one may be for a well-child visit and one may be for an ill-child visit. When the examination has been completed, the

---

EXAMPLE 9-1

Computer Template Questions

Chief complaint: Fever. The questions appearing in a pop-up screen might ask, "How long has the patient had a fever? What is the highest temperature reading?" "What other symptoms (chills, sweats, nausea, vomiting, rash, headache, pain) accompany the fever?"

---

software program may prompt the physician through a series of templates and screens to assist in the assignment of procedural codes.

When the diagnosis has been determined, a diagnostic screen appears. There are usually several diagnostic codes listed—those that were previously assigned and those relating to the current problem. The physician selects the appropriate one according to the description. With this data input, it is then possible for the system to generate either a paper claim for mailing or an electronic claim for transmission.

Electronic systems may also generate prescriptions, laboratory requisition forms, or specific written instructions for the patient to take home. There is less chance for error in reading or misinterpretation because all documents are legible.

In an electronic system, every examination room can be set up with a computer. Also, various electronic mobile devices exist that are used to input, store, and transfer data. As mentioned in Chapter 7, personal digital assistants (PDAs) are used to input information at remote locations. Also, graphic accelerators and iPods are now used to store and relay information that was previously difficult to digitize.

The physician can choose the typical language for normal findings already stored in the software or mark an insertion point for edited remarks and later dictate that section of the report. There may be a workstation in the hallway or at the physician's desk to finish notes after leaving the patient. The physician can release the report to be finalized by the medical transcriptionist, who reviews and edits it for accuracy of grammar and spelling, enters any information that has been dictated, and returns the report to the physician for final review and signature. With this system, the doctor does not have to spend time redictating each component of the report for each patient.

Electronic systems are continuing to improve and soon upcoming technology will enable the physician to make "mouse calls" to patients over the Internet for a fee. In some hospital settings, wireless networks are now in place where a wireless computer on a cart can be moved from room to room allowing nurses to view and input patient data (e.g., vital signs) directly into the electronic system. Efficiency and productivity are gained while storage space is saved.

Medical Record Organization Systems

The three basic types of medical record organization systems used by most physicians' offices are:

- Problem-oriented record
- Source-oriented record
- Integrated record

Problem-Oriented Record System

During the 1960s, Dr. Lawrence Weed developed a *problem-oriented medical record* (**POMR**) system. The system has been modified for use by individual disciplines, including the medical profession (Figure 9-1 and Figure 9-2).

The example in Figure 9-1 illustrates a form that includs identification data and lists in tabular form all of the patient's permanent and temporary problems, each one numbered and dated. The patient's continuing and temporary medications are cross-referenced (by number) to the problem for which they were prescribed, along with dosage information and the start and stop dates of the medication.

The example in Figure 9-2 indicates allergies and the patient's blood type and illustrates several **flow sheets** in the bottom portion of the form.

One flow sheet lists consultations, the specialty and name of the physician, and the date the appointments occurred. The type of problem is cross-referenced by number to the problem list shown in Figure 9-1. Another flow sheet lists immunizations and the dates they were received. A third one lists hospitalizations, the year they occurred, and the reason for the admission. There are also flow sheets for Pap tests, mammograms, and prostrate specific antigen (PSA) tests along with a tracking form for blood pressures.

Some data are hard to track in narrative progress notes; on the other hand, flow sheets, charts, or graphs allow the physician to quickly find information and perform comparative evaluations. These, however, do not replace documentation in the progress notes in the medical record. In addition to the types of flow sheets previously mentioned, they are commonly used to record blood sugar levels for diabetics, prothrombin levels for patients taking blood-thinning agents (e.g., Coumadin), weight for obstetric, obese, or undernourished patients, as well as medication refill information. They can be developed for any type of continuous problem, for example, cardiovascular cases (see Example 9-2 on page 270).

Using a problem-oriented medical record system helps the physician retrieve information quickly and handle large patient workloads. The POMR system permits evaluation of the physician's reasoning in assessing patients' conditions. There is less reliance on the physician's memory so errors are reduced, and the patient receives more efficient, continuous care. The disadvantage of this format is the time it takes to develop the problem list and to do the necessary repetitious recording.

Source-Oriented Record System

The *source-oriented record* (SOR) system is the most common paper-based management system. Documents are arranged according to sections, for exam-

PATIENT RECORD—COMPREHENSIVE FLOW SHEET (page 1)

Name: Morani   Betty   A.   **Account No.:** 00621

Address: 4040 Third St.   New Hill   XY   00421   **Telephone:** (555) 897-6543

Date of Birth: 6/20/45   **Sex:** F **Status:** M   **Social Security No.:** 111-XX-3333

Employer: Retired   **Occupation:** Hair stylist

Next of Kin: John Morani **Relationship:** H   **Telephone:** (555) 897-0060 work

Address: Same

Insurance: Medicare   **Policy No.:** 111-XX-3333A   **Group:**

Address: ABC Insurance Company Fiscal Intermediary   **Telephone:** (555) 499-0101

Date	PERMANENT PROBLEMS	Problem Number	Date	TEMPORARY PROBLEMS	Problem Number
10/98	Hypertension—essential	P-1	1/99	L. Rtinopathy	T-1
10/98	Diabetes mellitus—type II	P-2	3/03	Conjunctivitis	T-2
4/00	Atherosclerosis with cerebral vascular insufficiency	P-3	7/04	UTI	T-3
4/00	Hearing loss	P-4	11/06	Otitis media	T-4
1/02	Left bundle branch block	P-5			
1/02	Bilateral grade II retinopathy	P-6			

Date Start	CONTINUING MEDICATIONS	Date Stop	Problem Number	Date Start	TEMPORARY MEDICATIONS	Date Stop	Problem Number
10/98	Sinoserp 1 mg b.i.d.	10/00	P-1	3/03	Tetracycline 250 mg	10d	T-2
10/98	Orinase 0.5 gm daily	10/00	P-2	7/04	Amoxil 250 mg	10d	T-3
10/00	Hydrodiuril 50 mg am		P-1	11/06	Amoxil 250 mg	7d	T-4

Figure 9-1. Comprehensive flow sheet (page 1) used for problem-oriented medical record printed on or attached to inside front cover listing permanent and temporary medical problems and continuing/temporary medications

PATIENT RECORD—COMPREHENSIVE FLOW SHEET (page 2)

Name: Morani, Betty A.   **Allergies.:** Codeine

Acct No. 00621   Sulfa

Date of Birth: 6/20/45   **Blood Type:** A+

Physician: Fran Practon MD   **Health Care Directive.:** Yes

Date	CONSULTATIONS	Problem Number	✔	IMMUNIZATIONS	Dates			INFLUENZA Date
1/99	Ophth. – Dr. Metz	T-1		Haemophilus (b)				10/3/98
4/00	ENT – Dr. O'Farrell	P-4		Hepatitis A				9/18/99
1/02	Ophth. — Dr. Metz	P-6		Hepatitis B				9/03/00
			✔	Inactivated Polio	'51	'52		11/25/01
			✔	MMR	had			10/06/02
				Pneumococcal				9/18/03
			✔	Small Pox	'53			10/30/05
			✔	Varicella	had			9/09/06
Date	**HOSPITALIZATIONS**	**Problem Number**	✔	TB	'52	'98		
1950	T&A		✔	DPaT	'46	'59	'80	
1978	TAH							

Date	PAP TEST	Date	MAMMOGRAM	Date	PSA
10/98	Class I	10/98	Normal		
1/99	Class I	4/00	R Microcalcification		
4/00	Class I	1/02	R Microcalcification		
1/02	Class I	7/04	Normal		
3/03	Class I	11/06	Normal		
7/04	Class I				
11/06	Class I				

DATE	10/09	1/99	4/00	1/02	3/03	7/04	11/06			
BP	140/88	150/90	160/86	128/78	130/84	190/90	160/80			
DATE										
BP										

Figure 9-2. Comprehensive flow sheet (page 2) used for problem-oriented medical record printed on or attached to inside front cover listing various data for tracking purposes

ple, history and physical section, progress notes, laboratory, radiology, surgical operations, and so forth. Some SOR systems use color laminated tab dividers for each section, which make locating information quick and easy. The information in each section is sequenced in chronological order, with the most recent on top. Sequencing of the sections varies from practice to practice. The disadvantage of the SOR system is the lack of an overall picture of the patient's health or problem because documentation related to these issues is filed in different sections of the record.

EXAMPLE 9-2

Cardiovascular Flow Sheet

Patient's name: Clare McDonald				Physician: F. Practon, MD	
Normal Values ABC Lab	135–199	30–85	<130	L = < 3.7 M = > 3.7 H = > 4.7	35–160
Date	**Cholesterol**	**HDL**	**LDL**	**Cardiac Risk Ratio**	**Triglycerides**
1/18/2003	204	59	116	3.5	145
2/3/2004	232	61	160	3.80	57
2/17/2005	245	55	142	4.5	242
10/9/2005	256	62	178	4.1	80
2/16/2006	277	59	181	4.7	186
5/4/2007	266	50	186	5.3 Start Zocar 40 mg/d	149
9/14/2007	187	70	102	2.7	99

Integrated Record System

The *integrated record* system files all documents in chronological order without regard to their source. Trying to compare information from the same source, for example, laboratory test results, is difficult because they are scattered throughout the record.

RECORDKEEPING

With the appearance of computers and communication equipment, there are a variety of ways to keep records and record data. Following are four basic ways information can be entered into the medical record:

- *Physician hand enters data.* Entries in the patient's record are handwritten. Physicians have been held liable in a hospital setting when medication has been given to a patient in error

COMPLIANCE

Entries in the patient's record must be legible.

as a result of handwritten notes that were incorrectly read.

- *Physician dictates.* Although some physicians prefer to handwrite, the majority dictate their notes or comments. Dictation terminals may be available at the physician's desk, in the treatment room, or at office workstations. Portable equipment may be used by the physician when off site. The transcriptionist listens to voice recorded data and keys the information using a computer, word processor, or typewriter. The record or report is then reviewed and signed by the physician.

- *Physician keys data.* Data are entered via a remote device or terminal that is available in every examination room where the physician can key in information about the patient's visit. This information can be printed in the form of a progress note or medical report.

- *Medical assistant enters data.* A checklist, form, or template is used with common problems and procedures specific to the medical practice. The assistant fills in blanks or circles an abbreviation that represents phrases or complete sentences as the physician narrates findings and recommendations. The advantage of this system is that the medical record is completed before the physician leaves the examination room. The physician can review the input before leaving the room or at a later time (Figure 9-3).

Recordkeepers

In each medical practice, an individual should be named as the recordkeeper. In a small practice, this may be another duty of the administrative medical assistant. In a large medical practice, one person is usually in charge of all medical records. The larger the practice, the more duties the medical recordkeeper has. He or she may be in charge of overseeing the medical record system and all file clerks, documentation requirements, coding, internal audits, processing authorization requests for records, and obtaining patient records from other facilities. As mentioned in Chapter 3, this person would need to comply with all regulations regarding the use and transfer of private health information, including answering subpoenas.

Office policies vary, but records are usually sent to other physicians with no charge when the need has to do with continuation of care or transfer of care. When records are requested from patients for their personal use or for reasons that do not involve treatment (e.g., life insurance application) the physician's office usually charges for the copying and release of records (25 cents per page up to $25 for the entire record). Most offices notify insurance companies of the charge when signed requests are received and only release the records after the fee has been obtained. This saves billing insurance companies for miscellaneous fees and trying to collect small amounts of money.

Documenters

All individuals who provide health care services may be known as *documenters* because they chronologically record facts and observations about the patient and the patient's health.

The receptionist may record canceled or no-show appointments and messages, the insurance specialist may record authorization requests or alerts for patients who have been sent to a collection agency, and the clinical medical assistant may record vital signs, scheduled tests, and other clinical data; each taking the role of a documenter.

There are instances when the physician's title may change, depending on the specialty and services rendered. Because this can be a confusing issue and because it is important when submitting insurance claims, clarification of these various roles is detailed here.

- **Attending physician** refers to the medical staff member who is legally responsible for the care and treatment given to a patient.
- **Consulting physician** is a provider whose opinion or advice regarding evaluation and/or management of a specific problem is requested by another physician.
- **Ordering physician** is the individual directing the selection, preparation, or administration of tests, medication, or treatment.
- **Referring physician** is a provider who sends the patient for testing or treatment. It may also be the provider who transfers the management of a patient to another physician.
- **Treating** or **performing physician** is the provider who renders a service to a patient.

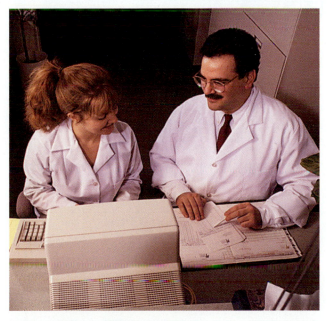

Figure 9-3. A medical assistant is shown checking with the physician to clarify information about a patient's condition before recording it in the medical record

Authentication of Documents

Each document must be authenticated by signature. The treating or attending physician must sign each progress note in the medical record as well as all test results and reports. In addition, all documenters must sign their name to the portion of the medical record that he or she documented. Initials are not recommended for progress notes, but if they are used for test results, telephone messages, chart corrections, and so forth, it is recommended that a staff signature and initial log be retained for legal purposes (Example 9-3). Stamped signatures are not allowed.

Manual Signatures

Handwritten or typed entries made during the continuing care of the patient should be signed by the treating or attending physician. For a chart to be admissible as evidence in court, the physician who dictated or wrote the entries must attest that the entries were true and correct at the time of writing. A physician's signature after the typed notes indicates this fact. If the physician is away from the office after dictating a document and the correspondence is urgent, there are two choices:

1. The assistant can sign the physician's name with his or her own initials after it.

2. A photocopy of the record (letter) may be sent, stating that the physician will sign and forward the original upon his or her return.

Electronic Signatures

In hospitals and large clinics, documents generated via computer may contain either electronic signatures or digital signatures. An *electronic signature* refers to a method of authenticating documents by the insertion of a facsimile of a person's actual handwritten signature or typed name that is affixed electronically at the end of a document. Because it can be altered, deleted, or forged by anyone with access privileges, an electronic signature creates obvious problems.

A *digital signature* is secure because it cannot be forged or altered without detection, and if the content of the signed document is altered, the signature is invalidated. To authenticate portions of the medi-

---

EXAMPLE 9-3

Signature/Initial Log for Office Staff

Data	Name	Position	Credential	Signature	Initials
January 3, 20XX	Gerald Practon	General Practitioner	MD = medical doctor	*Gerald Practon MD*	GP
January 3, 20XX	Fran Practon	Family Practice Physician	MD = medical doctor	*Fran Practon MD*	FP
January 5, 20XX	Suzanne Davenport	Office Manager	CMA = certified medical assistant	*Suzanne Davenport CMA*	SD
January 6, 20XX	Andrea Roddick	Administrative Medical Assistant	CMAS = certified medical administrative specialist	*Andrea Roddick CMAS*	AR
January 6, 20XX	Sondra Kovitz	Clinical Medical Assistant	RMA = registered medical assistant	*Sondra Kovitz RMA*	SK
January 6, 20XX	Beatrice Federrer	Medical Insurance Biller	CPC = certified professional coder	*Beatrice Federrer CPC*	BF

cal record using a digital signature, an individual has computer access and uses an identification encryption system such as a series of letters or numbers (alpha-numeric computer key entries), an electronic writing, or a biometric system (voice print, hand or fingerprint transmissions, facial, iris, or retinal scans).

Documentation Format

Documentation of patient progress notes can become voluminous. An organized system to dictate and record enables the physician and staff to locate certain sections quickly and find information. The following methods are used by physicians and have enjoyed some popularity because they were developed from acronyms that can be remembered easily.

SOAP Format

Figure 9-4 shows a progress note in a problem-oriented medical record that is divided into four sections using the **SOAP** format. The acronym is derived from the following:

S: *Subjective*—statements about how the patient feels and symptoms experienced. This would include comments by the patient about the history of present illness, responses to review of systems, and statements about the past, the family, and social history.

O: *Objective*—data from laboratory reports, x-rays, other diagnostic tests, and physical findings on examination by the physician. All objective data are seen (inspection and observation), heard

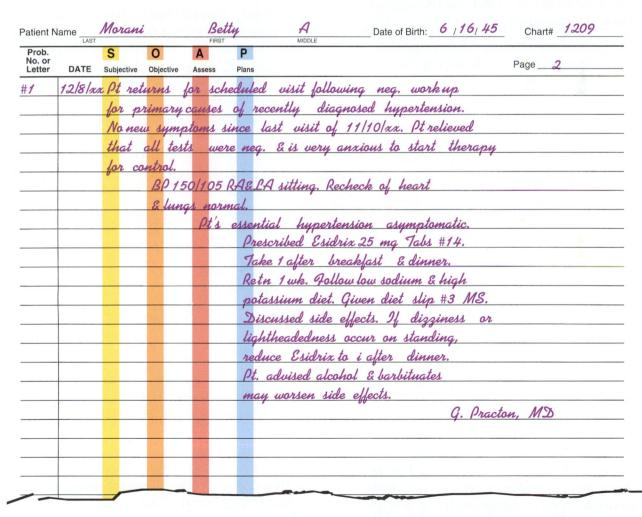

Figure 9-4. Progress note from a problem-oriented medical record with an example of the SOAP format. (Courtesy of Bibbero Systems, Inc., Petaluma, CA. Telephone: (800) 242-2376; Fax: (800) 242-9330; Web site: http://www.bibbero.com.)

(auscultation), felt (palpation), or measured as in diagnostic testing.

A: *Assessment*—analysis of the subjective and objective portions of the chart note used to attain a diagnosis.

P: *Plan*—therapeutic treatment plan and instructions to the patient by the physician. This includes further testing, medications, return visit, and outlook or prognosis of the case.

CHEDDAR Format

This format breaks down in further detail each element of the patient encounter. The **CHEDDAR** acronym is derived from the following:

C: *Chief complaint* stated by the patient as the main reason for seeing the doctor. This is usually a subjective statement.

H: *History of the present illness*, including social history and physical symptoms as well as contributing factors.

E: *Examination* by the physician.

D: *Details* of problems and complaints.

D: *Drugs and dosages* of the current medications the patient is taking.

A: *Assessment* of the diagnostic process and the impression (diagnosis) made by the physician.

R: *Return visit information or referral* to a specialist for additional tests.

Documentation Guidelines

A variety of formats of documentation (e.g., SOAP or CHEDDAR notes) are accepted by insurance companies as long as the information is discernible. Some physicians do not like to use printed forms; they prefer blank or ruled sheets for this purpose, especially if they dictate the history and physical examination findings for transcription purposes.

Other physicians prefer that the medical assistant interview patients and take the medical histories. Steps should be taken so that conversations of this nature are private and not overheard by others in the reception room or throughout the office. The data may also be obtained by questionnaire or checkoff list structured with specific questions or in outline form to be completed by the patient. These forms need to

be initialed by the physician and all positive findings expanded upon. They do not take the place of narrative documentation in the medical record.

The following guidelines should be adhered to in maintaining each patient's medical record. If a medical assistant is aware of documentation deficiencies, it is his or her responsibility to bring them to the physician's attention in a tactful manner.

1. Record the patient's name and date (month, day, and year) for each entry.

2. List each patient encounter in complete form, legibly, accurately, and in chronological order.

3. Enter all documentation in a timely fashion; state information objectively and be specific, including:
   - The reason for the encounter, with relevant history, physical examination findings, and prior diagnostic test results
   - The assessment, clinical impression, or diagnosis. Avoid generalizations (e.g., patient doing well). It is considered inadequate documentation to describe test results or conditions as "normal," "abnormal," or "within normal limits" if they relate to the body system being affected.
   - The plan for care
   - The date and legible identity of the observer

4. Use standard, approved abbreviations.

5. List all allergies and history of adverse reactions.

6. Record all immunizations or injections given to the patient.

7. Prominently display the patient's problem list, and document significant illnesses and medical conditions so the list is kept current.

8. Present rationale for ordering diagnostic and other ancillary services; if not stated, documented rationale should be easily inferred.

9. List the reasons for deviations from standard treatment.

10. Have past and present diagnoses accessible to the treating or consulting physician.

11. Identify appropriate health risk factors.

12. Include the patient's past medical history (serious illnesses, accidents, and operations).

13. Document smoking habits and/or history of alcohol or substance abuse.

14. Note the patient's medical condition on each visit, consisting of pertinent history, examination, assessment, and plan of action, including necessary follow-up by the attending physician.

15. Document all telephone conversations with or regarding the patient.

16. Document the patient's progress, response to and changes in treatment, and revision of diagnosis.

17. Support procedure and diagnostic codes reported on the health insurance claim form or billing statement with documentation in the medical record.

18. File the results of laboratory, x-ray, electrocardiogram (ECG), and other tests with the most recent report on top.

19. Read through written entries to verify that everything is legible.

20. Photocopy prescriptions written for the patient.

21. List the names of the staff members who assisted in any procedure.

22. Document any sample drugs that are given to the patient and the patient's agreement to accept the samples.

23. Indicate patient education and instructions.

24. Verify that each entry is signed or initialed by the author and include professional credentials.

25. Make all corrections using standard technique (see Figure 9-5 on page 277).

COMPLIANCE

Verify that each entry is signed or initialed by the author with his or her title or position and verify the initials are in the signature log.

Medicare Documentation Guidelines

In November 1994, the American Medical Association (AMA) and the Centers for Medicare and Medicaid Services (CMS), formerly the Health Care Financing Administration (HCFA), developed docu-

mentation guidelines for the Medicare program. They are referred to as the 1995 guidelines. Subsequently newer guidelines were developed in 1997. These policies affect reimbursement for procedure codes used for evaluation and management services and are routinely used by government programs and private carriers.

COMPLIANCE

Government programs and private insurance carriers have an obligation to those enrolled to ensure that services paid for have been provided and were medically necessary. Documentation must support the level of service and each procedure.

Physicians may use either the 1995 or 1997 guidelines but there is no formal requirement. However, Medicare and other claims processors and auditors may use them when reviewing documentation to determine that the reported services were actually rendered and that the level of service was provided.

When significant aberrant reporting patterns are detected by Medicare or other insurance carriers, then a review is conducted. Because these federal guidelines affect reimbursement, many medical practices have begun using these documentation policies for Medicare patients as well as those under private or managed care plans.

Documentation Terminology

Accurate words or phrases are of utmost importance when documenting a patient encounter and determining what charges to bill or verifying services that have been billed. Often a physician will list a normal situation or negative result by either dictating or writing "noncontributory" or "within normal limits (WNL)." Such phrases cannot be used when referring to an affected body area or to determine a diagnostic code assignment. These terms should not be used if the patient was not questioned or no examination was performed on the body part.

Likewise the term *negative* as in "chest x-ray, negative" does not indicate what service the physician provided. Instead state details such as "PA and lateral chest films were reviewed and no abnormalities were seen."

EXAMPLE 9-4

EXAMPLE 9-4

Documentation Terminology

A statement such as "All extremities are within normal limits" does not indicate how many extremities or which extremities were examined. Documentation must indicate which limb was examined and what it was examined for. For example, "The left lower extremity was examined for skin rash, and no abnormalities were found."

When describing the status of a condition, that is, acute or chronic, the word *acute* refers to a condition with a sudden onset that runs a short but relatively severe course. The word *chronic* means a condition persisting over a long period of time. However, the word *recurrent* may be preferred for certain ailments instead of *chronic*. For example, "chronic asthma" is listed in the diagnostic codebook as "recurrent asthma."

Documentation guidelines say "describe the condition" so if the physician states "controlled hypertension" or "controlled diabetes," this is stating a fact that describes the state of the diabetes and the reason for the visit (chief complaint). However, the patient should be questioned about blood sugar level results or diet, and the physician should document the response; then a finding has been identified supporting the state of the chronic condition.

Acronyms and Abbreviations

Abbreviations and symbols appear in chart notes because physicians need to document quickly and eliminate long words. In many instances, it would be difficult for a layperson to interpret a chart because of the physician's shorthand. The medical assistant needs to be familiar with all the abbreviations and symbols used by the physician and use standard acronyms and abbreviations that are commonly understood by the general medical community. Do not invent an abbreviation. Each medical office should develop a list of standard abbreviations applicable to the specialty. To assist in this task, each local hospital has its own list of abbreviations acceptable in its facility that might be available to staff physicians on request.

Official American Hospital Association policy states that "abbreviations should be totally eliminated from the more vital sections of the record, such as final diagnosis, operative notes, discharge summaries, and descriptions of special procedures." Many physicians are, however, unaware of this policy, and the final diagnosis may yet appear with abbreviations on the patient's record.

The current trend is to omit periods with specialized abbreviations, acronyms, and metric abbreviations as well as physicians' academic degrees (e.g., MD). Latin abbreviations are typed in lowercase letters with periods (e.g., b.i.d., a.m.), and many of these are pharmaceutical abbreviations (see Chapter 10). The patient care abbreviations are listed in Chapter 7, Table 7-1. The medical assistant can use a medical dictionary to look up abbreviations not included in this table.

Illustrations

Illustrations may be used by the physician to document an area of the body where a problem occurs. They may depict a finding, symptom, or procedure and may help educate the patient or verify a completed service. Physicians may either purchase or hand draw and label their illustrations. Illustrations that are used for some aspect of a patient encounter should be kept in the chart and must be legible, dated, and signed. Include the patient's name and date of birth on the drawing.

Digital Images

Some physicians (e.g., plastic surgeons, oral surgeons) may take photographs of the patient that become part of the medical record. These may be digital images that are imported while transcribing medical reports. These images may also consist of scans of various body organs or radiographic x-rays. A graphic may help the physician determine what corrective measures to take and also makes it easier for patients to understand their condition or disease because it gives more comprehensive detailed documentation. Microsoft Word or Corel WordPerfect word processing software has a feature that allows digital images to be imported into a document. If the document is an electronic medical record, the image can be attached so other physicians can view it. If photographs are part of the medical record, be sure to label them with the patient's name, date of birth, and date taken. Remember that if a patient's digital image is requested for publication, the authorization form must contain wording that indicates the digital image is to be used in this manner.

Measurements

Measurements that pertain to lacerations, lesions, burns, nerve and skin grafts, neoplasms, tattoos, cysts, injection material, and so forth, commonly appear in patients' medical records and operative reports. Most of the time, the metric system (e.g., centimeters) is used when measuring skin lacerations and lesions. Avoid using terms such as small, medium, or large. Documentation should consist of the location and site(s), the size(s), the number(s) of lesions treated, the method of destruction, and any extenuating circumstances. Reimbursement is affected by the size or area documented and subsequently reported on insurance claims.

Burns are listed by

1. Type (e.g., chemical)

2. Depth (first, second, or third degree)

3. Site (face, arm, leg, trunk)

4. Percentage of total body surface (TBS) affected

CORRECTING A MEDICAL RECORD

To alleviate confusion and prevent medicolegal problems, it is important to know how to correct chart notes as well as other records. Never erase or use correction fluid on handwritten or typed entries. If corrections need to be made on a patient's medical record, draw a line neatly through the incorrect entry so it remains readable. If there is adequate room above or below the original entry, insert the correct information there. Otherwise it may be inserted in the margin or after the conclusion of the note. The person making the correction writes "Corr.," the date, and his or her initials in the margin of the page as shown in Figure 9-5. If the correction is inserted at the end of the chart note, the person making the correction enters the date, writes or types "correction to chart note of 8-10-20XX (date of note being corrected)," enters the correction, and initials or signs at the end of the notation.

It is permissible when typing a chart note or medical report to use correction fluid or tape on typographical errors at the time of original entry, but one never obscures, erases, or puts self-adhesive typing strips

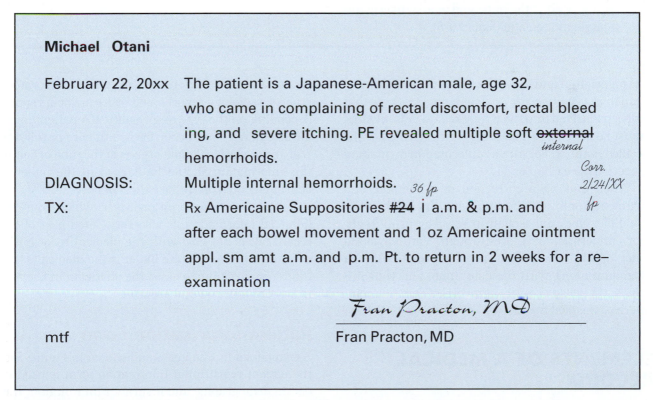

Figure 9-5. Typed chart note with examples of corrections made by physician Fran Practon (FP) on the day she read and signed entries

PROCEDURE 9-2

Correct a Medical Record

Objective: To insert a correction entry in a medical chart note using standard procedures.

Equipment/Supplies: Patient's medical record, reference documents for making correction (transcribed notes, telephone notes, physician's comments, correspondence), and pen.

Directions: Follow these step-by-step procedures, which include rationales, to learn this skill, which is presented in the *Workbook* (Job Skill 9-3) for practice.

Simple Correction

1. Draw a line neatly through the incorrect entry. It should remain readable because you do not want to suggest any altering or obliteration of a medical record.

2. Write or type the correct information where there is adequate space, either above or below the line being corrected.

3. Write "Corr.," the date, and your initials in the margin of the page (Figure 9-5).

Long Correction

1. If there is no room for the correction above or below the error, the correction must be made after the chart note.

2. Enter the corrected data.

3. Initial and sign at the end of the notation.

Correction with Addendum or Attached Document

1. If an addendum or attached document is necessary to correct the error or omission and there have been office visits after the error is found, date the entry with the current date and refer to the date of the chart note being corrected (e.g., "9/6/20XX Addendum to chart note of 8/10/20XX.").

2. Note in the original record where to find the addendum or attached document (e.g., "See addendum after chart note of 10/24/20XX.").

over an original entry to correct later. When the physician discovers an error, such as a progress note that has been inserted into the wrong record or is missing, it must be added as an addendum or corrected in the specified manner. For further information on making corrections, see Chapter 11.

When making a correction in a computerized document, maintain the original entry in the electronic file. Note the section in error by using highlight, underline, or score-through features found under "Tools." Enter the correct information as an addendum along with the date, time, and your initials. Never delete or key over incorrect data in a computerized medical record file.

ELEMENTS OF A MEDICAL RECORD

Patient records consist of a variety of documents, such as a patient information form and a medical history questionnaire, a history and physical report, prog-

ress notes, physiology reports (e.g., ECG), laboratory reports, radiology reports, and other medical reports depending on the type of speciality. If a patient has a durable power of attorney for health care or a living will and wishes to donate organs at the time of death, this information should be flagged in the patient's chart and noted on the face sheet or cover.

The patient's account or ledger, which contains financial information, is also considered part of the record but is not filed with the medical record; it is maintained in a separate file. It is the medical assistant's responsibility to assist the physician in keeping the records current and accurate.

Patient Information Form

As explained in Chapter 5 and shown in Figure 5-5, the patient registration information form is used to obtain demographic and insurance information. It is primarily a business record but also helps acquaint the physician with a patient's personal data and becomes part of the medical record.

Patient Medical History

The levels of evaluation and management (E/M) services are based on four types of history: problem focused (PF), expanded problem focused (EPF), detailed (D), and comprehensive (C). E/M services is a phrase used for various types of office visits when referring to documentation and appropriate procedure codes selected from the *Current Procedural Terminology* codebook. See Tables 14-4, 14-5, and 14-6 in Chapter 14.

When a patient comes in with a complaint of symptoms describing how he or she feels, this is called **subjective** information; that is, it cannot be measured and may be viewed differently by each individual. The history of the present illness is based on this subjective information. It is drawn from the patient's *own* words about the chief complaint (CC) and his or her response to questions asked. Depending on the specialty of the physician and the subjective symptoms, the medical history may vary. Each type of **case history** includes some or all of the following elements (Figure 9-6A).

Chief Complaint (CC)

The chief complaint (CC) is a concise statement, usually in the patient's own words, describing the **symptom**, problem, condition, or other factor that is the reason for the encounter. The symptom is any indication of the disease or disorder that is perceived or experienced by the patient. If more than one, list them in the order of importance. *The CC is required for all levels of history.* Complaints can also be **objective**; if a patient complains of something that can be seen, felt, heard, or measured (e.g., a rash or a bump), it is objective information.

History of Present Illness (HPI)

The chief complaint is followed by a detailed account of how the patient was injured or when he or she first noticed the illness, called history of present illness (HPI). The HPI is a chronological description of the development of the patient's present illness from the first sign or symptom or from the previous encounter to the present. It includes the following elements: location, quality, severity, duration, timing, context, modifying factors, and associated signs and symptoms (Example 9-5). When a symptom is demonstrable to an observer upon examination, it is an *objective symptom*, or, more generally, a **sign**.

If the patient has been treated by another physician for the same or a similar problem, this will be

---

EXAMPLE 9-5

Elements of History of Present Illness

If a patient has chest pain, the physician may describe (1) the location of the pain (e.g., midsternal), (2) the quality of the pain (e.g., dull, sharp, stabbing), (3) the severity of the pain to further define the magnitude of the problem usually using a scale of from 1 to 10, (4) the duration of the pain (when the symptom first occurred), (5) the timing or relationship to a specific place or time of day, (6) the context or when the pain occurs, (7) all remedies and interventions that have been tried to resolve the pain (modifying factors), and (8) any associated signs and symptoms (other problems that contribute to the pain).

---

discussed, along with the possible diagnosis and treatment prescribed.

Past, Family, and Social History (PFSH)

The PFSH consists of a review of the following areas:

Past History (PH)—The past history is a personal history, including usual childhood diseases (UCHD), previous illnesses, physical defects, operations, accidents or injuries, treatments, medications, drug reactions, immunizations, and allergies.

Medications include listing drugs the patient has taken recently or is currently taking. Allergies include any reactions the patient may have to drugs, food, or the environment. Allergies should be underlined in red in the medical record and placed on the front of the chart, boldly visible. Some medical practices list allergies at the top of each page in the patient's progress notes. Because new allergies may appear as individuals age, questions should be asked to verify allergies each time a patient is seen for an appointment.

Family History (FH)—The family history is a review of medical events in the patient's family, including diseases that may be hereditary or place the patient at risk. Notations are made regarding whether the mother and father are living and well (M & F, l & w), ages at death, cause of death, and similar information for siblings and grandparents. The place and circumstances of the patient's birth might also be noteworthy.

Social History (SH)—The social history is an age-appropriate review of past and current activities and occupational history (OH), habits, diet, alcohol, drugs, tobacco, marital history (MH), exercise, and recreational interests. Sexual activity and numbers of sexual partners are also noted.

Review of Systems (ROS)

A review of systems (ROS), or systemic review (SR), is an inventory of body obtained through a series of oral questions seeking to identify signs or symptoms the patient might be experiencing or has experienced that may reveal information related to the present illness (Figure 9-6A). The ROS should not be confused with the examination of body systems, which will follow. The ROS begins at the top of the body and continues down through each body system as questions are asked about previous medical problems.

The physician may use a check-off sheet or dictate ROS data with subheadings or in a single paragraph without subheadings. The medical assistant must be able to recognize the body part and divide the information as it is dictated. The following material contains descriptions of body systems and examples of words and phrases after each heading or subheading that may assist a medical assistant when keying or typing a history and physical examination report. Abbreviations that are commonly used and accepted are given where they are appropriate in the breakdown of systems and observations that follows:

Constitutional Symptoms—Physical makeup of a body, which includes the methods the body uses to function, actions of metabolic processes, manner and degree of reactions to stimuli, and power of resistance to disease organisms. For example, symptoms may consist of appearance, fever, weight loss or weight gain, or hot flashes.

Eyes—Assessment of the patient's perception of his or her vision functions. Symptoms and conditions concerning the eye and ocular adnexa are evaluated. These may include vision difficulties and problems such as lazy or wandering eye; glaucoma; scotoma; conjunctivitis; trachoma; pain; discharge; redness; limitation of visual fields; use of glasses, contact lenses, or intraocular lenses; blurring; double vision; seeing spots or rings around lights; watering; itch-ing; abnormal sensitivity to light; infection, tear duct problems, and so on.

Ears, Nose, Throat (ENT)—Because of intercommunication between the structures of the upper respiratory tract, the ears, nose, mouth, and throat are often reviewed together.

- *Ears*—Includes testing of the hearing and conditions such as hearing loss, discharge, dizziness, syncope, tinnitus (ringing in ears), and pain.

- *Nose*—Includes the sense of smell and conditions such as discharges, colds, allergies, chronic sinus congestion, and epistaxis (nosebleed).

- *Mouth and Throat*—Includes condition of teeth, dental hygiene, dentures, thyroid gland, movement of the neck, position of the trachea, and problems such as tender gums, sensitive tongue, difficulty in swallowing, hoarseness, sore throat, postnasal drip, and choking.

Cardiovascular (CV)—System that includes the heart and blood vessels. Symptoms include chest pain, angina, tachycardia, bradycardia, heart murmurs, palpitations, heart attacks, pitting or pedal edema, cool extremities, varicose veins, high blood pressure, hypotension, and so forth.

Respiratory—Exchange of oxygen is the main function of the lungs and respiratory system. Symptoms may include comments on dyspnea, orthopnea, two-pillow orthopnea, shortness of breath on exertion, wheezing, pneumonia, hemoptysis, and paroxysmal nocturnal dyspnea (PND).

Gastrointestinal (GI)—System that mechanically and chemically breaks food down to molecular size for absorption into the bloodstream to be used by the cells. The liver and gallbladder are also included in this system. Symptoms include comments on appetite, indigestion, melena, icterus, jaundice, anorexia, nausea, vomiting, hematemesis, flatus, borborygmus, flatulence, coffee-ground vomitus, stool color (black tarry or clay-colored), hematochezia, diarrhea, obstipation, dysphagia, change in weight or diet, change of bowel habits, and constipation.

Genitourinary (GU)—Review of the organs with urinary and reproductive functions. Symptoms include comments on urinary flow, incontinence, stress incontinence, burning and frequency during urination, dysuria, pyuria, nocturia, hematuria, oliguria, enuresis, sexually transmitted diseases (such as gonorrhea and syphilis), urgency or hesitancy during urination, dribbling, discharge, lumbar pain, and stones. Female: Notes on menarche (onset of menses), last menstrual period (LMP), menstrual flow, Pap smear, obstetric history (pregnancies, live births, abortions, e.g., gravida 3, para 2, aborto 1), and use of contraceptives. Female symptoms might include irregularity of menses, pain during intercourse, bleeding unrelated to menses, or problems associated with the onset of menopause; dysmenorrhea; menorrhagia; metrorrhagia, dyspareunia; and leucorrhea. Male symptoms might include impotence, white patches on the glans penis, and painful injury to the testes.

Musculoskeletal (MS)—System composed of the muscles, bones, and joints. Symptoms include pain, strains, sprains, stiffness, painful or swollen joints, limitation of movement, dislocations, fractures, and arthritis.

Integumentary (Skin and Breast)—System that pertains to the covering of the body (skin, hair, nails, sebaceous glands). Breasts are listed with this system because mammary glands are part of the integumentary system. Lumps found on self-examination and secretions from the nipples are symptoms of concern. Other symptoms include comments on eruptions, rashes, itches, scaling, dryness, and discolorations.

- *Hair*—Symptoms include notes on changes in the hair texture and distribution, hair loss, and excessive hair.

- *Head*—Symptoms include lumps, bumps, tenderness, swelling, or other abnormalities.

Neurological—Pertains to the central and peripheral nervous system. Symptoms might include loss of sensation (paresthesia) to a particular body part. Central nervous system disorders produce more severe symptoms such as headaches, vertigo, loss of consciousness, seizures, convulsions, paralysis, ataxia, or aphasia.

Psychiatric—System that deals with the interaction between the mind and body. Symptoms include comments on the emotional state of the individual (sadness, anxiety, depression, or thoughts of suicide).

Endocrine—System composed of glands and the interaction of hormones. Symptoms include over or under functioning of a gland and its hormone(s). For example, hypersecretion of thyroid hormone would produce symptoms of weakness, wasting, tremulousness, palpitations (cardiac arrhythmia), or bulging eyes.

Hematologic/lymphatic—Blood, blood-forming structures, and the lymphatics comprise this system. Symptoms include edema, swollen or tender lymph nodes, easy bruising, frequent infections, and fatigue.

Allergic/immunologic—Ability to fight disease is the focus of the immune system. Symptoms include allergic reactions, frequent infections, allergic rhinorrhea (runny nose), seasonal allergies, and allergies to food or medication or drugs.

Physical Examination

The physical examination (PE or PX) is objective (O) in nature; that is, it consists of findings the physician can discover by examination or through tests (Figure 9-6B). The thoroughness of the examination and the determination of what body systems will be covered depend on the patient's illness or injury and on the specialty of the physician. Sometimes a check-off list is used by the physician as each system is reviewed, and notes are made on a printed form as each system is examined, or keyed into a personal digital assistant (PDA). Then the physician dictates the entire physical examination for the patient's medical record. Rubber stamps or stencils showing different parts of the anatomy may be used by the physician to make notes and draw arrows to various organs. These stamps can be purchased from printing firms and can be used at the time of the initial visit as well as when progress notes are made.

If the patient is going to be admitted to the hospital and has had a physical examination one week before admission, the Joint Commission on Accreditation of Healthcare Organizations (JCAHO) permits a copy of the physical examination to become part of the hospital record instead of a new history and physical (H&P) on the date of admission. If the patient has had any new development or changes between the examination date and the admission date, then these are noted in the hospital record when the patient is admitted to the hospital.

During the PE, the physician goes through four basic procedures:

1. *Inspection*, or observation, of the patient's physical characteristics and body parts.

2. *Palpation*, or touching and feeling, various parts and organs of the body.

3. *Percussion*, or striking, parts of the body with short, sharp blows, during which attention is

Larson, Vivian P.   80-02-41
February 12, 20XX

HISTORY

CHIEF COMPLAINT:

Pain and restriction of motion of the right arm and a cut on the head.

PRESENT ILLNESS:

This 65-year-old Caucasian female was walking on the street when she slipped on some loose gravel and fell, landing on her right arm and striking her head against the curb. She sustained a laceration of her scalp and an injury to her right shoulder. She went home to change her clothes and started experiencing dizziness and blurred vision. She then went to the University Hospital Emergency Room by automobile where an x-ray of her right arm revealed a fracture involving the greater tuberosity of the humerus and a-CAT-Scan of her head revealed a subdural hematoma.

PAST HISTORY:

The patient states that her general health has always been good except that in recent years she has suffered from spastic colitis. She had a flare-up of this condition about six months ago. Operations: T & A at age 13. A total abdominal hysterectomy in 1956. Social History: She smokes cigarettes occasionally and drinks alcohol socially only. Allergies: No known allergies.

FAMILY HISTORY:

Her father died at age 72 of a cerebrovascular accident. Her mother died at age 74 of a myocardial infarction. Three brothers, all deceased, two with cancer (age 67 and 71), and one with heart disease (age 60). Two sisters, alive and well, one has heart problems. No family history of tuberculosis or diabetes.

REVIEW OF SYSTEMS:

GENERAL: No fever, no chills, no night sweats, or weight loss.
HEENT: Blurred vision, headache, and head pain. No earaches, deafness, sore throats, hoarseness, or difficulty in swallowing.
CR: No chest pains, tachycardia, or ankle edema. No shortness of breath, chronic cough, or wheezing.
GI: Appetite good, slight nausea, no vomiting, diarrhea, constipation, or melena.
GU: No dysuria, hematuria or pyuria.
CNS: Dizziness reported. No fainting or seizures.
GYN: No spotting since her hysterectomy.

PHYSICAL EXAMINATION

GENERAL

This patient is a well-nourished, well-developed, 65-year-old Caucasian female who is awake, alert, and experiencing head pain, headache, dizziness, blurred vision, and slight nausea. She also is experiencing pain in her right shoulder when she attempts to move her right arm. Height 5'8". Weight: 155 lb. Blood pressure: 170/90. Temperature: 99°. Pulse: 100. Respirations: 20.

HEENT:

The pupils are dilated, equal, and react slowly. Extraocular movements are normal. Nasopharynx is clear. Upper and lower dentures. Ears are clear. There is a laceration measuring 2.3 cm on occipital region of scalp.

Figure 9-6 A. The first page of a medial history and results of a physical examination prepared in full block report style

Larson, Vivian P.   80-02-41
February 12, 20XX
Page 2

NECK:

Supple with a full range of painless motion. Thyroid is not enlarged. No lymphadenopathy and no venous engorgement.

CHEST:

Symmetrical with normal expansion. Breasts: No atrophy and no masses. Lungs: Clear to auscultation. Heart: Normal sinus rhythm, no murmurs, and no enlargement.

ABDOMEN:

Soft and nontender and somewhat obese. Liver, kidneys, and spleen are not palpable.

GENITALIA:

Normal external female.

RECTAL:

Deferred.

NEUROLOGICAL:

No motor deficits. Dizziness experienced without relation to head movement. Patient is oriented to person, place, and time. Slight drowsiness occurring.

MUSCULOSKELETAL:

There is a small bruise over the anterior aspect of the left knee. The hips, knees, and ankle joints are otherwise normal. Good peripheral pulses. The right upper arm is moderately swollen and discolored. There are no other gross deformities. The patient has considerable pain with any attempt at either active or passive movement of the right shoulder.

DIAGNOSIS:

1. Laceration—occipital region of scalp measuring 2.3 cm.
2. Subdural hematoma.
3. Relatively undisplaced fracture proximal right humerus (greater tuberosity).
4. Hypertension.

TREATMENT PLAN:

Suture scalp wound. Fracture treatment (without manipulation) with right arm placed in a long arm fiberglass cast. Admit patient to hospital observation unit directly from Emergency Department. Place patient under head trauma precaution and monitor blood pressure every hour.

Gerald Practon, MD
_____
Gerald Practon, MD
mtf
D: 2-12-XX
T: 2-13-XX

Figure 9-6 B. The second page of a medical history and results of a physical examination prepared in full block report style

Table 9-1. List of Body Areas and Organ Systems for Purposes of Examination

Body Areas	Organ Systems
Head, including the face	Constitutional (vital signs, general appearance)
Neck	Eyes
Chest, including the breasts and axillae	Ears, nose, mouth, and throat
Abdomen	Respiratory
Genitalia, groin, buttocks	Cardiovascular
Back, including the spine	Gastrointestinal
Each extremity	Genitourinary
	Lymphatic
	Musculoskeletal
	Skin
	Neurologic
	Psychiatric

fixed on the resistance of the tissues under the fingers and on the sound elicited to determine tissue size, density, and location.

4. *Auscultation,* or listening, to sounds of the internal parts of the body with the aid of a stethoscope.

Levels of Examination, Body Areas, and Organ Systems

The levels of E/M services are based on four types of examination that are defined as follows:

- *Problem focused (PF):* A limited examination of the affected body area or organ.

- *Expanded problem focused (EPF):* A limited examination of the affected body area or organ system and other symptomatic or related body areas or organ systems.

- *Detailed (D):* An extended detailed examination of the affected body area or organ system and other symptomatic or related body areas or organ systems.

- *Comprehensive (C):* A general multisystem examination or complete examination of a single organ system and other symptomatic or related body areas or organ systems.

The extent of the examination and what is documented depends on clinical judgment and the nature of the presenting problem or problems. They range

from limited examinations of single body areas or complete single organ system examinations to general multisystem examinations.

Table 9-1 lists the body areas and organ systems that are recognized for purposes of examination. See Chapter 16 (Tables 16-4, 5, 6) for more information.

Constitutional (or General)—Includes assessing the patient's vital signs (sitting, standing, or supine blood pressure), pulse rate and regularity, respiration, temperature, age, height, weight, race, and general appearance (development, nutritional state, body habitus, deformities, grooming, and emotional condition of the patient).

EXAMPLE 9-6

Constitutional Examination

In this section of the physical examination, physician comments might include statements such as "appearing younger" or "appearing older than the stated age"; description of whether the patient is a well-developed and well-nourished male or female; body type; alertness; general state of health; whether in acute distress, in no distress, conscious, coherent, euphoric, lethargic, distracted, well oriented, or agitated.

Eyes—Includes inspection of the patient's vision, ocular adnexa (area around the eye), conjunctivae, lids; examination of the pupils and irises (reaction to light and accommodation, size, and symmetry); ophthalmoscope examination of optic disks (size, C/D ratio, appearance, and posterior segments [e.g., vessel changes, exudates, hemorrhages]); extraocular movements (EOMs); and fundi (back portion of the interior of the eyeballs).

EXAMPLE 9-7

Eye Examination

Dictation may include description of the sclerae, cornea, conjunctivae, and lids; whether pupils and irises are equal, round, react to light, and accommodation (PERRLA or PERLA); whether there are silver wire arterioles; presence of Keith-Waggoner I or II (KW I or II) changes; any retinopathy, hemorrhages, exudates, papilledema, or arteriovenous (AV) nicking; disc margins (whether flat or choked); scotoma, diplopia, arcus senilis, and aphakia.

Ears, Nose, Mouth, and Throat—Includes inspection of the external auditory meatus (external ear canals); tympanic membranes (TMs—eardrums); ossicles; airway, nasal septum, lips, gums, oral hygiene; tongue; oral and buccal mucosa, salivary glands; tonsils, palate, uvula, and posterior pharynx.

EXAMPLE 9-8

Examination of Ears, Nose, Mouth, and Throat

Documentation about ears may indicate presence of otitis media, tinnitus, cerumen (earwax); ear discharge; and hearing. Comments on nose, mouth, and throat would include if there is a patent airway, a deviated nasal septum, whether there is rhinorrhea, or allergic rhinitis. Inspection of teeth would mention whether edentulous or presence of dentures (upper and lower plates) or carious; tongue midline and whether uncoated or coated.

Neck—Includes inspection of contour; mobility (whether supple, crepitus) or any limitation of motion of the cervical spine; examination of the thyroid (size, shape, enlargement, tenderness, mass, or nuchal rigidity); position of the trachea (midline, mobile); and carotid pulses (full, equal bilaterally).

EXAMPLE 9-9

Neck Examination

Physician may describe the presence of enlarged lymph nodes (whether shotty), any cervical lymphadenopathy, euthyroidism, thyromegaly, any carotid bruit, venous distention, hepatojugular reflux (jugular vein distention), and venous engorgement.

Respiratory—Includes assessment of respiratory effort (intercostal retractions, use of accessory muscles, diaphragmatic movement), auscultation of lungs (breath sounds, adventitious sounds, rubs, rhonchi, wheeze, stridor), percussion of chest (dullness, flatness, hyperresonant or hyporesonant), palpation of chest (tactile fremitus), lung fields, and bronchovesicular and vesicular function.

EXAMPLE 9-10

Examination of Respiratory System

Physician would mention whether lungs are clear to inspection, palpation, percussion and auscultation (IPPA); whether rales are sibilant, musical, bubbling, or coarse; and whether at base or apex.

Cardiovascular—Includes palpation of the heart (location, size, thrills); auscultation of the heart with notation of abnormal sounds and murmurs; assessment of rhythm, either normal sinus rhythm (NSR) or regular sinus rhythm (RSR), borders, silhouette, heart rate; rubs, gallops, heaves, lifts; examination of carotid arteries (pulse, amplitude, bruits), abdominal aorta (size, bruits), femoral arteries (pulse amplitude, bruits), pedal pulses (pulse amplitude), and extremities for edema or varicosities.

Chest—Inspection of breasts (shape, whether symmetrical, nipple discharge); palpation of breasts and

EXAMPLE 9-11

Cardiovascular Examination

Physician comments may contain words and phrases, such as A2 to P2 point of maximal impulse (PMI) at the fifth intercostal space; midclavicular line (MCL); left border of cardiac dullness; systole, asystole, diastole; arrhythmia; murmurs grades II through VI (ejection, faint diastolic, harsh, soft blowing, and apical low-pitched); any physiological splitting of P2; precordium; any palpitation or opening snap.

axillae (masses or lumps, tenderness), expansion (whether equal), thorax (whether bony).

Gastrointestinal (GI) (Abdomen)—Examination of abdomen; palpation of liver, spleen, and kidneys (LSK); hernia (absence or presence) symmetry, shape, and contours; scaphoid. Examination (when indicated) of anus, perineum, and rectum, including sphincter tone, presence of hemorrhoids, rectal masses. Obtain stool sample for occult blood test when indicated.

EXAMPLE 9-12

Gastrointestinal (Abdomen) Examination

Physician may include statements about presence of masses, rebound tenderness, rigidity, guarding, any ascites; peristalsis; bowel sounds (tinkles, gurgles, rushes, borborygmus); any suprapubic tenderness, costovertebral angle (CVA) tenderness or tenderness at McBurney's point; any visceromegaly, hepatosplenomegaly, or organomegaly; any hernias (whether inguinal, reducible, femoral, ventral, incisional, umbilical); right costal margin; left costal margin; liver (two fingerwidths below the costal margin); quadrants (right upper, left upper, right lower, left lower).

Genitourinary/male—Examination of scrotal contents, penis, digital rectal examination of prostate gland.

EXAMPLE 9-13

Genitourinary Male Examination

Physician may include comments on whether testes is descended, penis is circumcised or uncircumcised, whether prostate is tender, boggy, firm, nodular, enlarged; whether scrotum contents show hydrocele, spermatocele, tenderness of cord, or testicular mass.

Genitourinary/female—Pelvic examination (with or without specimen collection for smears and cultures), examination of external genitalia (general appearance, hair distribution, lesions), vagina (general appearance, estrogen effect, discharge, lesions, pelvic support, cytocele, rectocele), examination of urethra (masses, tenderness, scarring), examination of bladder (fullness, masses, tenderness), cervix (general appearance, lesions, discharge), uterus (size, contour, position, mobility, tenderness, consistency, descent or support), and adnexa/parametria (masses, tenderness, organomegaly, nodularity).

EXAMPLE 9-14

Genitourinary Female Examination

Physician may include comments on external genitalia (vulva, labia, perineum); vaginal discharge; size and motion of cervix (i.e., retroflexion or anteflexion); uterine size; adnexal masses; whether parous, nulliparous, or marital introitus; results of bimanual or speculum examination; adnexal regions; uterine fundus; any cystocele or urethrocele; condition of Bartholin's duct, urethra, and Skene's duct (BUS), whether well epithelialized.

Lymphatic—Examination by palpation of two or more areas (neck, axillae, groin, other).

Musculoskeletal—Examination of gait and station; inspection and palpation of digits and nails; examination of joints, bones, and muscles of one or more of the following six areas: (1) head and neck; (2) spine, ribs,

---

EXAMPLE 9-15

Lymphatic System Examination

Physician may include comments about lymph nodes on palpation in neck (cervical), arm pit (axillary), and groin (inguinal).

---

and pelvis; (3) right upper extremity; (4) left upper extremity; (5) right lower extremity; and (6) left lower extremity. Examination of the spine (cervical, C1 to C7; thoracic, or dorsal, T1 to T12; lumbar, L1 to L5; sacrum, S1 to S2), lumbosacral spine, sacrococcygeal spine, and coccyx.

EXAMPLE 9-16

Musculoskeletal Examination

Physician may include comments about fingers and nails, such as clubbing, cyanosis, inflammation, petechiae, ischemia, infection, and nodes. Examination of these areas includes inspection and palpation, range of motion, dislocation or subluxation or laxity, muscle strength and tone (e.g., flaccid, cog wheel, spastic), atrophy, abnormal movements; color; temperature; any edema (whether pitting, pedal, pretibial); varicosities, clubbing, or cyanosis; pulses (pedal, peripheral, radial, femoral, popliteal, dorsalis pedis); and any intermittent claudication or stasis dermatitis. Examination of the spine would render a description of any scoliosis, lordosis, or kyphosis.

Skin—Inspection and palpation of the skin and subcutaneous tissues.

Neurologic—Test of cranial nerves with notations of any deficits for cerebral and cerebellar function; examination of deep tendon reflexes (DTR) (biceps, triceps, knee jerk, ankle jerk); examination of sensation (touch, pin, vibration, proprioception).

Psychiatric—Description of patient's judgment and insight; assessment of mental status, including orientation in all three spheres to time, place, and person, recent and remote memory, mood, and affect (depression, anxiety, agitation).

EXAMPLE 9-17

Examination of the Skin

Physician may include description of the skin—warm, dry, moist; turgor; pallid, jaundiced, icteric, cyanotic, rashes, lesions, ulcers, induration, subcutaneous nodule, tightening. Description of the head includes shape (whether normocephalic [normal, without lumps] or exostotic [with bumps]); color and texture of the skin and hair (e.g., whether there is alopecia [balding]).

EXAMPLE 9-18

Neurologic Examination

Physician comments may include notation of pathological reflexes (Hoffman, Babinski, Brudzinski, Gonda, Hoffmann, Kernig, Romberg, Homan, Strunsky); ankle clonus; any lingual, facial, or palatal weakness; clear sensorium; station; and gait (e.g., whether broad-based, ataxic gait).

Complexity of Medical Decision Making

Medical decision making is the thought process that the physician goes through. It refers to the complexity of establishing a diagnosis and selecting a management option. The levels of E/M services recognize four types of medical decision making:

- Straightforward (SF)
- Low complexity (LC)
- Moderate complexity (MC)
- High complexity (HC)

The following three elements are considered to qualify for a level of decision making:

Management Options

The number of diagnoses or management options is based on the number and types of problems addressed during the visit, the complexity of establishing a diagnosis, and the management decisions made by the doctor.

Amount and Complexity of Data

The amount and complexity of data to be reviewed is based on the amount and complexity of diagnostic testing ordered or reviewed. A decision to obtain and review old medical records or to obtain history from sources other than the patient increases the amount and complexity of data to be reviewed.

Risk

The risk of significant complications, morbidity, comorbidities, or mortality levels are based on (1) significant complications, (2) other conditions associated with the presenting problem(s) (morbidity), (3) underlying diseases or other conditions present at the time of the visit (comorbidity), (4) the risk of death associated with the problem (mortality), (5) the diagnostic procedure(s), and (6) the possible management options (treatment rendered—surgery, therapy, drug management, procedures, and supplies).

The final section of the history and physical examination report consists of stating the diagnosis, the recommended treatment, and the prospect of recovery.

Diagnosis

The **diagnosis** is an impression, assessment, or final conclusion of the nature of the disease or illness based on history, physical examination findings, and, sometimes, diagnostic tests such as x-rays, laboratory tests, or electrocardiogram (ECG).

Treatment

This is a recommended plan or treatment for the diagnosis. It might include admission to the hospital, physical therapy, additional tests, medication to be given with dosage, and scheduling a future appointment.

Prognosis

Prognosis is a probable outcome of the disease or injury and the prospect of recovery. It includes an estimate of partial or total disability in an accident or industrial case.

Progress or Chart Notes

After the initial visit, the history and physical examination are recorded on the chart, and each subsequent patient visit is documented with progress notes chronologically entered in the medical record during the visit or as soon as possible after the patient leaves the office (see Figures 9-4, 9-5, and 9-7). For clarity and readability, it is preferred that progress notes be typed and not be handwritten. Chart notes contain information documenting each patient encounter, whether in the office, at home, in a skilled nursing facility, in the emergency room, or at the hospital. The medical assistant must check with the physician daily to find out if patients have been seen at other sites, so patient records can be pulled, entries can be made, and charges can be posted. Prescription refills need to be noted in the record, specifying frequency and dosage. If a patient is referred for a consultation, this must be stated. Telephone conversations are noted if medical advice is requested or given. Appointment

---

Goldberg, Arlene   No. 0697

1-7-XX   Wt: 169 lbs   BP: 136/72
1-7-XX   CC: Malaise, anorexia, epigastric pressure with sensation of fullness, nausea, headache, vertigo, and vomiting.
              PE: Abdomen tender and rigid; esophagitis with pain and dysphagia; and severe epigastric pain.
              Dx: Acute gastritis.
              Plan: Discontinue alcohol, IM inj Prochlorperazine, 10 mg.
              Gave Rx for 20 Meperidine, 50 mg, q4h, orally. Retn 4 days.

                                          Gerald Practon, MD
                                          _____
                                          Gerald Practon, MD
mtf

Figure 9-7. Typed chart note signed by the physician

cancellations that are not rescheduled, no-shows, and the refusal of a patient to cooperate with instructions should also be documented on the patient's chart.

Chart notes, as part of the record, may be requested to be seen by attorneys, other physicians, and insurance companies, and may be used as evidence during litigation; therefore, they must be neat, accurate, and complete. Notes must be current, with no omissions, dated, and signed or initialed by the physician. They should be typed single-spaced or handwritten, with a line at the end of the note for the physician's signature or initials.

Self-Adhesive Chart Notes

Some companies manufacture pressure-sensitive paper in single sheets or as continuous sheets that are perforated at various intervals. A series of chart notes for different patients can be typed on the paper and the notes are placed on the physician's desk for initialing. Finally, each note can be carefully separated at perforations or cut apart. Take care when dividing the notes for placement because brief notes can easily be placed on the wrong patient's chart. The backing is peeled off and each note is secured in the next available blank space of the patient's progress sheet so information previously entered is not obliterated. This eliminates the time-consuming work of obtaining each medical record and locating the proper page to type in the information.

Electronic Progress or Chart Notes

In electronic record management, chart notes may be dictated or transcribed directly into the computer system. New chart notes are printed, signed, and added to the previous notes in the hard copy record. If passwords are used for restricted access, electronic or digital signatures may be acceptable.

Medical Reports

A **medical report** is a permanent, legal document in either letter or report format that formally states the elements performed and the results of an examination and recommended treatment. Consultations are a type of medical report.

Laboratory Reports

Laboratory tests may be performed in the physician's office laboratory (POL), by an outside freestanding lab, or by a hospital laboratory, which sends test results to the physician's office. In the report, when normal value ranges are indicated, the medical assistant can circle, underline in red, or highlight those of the patient's values that appear higher or lower than the norms, thus calling them to the physician's immediate attention. Other laboratory reports may present abnormal values that can be easily identified (Figure 9-8). Then the **laboratory report**, along with the patient's chart, may be placed on the physician's desk. The medical assistant should never *interpret* a laboratory report to the patient in person or over the telephone. The physician must initial all laboratory reports before they are filed in patients' medical records.

Laboratory Log

When patients or their specimens are sent to an outside laboratory, it is important to be sure that the test has been done, the report has been received, the physician has read it, and the proper response has been made (i.e., file it or have the physician telephone the patient if there are abnormal results). Maintaining a log in a notebook, calendar book, or using a preprinted form with columns is quick and easy—more important, it is imperative if trying to identify which patient's laboratory results are pending (see Figures 9-9 and 9-10). Enter each report that is received and identify if a report is missing.

Radiographs (X-Ray Films)

Some physicians take x-rays in their offices and store the x-ray films in a separate file using a numeric system because of their size. Other physicians send their patients to a radiology group or hospital radiology department to have films taken, and these films are kept by the facility. The findings are sent to the physician in the form of an **x-ray report** to be included in the patient's medical record. If the physician takes the films and dictates the findings, the results may be included in the patient's initial history and physical examination report, progress note, or dictated in letter form.

Electrocardiograms

Some offices perform electrocardiograms (ECGs or EKGs) on patients. Special cards are available to mount the strips of paper on which ECGs are recorded. The original ECG record, if mounted on a card, is stored separately. A copy of the ECG and written interpretation is placed in the patient's record.

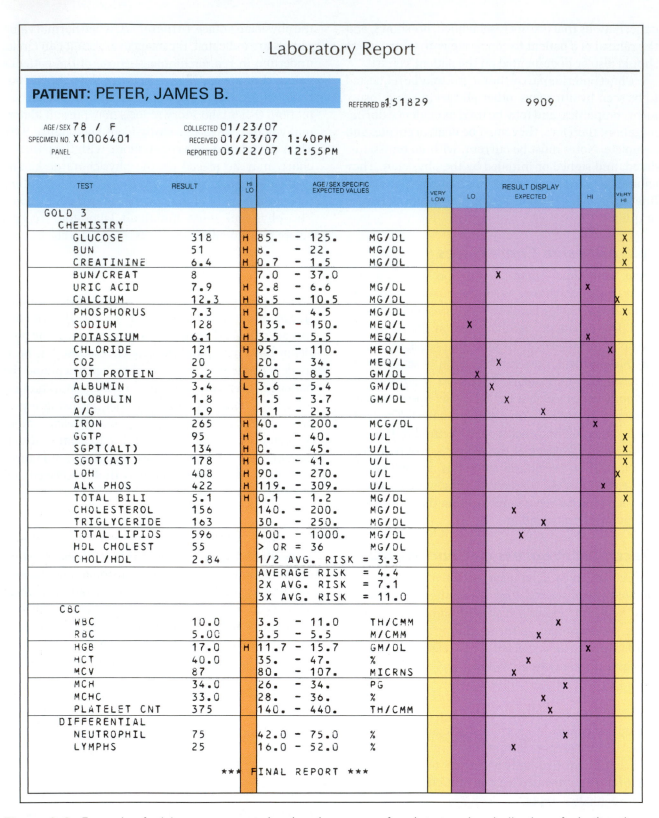

Laboratory Report

PATIENT: PETER, JAMES B.

REFERRED BY 151829   9909

AGE/SEX 78 / F   COLLECTED 01/23/07
SPECIMEN NO. X1006401   RECEIVED 01/23/07 1:40PM
PANEL   REPORTED 05/22/07 12:55PM

TEST	RESULT	HI/LO	AGE/SEX SPECIFIC EXPECTED VALUES			VERY LOW	LO	RESULT DISPLAY EXPECTED		HI	VERY HI
GOLD 3											
CHEMISTRY											
GLUCOSE	318	H	85.	- 125.	MG/DL						X
BUN	51	H	8.	- 22.	MG/DL						X
CREATININE	6.4	H	0.7	- 1.5	MG/DL						X
BUN/CREAT	8		7.0	- 37.0				X			
URIC ACID	7.9	H	2.8	- 6.6	MG/DL					X	
CALCIUM	12.3	H	8.5	- 10.5	MG/DL						X
PHOSPHORUS	7.3	H	2.0	- 4.5	MG/DL						X
SODIUM	128	L	135.	- 150.	MEQ/L		X				
POTASSIUM	6.1	H	3.5	- 5.5	MEQ/L					X	
CHLORIDE	121	H	95.	- 110.	MEQ/L					X	
CO2	20		20.	- 34.	MEQ/L			X			
TOT PROTEIN	5.2	L	6.0	- 8.5	GM/DL		X				
ALBUMIN	3.4	L	3.6	- 5.4	GM/DL			X			
GLOBULIN	1.8		1.5	- 3.7	GM/DL			X			
A/G	1.9		1.1	- 2.3					X		
IRON	265	H	40.	- 200.	MCG/DL					X	
GGTP	95	H	5.	- 40.	U/L						X
SGPT(ALT)	134	H	0.	- 45.	U/L						X
SGOT(AST)	178	H	0.	- 41.	U/L						X
LDH	408	H	90.	- 270.	U/L						X
ALK PHOS	422	H	119.	- 309.	U/L					X	
TOTAL BILI	5.1	H	0.1	- 1.2	MG/DL						X
CHOLESTEROL	156		140.	- 200.	MG/DL			X			
TRIGLYCERIDE	163		30.	- 250.	MG/DL				X		
TOTAL LIPIDS	596		400.	- 1000.	MG/DL			X			
HDL CHOLEST	55		> OR = 36		MG/DL						
CHOL/HDL	2.84		1/2 AVG. RISK = 3.3								
			AVERAGE RISK = 4.4								
			2X AVG. RISK = 7.1								
			3X AVG. RISK = 11.0								
CBC											
WBC	10.0		3.5	- 11.0	TH/CMM				X		
RBC	5.00		3.5	- 5.5	M/CMM				X		
HGB	17.0	H	11.7	- 15.7	GM/DL					X	
HCT	40.0		35.	- 47.	%				X		
MCV	87		80.	- 107.	MICRNS			X			
MCH	34.0		26.	- 34.	PG				X		
MCHC	33.0		28.	- 36.	%				X		
PLATELET CNT	375		140.	- 440.	TH/CMM				X		
DIFFERENTIAL											
NEUTROPHIL	75		42.0	- 75.0	%				X		
LYMPHS	25		16.0	- 52.0	%			X			
			*** FINAL REPORT ***								

Figure 9-8. Example of a laboratory report showing the names of each test and an indication of whether the results are low, in the expected normal range, or high

Outside Test Log

Date Ordered	Patient Name	Test Ordered	Facility Name	Date of Test	Date Report Rec'd	Test Results to Patient (Date & Initial)
1/6/XX	Kim Chang	CBC c̄ Sed Rate	ABC Lab	1/7/XX	1/9/XX	✓
1/6/XX	Bruce Johnson	UGI	College Hosp.	1/4/XX	1/17/XX	
1/7/XX	Joe Felipe	3 hr GTT	College Hosp.	1/8/XX	1/11/XX	✓
1/8/XX	Lori Carr	Serum Beta HCG Quan	ABC Lab	1/10/XX		

Figure 9-9. Example of entries made in a test log showing when tests have been ordered and reports received

June	22
Maria DiPetro	treadmill—College Hosp
Cecilia Chung	protime—ABC Lab

Figure 9-10. Example of entries made on the page of a flip calendar used as a tickler file to track tests

ABSTRACTING FROM MEDICAL RECORDS

An **abstract** of data is required to complete reports, forms, and insurance claims. During this process, information is extracted from various places in the medical record and used to answer questions, fill in blanks on forms, or compose a summary. The summary should include such information as the patient's name, address, birth date, height, weight, marital history, social history, objective findings on physical examination, laboratory results, x-ray findings, diagnosis, anticipated further treatment, and prognosis.

For industrial or work-related injuries or illnesses, initial medical reports and subsequent **progress reports** are submitted until the patient has fully recovered, or until the condition is declared permanent and stationary.

AUDIT OF MEDICAL RECORDS

To perform an **audit** of medical records is to periodically examine or review a group of patient records. The purpose of an audit is to verify that good record-keeping is in place, that documentation is valid for the level of service provided and billed, and that proper medical care is being provided.

Internal Review

When an audit is done by the medical office staff, this process is called an *internal review,* and records may be picked at random. There are two types of internal reviews: the *prospective review,* which is done before billing is submitted, and the *retrospective review,* which is done after billing insurance carriers. Worksheets may be used, which separate the components of the medical record to check off various items and to simplify and expedite the process.

Table 9-2 presents some of the important and most error-prone areas when reviewing documents during the process of performing an internal review.

PROCEDURE 9-3

Abstract Data from a Medical Record

Objective: To abstract data from a medical record.

Equipment/Supplies: Patient's medical record, form to insert abstracted data, and pen or pencil.

Directions: Follow these step-by-step procedures, which include rationales, to learn this skill, which is presented in the *Workbook* (Job Skill 9-4) for practice.

1. Read and review the patient's entire medical record thoroughly to become familiar with all aspects of the case.

2. Answer the following questions to see if you understand all aspects of this patient's medical record.

   a. Did this patient have surgery, and, if so, what was performed?

   b. What is the patient's diagnosis?

   c. Was any medication prescribed?

   d. Does the patient's past history show anything of consequence?

   e. Does this patient have any drug or food allergies?

   f. What is the etiology (cause) of this disease, injury, or illness?

   g. What is the prognosis for this patient's case?

   h. Was any laboratory work performed or ordered?

   i. Were any x-rays performed or ordered?

3. Define all abbreviations listed in the patient's progress notes or history and physical examination.

4. What documents helped you find the answers to these questions?

Table 9-2. Internal Medical Record Review

1. Confirm that the patient's name or identification number is listed on each page of documentation for the date of service reviewed.

2. Make sure dates are recorded for all entries and that the date of service matches the date on the insurance claim form.

3. Look to see if all chart entries are signed or initialed by the attending physician.

4. Check to see if allergies and adverse reactions are noted prominently so patients are not prescribed medications they will have allergic reactions to.

5. Be sure evaluation and management procedures codes conform correctly to either 1995 or 1997 documentation guidelines.

6. Check for documentation of a request from a third party when a consultation is billed.

7. Determine if handwritten progress notes or other hand entries are legible to an outside reviewer.

8. Check to see if proper consent forms and authorization forms for release of records are in place and signed by the patient within the past year.

9. Verify that selected *CPT* codes representing procedures and services are correct, and make sure medical necessity is documented.

10. Verify that the documented diagnosis is consistent with the current *ICD-9-CM* diagnostic codes on the insurance claim form and that they match the treatment plan, and are documented for the correct date of service.

External Audit

Government programs, managed care organizations, and private insurance carriers that have a contract with a physician have the right to do an *external audit* of medical records. This usually occurs as the result of unusual billing patterns by a medical practice and after insurance claims have been submitted and paid. During the external audit, charts may be selected by the insurance carrier. Elements in the medical record are categorized and awarded points according to the extent of the documentation. For example, the history would be one category. Other categories might include the extent of the physical examination, com-

plexity of medical decision making, time, and so forth. No points are given when elements are missing. This system shows where deficiencies occur in documentation and whether billed diagnostic and procedures codes are substantiated. Investigators may question the patient, review the medical documentation and financial records, and interview the staff and all physicians who participated in the care of the patients' cases being audited. If improper coding patterns are discovered, the physician may have to refund monies or may be penalized.

Table 9-3 lists where you can find documents in a medical record.

Table 9-3. Examples of Documents Found in a Medical Record

Title	Chapter	Figure/Example Number	Page Number
Patient Information/Registration Form	5	Fig. 5-5	138
Telephone Message Slips	6	Fig. 6-4 & 6-5	181
SOAP Chart Note	9	Fig. 9-4	273
Correction to Chart Note	9	Fig. 9-5	277
Medical History	9	Fig. 9-6A	282
Physical Examination	9	Fig. 9-6A/B	282–283
Chart Note Example	9	Fig. 9-7	288
Laboratory Report	9	Fig. 9-8	290
Flow Sheets	9	Fig. 9-1, 9-2 and Example 9-2	268–270
Prescriptions	10	Fig. 10-6	313
Drug Flow Sheet	10	Fig. 10-8	322
Insurance Card	16	Fig. 16-11	533

STOP AND THINK CASE SCENARIO

Physician Roles and Titles

Scenario: Kay Lenzer has been under the care of Dr. Practon for her annual physical examinations. She falls at home, suffering a compound fracture of her left tibia. Dr. Practon determines that the fracture requires treatment by a specialist and sends her to Dr. Skeleton, an orthopedic surgeon, who orders x-rays and performs surgery to stabilize the fracture. During the recovery phase, Ms. Lenzer develops a peculiar skin rash and Dr. Skeleton sends her to a dermatologist, Dr. Cutis, for an opinion about the skin ailment.

Critical Thinking: What roles do the following physicians play and what are their correct titles? Remember, a physician can wear more than one hat and take on more than one role.

Dr. Practon: _____

Dr. Skeleton: _____

Dr. Cutis: _____

STOP AND THINK CASE SCENARIO

Chart Documentation

Scenario: You are the administrative medical assistant and have the certification of "CMA." It is Friday, October 16, 20XX at 2:00 p.m. and an established patient, Mrs. Beverly Brooks stops by the office and wants to see Dr. Fran Practon. Neither doctor is in the office this afternoon and the patient complains that they are never there when she needs them. She refuses to tell you what is wrong or to see the doctor on call, go to an urgent care center, or go to the hospital emergency room; she just says she is not feeling well. She left upset and would not schedule an appointment or answer questions as to when she would be home to receive a telephone call.

Critical Thinking: Write a narrative chart note describing the interaction that will serve both as a message and as documentation for the medical record. _____

_____

_____

_____

_____

_____

_____

_____

_____

_____

FOCUS ON CERTIFICATION*

CMA Content Summary

- Medical terminology
- Body systems
- Releasing patient information
- Living wills
- Medical records (types)
- Scanners
- Making corrections in records

RMA Content Summary

- A/P body systems
- Medical terminology
- Abbreviations
- Documentation of patient encounters
- Confidentiality
- Chart and records management
- Chart systems

- Transcription format
- Encryption and passwords

CMAS Content Summary

- Medical terminology
- Structure and function of body systems
- Diseases of body systems
- Chart patient information
- Patient record systems
- Documents and charts (paper and computerized)
- Chart contents
- Correct medical records
- Audits
- Confidentiality
- Confidentiality of computer-stored information

REVIEW EXAM-STYLE QUESTIONS

1. One advantage of a paper-based medical record system is:

   a. management costs are reasonable

   b. they are easy to move

   c. they are easy to store

   d. people feel secure with a piece of hard copy information in hand

   e. they are less vulnerable to security threats

2. A flow sheet:

   a. takes the place of listing data in the medical record

   b. can be used instead of dictating such things as lab results, blood pressure, and immunizations

   c. can be used to help view continuous problems and comparative values

   d. is one of the three basic medical record organizational systems

   e. is no longer allowed according to HIPAA

3. Documents are arranged according to sections in the:

   a. flow sheet

   b. POMR system

   c. SOR system

   d. Integrated Record system

   e. SOAP format

---

* This textbook and accompanying Workbook *meet the entry-level administrative and general competencies for the CMA outlined by the* AAMA Examination Content Outline and Role Delineation Study *and for the RMA and CMAS outlined by the AMT Competencies and Examination Specifications (see Competency Grid in Appendix B).*

4. In a patient medical record, data can be:

   a. hand entered by the physician

   b. dictated by the physician

   c. keyed into the system by the physician

   d. entered by the medical assistant

   e. all the above

5. Documenters of the medical record:

   a. should be only physicians in the medical practice

   b. are all individuals who provide health care services

   c. need to be licensed health care providers

   d. have to be the attending or ordering physician

   e. all of the above

6. The provider who renders service to the patient in an office setting is referred to as the:

   a. attending physician

   b. consulting physician

   c. ordering physician

   d. referring physician

   e. treating physician

7. The difference between an electronic signature and a digital signature is:

   a. the digital signature is a facsimile of a person's actual handwriting and an electronic signature is a series of letters or numbers that cannot be altered

   b. the digital signature is a series of letters or numbers that cannot be altered and an electronic signature is a facsimile of a person's actual handwriting

   c. the electronic signature is affixed electronically to the end of the document and the digital signature is a facsimile of a person's actual handwriting

   d. the digital signature is secure and cannot be forged and the electronic signature uses an encryption system to make it secure

   e. the electronic system uses such things as a voice print, hand print, or fingerprint and the digital system uses a biometric system

8. The acronym SOAP stands for:

   a. Subjective, Operative, Action, Plan

   b. Sensible, Operational, Analogy, Plan

   c. Subjective, Objective, Assessment, Plan

   d. Subjective, Objective, Appraisal, Program

   e. Secure, Object, Aim, Purpose

9. An example of subjective information would be:

   a. laboratory test

   b. EKG

   c. blood pressure

   d. temperature

   e. pain

10. When an error in a medical record is discovered, the first step is to:

    a. draw a single line through the incorrect entry

    b. use white out to obscure the incorrect entry

    c. use correction tape to obliterate the incorrect entry

    d. draw a heavy line through the incorrect entry

    e. erase the incorrect entry

11. The HPI is:

    a. the patient's family history: all illnesses, diseases, and a list of deceased relatives

    b. the chief complaint; reason for the visit

    c. a chronological description of the development of the patient's present illness

    d. a review of all body systems from top to bottom

    e. the patient's social history including smoking, alcohol consumption, and sexual practices

12. During a comprehensive physical examination, in what order does the physician examine the body?

    a. Examines the body area mentioned in the chief complaint first

    b. Examines the body starting at the feet and working toward the head

c. Examines all areas that do not look normal first

d. Examines the body starting at the head and working toward the feet

e. Examines the body starting in the core (chest and stomach) first and works toward the extremities and head

13. The complexity of medical decision making is dependent on which three items?

a. The level of (1) personal, (2) family, and (3) social history.

b. The (1) number of diagnoses and management options, (2) amount and complexity of data to be reviewed, and (3) the risk of complications, morbidity and comorbidities or mortality.

c. The (1) diagnoses, (2) treatment, and (3) prognosis.

d. The (1) review of systems, (2) body areas examined, and (3) organ systems examined.

e. The level of (1) history, (2) physical examination, and (3) number of diagnoses.

14. A type of internal review, where medical staff look at medical records to verify that good recordkeeping is in place and that documentation is valid before billing is submitted is called a/an:

a. self-audit

b. retrospective review

c. external review

d. external audit

e. prospective review

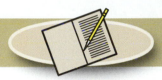

WORKBOOK ASSIGNMENT

To develop competency-based job skills, refer to the *Workbook* and complete the:

- Abbreviations and Spelling Review
- Review Questions
- Critical Thinking Exercises
- Job Skill activities, which are outlined at the beginning of this chapter under "Performance Objectives in the *Workbook*."

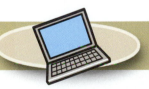

COMPUTER ASSIGNMENT

To review the concepts you have learned in this chapter, insert the *Student Practice* CD-ROM into a computer and work through the *StudyWARE* activities and games. Answer the review questions in the practice mode and read the feedback, studying the questions you have missed. Take the chapter quiz until you achieve a minimum score of 90 percent. Successfully completing the *Critical Thinking Challenge* at the end of this course will help you think through scenarios and develop problem solving skills.

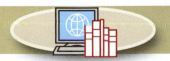

RESOURCES

Books

Dorland's Illustrated Medical Dictionary
Updated periodically—available on CD-ROM
W. B. Saunders/Elsevier Science
Philadelphia, PA
(800) 545-2522

Medical Abbreviations and Eponyms, 2 ed.
Sheila B. Sloane
W. B. Saunders/Elsevier Science
Philadelphia, PA
(800) 545-2522

Internet

American Health Information Management
Association (AHIMA)
Web Site: http://www.ahima.org
SEARCH: electronic medical records
health records
Medem—Offering online consultations for
physicians and patients
Web site: http://www.medem.com
SEARCH: For physicians—iHealthRecords for
Your Patients
Office of the Inspector General (OIG) and Federal
Bureau of Investigation
OIG national hotline: (800) HHS-TIPS
Web Site: http://www.cms.gov

Remote Digital Devices
SEARCH: PDA Resources for Health
Professionals

Magazine

ADVANCE for Health Information Professionals
Information on medical records, medical recordkeeping, medical transcription, diagnostic, and
procedure coding (published biweekly—free
subscription).
(800) 355-1088

CHAPTER 10

Drug and
Prescription Records

OBJECTIVES

After reading this chapter and learning step-by-step procedures to gain job skills,* you should be able to:

Learning Objectives

▌ Define the five schedules of controlled substances.

▌ Understand when and how to renew a physician's narcotic license.

▌ Explain the three types of drug names.

▌ Name the components of a prescription.

▌ Define terms and abbreviations pertaining to drugs.

▌ Determine classifications of drugs based on their function.

▌ Document telephone calls regarding prescriptions in the medical record.

▌ State the prevention measures used to track prescription refills and avoid prescription errors.

▌ Describe the methods used to store, control, and dispose of drugs.

Performance Objectives (Procedures) in This Textbook

▌ Use a *Physicians' Desk Reference* to spell and locate drug information (Procedure 10-1).

▌ Read and interpret a written prescription (Procedure 10-2).

▌ Record medication in a patient's chart and on a medication log (Procedure 10-3).

Performance Objectives (Job Skills) in the Workbook

▌ Spell drug names (Job Skill 10-1).

▌ Determine the correct spelling of drug names (Job Skill 10-2).

▌ Use a *Physicians' Desk Reference (PDR)* (Job Skill 10-3).

This textbook and the accompanying Workbook meet the educational components for entry-level administrative and general competencies outlined by CAAHEP and ABHES.

■ Translate prescriptions (Job Skill 10-4).

■ Record prescription refills in medical records (Job Skill 10-5).

■ Write a prescription (Job Skill 10-6).

■ Interpret a medication log (Job Skill 10-7).

■ Record on a medication schedule (Job Skill 10-8).

OUTLINE WITH LECTURE NOTES

History of Drug Laws

The Harrison Narcotic Act

_____

_____

_____

_____

The Volstead Act

_____

_____

_____

_____

The Marijuana Tax Act

_____

_____

_____

The Food, Drug, and Cosmetic Act

_____

_____

_____

_____

The Drug Enforcement Administration

_____

_____

_____

_____

Controlled Substance Act

_____

_____

_____

_____

The Omnibus Budget Reconciliation Act (OBRA)

_____

_____

_____

_____

The Compassionate Use Act

_____

_____

_____

_____

_____

Drug Names

Chemical Name

_____

_____

_____

_____

Brand Name

_____

_____

_____

_____

Generic Name

_____

_____

_____

_____

Drug References

Physicians' Desk Reference

_____

_____

_____

_____

Other Drug Reference Books

_____
_____
_____
_____

Understanding Prescriptions
Routes of Administration

_____
_____
_____
_____

Components of a Prescription

_____
_____
_____
_____

Authorizing Prescriptions

_____
_____
_____
_____

Prescription Abbreviations

_____
_____
_____
_____

Prescription Drugs and the Role of the Medical Assistant
Pharmaceutical Representative

_____
_____
_____
_____

Drug Classifications

_____
_____
_____

Medication Instructions

_____
_____
_____

Medication Refills

_____
_____
_____

Charting Prescriptions

_____
_____
_____

Drug Abuse Prevention Measures

_____
_____
_____

Drug Side Effects and Adverse Reactions

_____
_____
_____
_____

Control and Storage of Drugs
Disposal of Drugs

_____
_____
_____
_____

KEY TERMS

brand name
chemical name
Drug Enforcement Administration (DEA)
generic name

inscription
official name
pharmaceutical
pharmaceutical representative

(continues)

pharmacist
Physicians' Desk Reference (PDR)
prescriptions
shelf life

signature
subscription
superscription
transcription

HEART OF THE HEALTH CARE PROFESSIONAL

Service

When patients are prescribed medications, they need to take them regularly. As medications run out, patients rely on the medical assistant to handle the prescription renewal in an expedient manner. Efficiently completing this important responsibility will serve the patient in ways you may never fully realize.

HISTORY OF DRUG LAWS

Federal drug laws are designed to minimize the availability and diminish the opportunity for abuse of controlled substances; a prescription drug may or may not be considered a "controlled substance." State laws vary from state to state; as a rule, a state can add restrictions to the federal laws, but almost never reverse or reduce them. Pharmacies and doctors must conform to all applicable laws within their jurisdiction.

The Harrison Narcotic Act

The United States became increasingly involved in world affairs after the Spanish-American War. During the Roosevelt and Taft administrations an Episcopalian Bishop, the Reverend Charles Brent, who had been assigned to the Philippines after they were colonized, began to address the opium problem among that population and convinced the State Department to call for an international conference dedicated to the eradication of worldwide drug traffic.

The State Department's efforts were headed by Dr. Hamilton Wright who enlisted the help of Representative Francis Burton Harrison to introduce legislation to control the prescription, sale, and possession of drugs such as cocaine, heroin, morphine, and opium within the United States. In June 1914, the Harrison Narcotic Act was passed as the beginning of a long history of narcotic control legislation. The act called for all doctors, pharmacists, and vendors to register and submit paperwork for all drug transactions, but it was also used to shut down legitimate medical practices as well as dope clinics that were in violation.

The Volstead Act

In 1919 Congress passed the National Prohibition Act. Authored by Andrew Volstead, it was also known as the Volstead Act. The law prohibited the manufacture, transportation, and sale of beverages containing more than 0.5 % alcohol. This Act did not address pharmaceutical substances, but it was a precursor of regulations that were to come.

The Marijuana Tax Act

During the 1930s there was disagreement among the medical profession as to the dangers of marijuana. The pharmaceutical manufacturers managed to keep cannabis out of the Harrison Act; alcohol was illegal, but marijuana was legal. The Treasury Department's Prohibition Unit hired Harry J. Anslinger, the first federal commissioner of narcotics to be in charge of improving the effectiveness and enforcement of the Volstead Act. At this time many civil organizations and local law enforcement officials began to pressure the federal government to outlaw marijuana. Hearings were held by Congress to consider the evidence for federal-level prohibition and the Marijuana Tax Act was passed in 1937, which required a transfer tax for all who sold marijuana.

The Food, Drug, and Cosmetic Act

The Food, Drug, and Cosmetic Act of 1938 was aimed at controlling cosmetics and medical devices and required the first labeling of drugs with adequate directions for safe use. It also mandated pre-market approval from the Food and Drug Administration (FDA) for all new drugs.

In 1951 the Durham-Humphrey amendment to the Food, Drug, and Cosmetic Act changed over-the-counter availability for the most effective therapeutic agents and mandated prescription status.

Today, the FDA is under the jurisdiction of the U.S. Department of Health and Human Services (HHS [formerly the Department of Health, Education, and Welfare]) and has the responsibility to patients as consumers to enforce all drug legislation, thereby protecting the public and keeping them informed of the potential dangers of drugs. It also determines which drugs are prescription and which can be distributed over the counter. It ensures that drugs are safe before it permits them to be marketed and guarantees the identity, strength, and quality of drugs shipped in interstate commerce. As a result, the drugs used in the United States are standardized. Information on new drugs is gathered and published periodically by the FDA.

The Drug Enforcement Administration

With the social changes and political upheavals of the 1960s, intolerance of drug use changed. Debates increased about the decriminalization and legalization of drug use, and President Nixon launched a vigorous campaign to sway the public against these forces, calling for a "War on Drugs." The **Drug Enforcement Administration (DEA)** was established as well as the National Institute for Drug Abuse.

The DEA, which is part of the U.S. Department of Justice, regulates the manufacturing and dispensing of dangerous and potentially abused drugs.

The Controlled Substance Act

The Comprehensive Drug Abuse and Control Act, which replaced the Harrison Narcotic Act, Food, Drug, and Cosmetic Act, and the Durham-Humphrey laws, is commonly referred to as the Controlled Substances Act (CSA) of 1970 (Title II). It is a federal law that requires the pharmaceutical industry to maintain physical security and strict recordkeeping for certain types of drugs in order to limit and control access to drugs that intoxicate or can make a person "high," such as depressants, hallucinogens, narcotics, and stimulants. Other drugs of abuse such as anabolic steroids used by athletes to increase muscle mass are also controlled through this Act. This Act allows for finer control of drugs by using five categories to classify drugs according to their dangerousness and apply restrictions to the highest categories. Most states have passed laws that mirror the Controlled Substances Act; however, state schedules may vary from federal schedules.

Schedule of Controlled Substances

A note on a June calendar will signal the assistant to remind the physician to renew the narcotic license. If the physician is late in renewing, there is a three-month grace period after a registration expires during which controlled substances can be prescribed. The physician must keep a record of all drugs dispensed under the act for two years.

Controlled drugs, which include both narcotics and certain nonnarcotics are divided into five schedules on the basis of their potential for abuse, accepted medical use, and safety. Substances found in Schedule I have a high potential for abuse, no accredited medical use, and a lack of accepted safety. The potential for abuse decreases for drugs found in Schedules II to V, therefore, control varies depending on which schedule the drug is placed.

All scheduled drugs must have the physician's federal DEA license number; however, some drugs in Schedule V do not require a prescription.

A controlled substance label and packaging must clearly show the drug's assigned schedule. This is written to the right of the drug name as shown in Figure 10-1.

To prevent unauthorized use of controlled substances, the nine-digit (alphanumeric) DEA number issued must appear on all the physician's narcotics prescription blanks, purchase orders, and any other documents of transfer for Schedules III, IV, and V substances. Schedule II substances must be ordered with a federal triplicate order form (DEA-222). In some states, when ordering Schedule II substances from out-of-state companies, a copy of the purchase agreement (not the federal triplicate order form) must be sent within 24 hours of placing the order to the office of the state attorney general.

Physician Narcotic License

If a physician administers, prescribes, or dispenses drugs listed in the Controlled Substances Act, he or she must be registered with the DEA. Physicians are

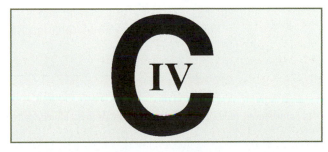

Figure 10-1. Large "C" stands for "controlled substance." The Roman numeral written inside indicates the assigned schedule number, IV. It is important to note that a "C" with the Roman numeral IV inside does not mean that the drug is to be given intravenously.

Table 10-1. Five Schedules of Controlled Substances

Schedule	Use and Abuse	Examples of Substances
I	High abuse potential Limited medical use; with special permission these drugs can be used for research Use leads to severe dependence Must be ordered on a DEA form only by certain qualified medical researchers	Heroin LSD Marijuana Mescaline Peyote
II	High abuse potential Limited medical use in the United States Severe psychic and/or physical dependence DEA order form for Rx (triplicate) handwritten by physician, no refills No refills by telephone Rx must be filled within 7 days In emergency, physician may telephone or fax Rx but written Rx must go to pharmacy prior to distribution Records retained in separate file	Cocaine Fentanyl Methadone Methamphetamine (injectable liquid) Opium
III	Lower abuse potential than in Schedules I and II Moderate to low physical dependence May contain limited quantities of substances from Schedules I and II Written or verbal (phoned in) Rx by physician only Refillable up to five times in 6 months	Amphetamine Anabolic steroids Barbiturates (short acting) Codeine combinations (e.g., Tylenol w/codeine, Fiorinal w/codeine) Methamphetamine (non-liquid)
IV	Lower abuse potential than in Schedule III Limited physical or psychological dependence **Rx may be written by health care worker but signed by physician*** **Rx may be phoned in by health care worker under order of the physician*** Refillable up to five times in 6 months	Darvon Librium Meprobamate Phenobarbital Serax Valium Xanax
V	Lower abuse potential than in Schedule IV Limited physical or psychological dependence State laws vary—may require Rx or may be sold over the counter Purchaser must be 18 years old and sign Exempt Narcotic Registration Form with the pharmacist	Antibiotics Cardiac preparations Cough syrups containing codeine and similar narcotics Donnagel Hormones Lomotil Preparations for diarrhea (e.g., paregoric mixture)

*In some states, medical assistants are allowed to handwrite prescriptions under the direction of the physician.

required to register on June 30 of each year with the DEA Registration Branch, PO Box 28083, Central Station, Washington, DC 20005. In some states, a physician with offices in more than one DEA region must also contact the district or regional branches and register at each. If drugs are administered and dispensed only at a main office, then registration at the DEA regional branch near the principal office is sufficient.

The Omnibus Budget Reconciliation Act (OBRA)

In 1990 Congress enacted the Omnibus Budget Reconciliation Act (OBRA), which included provisions that directly affect Medicaid pharmacy programs and providers. Effective since 1993, pharmacies have been responsible for the following:

- *Prospective Drug Utilization Review (ProDUR)*—Requires evaluation of drug therapy problems, therapeutic duplication, drug-disease contraindications, multiple drug interactions (including over the counter drugs), incorrect drug dosage, duration of drug treatment, drug-allergy interactions, and evidence of clinical misuse and abuse.

- *Patient Counseling Standards*—Governs patient counseling, which involves the pharmacist offering to discuss the unique drug therapy regimen of each Medicaid recipient when filling prescriptions.

- *Maintenance of Patient Records*—Requires pharmacy providers to obtain, record, and maintain basic patient information such as name, address, telephone number, age, gender, history, disease states, known allergies, drug reactions, and a comprehensive list of medications.

- *Drug Use Review Board*—Requires that state Medicaid programs maintain a board; individual states may require the board be comprised of specific types of professionals.

Because of this federal mandate directed at Medicaid patients, pharmacies across the nation have begun to include similar provisions for non-Medicaid patients as well.

The Compassionate Use Act

Recently evidence was brought forth that marijuana has some clinical use in the treatment of several conditions such as decreasing nausea in patients undergoing chemotherapy, decreasing intraocular pressure in patients with glaucoma, and improving appetite in anorexic patients suffering from AIDS. Cannabis, the main substance in marijuana was already available in oral form as a schedule II controlled substance known by the brand name Marinol when the National Organization for the Reform of Marijuana Laws (NORML) joined forces with other groups to repeal the prohibition of marijuana for medical use at the state level. Each state has the option of passing such laws; however, federal laws that have not approved legalizing marijuana still prevail and can override state laws that are in place.

DRUG NAMES

When communicating with patients, typing medical reports, or writing information on patients' charts, the assistant needs to understand that drugs have more than one name and must be extremely careful about the exact name and spelling. The assistant needs to know the three categories where drug names are found and be able to locate specific information under each category in reference books.

Chemical Name

The **chemical name** is one that indicates the chemical content of the drug. It is usually very long and not commonly referred to by that name.

EXAMPLE 10-1

A Drug's Three Name Types

Brand Name	Chemical Name	Generic Name
Dopar Larodopa capsules Larodopa tablets Sinemet	(1)-3(3,4-Dihydroxphenyl)-L-alanine	levodopa

Brand Name

The **brand name** is one that indicates ownership by a manufacturer and serves as a trademark protected from competition. A superscript ® to the right of the name indicates that the trademark has been registered with the U.S. Patent and Trademark Office. A ™ to the right of the name indicates it is being used as a trademark but is not federally registered. Brand names are chosen to be easier to spell and pronounce for marketing purposes. They begin with a capital letter when written, with a few exceptions, such as pHisoHex. Most hyphenated brand names have capital letters after the hyphens such as Ser-Ap-Es or Cytosar-U. There are also names, such as NegGram, that contain no hyphen but nonetheless have a capital letter in the middle of the word. Some drug names, such as penicillin, may appear either capitalized or not; however, specific types of penicillin, such as PenicillinV, are capitalized.

Generic Name

When a patent expires from the pharmaceutical company that originally manufactured a drug, it may then be manufactured by a number of pharmaceutical companies; known as a generic. At that time the drug may be given a **generic name** that is slightly different with each manufacturer and is the established, nonproprietary **official name** by which a drug is known as an isolated substance, irrespective of its manufacturer. A drug is licensed under its generic name, and it also may be given a *brand name* by its manufacturer. The generic name is assigned by the United States Adopted Names (USAN) Council. When typed or written, a generic drug name is not capitalized, unless the generic name is identical to the brand name.

Patients are often confused about generic drugs and may think that because the price is greatly reduced that the generic drug is a different drug than the brand name. Federal law mandates that the generic drug be manufactured according to the same chemical formula so they are essentially identical; only the "fillers" (powders and liquids in which the chemicals are suspended) may differ.

Other drugs may be evaluated by the FDA and released as over-the-counter (OTC) drugs at a lower strength, while remaining in prescription form at a higher strength (e.g., ibuprofen/Motrin). This may cause confusion for the patient, so the medical assistant needs to have current reference books and keep up-to-date with the latest drug releases.

Legislation in some states allows patients to request generic drugs if the prescription does not specify a particular brand. In some states, pharmacists can substitute generic for brand-name drugs if they get the patient's and the physician's permission and if the substitution does not increase their dollar profit. For example, the generic drug oxytetracycline HCL might be substituted for its brand-name counterpart Terramycin. Generic drugs are almost always less expensive; therefore, it is likely that more patients will request generic drugs on their prescriptions now that the law requires physicians to comply with such requests.

Generic drugs are also used on many drug formularies developed by insurance companies for managed care plans to help keep health care costs down. A *drug formulary* is a listing of a wide range of drugs, preapproved by a third-party organization. If the physician follows the formulary, the patient can usually buy the medication with only a small copayment. If the physician does not follow the formulary, or feels that a medication that is needed is not included on the formulary, the cost to the patient is usually much higher.

DRUG REFERENCES

It was determined in the mid-1800s that there was very little uniformity in the strength of drugs. The *United States Pharmacopeia (USP)* was published around this time to provide drug standards for identification, to indicate the purity of drugs, and to ensure uniformity of strength.

The American Pharmaceutical Association sponsors another book entitled *National Formulary (NF)*, which contains formulas for drug mixtures. Drugs selected for this reference book are chosen on the basis of therapeutic value.

PATIENT EDUCATION

Many pharmaceutical companies offer free medicine for low-income patients and disabled Medicare patients. Check with pharmaceutical representatives to obtain information or look at the Directory of Prescription Drug Patient Assistance Programs on the Internet; Web site: http://www.pharma.org/patients.

Physicians' Desk Reference

A useful reference book, which most physicians have in their libraries, is the *Physicians' Desk Reference (PDR)*, published annually with supplements provided during the year by Thomson PDR, Montvale, NJ 07645 (Figure 10-2). This reference book, which provides essential prescription information on major **pharmaceutical** products, is invaluable to the physician and medical assistant. However, it lists only those drugs that the pharmaceutical companies pay to have listed, and, therefore, not all drugs are included. It is now available for free download (mobilePDR) to MDs, DOs, NPs, and PAs practicing medicine in the United States as well as U.S. medical students and residents.

Prior to 1994, the *PDR* was divided into seven sections. A separate (yellow) section listing generic and chemical names was included. These were later integrated into the (white) brand/generic name index. The sections may vary in color designation and titles with different editions but, in addition to the brand/generic name index, a manufacturer's index typically lists manufacturers' names alphabetically; a product category index lists drugs according to the type of agent (e.g., antidiabetic, gastrointestinal); a diagnostic product information section provides comprehensive product information when products do not include an official package circular; and a product identifi-

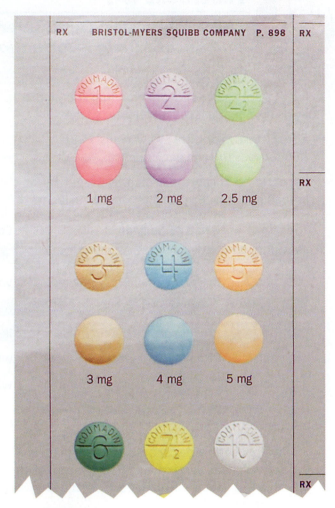

Figure 10-3. Sample from *Physicians' Desk Reference*, Product Identification Section of Coumadin® medication (brand name), showing various strenthgs the pill comes in and the color and shape of each pill. (Courtesy of Thomson Healthcare.)

cation guide distinguishes certain pills that come in different shapes and colors (Figure 10-3). This section can be particularly helpful to the medical assistant. For example, a patient who regularly takes Coumadin has called for the results of her weekly Prothrombin test. The physician has changed the dosage from 2.5 to 2 mg. The patient has been on a variety of dosages, including 1 mg, 3 mg, and 4 mg, and she indicates that she has leftover pills. The patient asks what color the new dosage is in order to determine whether she already has that level on hand. The assistant can refer to this guide to identify the medication and have assurance that the instructions will be correct.

Previous editions of the *PDR* may be helpful in locating a medication a patient may have used in the past that is no longer listed and also for training and use in the classroom.

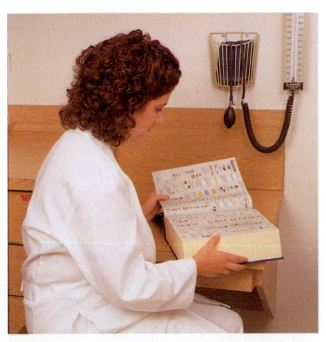

Figure 10-2. The medical assistant is using the *Physicians' Desk Reference* to obtain information about a drug

PROCEDURE 10-3

Use a Physicians' Desk Reference (PDR) *To Spell and Locate Drug Information*

Objective: To obtain the correct spelling of a drug name or search for drug information by using a pharmaceutical reference book.

Equipment/Supplies: *Physicians' Desk Reference (PDR)* and pen or pencil.

Directions: Follow these step-by-step procedures, which include rationales, to learn this skill. Three exercises are presented in the *Workbook* (Job Skills 10-1, 10-2, 10-3) to practice this skill.

1. The 2007 edition of the *PDR* is divided into six, alphabetized sections used for ease in identification and quick reference. They are described in the following table.

Section	Name of Section	Color	Use
Section 1	Manufacturers' Index	dark gray	Contact drug company
Section 2	Brand and Generic Name Index	white	Spell drug names
Section 3	Product Category Index	dark gray	Categories
Section 4	Product Identification Guide	light gray	Identify pills
Section 5	Product Information	white	Details about drugs
Section 6	Diagnostic Product Information	white	Comprehensive product information for drugs without circulars

2. The first section lists the *drug manufacturers* in alphabetic order and includes the manufacturer's name, address, and telephone number. It can be used if you need to contact a drug company.

3. Find the name of the drug being researched in the second section that lists each product by *brand* and *generic name* with a reference listing the page number where a description of each product may be found. This is the most commonly used section for looking up a drug name or finding a medication. Write down the page number where the information can be found in the *Product Information* section.

   Spelling: If the physician writes or dictates an unfamiliar drug name, the assistant can use this section for proper spelling and capitalization. Write each letter using uppercase (capitals) and lowercase letters for the drug name when spelling it out.

4. Locate the page number (shown in the *Brand and Generic Name Index*) in section 5, *Product Information*. This is the largest section and lists over 2,500 drugs and products alphabetized by manufacturer and then by product name within each manufacturer's list. The generic name of the drug appears in parentheses below the brand name. This section contains detailed information on use, dosage, composition, actions, and side effects.

5. Go to the third section, which lists *product categories*. This section is useful as a reference if the assistant has difficulty understanding the name of a drug but knows the category (e.g., antihistamine, antibiotic, laxative). A list of drug classifications and their functions may be found in Table 10-5 on page 318.

6. Next look at the fourth section, which is the *Product Identification Guide*. It has full-color reproductions of the actual size and color of tablets, capsules, bottles, tubes, and packages. If a patient calls and is confused about what pill to take, this section may help identify the medication.

7. Last, look at the sixth section, *Diagnostic Product Information* and notice how many or few drugs are listed with comprehensive information. Drugs listed here do not have official package circulars that provide this information.

Other Drug Reference Books

Many drug reference books that are smaller than the *PDR* that were originally developed for nurses may be useful to the medical assistant. Such drug handbooks provide an alphabetized index of drug names by generic and brand. A modified description of the following is usually included:

1. How supplied (e.g., capsules, tablets, solutions)
2. Mechanism of action (pharmacokinetics)
3. Route, indication, and dosage
4. Adverse reaction
5. Contraindications (interactions and precautions)
6. Nursing considerations

Over-the-Counter Drugs

There is a reference book for nonprescription drugs entitled *Physicians' Desk Reference for Nonprescription Drugs*. Although much smaller, this book is similar in design to the *PDR* and is helpful when looking up over-the-counter (OTC) drugs. Figure 10-4 illustrates an example of a drug bottle identifying the label contents and product information for the safe and effective use of an over-the-counter drug.

Word Books

Excellent tools to help in spelling of medications are word books of brand and generic drug names. They are inexpensive, compact, and provide a simple arrangement for locating terms quickly because the words are listed alphabetically and detailed drug information is not included. Some books, by use of color or symbol, show whether a word represents the generic or brand name and what type of drug it is (narcotic, laxative, diet aid, hormone, and so forth).

UNDERSTANDING PRESCRIPTIONS

Multiskilled allied health professionals may be involved with preparing and reading prescriptions, explaining to patients the components of a prescription, as well as authorizing refills for medications that are in Levels IV and V of the Controlled Substance Schedule; refer to individual state laws regarding this. In order to understand a medical prescription, the medical assistant must be knowledgeable of

---

PATIENT EDUCATION

Instructing the patient on how to read label information on a nonprescription bottle of medication may be a task assigned to the medical assistant. In addition, educating the patient about generic drugs is an important job, eliminating confusion and saving the patient money for the purchase of medications.

---

the various routes used to administer medication, know prescription abbreviations, and be familiar with common errors found when writing or reading prescriptions.

Routes of Administration

Medication may be administered in various ways depending on how fast the drug is to be absorbed into the body system. Also, convenience of administration is a factor. See Table 10-2 for an overview of different ways medication can be given.

Components of a Prescription

All **prescriptions** follow a specific format, the components of which are shown in Figure 10-5 on page 312. A prescription is an order to prepare medications written by a physician, directed to a pharmacist. Each is preprinted with the physician's name, address, telephone number, and often the DEA narcotic number and state license number at the top. If the prescription is not preprinted with the physician's narcotic number and if the prescription contains a narcotic, the DEA number must be listed. A space is provided for the patient's name, address, and date to be completed by the physician. In the remaining space, the physician writes the four standard components of the prescription:

1. **Superscription**—The first element of a prescription, represented by either the word "recipe" (Latin for "take") or by the familiar symbol "Rx." This is usually imprinted on the prescription pad.
2. **Inscription**—The name of the drug or medication (generic or brand name), the quantity of ingredients, and the dosage amount and/or dose strength (DS for double strength). The amount of active drug in each capsule, tablet, or suppository is usually given in milligrams. The strength of creams, ointments,

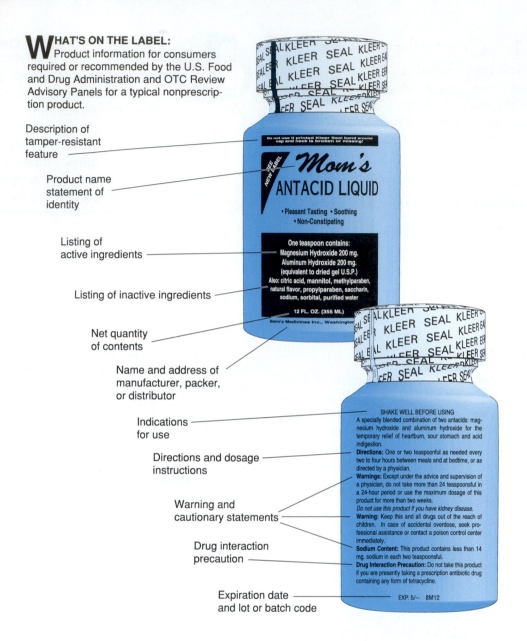

WHAT'S ON THE LABEL: Product information for consumers required or recommended by the U.S. Food and Drug Administration and OTC Review Advisory Panels for a typical nonprescription product.

Description of tamper-resistant feature

Product name statement of identity

Listing of active ingredients

Listing of inactive ingredients

Net quantity of contents

Name and address of manufacturer, packer, or distributor

Indications for use

Directions and dosage instructions

Warning and cautionary statements

Drug interaction precaution

Expiration date and lot or batch code

(Label text, top bottle)

Do not use if printed Kleer Seal band around cap and neck is broken or missing!

Mom's ANTACID LIQUID

• Pleasant Tasting • Soothing • Non-Constipating

One teaspoon contains:
Magnesium Hydroxide 200 mg.
Aluminum Hydroxide 200 mg.
(equivalent to dried gel U.S.P.)
Also: citric acid, mannitol, methylparaben, natural flavor, propylparaben, saccharin, sodium, sorbital, purified water

12 FL. OZ. (355 ML)

Balm's Medicines Inc., Washington

(Label text, bottom bottle)

SHAKE WELL BEFORE USING
A specially blended combination of two antacids: magnesium hydroxide and aluminum hydroxide for the temporary relief of heartburn, sour stomach and acid indigestion.
Directions: One or two teaspoonful as needed every two to four hours between meals and at bedtime, or as directed by a physician.
Warnings: Except under the advice and supervision of a physician, do not take more than 24 teaspoonful in a 24-hour period or use the maximum dosage of this product for more than two weeks.
Do not use this product if you have kidney disease.
Warning: Keep this and all drugs out of the reach of children. In case of accidental overdose, seek professional assistance or contact a poison control center immediately.
Sodium Content: This product contains less than 14 mg. sodium in each two teaspoonful.
Drug Interaction Precaution: Do not take this product if you are presently taking a prescription antibiotic drug containing any form of tetracycline.

EXP. 5/--   8M12

Figure 10-4. Components of an over-the-counter drug label

and topical liquid medicines is usually given as a percentage. The strength of oral liquid medications is given as milligrams per milliliter.

3. **Subscription**—Directions to the pharmacist on the total quantity of the drug to be given for the prescription and the form of the medication (e.g., capsules, tablets).

4. **Signature** or **transcription**—Instructions to the patient, which are included on the label, so the patient will know how to take or apply the medication. The instructions are often written in Latin abbreviations, which the pharmacist must translate. Sometimes written instructions are supplemented with verbal directions to

the patient; for example, whether to take the medication around the clock or during waking hours only.

The physician's signature is required in ink or indelible pencil. At the bottom of the prescription, is a space where the physician can indicate how many more times the prescription may be filled (e.g., "Repeat _____ times" or "Rep. 0-1-2-3 PRN").

Prescription forms may have a line with a check box that states, "Do not substitute," referring to the substitution of a generic drug for the specified brand-name drug. In some states the physician must not only check the box or statement but also initial or sign in that area to signify no substitution. Some physi-

Table 10-2. Drug Routes

Drug Route of Distribution	Method of Administration
Buccal	Medication placed between the cheek and gum
Endotracheal	Medications administered through the trachea (windpipe) and absorbed through the lung
Inhalation	Medication administration by means of a special apparatus such as an inhalator, vaporizer, atomizer, nebulizer, intermittent positive-pressure machine, or respirator that enables the patient to draw air or other substances into the lungs by breathing through the nose or mouth
Injection	Medication administration either directly into the bloodstream or into the tissues
Intra-articular	Administration into a joint
Intradermal	Administration just beneath the outer layer of the skin (e.g., allergy and tuberculosis skin testing)
Intramuscular	Administration into large muscles (e.g., antibiotic injections)
Intrathecal	Administration into the subarachnoid or subdural space of the brain or spinal cord
Intravenous	Administration into a vein for immediate access to the bloodstream
Instillation	Medication in liquid form administered in drops
Inunction	Applying an ointment with friction (i.e., rubbing it into the skin for absorption)
Nasal	Medication administered through the nose, such as drops or sprays
Ophthalmic	Medications administered to the eye. Liquid drops, ointments, or implantable devices (e.g., medication disc) that continually release medication can be used.
Oral	Medications given by mouth, which may be either liquid or solid in the form of tablets, lozenges, pills, or capsules. Pills and capsules are swallowed and absorbed by the body. Tablets and lozenges are held in the mouth and absorbed through mucous membranes.
Otic	Medication administered through the ear (e.g., drops)
Parenteral	Describing all methods of giving medications by means of a needle or cannula introduced through the skin (e.g., subcutaneous, intradermal, intramuscular)
Rectal	Medications given via the rectum such as suppositories, ointments, or enemas dissolved and absorbed by the mucous membranes of the rectum
Sublingual	Medication placed under the tongue
Topical	Substances applied to the skin such as unguents, ointments, creams, sprays, emulsions, powders, plasters, liniments, or liquids for washing
Transdermal	Delivering medication through the skin by means of a dosage-regulator membrane (patch); also known as transcutaneous delivery
Urethral	Medication administered into the bladder using a catheter
Vaginal	Medications absorbed via the vagina, such as suppositories and creams

cians either handwrite or have a section on their prescription forms that states, "Dispense as written," or "Brand medically necessary."

The patient can still ask for a generic drug, even though the physician has requested a brand name. However, in this case, the pharmacist may call the physician for approval to dispense the generic drug. Other prescriptions may include the statement "Generic drugs are permissible."

State Prescription Regulations

Certain states have mandates over and above those required by federal law. In January 2005 California state law mandated replacing triplicate forms with new California Security prescription forms that are now required for all Schedule II, III, and IV drugs and some Schedule V drugs. The tamper-resistant security forms have special features required by the California Board of Pharmacy.

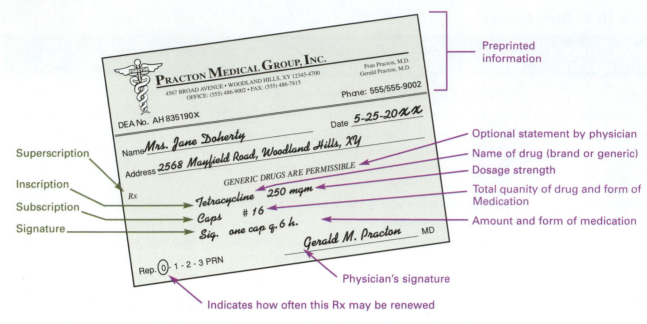

Figure 10-5. A completed prescription with components identified

Florida and Mississippi have special prescription form requirements for state Medicaid prescriptions. New Jersey has a state-approved prescription paper printer, and prescription pads in New York can only be purchased directly from the state. Some of the security features for states that have special requirements include:

- Colored background—which is harder to copy

- Resistant paper—resists erasures and alterations

- Copy alerts—the word "VOID" appears when photocopied

- Tracking devices—identification and batch numbers

- Thermocratic ink—on reverse side that reveals the word "SAFE" when rubbed

Check laws within your state to see if special forms or requirements are necessary.

Authorizing Prescriptions

Because the prescription is a legal document, many physicians prefer to write out all orders themselves. If the writing is illegible, it is the pharmacist's responsibility to telephone the physician to make certain of the drug ordered. Table 10-1 on page 304 outlines which schedule of drugs may be written by a health care worker and signed by the physician.

In Iowa and Texas, physicians must call pharmacies themselves with new prescriptions or to authorize refills for controlled substances; pharmacists can no longer accept those orders from office personnel.

Electronic Prescription Programs

Electronic prescription programs have been developed and are in operation throughout the country to transmit orders to pharmacies. Upon receiving the information via computer or fax and filling the prescription, the pharmacy then sends a message marked "filled" to record that the order has been completed. The advantages include less telephone time, accuracy (not having to clarify handwriting), reduction of errors, and efficiency. Handwritten faxes should never be used for medication orders because of potential problems interpreting the physician's handwriting as well as the inherent difficulty of reading faxes. Because 99 percent of pharmacies are fully computerized, it is important to understand this automated technology.

E-Prescribing—The Centers for Medicare and Medicaid Services (CMS) are establishing standards for electronic prescribing (e-prescribing) and would like to make the system mandatory for participating drug plans by the year 2009. Prescriptions can be entered into a software application during patient examinations using a portable computer such as a laptop or hand-held device, which then electronically transmits the request to a pharmacy's software program.

A refill request goes directly into the pharmacy system and automatically checks on the availability of refills. The software system routes a request to the physician's system if a refill is not available. E-prescribing allows the physician to look up drugs in a formulary provided by insurance carriers, has automated drug interaction checks, and can include individualized allergy alerts. The patient's full drug history can be viewed, including drugs that have been prescribed by other physicians. Other software can let the physician know if the patient fails to refill a drug or pick up medication after it is ordered. It alleviates illegible written prescriptions and expedites the filling and refilling process.

Preprinted and Duplicate Prescriptions

In some practices, physicians have found it efficient to use preprinted prescriptions for certain drugs; however, too many prescriptions in this format can result in wasted time sorting through the pads to find the right one.

Federal law does not require that a physician keep a copy of a patient's prescription, but it is a good idea in the event a physician is questioned about a prescribed medication. Prescription pads that have carbonless (NCR) paper can be obtained, allowing for a duplicate copy to be retained for the patient's medical record. Because these are small sheets and can be easily misplaced, shingle them with tape onto large, colored sheets for easy reference. The first copy is placed on the bottom of a large sheet and, as each subsequent prescription is written, it is taped on top of the previous one about one-half inch above it, as shown in Figure 10-6. The patient's name and account number are typed in the upper right corner of the large sheet.

Prescription Abbreviations

All medical assistants should know prescription terms and abbreviations because they will use them when communicating with patients and pharmacy staff, when taking dictation, and for understanding instructions on the administration of medications (Table 10-3). The Latin abbreviations are a kind of

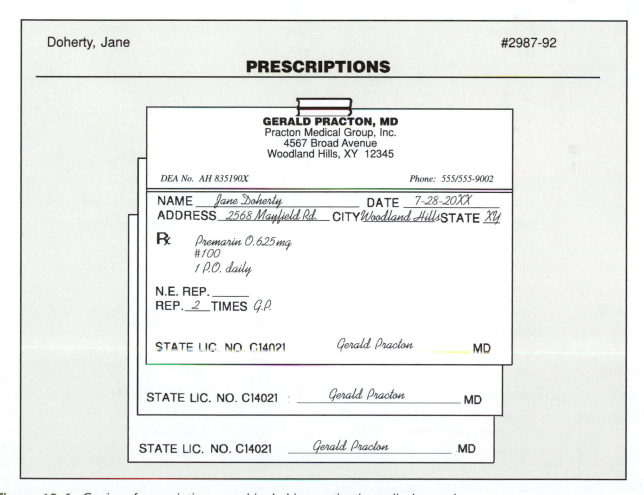

Figure 10-6. Copies of prescriptions are shingled in a patient's medical record

Table 10-3. Common Prescription Abbreviations* and Symbols

$\bar{a}$	before	N.E. or ne	negative
$\bar{aa}$	of each	noct.	night
a.c.	before meals	NPO or n.p.o.	nothing by mouth
ad lib.	as much as needed	O_2	oxygen
a.m. or AM	morning	o.d.	once a day
ante	before	o.h.	every hour
aq.	aqueous/water	oint	ointment
b.i.d.	two times a day	o.m.	every morning
caps	capsule	o.n.	every night
$\bar{c}$	with	OTC	over-the-counter (drugs)
$\bar{cc}$	with meals	oz	ounce
comp. or comp	compound	$\bar{p}$	after
d	day	p.c.	after meals
DC or D/C	discontinue	p.o.	by mouth (per os)
dos.	doses	p.r.	per rectum
DS	double strength	p.r.n. or PRN	whenever necessary
DSD	double starting dose	q.	every
elix.	elixir	q.a.m.	every morning
emul.	emulsion	q.h.	every hour
et	and	q.h.s.	every night
ext.	extract	q.i.d.	four times a day (not at night)
garg.	gargle	q. n.	every night
gm or g	gram	q.p.m.	every night
gr	grain	q.2 h.	every two hours
gt.	drop	q.3 h.	every three hours
gtt.	drops	q.4 h.	every four hours
h.	hour	rep, REP	let it be repeated; Latin repeto
h.s.	before bedtime (hour of sleep)	Rx	take (recipe), prescription
ID	intradermal	$\bar{s}$	without
IM	intramuscular	SC or subq	subcutaneous
inj.	injection; to be injected	sat.	saturated
IV or I.V.	intravenous	Sig.	write on label; give directions on prescription
kg	kilogram		
liq	liquid	SL	sublingual
M or m.	mix	sol.	solution
mcg	microgram	SR	sustained release
mg or mgm	milligram (used instead of "cc" for cubic centimeter)	ss	one-half
		stat or STAT	immediately
ml	milliliter	syr.	syrup

Many of these abbreviations are derived from Latin; they are usually typed in lowercase and with periods. Periods are especially important, if without periods an abbreviation would spell a word; for example, b.i.d. without periods is bid.

Table 10-3 (*continued*). Common Prescription Abbreviations and Symbols

tab.	tablet	X or x	times (X10d/times ten days)
t.i.d.	three times a day	i, ii, iii, iv; viii, etc.	1, 2, 3, 4; 8, etc.
top	topically	5″, 10″, 15″	5 , 10 , 15 minutes, etc.
Tr. or tinct.	tincture	5°, 10°, 15°, or 5′, 10′, 15′, etc.	5 hours, 10 hours, 15 hours, etc.
tsp	teaspoon	ʒ or dr.	dram (drachm)
vag.	vagina	ʒ or oz.	ounce

shorthand that speeds writing or taking messages and relaying them to the physician.

Common Errors and Dangerous Abbreviations to Avoid

Because handwriting is sometimes difficult to decipher and poor penmanship is common, errors can occur when reading and filling a prescription.

The Joint Commission on Accreditation of Healthcare Organizations (JCAHO) publishes standards that must be met by all hospital facilities. To make sure that standard protocols are in place and followed, JCAHO surveys hospital facilities and issues sanctions in the areas of noncompliance. As of this date, JCAHO has not issued a comprehensive list of approved abbreviations for Health Information Management (HIM) departments; however, they did publish National Patient Safety Goals in 2004. Goal 2b states, "Standardize the abbreviations, acronyms, and symbols used throughout the organization, including a list of abbreviations, acronyms, and symbols not to use." JACO has published its own list of prohibited abbreviations that may not be used in patient charts, written orders, or notes. Although physician outpatient practices are not bound by JCAHO standards, physicians must comply in inpatient settings and it makes sense to follow these recommendations to avoid abbreviations that are easily misunderstood on medical records. Read through Table 10-4 to view examples of recommendations to follow and some abbreviations to avoid in order to prevent misreading and misinterpreting prescriptions. Abbreviations shown with an asterisk sign (*) are prohibited by JCAHO. Since many of these abbreviations have been long used by members of the health care community, a list of approved abbreviations needs to be in place. Also, a list of abbreviations to avoid needs to be printed for office use and staff members need to be educated regarding the dangers of their use.

Formatting Errors

When writing multiple medication names and dosages in a patient medical record, it is advisable to write them in list form instead of paragraph form. Lists are easier to read and locate data without error (see Example 10-2).

PRESCRIPTION DRUGS AND THE ROLE OF THE MEDICAL ASSISTANT

The administrative medical assistant's responsibility with regard to drugs and prescriptions is to assist the physician by being knowledgeable about federal and state statutes on medications, to help patients, and to

---

EXAMPLE 10-2

Medication Formatting for Medical Records

Paragraph Form:

The patient is on Premarin 0.625 mg daily, Calcium 500 mg b.i.d., Zocor 40 mg at bedtime, Verapamil 180 mg SR q.a.m., Ambien 5 mg at bedtime, and Lasix 20 mg daily.

List Form:

MEDICATIONS

Premarin 0.625 mg daily

Calcium 500 mg b.i.d.

Zocor 40 mg at bedtime

Verapamil 180 mg SR q.a.m.

Ambien 5 mg at bedtime

Lasix 20 mg daily

Table 10-4. Common Errors and Dangerous Abbreviations to Avoid

When Penmanship is Poor, This . . .	. . . Can be Misread As This . . .	. . . So Write This Instead or Use This Guideline
1.0 mg	10 mg	"1 mg"
.3 mg	3 mg	"0.3 mg"
10000	100000	Insert comma (10,000)
6 units regular insulin/ 20 units NPH insulin	120 units of NPH	Never use a slash
*AD (right ear)	AD (*atrium dextrum* = right atrium)	right ear
*AS (left ear)	AS (aortic sac)	left ear
*AU (each ear)	AU (*ad usum*) according to custom	each or both ears
BT (bedtime)	BID (twice daily)	"h.s." (before bedtime)
*cc	U (units)	"ml"
D/C	Discharge or discontinue	Discharge or discontinue
*DPT	Demerol-Phenergan-Thorazine or diphtheria-pertussis-tetanus	Completely spell out drug names
Every 3–4 hours	Every 3/4 hour	"every 3 to 4 hours"
HCl	KCl	Completely spell out drug names (hydrochloric)
HCT	Hydrocortisone or hydrochlorothiazide	Completely spell out drug names
1U	*IU (International unit)	"unit" or international unit
*MgSO$_4$, *MSO$_4$, MS	Magnesium sulfate or morphine	Spell out term
o.d. or *OD (every day)	OD "right eye" (oculus dexter)	"daily" or "right eye"
OU (each eye)	OU (outer upper)	each eye
per os	*OS (left eye)	"po" "by mouth" or "left eye"
q.d. or *QD	q.i.d. (4 times a day)	"daily" or "every day"
qn	qh (every hour)	"nightly"
qhs	Every hour	"nightly"
q6PM	Every six hours	"6 p.m. nightly"
q.o.d. or *QOD	q.d. (daily) or q.i.d. (four times daily)	"every other day"
SC, *sc, *sq	SL (sublingual)	"subcut," "subQ," or "subcutaneous"
sub q	Every	"subcut," "subQ," or "subcutaneous"
TIW or tiw	Three times a day	Do not use this abbreviation
*U or *u	Zero (0), 6, cc, or a four (4), causing a 10-fold overdose or greater (e.g., 4U seen as "40" or 4u seen as "44")	"unit" (Do not abbreviate)
*ug	microgram	"mcg"
x3d	three doses	"for three days"
1.0 Zero after a decimal point	10 mg (if the decimal point is not seen)	Do not use terminal zeros for doses expressed in whole numbers
.5 mg No zero before decimal dose	5 mg	Always use zero before a decimal when the dose is less than a whole unit

*Abbreviations prohibited by the Joint Commission.

PROCEDURE 10-2

STEP 1 2 3

Read and Interpret a Written Prescription

Objective: To read and accurately interpret a written prescription.

Equipment/Supplies: Patient's prescription, abbreviations (Table 10-3), and pen or pencil.

Directions: Follow these step-by-step procedures, which include rationales, to learn this skill, which is presented in the *Workbook* (Job Skill 10-4) for practice.

1. Read the patient's name on the prescription to verify spelling, accuracy, and legibility.

2. Read the patient's address to check that it is inserted.

3. Confirm the date written on the prescription.

4. Review the inscription (brand or generic drug name).

5. Confirm that the drug dosage strength is listed and correct.

6. Look at the subscription (form of the medication—capsules, tablets) and the quantity (number or amount) of the drug prescribed for legibility.

7. Read the signature or transcription— directions to the patient on how to take or apply the medication and what time(s) to take or apply it. Translate the Latin into common English.

8. Validate that the renewal or refill times are indicated and note the number allowed.

9. Check the prescription for the physician's signature and indicate who prescribed the medication.

---

record drug information. It is beyond the scope of the medical assistant's training to give advice, administer, dispense, or prescribe medication. This also includes over-the-counter (OTC) medication, herbs, and drug samples.

Pharmaceutical Representative

Pharmaceutical representatives or "detail rep's" may schedule an appointment to visit the physician and leave drug samples and literature. Detail reps are often allowed into the back office to view medi-

cation samples to determine the need for additional samples prior to writing up the order for the physician to sign. In some clinics, representatives must sign in at the front desk. Others do not allow representatives to meet with the doctors during office hours. Instead they create a drop box for pamphlets; however, if samples are left, the physician, nurse practitioner, or physician's assistant must sign for them. In lieu of having drug samples on hand, some medical practices establish a voucher system. Vouchers are distributed to patients, which are then given to the pharmacist for free medication.

COMPLIANCE

According to an anti-kickback statute, physicians commit a felony if they knowingly and willfully offer, solicit, pay, or receive payment in exchange for drug referrals payable under Medicare, Medical Assistance, or other government health programs. Payment can be in the form of money, vacations, tickets to sporting events, and so on. Violations are punishable by fines, imprisonment, or exclusion from the Medicare program.

Drug Classifications

If sample medications are kept in the office, the medical assistant must make sure that they have not expired and are organized so that all physicians can easily find them to give to patients. They can be located quickly if they are organized alphabetically or grouped by type of substance in drawers, bins, or on shelves. Headings, following classifications such as those listed in Table 10-5 may be used to group drugs according to their type of use. The choice and number of identifying labels depends on the medical specialty and the supply of medications kept on hand.

Table 10-5. Drug Classification and Their Functions

Drug Category	Drug Use
Analgesic	Given to relieve pain without loss of consciousness
Anesthetic	Causes loss of sensation and insensibility to pain or touch. A *general anesthetic* produces insensibility to pain in all parts of the body and unconsciousness. A *local anesthetic* produces insensibility to pain at the site of application
Antacid	Neutralizes acidity, especially in the digestive tract
Antibiotic	Used to kill living microorganisms that cause infection
Anticholinergic	Blocks the passage of impulses through the parasympathetic system
Anticoagulant	Used to prevent blood clotting
Anticonvulsant	Relieves or prevents convulsions
Antidepressant	Used to relieve symptoms of depression. Antipsychotic drugs, antianxiety agents, psychomotor stimulants, and lithium also treat depression.
Antiemetic	Prevents or relieves vomiting
Antihistamine	Used to treat allergy symptoms
Anti-inflammatory	Used to reduce or relieve inflammation; may be a steroid or nonsteroid agent
Antipyretic	Given to reduce fever
Antiseptic	Substance that prevents the growth or arrests the development of microorganisms
Antitussive	Used to relieve a cough
Astringent	Substance that produces shrinkage of mucous membranes or other tissues and decreases secretion
Bronchodilator	Used to dilate bronchial tubes
Carminative	Expels flatus (gas) from the stomach and the intestines
Cathartic	Increases and hastens the evacuation of the bowel; a laxative
Coagulant	Drug or substance that causes blood or fluid to clot
Contraceptive (pharmaceutical)	Prevents conception; oral contraceptives are commonly known as "the Pill"
Decongestant	Decreases congestion or swelling
Disinfectant	Substance that destroys bacteria on objects, places, and materials; not used on the living body because of its capacity to destroy living tissue
Diuretic	Increases the excretion of urine
Emetic	Causes vomiting
Expectorant	Used to increase secretion and aid in expelling mucus from the respiratory tract, or to modify such secretions
Hemostatic	Used to decrease and control bleeding
Hypnotic	Produces sleep; a soporific
Laxative	Mild cathartic that produces one or two bowel movements without discomfort
Miotic	Causes the pupil of the eye to contract
Mydriatic	Causes the pupil of the eye to dilate
Narcotic	Relieves pain and produces sleep or stupor

(continues)

Table 10-5 (*continued*). Drug Classification and Their Functions

Drug Category	Drug Use
Ointment	Soft, fatty substance having soothing or healing action
Placebo	An inactive preparation given in place of an actual drug to gratify the patient or as a control in pharmaceutical studies of drugs
Prophylactic	Prevents the development of a disease; such as a vaccine, a vitamin, a hormone, or an immunologic preparation
Sedative	Exerts a soothing or tranquilizing effect; a tranquilizer
Solution	Liquid with ingredients dissolved evenly
Stimulant	Temporarily increases activity or hastens actions in the body or any of its organs
Suspension	Preparation with undissolved ingredients that must be shaken well before using
Therapeutic drugs	Administered to combat a specific disorder
Tranquilizer	Reduces anxiety without clouding consciousness; a sedative
Vaccine	Suspension of infectious agents or some part of them used to convey resistance to infectious disease
Vasoconstrictor	Causes constriction of blood vessels
Vasodilator	Causes dilation of blood vessels

Medication Instructions

Pharmacists are encouraged by the FDA to provide printed instructions with every new prescription.

Some physicians ask their medical assistants to instruct patients about drug dosages and drug schedules. Such instructions supplement physician orders and do not replace directions given to patients by pharmacists. Past studies indicate that poor interpersonal communication is the cause of multiple medication errors. Be alert to discern whether the patient understands the directions given. Elderly patients may have difficulty hearing and seeing and may be reluctant to admit they are confused or do not comprehend.

Patients forget approximately 50 to 75 percent of what they have been told after leaving the office. Personal instructions will help prevent confusion when several medications are to be taken at various times and if there are similarities in drug names.

According to the Food and Drug Administration (FDA), among older adults, 17 percent of all hospitalizations are caused by side effects of prescription drugs. This is six times more than for the general population. Errors may also be made when a prescription is written, filled, or taken at home.

One common error occurs when patients confuse medications with names that sound alike, such as Lanoxin (for heart failure) and Levoxine (for hypothyroidism). Ask the patient to verify the drug by bringing it in, taking it to the pharmacy, or using the product identification section in the *Physicians' Desk Reference* (see previous section), if there is any confusion.

Medication Schedule Card

Some practices use patient medication schedule cards (Figure 10-7) to help patients keep track of their medicines. These cards are also useful if the patient has an emergency or sees a specialist and the primary care physician does not have an opportunity to supply medical records.

Drug Dispensing Containers

Various drug dispensing containers are sold at pharmacies or provided by pharmaceutical representatives to aid patients in separating their medications according to the days of the week and times of day they need to take them. If a friend or family member assists the patient in preparing and administering the medication, that person should be included when instructions are given. Medicine spoons and cups should be clearly marked; tableware and drinking glasses vary in capacity and do not provide accurate measurement.

PRACTON MEDICAL GROUP, INC.
4567 Broad Avenue
Woodland Hills, XY 12345-4700
Tel. 555/486-9002

With so many potent medicines available today, the possibility of undesirable effects of single drugs, or adverse interactions of multiple drugs, is always present. If there is any question of side effects of drugs, or their potential toxicity, feel free to call and discuss this with your physician.

Patient's name:

Gloria V. Smith

Please bring this card with you for each appointment.

Your primary physician is:

Gerald Practon, MD

It is vital that you, and all health care professionals involved in your care, know exactly the names and dosages of ALL medicines you are currently taking. Please keep this card with you and show it to your doctor or dentist, during office visits, and to your pharmacist when prescriptions and/or over-the-counter preparations are purchased.

MEDICATION SCHEDULE

Name of Medication	Strength	Times to be Taken Each Day						
		AM		Noon		PM		Bed
Lasix	*40 mg*	1		1		1		
Sonata	*5 mg*							1

If you have any questions or problems with medications, please call (555) 486-9002

Figure 10-7. Example of a medication schedule card given to a patient with some medications recorded

Medication Log

Some offices use a drug flow sheet or medication log for all medications the patient takes, including drugs prescribed by the attending as well as other physicians. This is useful for patients on multiple medications and shows, at a quick glance, the usage habits of a patient or whether a drug might be contraindicated (Figure 10-8). It includes patient name, date of birth, date prescribed, name of medication, dosage, amount prescribed, directions, whether the medication is taken regularly or as needed, telephone or written order, name of the pharmacy, and the physician's initials indicating approval. Flow sheets can be easily checked to see the frequency of drug refills; however, they should never replace the physician's initial documentation in the medical record.

Medication Refills

Often a separate pharmacy line is designated for prescription refills. The medical assistant must obtain the following information from the patient before a refill can be processed.

1. Name and telephone number of the patient in case the physician needs to talk with the patient before prescribing the medication or renewing the prescription

2. Name and spelling of the medication

PATIENT EDUCATION

When instructing patients about proper guidelines for taking prescription medication*, include the following:

1. Speak directly to the patient and ask him or her to repeat the directions to be sure that he or she clearly understands them.

2. Write the name of the medication, dosage, and directions for the patient.

3. Advise the patient to take the medication exactly as prescribed, at the right times, and in the correct amounts.

4. Instruct the patient about special precautions when taking certain medications. For example, Coumadin is a blood thinning agent, so blood samples must be tested regularly to avoid blood clots or blood loss.

5. Tell the patient to inform the physician if any new symptoms or adverse effects develop when taking the drug.

6. Instruct the patient to take the medication for the prescribed duration of time, even if he or she begins to feel improved. If the patient has been prescribed antibiotics, instruct the patient to:
   a. Always finish the complete prescription, even if symptoms subside and the patient is feeling better.
   b. Call and inform the doctor's office if, for any reason, the patient stops using the medication.
   c. Report all symptoms immediately if any adverse reactions occur.

7. Ask the patient to tell the physician if he or she decides not to take the medication.

8. Inform the patient not to take other medications, such as over-the-counter drugs, without first asking the physician.

9. Warn the patient not to take any medications that are prescribed for someone else and not to share their medication with anyone else, not even family members.

10. Teach the patient to store the medication in an appropriate place, such as away from the reach of children, in the refrigerator, or in a dark, cool place.

11. Instruct the patient to discard unused portions of prescription medications and medications that have expired dates.

12. Caution patients about taking medications that could cause sleepiness, interfere with concentration, or affect the ability to drive or operate machinery.

*Instructing patients about taking prescription medication should be done only at the direction of the physician.

3. Dosage strength (e.g., milligrams)

4. Number of tablets or capsules in the prescription

5. Prescription number

6. Name and telephone or fax number of the pharmacy. If the prescription approval is faxed, the form may list the birth date, Social Security number, medical insurance number, and the patient's telephone number.

7. How many refills remain on the prescription

Prescriptions for federally controlled substances must be handed directly to the patient by the physician or in some states may be prescribed by the physician over the telephone as long as the DEA number is given and a follow-up written prescription is sent immediately to the pharmacy. In such cases, the assistant might advise the patient by saying, "I'm sorry, Mr. Wayne, but that drug cannot be prescribed over the telephone. Could you please come into the office to pick up the prescription this afternoon?"

To eliminate the possibility of errors when telephoning in a prescription, ask the pharmacist to read back each prescription. If unsure of the pronunciation, spell the name of the medication. If the medical assistant handles the medication refills, advise the pharmacist of the office protocol regarding pharmacy call-backs and instruct patients about office procedures. Individual office policies vary, but the following

MEDICATION LOG

PATIENT NAME: FOLEY, Mary Beth   DATE OF BIRTH: 9-30-52

ALLERGIES: NKA

DATE	MEDICATIONS	DOSE	#	INSTRUCTIONS (SIG)	PRN REG	TEL WRIT	PHARMACY	DR. SIG.
8/5/XX	Amitriptyline	100 mg	90	i p.o. bedtime	R	T	ABC Pharm	GP
10/28/XX	Amitriptyline	100 mg	90	i p.o. bedtime	R	T	ABC Pharm	GP
9/23/XX	Glucotrol	10 mg	30	i p.o. a.c./a.m.	R	T	ABC Pharm	GP
9/23/XX	Verapamil SR	240 mg	30	i p.o. q.a.m.	R	T	ABC Pharm	GP
10/7/XX	Glucotrol	10 mg	90	i p.o. a.c./a.m.	R	W	mail order pharmacy	GP
10/7/XX	Tetracycline	250 mg	30	i p.o. T.I.D. p.r.n. yellow sputum	P	T	ABC Pharm	GP
10/16/XX	Verapamil SR	240 mg	90	i p.o. q.a.m.	R	W	mail order pharmacy	GP

Figure 10-8. Medication log, also called drug flow sheet, showing recorded medications

---

EXAMPLE 10-3

Prescription Call-Back Protocols

A. Call-backs are made after 4:00 p.m.

B. Call-backs are made twice a day.

C. Refills will be faxed at the end of the day.

---

are a few common protocols. If the patient is taking an ongoing medication:

- Instruct the patient to call the office two working days in advance to request a refill.
- Instruct the patient to call the pharmacy where the prescription was originally filled two working days in advance to request a refill. The pharmacy will then call the office to get an approval and have time to refill the medication.
- For a mail-order pharmacy, initially give the patient two written prescriptions, one for a 30-day supply and one for a 3-month supply. Instruct the patient to fill the 30-day

prescription locally and begin taking the medication. The patient should then send the other prescription to the mail-order pharmacy. When the patient receives the mail-order prescription, the other medication should be put aside to use as a backup if the mail order is delayed or if the patient forgets to allow for enough delivery time. The patient should begin taking the mail-order medication and mark the calendar to allow for a two-week turnaround processing time for future refills.

PATIENT EDUCATION

Advise patients about office policies for prescription refills. Instruct patients to bring in their medications in the original bottles every time they see the physician or when they are admitted to the hospital. Encourage patients to call with questions regarding their medications.

EXAMPLE 10-4

Record of Prescription Refill in a Patient's Chart

Scenario A: On January 12, 20XX, Marjean Hope called at 10:15 in the morning to request a refill of her Lorazepam prescription, 30 tablets at a strength of 0.5 mg. The medical assistant looked at her chart, which showed that her last refill was a month ago and that she was scheduled to see the doctor in one week. Approval for a refill was telephoned to ABC Pharmacy.

Chart note entry for Marjean Hope: January 12, 20XX—Refill Lorazepam 0.5 mg, #30 tabs, ABC Pharmacy

Scenario B: Patient Mindy Jones called on July 7, 20XX, asking for a written prescription for Diovan HCT tabs for her mail order pharmacy (WellCheck). She said the strength is 160/12.5 and she takes one a day. Dr. Gerald Practon always gives her ninety pills with three refills. The chart was pulled and Dr. Practon verified the request and wrote the prescription.

Chart note entry for Mindy Jones: July 7, 20XX—Written Rx for Diovan HCT tabs 160/12.5, #90 1 q. day, X3 refills (WellCheck Pharmacy)

Charting Prescriptions

The medical assistant must see that oral prescription orders and refills are promptly committed to writing and recorded in patients' medical records. The items to record are the date of refill approval, name of the medication, dosage strength, and number of tablets or capsules.

Adding the telephone number of a patient's **pharmacist** to the chart and ledger card is also a good idea, because it provides the assistant with a ready reference for telephoning a prescription refill.

Drug Abuse Prevention Measures

Physicians may be approached by people who exhibit varying extremes of drug-seeking behavior. The medical assistant must be able to recognize those patients who might be drug misusers or abusers. One indication might be an unfamiliar patient's statement that a

PROCEDURE 10-3

Record Medication in a Patient's Chart and on a Medication Log

Objective: To record medication in a patient's medical record and on a medication sheet.

Equipment/Supplies: Patient's medical record, progress sheet, medication log sheet, and pen.

Directions: Follow these step-by-step procedures to learn this skill, which is presented in the *Workbook* (Job Skills 10-5 and 10-6) for practice. The rationale for each step is to comply with CMS documentation guidelines.

1. Write the date of the chart entry.

2. State if it is a new prescription or a refill.

3. Insert the name of the medication.

4. Include the dosage.

5. List the amount given.

6. Write the directions.

7. Sign or initial the chart entry with your professional title.

8. Write the date of the prescription on the medication log.

9. List the name of the medication, dose, amount, instructions or directions (signature) to the patient, and whether taken regularly or as needed.

10. Indicate the telephone or written order and name of the pharmacy.

11. Sign or initial the log entry.

controlled substance being requested was previously prescribed by another physician. Another hint might be an unfamiliar patient's statement that he or she is the patient of another physician for whom the physician occasionally covers and that the patient wishes to have a prescription for a controlled substance renewed. In such situations, the assistant should ask the patient for the name of his or her regular physician and attempt to verify the story. A patient's hesitancy in answering or avoiding questions can also indicate a problem.

Good documentation in the medical record is the best way of tracking a patient's drug use habits. The medical record should always be consulted, not only to verify that the medication was prescribed, but to check the correct dosage and amount (number of pills) prescribed. This will help verify if the patient has been taking the medication correctly and whether it is the proper time frame for a refill. Drug flow sheets are useful for such tracking purposes, and sometimes pharmacies can be helpful in alerting the office staff if a patient has prescriptions from more than one physician for the same medication.

Protecting Prescription Pads

A prime target of drug abusers is the prescription pad. Some medical practices use computer-generated prescriptions. To discourage anyone from photocopying these prescription sheets, special paper is used, which, if copied, shows the word "copy" in bold relief on the photocopy. The assistant can protect the prescription pads in the office by:

1. Storing unused prescription pads in a safe place, preferably under lock and key, so they cannot be stolen easily

2. Minimizing the number of pads in use at one time; if the physician can carry a pad in his or her pocket where it is easily accessible at all times, pads in use could be limited to one

3. Not leaving prescription pads in unattended office areas or examining rooms and making sure the physician does not leave them in a car, where they may be easily taken by unauthorized persons

4. Having prescription blanks numbered consecutively by printers so that if one is missing, it will be noticed quickly. They can also be printed in colored ink that is not reproducible, and the DEA number can be omitted. Prescription blanks for

nonrestricted medications should have a printed statement centered across the prescription that reads "Rx not valid for narcotics, barbiturates, or amphetamines" or "not valid for Schedules II and III drugs"; the placement is important so the message cannot be cut off.

5. Asking the physician to avoid signing prescription blanks in advance

6. Making sure the physician writes and signs prescription orders in ink or indelible pencil to prevent alterations. For example, if the prescription does not have a place for "zero" refills, the medical assistant should make sure the physician indicates that there are no refills.

7. Checking to make sure the amount of medication prescribed is written out or in Roman numerals, as well as expressed in an Arabic numeral, thus preventing changes; for example, "30 (thirty or XXX) tablets" cannot be changed to "80 tablets"

8. Not permitting prescription blanks to be used as memo pads for notes; drug abusers can erase notes and use the blanks to obtain drugs

9. Obtaining tamper-proof prescription pads that are tinted so erasures or white correction ink are easily detected. The prescription copies appear with the word "void" printed across them.

If a pad is missing, it might be wise to clip the left or right lower corner of the remaining pads, then notify local pharmacists to reject any whole sheets. Some communities have set up a telephone network for stolen prescription blanks, in which one pharmacist calls two pharmacists, those two each call two, and so forth until the entire community knows about the problem in a short time.

Drug Side Effects and Adverse Reactions

The assistant must be aware that medication taken in the correct dosage may produce side effects. Also, food, beverages, and other drugs taken in conjunction with prescribed medication may produce adverse reactions. The patient should be asked every time medication is prescribed if he or she has allergies to any or medication, because an individual may have developed one since the last time seen. Legally, the assistant is not permitted to tell the patient to stop

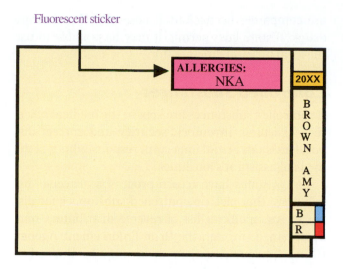

Fluorescent sticker

ALLERGIES:
NKA

20XX

B
R
O
W
N

A
M
Y

B
R

Figure 10-9. A fluorescent sticker on a file folder alerts the physician to a patient's drug allergies

the medication; this falls under medical care. In case a patient should take an overdose of medication, the telephone numbers of the nearest fire department and poison control center should be kept close at hand in the physician's office.

Information about a patient's previous adverse side effects from drugs should always be recorded in a prominent place near the front of the medical record. Brightly colored "ALERT TAGS" (Figure 10-9) may be used on the front cover of the patient's chart to bring this information to the attention of anyone handling the record. If the patient does not have any allergies to medications, the abbreviation NKA (no known allergies) should be inserted, indicating that the patient has been questioned regarding allergic reactions. Be sure to ask the physician if a patient should be questioned regarding food allergies and "natural" medication or herbs.

PATIENT EDUCATION

When a patient is taking a prescribed or over-the-counter drug, instruct him or her to call the office when experiencing one or more of the following complaints: *dizziness, drowsiness, nausea, vomiting, rash, respiratory trouble, sleeplessness, headache, blurred vision, hemorrhaging, constipation, or appetite or weight loss.* The medical assistant should then bring the situation to the physician's immediate attention.

CONTROL AND STORAGE OF DRUGS

The medical assistant can help the physician avoid potential liability by setting up a systematic plan for the management and storage of all drugs. The clinical assistant who handles the medications daily is usually delegated the task of keeping an inventory—evaluating needs and jotting down in a notebook the names of drugs that are running low. The administrative assistant follows through by contacting the medical supply company, pharmacy, or sales representative to place the order. A small file of calling cards arranged alphabetically by company name will speed contacting a particular company or pharmaceutical representative for a drug; the sales representative's name can be written on each card if it is not printed. All controlled drugs (Schedules I–V) should be kept under lock and key.

Pharmaceutical companies often provide notebooks to facilitate the ordering of items they handle. When the sales representative visits the office periodically, he or she checks off any items written in the notebook by the assistants and then places the order or fills the order and stocks the drugs. Periodically check the expiration dates (i.e., **shelf life**) of drugs and remove outdated ones because the physician might be held liable if a patient took an expired medication and had an adverse reaction. To determine when medications lose their potency or deteriorate, the expiration dates are printed on the labels. When stocking recently received drugs, place them behind the oldest dated drugs to ensure using drugs before they expire. Certain drugs must be refrigerated; others, kept in dark, dry cabinets. Be sure to follow specific storage instructions.

Disposal of Drugs

Drugs should be discarded immediately when expired or if labels are detached or become illegible. Never throw medications where unauthorized people might have access. Types of wastes that might be encountered by medical office personnel are referred to as hazardous, medical, and universal wastes.

Hazardous wastes are solid, liquid, or gas wastes that can cause death, illness, or injury to people or destruction of the environment if improperly treated, stored, transported, or discarded. Substances are considered hazardous wastes if they are ignitable (capable of burning or causing a fire), corrosive (able to corrode steel or harm organisms because of acidic properties), reactive (able to explode or produce toxic cyanide or sulfide gas), or toxic (containing substances that are poisonous). Mixtures, residues, or materials containing hazardous wastes are also considered hazardous wastes. Examples of hazardous wastes that might be found in a medical office are copier toner, fluorescent bulbs, batteries, pesticides, spilled chemicals, toilet bowl cleaners, mercury, x-ray film, nitrates, hydrogen peroxide, sulfuric acid, compressed gas cylinders like oxygen and spray cans, UV germicidal lamps, and cloths used to clean solvent spills.

Medical waste, also called biomedical waste, is any solid waste generated in the diagnosis, treatment, or immunization of human beings or animals, in research pertaining thereto, or in the production of testing of biologicals. Medical waste includes, but is not limited to, soiled or blood-soaked bandages, discarded surgical gloves, discarded surgical instruments, needles used to draw blood and give injections, cultures, swabs used to inoculate cultures, removed body organs (tonsils, appendixes, limbs), and lancets.

Universal wastes are lower risk hazardous wastes that are generated by a wide variety of people rather than by the industrial businesses that primarily generate other hazardous wastes.

Uncontrolled Substances

It is not recommended to discard drugs in trash bins or flush even small quantities of drugs down the toilet because trace amounts of chemicals have been found in drinking water. Expired drugs may be discarded with the hazardous or medical waste depending on county, state, or federal laws; the strictest law prevails. Incineration may be another option and there are companies licensed to dispose of and incinerate drugs. If state laws permit, it may be possible to use the local hospital's incinerator.

Controlled Substances

If controlled substances are kept in the medical office, recordkeeping, inventory, security and correct disposal methods are all important responsibilities of the medical assistant's job duties.

Most states have return processors (reverse distributors) that pick up controlled substances for disposal. An unofficial list of reverse distributors may be obtained through the Drug Enforcement Agency (DEA). In some situations drugs may be shipped to a disposal site and the medical assistant may obtain DEA Form 41, Inventory of Drugs Surrendered, from the nearest DEA office. Complete the form and have the physician sign it to verify its accuracy. Call the nearest DEA office for instructions prior to using this method because not all offices have facilities for storing and destroying controlled substances. To ship the drugs, use Registered Mail. Drugs may also be personally delivered to an Environmental Protection Agency (EPA) approved incinerator; notify the DEA 14 days in advance. Two responsible individuals from the medical practice must accompany the controlled substances and actually witness their being rendered irretrievable. After they are destroyed, the DEA (or whoever destroyed them) should supply a receipt. File the receipt in a safe place.

Regardless of the procedure followed, all federal, state, and local requirements for the handling of controlled substances and for waste disposal must be followed.

STOP AND THINK CASE SCENARIO

Determine Correct Medication

Scenario: An established patient, Charlie Gutierrez, is seen for an evaluation of a red rash-like dermatitis on both feet. Dr. Practon hands the patient a written prescription. As the patient is leaving the office, Mr. Gutierrez hands you the prescription and asks you what it says. In reading it, the handwritten name of the medication looks like either Lamictal or Lamisil.

Critical Thinking:

1. What would you do to determine the correct medication?

_____

_____

_____

_____

2. What are some preventive measures to help avoid cases of mistaken drug identity?

_____

_____

_____

_____

STOP AND THINK CASE SCENARIO

Determine Food and Drug Allergies

Scenario: An established patient, Sonja Tucker, is seen for an evaluation of severe back and side pain. It is suspected she may be passing a kidney stone, so Dr. Practon orders an intravenous pyelogram, which will require radiographic contrast material. You notice an alert tag on her medical record that states she is allergic to shellfish.

Critical Thinking:

1. What else might the patient also be allergic to?

_____

_____

_____

2. What should you say to Dr. Practon in this situation?

_____

_____

_____

3. Are there additional questions you might ask the patient?

_____

_____

_____

FOCUS ON CERTIFICATION*

CMA Content Summary

- Medical abbreviations
- Facility accreditation
- Controlled substances
- Drug enforcement administration
- Computer database
- Restocking supplies
- Classes of drugs
- Drug forms
- Drug action/uses
- Side effects/adverse effects
- Substance abuse
- Prescriptions
- Maintaining medication records
- Medication disposal

RMA Content Summary

- Medical terms and abbreviations
- Patient instruction
- Documentation of medications
- Chart medication information
- Maintain inventory
- Prescriptions
- Drug Enforcement Administration
- Drug categories
- Routes of administration
- *Physicians' Desk Reference*

CMAS Content Summary

- Medical terminology
- Chart information (paper/computerized)
- Pharmacology concepts

REVIEW EXAM-STYLE QUESTIONS

1. The drug law that mandates drugs be put into five different schedules according to their dangerousness is the:

   a. Harrison Narcotic Act

   b. Volstead Act

   c. Food, Drug, and Cosmetic Act

   d. Controlled Substance Act

   e. Compassionate Use Act

2. The drug law that called for registration of all doctors, pharmacists, and vendors to submit paperwork for all drug transactions is the:

   a. Harrison Narcotic Act

   b. Volstead Act

   c. Food, Drug, and Cosmetic Act

   d. Controlled Substance Act

   e. Compassionate Use Act

This textbook and accompanying Workbook meet the entry-level administrative and general competencies for the CMA outlined by the AAMA Examination Content Outline and Role Delineation Study and for the RMA and CMAS outlined by the AMT Competencies and Examination Specifications (see Competency Grid in Appendix B).

3. The first federal commissioner of narcotics was:

    a. Reverend Charles Brent

    b. Hamilton Wright

    c. Francis Burton Harrison

    d. Andrew Volstead

    e. Harry J. Anslinger

4. Less expensive drugs manufactured with the same chemical formula as the original drug whose patent has expired are called:

    a. brand name drugs

    b. generic drugs

    c. chemical duplicates

    d. pharmaceutical substitutes

    e. Class B drugs

5. A useful reference book that most physicians have in their libraries is the:

    a. *United States Pharmacopeia*

    b. *National Formulary*

    c. *Physicians' Desk Reference*

    d. *Physicians' Desk Reference for Nonprescription Drugs*

    e. word book

6. The administration route for medication placed under the tongue would be called:

    a. sublingual

    b. otic

    c. buccal

    d. transdermal

    e. oral

7. The component of a prescription labeled "signature" is:

    a. the recipe

    b. where the name of the drug or medication goes

    c. where the instructions to the patient are written

    d. where the physician signs his or her name

    e. the directions to the pharmacist

8. When "e-prescribing" a drug:

    a. colored prescription pads are used

    b. tamper-proof prescription pads are used

    c. resistant paper is used

    d. thermocratic ink is used

    e. prescriptions are entered into software applications and transmitted electronically

9. The abbreviation "q. i. d." means:

    a. four times a day

    b. three times a day

    c. two times a day

    d. morning, noon, and night time

    e. every afternoon

10. A pharmaceutical representative is also called a:

    a. sales person

    b. sales representative

    c. pharmacist

    d. detail representative or person

    e. medical representative

11. What device can be used when a patient has difficulty remembering when to take medications?

    a. medication schedule card

    b. drug dispensing container

    c. medication alert bracelet

    d. drug flow sheet

    e. both a and b

12. The following procedure(s) is typically followed when prescribing narcotics:

    a. The physician writes an order for the narcotic on a triplicate prescription form.

    b. The physician writes an order for the narcotic on a regular prescription form.

    c. The physician telephones in the order for the narcotic prescription.

    d. The physician writes the prescription on a "narcotics only" prescription form.

    e. all of the above

13. To educate a patient about possible drug side effects, advise the patient to:

    a. stop taking the medication if a side effect is suspected

    b. throw away the medication if a side effect occurs

    c. call the office if one of the typical symptoms occurs (e.g., dizziness, nausea, headache)

    d. go directly to the emergency room

    e. wait until the next office visit and advise the physician

14. Which of the following statements is correct?

    a. All Schedule I drugs should be kept under lock and key.

    b. All Schedule I and II drugs should be kept under lock and key.

    c. All Schedule I, II, and III drugs should be kept under lock and key.

    d. All Schedule I, II, III, and IV drugs should be kept under lock and key.

    e. All Schedule I, II, III, IV, and V drugs should be kept under lock and key.

15. Uncontrolled substances may be discarded by:

    a. throwing them in a waste receptacle

    b. flushing them down the toilet

    c. discarding them with hazardous medical waste

    d. contacting a reverse distributor for pick up

    e. shipping them to the DEA

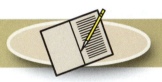

WORKBOOK ASSIGNMENT

To develop competency-based job skills, refer to the *Workbook* and complete the:

- Abbreviation and Spelling Review
- Review Questions

- Critical Thinking Exercises
- Job Skill activities, which are outlined at the beginning of this chapter under "Performance Objective in the *Workbook*."

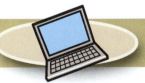

COMPUTER ASSIGNMENT

To review the concepts you have learned in this chapter, insert the *Student Practice* CD-ROM into a computer and work through the *StudyWARE* activities and games. Answer review questions in the practice mode and read the feedback, studying the questions you have missed. Take the chapter quiz until you acheive a minimum score of 90 percent. Successfully completing the *Critical Thinking Challenge* at the end of this course will help you think through scenarios and develop problem solving skills.

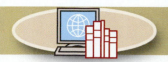

RESOURCES

Books

2007 PDR® Nurse's Drug Handbook™
George R. Spratto, Adrienne L. Woods (published annually)
Delmar Cengage Learning
Executive Woods
5 Maxwell Drive
Clifton Park, NY 12065-2919
(800) 347-7707

Physicians' Desk Reference (published annually)
Thomson Healthcare
Montvale, NJ 07645-1742
(800) 432-4570

Physicians' Desk Reference for Nonprescription Drugs (published annually)
Thomson Healthcare
Montvale, NJ 07645-1742
(800) 432-4570

Saunders Pharmaceutical Word Book (published annually)
Drake and Drake
Elsevier Science
6277 Sea Harbor Drive
Orlando, FL 32821-9989
(800) 545-2522

Internet

To obtain information on drugs, including newly approved drugs and developments in drug therapy, the following Web sites may be useful:

Be Med Wise®—information on nonprescription products with quiz
Web site: http://www.bemedwise.org

Directory of Prescription Drug Patient Assistance Programs—Click on the Patient Assistance Programs link.
Web site: http://www.phrma.org

Drug Enforcement Agency—Drug information
Web site : http://www.usdoj.gov/dea

Drugs.com™—Pill identifier
Web site: http://www.drugs.com

Food and Drug Administration—Click on "Information for Consumers" for an alphabetized index, which includes A = anthrax, B = buying medicine online, C = cancer/cellular phones, and so forth.
Web site: http://www.fda.gov

Institute for Safe Medication Practices—
Confused drug names
High-Alert Medications
Error-Prone abbreviations, symbols, and dose designations
Web site: http://www.ismp.org

The Medical Letter—Critical appraisals of new drugs, comparative reviews of older drugs
Web site: http://www.medletter.com

National Council on Patient Information and Education (NCPIE)
Web site: http://www.talkaboutrx.org

Personal Injury Lawyer America—Drug recalls
Web site : http://personalinjurylawyeramerica.com/medical/drugs.htm

The Prescriber's Letter—New developments in drug therapy
Web site: http://www.prescribersletter.com

UNIT 4

Written Communications

CHAPTER 11

Written Correspondence

OBJECTIVES

After reading this chapter and learning step-by-step procedures to gain job skills,* you should be able to:

Learning Objectives

Name office equipment used in written communications.

Identify ergonomic factors that affect the medical assistant's work environment.

State various functions word processing software can perform.

Describe different letter formats and punctuation styles.

List the parts of a letter.

Assemble reference materials that aid in writing effective letters.

Identify types of memos and describe proper format.

Demonstrate proper editing and proofreading techniques.

Operate a photocopy machine and state solutions to common copier problems.

Performance Objectives (Procedures) in This Textbook

Work at a computer station and comply with ergonomic standards (Procedure 11-1).

Compose, format, key, proofread, and print business correspondence (Procedure 11-2).

Proofread a business document (Procedure 11-3).

Transcribe a dictated document (Procedure 11-4).

Prepare documents for photocopying (Procedure 11-5).

Performance Objectives (Job Skills) in the *Workbook*

Spell medical words (Job Skill 11-1).

Key a letter of withdrawal (Job Skill 11-2).

*This textbook and the accompanying Workbook *meet the educational components for entry-level administrative and general competencies outlined by CAAHEP and ABHES.*

■ Edit written communication (Job Skill 11-3).

■ Compose and key a letter for a failed appointment (Job Skill 11-4).

■ Compose and key a letter for an initial visit (Job Skill 11-5).

■ Compose and key a letter to another physician (Job Skill 11-6).

■ Compose and key a letter requesting payment (Job Skill 11-7).

■ Key an interoffice memoranda (Job Skill 11-8).

■ Key memoranda from handwritten notes (Job Skill 11-9).

■ Abstract information from a medical record, compose, and key a letter (Job Skill 11-10).

■ Key a two-page letter (Job Skill 11-11).

OUTLINE   WITH LECTURE NOTES

Written Communication
Equipment Used for Written Correspondence

_____

_____

_____

Letter Standards, Styles, and Components
Letter Styles

_____

_____

_____

Parts of a Letter

_____

_____

_____

_____

Composing Letters
Reference Material

_____

_____

_____

Outline and Tone

_____

_____

_____

_____

Introduction, Body, and Closing

_____

_____

_____

Characteristics of a Letter

_____

_____

_____

_____

Sample Letters

_____

_____

_____

Types of Letters

_____

_____

_____

_____

Corrections in Business Correspondence
Text-Editing Features

_____

_____

_____

Envelope Enclosures
Folding Enclosures

_____

_____

Medical Transcription

Transcription Procedures and Equipment

_____

_____

_____

Photocopying Procedures

_____

_____

Multifunction Devices

_____

_____

_____

Photocopy Machine

_____

_____

_____

KEY TERMS

edit
elite (E) type
ergonomics
form letter
full block letter style
interoffice memorandum
mixed punctuation
modified block letter style
open punctuation

photocopy
photocopy machine
pica (P) type
proofreading
simplified letter style
thesaurus
transcriptionist
word processing
word processing log

HEART OF THE HEALTH CARE PROFESSIONAL

Service

Communicating in written form is a special talent, and written words said "just right" can set the mood to induce positive action. Patients appreciate a goodwill message, short note, or comment directed personally. Developing written communication skills will help you serve patients' needs.

WRITTEN COMMUNICATION

Letter writing was the primary mode of personal and business communication before the onset of newspapers, telegrams, telephones, fax, and e-mail. At that time, many people maintained diaries, journals, and personal letter records. Today, because it is fast and convenient, most correspondence is via fax or e-mail.

There are times, however, when only professionally typed correspondence on business letterhead can convey the desired message and tone. If letters of an official or legal nature must be sent by fax or e-mail, the original should always be prepared on letterhead with original signatures and also sent via mail.

Equipment Used for Written Correspondence

Handling medical communications requires composing written materials that clearly transmit the physician's ideas and office policy. It also requires expertise in operating computer equipment and a variety of business machines. Responsibilities assigned to the medical assistant involve composing and keying or typing routine letters, transcribing medical data, duplicating directives, and generating financial reports. Professionally written and accurately keyed office communications are indications of an orderly, well-run professional office.

Computer Equipment

Computer software is programmed to permanently store data on the hard drive, which can be duplicated and transferred to other data-storing media, such as floppy disks, Zip disks, CDs, or flash drives. In fact, technological advances are moving us toward a paperless society. Computer equipment is becoming more reasonably priced so medical offices that previously could not afford to be computerized are now jumping into the electronic age.

Ergonomics—Many companies design office systems to meet the needs of the human body, and this science is known as **ergonomics** (Figure 11-1). When the medical assistant works at a computer in one

Sitting Diagram

This is the general diagram of the recommended sitting posture for computer users. Keep in mind that fixed postures contribute to the risk of cumulative trauma injury. Variety of posture is crucial, as is the habit of standing up often. The body needs movement. Nothing counts more than comfort, and this illustration is simply a tool to understand what is happening in your body at the computer. Keep these principles in mind as you develop a repertoire of comfortable postures to use throughout the workday, knowing that slumped and leaning postures demand more work from the body and lead to early fatigue.

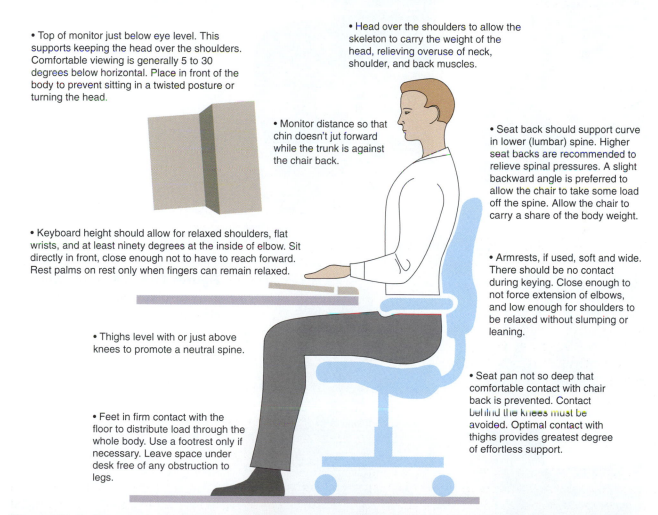

• Top of monitor just below eye level. This supports keeping the head over the shoulders. Comfortable viewing is generally 5 to 30 degrees below horizontal. Place in front of the body to prevent sitting in a twisted posture or turning the head.

• Head over the shoulders to allow the skeleton to carry the weight of the head, relieving overuse of neck, shoulder, and back muscles.

• Monitor distance so that chin doesn't jut forward while the trunk is against the chair back.

• Seat back should support curve in lower (lumbar) spine. Higher seat backs are recommended to relieve spinal pressures. A slight backward angle is preferred to allow the chair to take some load off the spine. Allow the chair to carry a share of the body weight.

• Keyboard height should allow for relaxed shoulders, flat wrists, and at least ninety degrees at the inside of elbow. Sit directly in front, close enough not to have to reach forward. Rest palms on rest only when fingers can remain relaxed.

• Armrests, if used, soft and wide. There should be no contact during keying. Close enough to not force extension of elbows, and low enough for shoulders to be relaxed without slumping or leaning.

• Thighs level with or just above knees to promote a neutral spine.

• Seat pan not so deep that comfortable contact with chair back is prevented. Contact behind the knees must be avoided. Optimal contact with thighs provides greatest degree of effortless support.

• Feet in firm contact with the floor to distribute load through the whole body. Use a footrest only if necessary. Leave space under desk free of any obstruction to legs.

Figure 11-1. Ergonomic workstation illustrating possible adjustments for proper computer-operator position to avoid injury and strain to the body. (Courtesy of Gary Karp, Ergonomics Consultant, Onsight Technology Education Services, San Francisco, CA.)

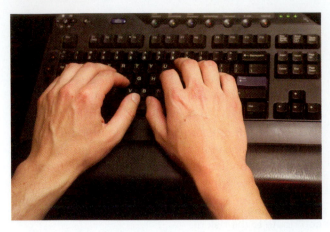

Figure 11-2. Keyboard with built-in wrist support

position hour after hour performing repetitive movements, injuries can occur. These problems are known as cumulative trauma disorders (CTDs) or repetitive stress injuries (RSIs). It is important that the computer keyboard have wrist support (Figure 11-2). Other office tasks may require bending and carrying heavy objects. Figures 11-3 and 11-4 illustrate the correct methods to execute these movements to avoid strain and injury to the body.

Electronic Typewriter

Although most offices use computers, the office may also be equipped with an electronic typewriter.

Typing elements for electronic typewriters are available in a variety of type styles, but the two most

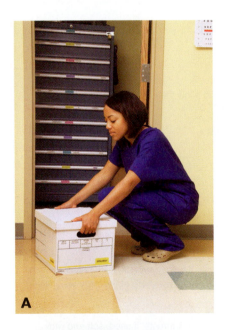
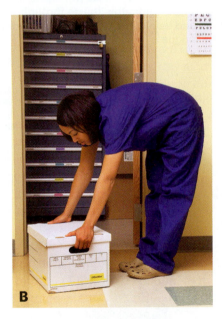

Figures 11-3 A & B. (A) Always bend from the hips and knees. (B) Never bend from the waist.

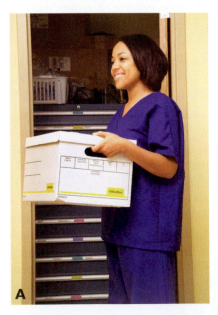
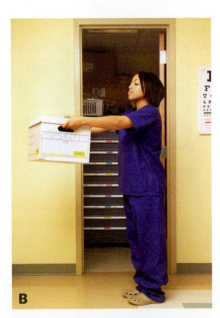

Figures 11-4 A & B. (A) When carrying heavy objects, hold them close to the body. (B) Never carry heavy objects out in front of your body.

traditional styles are **pica (P)** and **elite (E)**. If the typewriter is dual-pitch, the typing element can be changed at the touch of a switch from pica type with 10 characters to the horizontal inch to elite type with 12 characters to the horizontal inch. Correspondence might appear more professional when set with the elite type, while reports with numbers might be done on the larger pica type. Most electronic typewriters with memory capabilities and a screen (monitor) use a single microfloppy disk (three inch) for storing information for retrieval. It is important to note that manufacturers usually produce their own disks, which cannot be read on other manufacturers' machines. Offices with computer systems may also have electronic typewriters for the completion of forms.

Word Processing Software

Word processing is an automated communication system that uses computer memory with specific software installed to produce a variety of documents. Refer to Figure 11-5 for an illustration of some word processing software features, such as margin controls, centering text, indentions, and boldface.

Word processing systems increase secretarial productivity and lower office costs.

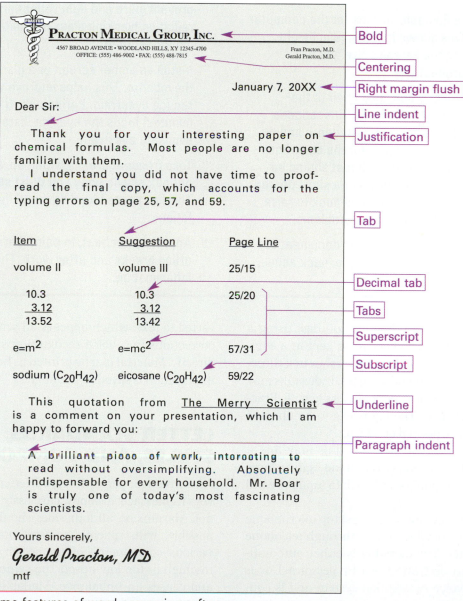

Figure 11-5. Some features of word processing software

PROCEDURE 11-1

Work at a Computer Station and Comply with Ergonomic Standards

Objective: To avoid on-the-job injuries while using a computer by instituting ergonomic principles.

Equipment/Supplies: Computer terminal with monitor, keyboard, wrist support, office chair, footrest, ergonomic mouse or trackball, and copyholder.

Directions: Follow these step-by-step procedures, which include rationales, to practice this skill. This may be done at home or in the classroom.

1. Select an adjustable surface for the computer to sit on. This allows for change in height according to the person's size and will increase productivity.

2. Adjust a properly designed chair to the individual's height and build. This reduces fatigue and tension. Both seat depth and tilt, as well as lumbar support for the chair back should be considered. Both feet should be able to be flat on the floor. For a short person, a small footstool or telephone book to raise the feet will help avoid back problems.

3. Use a copyholder to place the document at eye level. This prevents fatigue, neck aches, backaches, and eyestrain.

4. Place the computer keyboard low so the arms relax comfortably. Forearms should be parallel to the floor and wrists kept straight to prevent frozen shoulders and carpal tunnel syndrome. Installation of a hand and wrist support is also useful.

5. Place the computer monitor at or below eye level. It should be approximately 18 to 24 inches from the eyes; charts and written material should be 15 to 20 inches.

6. Eliminate low-frequency radiation and prevent glare and light reflection by installing radiation blocking glass or plastic over the monitor screen.

7. Install an amber screen or a glare guard over the monitor. This helps improve vision and reduce eyestrain. Periodically (i.e., every 10 minutes) focus the eyes on distant objects to eliminate eyestrain.

8. Take frequent breaks, stand up, and periodically do body and wrist stretches. This increases blood flow and decreases fatigue.

9. Apply ice, not heat, to painful areas during office breaks and after work. This prevents inflammation.

Stored documents can be saved on disk using a **word processing log**. The log can be kept in a computer file labeled "Practice Form Letters" or in a three-ring notebook containing hard copies. Index tabs may be used to locate specific types of letters (e.g., F. Practon Collection Letters). The log needs to be updated each time items are deleted or added.

Large medical groups and hospitals may find it economically advantageous to combine high-volume transcription and typing tasks in a data input or word processing center.

The physician dictates into a desktop microphone attached to a to a portable unit, or through telephone lines to the center. The dictation is either automatically recorded to be transcribed by personnel or is received into a voice recognition system and is con-

verted to text, which appears on screen. Editing and corrections in a voice recognition system are keyed directly. Material can be printed as hard copy, and the information is saved in memory.

LETTER STANDARDS, STYLES, AND COMPONENTS

An attractive, perfectly typed letter effectively conveys its message; a sloppy, carelessly keyed letter does not. Margins on all four sides should be as equal as possible, with spacing adjustments made between various components of the letter. Material placed too high or too low upsets the symmetry of the page and causes an imbalance. Mailability standards for

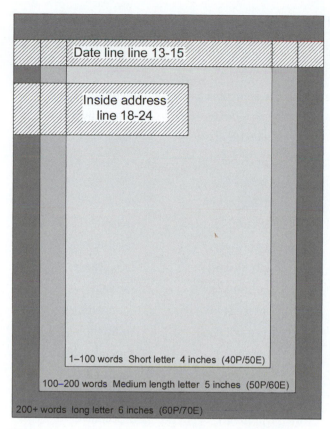

Date line line 13-15

Inside address
line 18-24

1–100 words Short letter 4 inches (40P/50E)

100–200 words Medium length letter 5 inches (50P/60E)

200+ words long letter 6 inches (60P/70E)

Figure 11-6. Reduced version of a visual guide used for letter placement. Word processing software defaults to margins indicated by the dark grey screen. (P = pica, E = elite)

a keyed communication require a perfect letter with balanced margins (Figure 11-6) and without grammatical or keyed errors. An unmailable letter is one with an uncorrectable error, a poor correction, or a grammatical mistake. A letter should not be mailed if it has any one of the following:

1. Misspelled word

2. Word incorrectly divided at the end of the line

3. Keyed error or a poorly corrected error

4. Unbalanced margins; any of the four

5. Special lines omitted, such as a date line or a signature line

6. City name abbreviated, such as "L.A." for "Los Angeles" or "N.Y." for "New York City"

Study the words listed in Table 11-1, which are some of the most commonly misspelled words in medical office correspondence.

Letter Styles

The most common letter styles are (1) **full block style**, which has all lines aligned at the left margin and adapts best to computerized preparation, as shown in Figure 11-7; (2) **modified block format**, which has the date and closing lines beginning at the center of the page, as shown in Figure 11-8 (note: this figure also labels the parts of a letter); and (3) impersonal **simplified style** (of the Administrative Management Society), which eliminates both the salutation and the complimentary close and includes a subject line typed in all capital letters a triple line space after the inside address. In the simplified format, reference initials and notations are keyed in lowercase, two lines below the signature line, as in other styles. The simplified style is rarely used by physicians, because it is too impersonal. It is used in situations in which form letters are sent in the corporate setting. The physician's preference determines the letter style used in a particular office.

Letter Punctuation Styles

Letters have two types of punctuation styles—open punctuation and mixed punctuation. **Open punctuation** is a style in which no punctuation mark is used after the salutation or complimentary close, as shown in Figure 11-8. **Mixed punctuation** is a style in which a colon or a comma is used after the salutation and complimentary close, as shown in Figure 11-7.

Margins

Right and left margins may be changed according to whether a letter is short or long. Most of the time the default (preset) feature of the word processing program is used to keep side margins of letters consistent in dimension (Figure 11-9). This default is usually set at 1 or 1.25 inches and is ideal for long letters. Side margins for short letters might be increased in width and set at two inches.

Defaults are also in place for top and bottom margins, usually set at one inch. If there is a second page to the letter, the bottom margin of the first page can be increased up to two inches (12 lines) so that material can be better spaced on the additional page.

Word processing programs also have a justification feature, which automatically justify both margins while keying, if desired. *Justify* means to space words on each line of text so that the ends of the lines are flush at the right and left margins.

Table 11-1. Words Commonly Misspelled in Medical Office Correspondence

abnormally	consensus	inadvertently	particular	reiterated
abrupt	convalescent	incision	penicillin	repetition
abscess	cough	indispensable	permissible	reviewed
absorbent	cycle	infectious	perseverance	rheumatism
acceptable	deficiency	inoculate	persistent	rhythm
accessible	definitely	insomnia	personal	schedule
accidentally	delinquent	interfered	personnel	seizure
accommodation	demise	intermittent	perspiration	senility
acknowledgment	described	interpret	pharmaceutical	separate
acuity	diagnosis (sing.)	irritated	pharmacy	severity
administration	diagnoses (plur.)	jeopardize	physician	significance
admissible	diaphragm	judgment	precaution	specialist
admittance	diarrhea	labeling	precede	successful
affect (influence)	disappointed	laboratory	prescription	sufficient
alcohol	disease(s)	liquefy	prevalent	superintendent
analysis	effect (result) (noun)	markedly	principal (chief)	supersede
analyze	eligible	muscle	principle (rule)	surgeon
appointment	evidence	necessary	probably	susceptible
bandage	exertion	ninety	procedure	suture
behavior	existence	noticeable	profession	symptom
beneficial	experience	nourishment	prognosis	technique
benefited	explanation	observation	pursue	temperature
brochure	facility	occasionally	quantity	thorough
cancel	fracture	occurrence	receiving	transferred
canceled	height	occurring	recognize	unconscious
capsule	hemorrhage	omission	recommend	urinalysis
carcinoma	hygiene	omitted	recovery	vaccine
cartilage	illegible	opinion	recurrence	visible
comparative	immediately	opportunity	referral	vitamin
conscious	immunity	paralyzed	referring	weight

Parts of a Letter

Refer to the following letter parts in Figure 11-8.

Letterhead (1)

Letterhead lines are designed in an attractive format and are positioned in the upper two inches of a sheet of bond paper. They generally include the medical practice name, physician's name and title, address, telephone number, fax number, and possibly e-mail address (Example 11-1). They should be engraved or

EXAMPLE 11-1

Letterhead Format

PRACTON MEDICAL GROUP, INC.

4567 Broad Avenue

Woodland Hills, XY 12345-4700

Office: (555) 486-9002—Fax: (555) 488-7815

Fran Practon, M.D. • Gerald Practon, M.D.

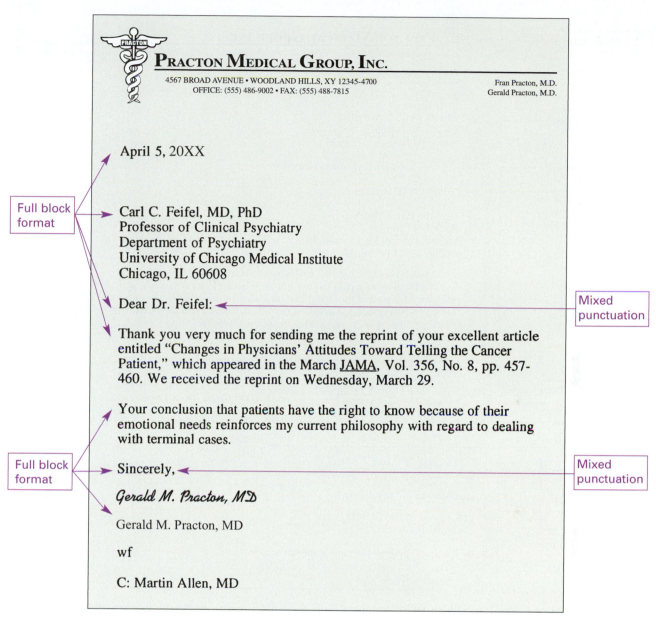

Figure 11-7. Letter in full block style with mixed punctuation

printed on a type of bond paper that has a crisp surface and is receptive to both ink and printed copy. The return address on the envelope may match the letterhead format in miniature. Plain or printed bond paper is used for continuation sheets.

Date Line (2)

The date line is keyed 13 or 14 line spaces from the top of the paper or 3 spaces below the letterhead, depending somewhat on the size and position of the letterhead. Do not abbreviate the month or show the date in numbers only (e.g., 1/28/XX). Example 11-2 shows acceptable date line formats.

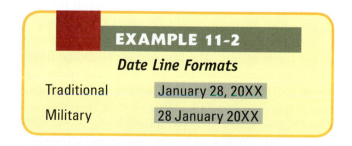

EXAMPLE 11-2

Date Line Formats

Traditional	January 28, 20XX
Military	28 January 20XX

Inside Address (3)

The inside address consists of the name and address of the individual, the firm, or the medical facility that the letter is being sent to, and may include the correspon-

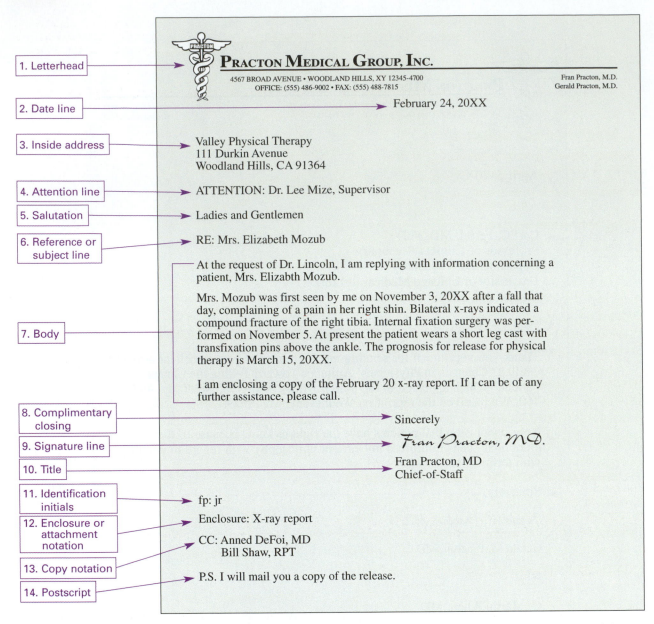

Figure 11-8. Letter in modified block style (numbers 2, 8, 9, and 10) with open punctuation and special notations for various parts of a letter

dent's title, position, department, or office. It is keyed exactly as it appears on the recipient's letterhead or return address, beginning four to eight line spaces below the date line. The first line includes the name of the addressee. Never use "Dr." before the name of a physician; instead use "M.D." after the name. The position and firm or institution name follow; then the post office box number or street number and name; and last, the city (always spelled in full), state (using two-letter standard abbreviations), and five- or nine-digit ZIP code. If the letter is being sent to a foreign country, the name of that country is keyed in all capital letters as the last line of the address. The inside address

of a letter and the envelope address usually match in style and format. Example 11-3 shows acceptable formats for the inside address.

Attention Line (4)

The attention line is used when the correspondence is addressed to an organization or to a particular person within the organization (Example 11-4). It usually precedes the salutation, starting at the left margin and a double line space below the last line of the inside address. Unless it is absolutely necessary, the use of the attention line should be avoided and the

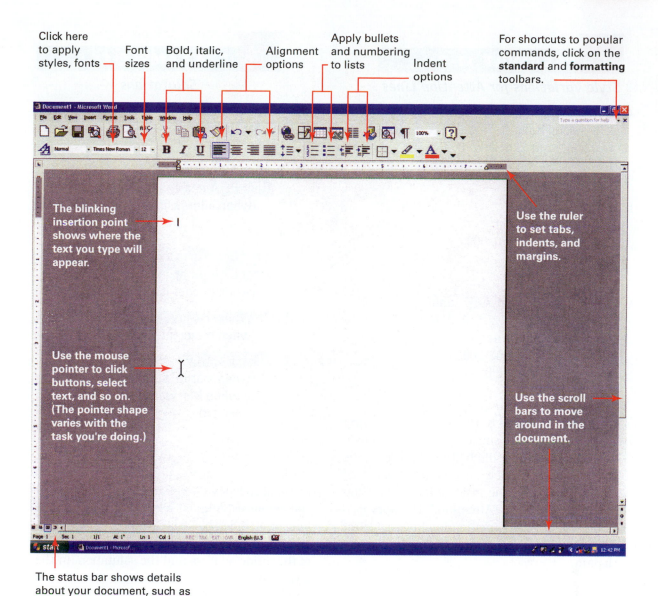

Figure 11-9. Computer screen showing format features of a word processing program. The blinking insertion point shows where the left margin is set.

EXAMPLE 11-3

Inside Address Formats

A. Dr. Benjamin Wong
Chief of Staff
Memorial Hospital
2211 East Eighth Avenue
Indianapolis, IN 46205-0000

B. Lillian Frank, M.D.
126 North Bender Road, Suite B
Miami, FL 33136-2021

C. James Mozby, D.D.S.
P.O. Box 2338
Toledo, OH 43503-0000

D. Guy DePetridiantonio, M.D.
14017 Via Vento
Rome 4LI 7523
ITALY

EXAMPLE 11-4

Style Variations for Attention Lines

A. Carter Laboratory
198 Upjohn Road
Mission, Kansas 66202-0000
ATTENTION: MEDICAL DIVISION
Dear Sir or Madam:

B. United Pharmacy
198 260 Main Street
Somerset, NJ 40001-000
Attn: Ann Talbot
Dear Ms. Talbot:

C. Attention: Art West, M.D., and
Jean Coe, M.D.
One North 14th Street
Las Vegas, NV 89102-0000
Dear Drs. West and Coe:

EXAMPLE 11-5

Salutations

A. **Open Punctuation**
Dear Dr. McGuirer
Dear Doctors

B. **Mixed Punctuation**
Dear Dr. Ames and Dr. Rulfo:
(when addressing two physicians)

or

C. Dear Drs. Ames and Rulfo:
Dear Sir or Madam:
(when gender is unknown)

D. To Whom It May Concern:
(when recipient is unknown)

E. Dear Ms. Troy:
(when marital status is unknown
or when Ms. was used on letter
received)

letter should be addressed to the person(s) receiving it. The U.S. Postal Service suggests that on the envelope the attention line should be the first line of the address, and for consistency, it would then be placed in the same position in the inside address. A colon is optional after the word "Attention." The appropriate salutation to use with an attention line in a letter addressed to a company or a medical facility is "Dear Sir or Madam."

Salutation (5)

The salutation, or greeting, is placed a double line space below the last line of the inside address or a double line space below the attention line. In *open punctuation*, there is no punctuation after the salutation. In *mixed punctuation*, the salutation is followed by a colon (Example 11-5). "Ms." is used when a woman's title is not known or as a substitute for "Miss" or "Mrs." Many professional women either do not like to have a title or prefer Ms. The best clue is what the letter writer uses to identify herself. "Dear Madam or Sir" is used when it is not known whether the addressee is a man or a woman.

Reference or Subject Line (6)

The reference or subject line draws the reader's attention to a subject or, in medical correspondence, to a patient's name or account number. It is customarily positioned a double line space after the salutation. In

block style, it is always positioned at the left margin; in modified block style, it may be centered or, for special emphasis, aligned with the left edge of the date line. In modified block style, another placement variation is to type the subject line between the last line of the inside address and the salutation, in the same style and position as the attention line. An attention line and a subject line can be keyed in the same style if both appear in a letter (Example 11-6).

Body (7)

The body of the letter contains the message to be conveyed to the recipient, and it should begin two lines below the salutation or two lines after the reference or subject line if there is one. In block style, all paragraphs begin at the left margin. Paragraphs are single-spaced internally, with double-spacing separating the paragraphs. Extremely short letters can be double-spaced with indented paragraphs.

Complimentary Close (8)

At the conclusion of a letter, one to three complimentary words are typed a double line space below the last line of the body of the letter, indicating that the sender has concluded the message; only the first letter is capitalized (Example 11-7). The closing line is fol-

---

EXAMPLE 11-6

Reference or Subject Lines

A. **Block Style**
Dear Dr. McMurtry:
RE: Faith Upton

B. **Modified Block Style**
Dear Miss Allison:
Refer to: Policy No. 5682

or

C. Dear Dr. Arthur:
SUBJECT: AMA Meeting

D. ABC Laboratory
2340 Main Street
Any City 50201-6912
Dear Madam or Sir:
Re: Nancy Smith, Office Manager

---

lowed by a comma if a colon has been used after the salutation in keeping with the *mixed punctuation* format; in *open punctuation*, no punctuation follows the closing.

EXAMPLE 11-7

Complimentary Close Phrases

A. **Mixed Punctuation**
Sincerely,

B. **Open Punctuation**
Cordially

Signature Line (9)

The signature line includes the first and last names of the person responsible for writing the letter and his or her credential (e.g., MD). It is keyed three to five line spaces below the complimentary close to allow space for the handwritten signature. The space may be reduced or increased to improve letter placement. The signature line uses complete names rather than initials so the reader can determine the title to use in response. Thus, a male medical assistant always spells out his first name to enable the correspondent to address a reply to "Mr." A female includes a cour-

---

EXAMPLE 11-8

Signature Lines

A. *John D. Carter, MD*
John D. Carter, MD
Chief of Surgery

B. *(Ms.) Kim Hall*
Kim Hall, CMT

C. *Roberta Avila, MD*
Roberta Avila, MD, PhD
Director, Medical Research

D. *Bryon Avery*
Bryon Avery

E. *(Mrs.) Sally Hartman-Fox*
Sally Hartman-Fox, CMA-A
Office Manager

F. *(Mrs.) Marsha Cole*
Marsha Cole
Secretary to Dr. Blake

---

tesy title (e.g., "Miss," "Mrs.," or "Ms.") enclosed in parentheses in her handwritten signature. Example 11-8 shows variations in signature lines.

Title Line (10)

A business or professional title associated with the person who has written the letter is keyed on the line below the signature line or immediately after the signature and preceded by a comma. Title lines are highlighted in Example 11-9.

EXAMPLE 11-9

Title Lines

A. Marilyn Smythe, DDS
Chairman, Dental Department

B. Robert Belasco, MD, Administrator

Identification or Reference Initials (11)

Identification initials to distinguish the writer and the person who has keyed the letter are inserted a double line space below the signature or title lines (Exam-

EXAMPLE 11-10

Dictator (Writer) and Typist's Reference Initials

A. Dg   [typist]

B. ABJ   [typist]

C. RBCJr:lm   [dictator and typist]

D. MF:CFP   [dictator and typist]

E. KL/me   [dictator and typist]

ple 11-10). If both the writer's initials and the initials of the person who keyed the letter appear, include a colon or slash in between. The trend is to omit the dictator's initials if the name has been keyed in the signature block or if it appears in the letterhead. (The assistant should be careful to avoid humorous or confusing three-letter combinations.)

The fact that a letter is dictated or written by someone other than the person who signs it is indicated by the writer's name or initials followed by the typist's initials (rather than the signer's and the typist's). Example 11-11 shows two ways to identify the person who wrote the letter.

EXAMPLE 11-11

Writer's Identification Initials and Typist's Reference Initials

A. *James B. Moore, MD*
James B. Moore, MD
MHJ:bt

B. *Mary T. Washington, MD*
Mary T. Washington, MD
ATMcGuire/lw

Enclosure or Attachment Notation (12)

The enclosure notation is a courtesy to the correspondent to affirm that separate material is enclosed with the letter. The word "enclosure" or an abbreviation is keyed either a single or double line space below the identification initials. It is appropriate to list the enclosures or particular attachments when several items

are included. When an enclosure is large or bulky, it may be best to indicate that the enclosure will be sent separately. (See Example 11-12.)

EXAMPLE 11-12

Enclosure or Attachment Notations

A. Attachments (2)

B. Enclosures 2

C. Enc.

D. 2 encls.

E. 1 Enclosure

F. Enclosures: Pathology report
                    Operation schedule

G. Check enclosed

H. Enclosure–Software

I. Enclosure sent separately

Copy Notations (13)

When several copies have been made to be mailed to people other than the person whose name appears on the inside address, a copy notation is keyed at the bottom of the letter (a single or double line space below the enclosure notation) to indicate the names of the people who have received a copy. "Copy," "CC," or "C" indicates that courtesy copies have been mailed or made for distribution to the named people; names or initials are given in alphabetic order (see Example 11-13). Never key a copy notation without a name following it.

EXAMPLE 11-13

Copy Notations

A. c: Al Moore

B. bc: Carol Yu, MD

C. Copies to Dr. Alcott
              Dr. Sowell

D. BCC: Hal Ames

E. cc: James More, MD
        Carolyn Shaw, RPT

The notation "bcc," "bc," or "BCC" is used for *blind* copies, when the writer sends a copy of the correspondence to a third party without the knowledge of the person receiving the original letter. For blind copies, do not make a copy notation on the original, but make a notation on the file copy with the name of the recipient following it. Mark a photocopy of the original letter with "bcc" to indicate that a blind copy was sent. When letters are done on a word processor or computer, copies can be made automatically by instructing the printer to print as many as are needed.

Postscript (14)

A postscript is an afterthought or a statement made for emphasis (Example 11-14). It is keyed a double line space below the last keyed line and may be preceded by "P.S.," if desired.

EXAMPLE 11-14

Postscripts

A. P.S. Don't forget the Thursday AMA meeting! [Reiteration]

B. P.S. I spoke to the hospital electrician who said that nine plugs will be adequate. [Afterthought]

COMPOSING LETTERS

A medical assistant who can independently compose letters for the physician possesses a skill that is an asset to the practice. Letter-writing tasks often involve the abstraction of medical data from patients' charts in reply to requests for information. Letters written over the assistant's signature will deal with patient appointments, insurance, and routine business matters. Letters written by the assistant for the physician's signature will usually concern medical matters and should emulate as much as possible his or her usual degree of formality and professional style.

Reference Material

Useful references for letter writing include an English grammar reference book for punctuation and correct use of grammar, a medical dictionary for spelling and definitions, a secretarial manual for style and format, and a thesaurus. A **thesaurus** ("treasury" in Greek) is an alphabetic listing of synonyms and antonyms used to find alternative words to express the same or opposite ideas. It is a useful tool for preventing words in letters from sounding repetitious. These reference materials are available in printed form, as part of word processing software programs and via the Internet (See Resources). A reference folder of well-written sample phrases, paragraphs, or letters can be assembled to save time and effort when similar letters are being prepared.

Outline and Tone

Before beginning to outline the content of a letter, the assistant should try to visualize the person receiving the correspondence and anticipate what the recipient needs or wants to know. Picture the reader and ask, "What would I say if the person was on the telephone or across the desk?" Proceed to write the letter as though talking with the recipient, using conversational language when writing to a familiar person. More reserved language may be used when writing to an unknown recipient. The trend when writing business letters is to use a personalized approach. Eliminate the use of formal words or artificially worded phrases, and keep the number of words to a minimum, which will increase clearness and avoid the possibility of overwhelming the reader with more words than are needed. Simplicity, clarity, and conciseness are basic standards for every medical communication.

Use gender-neutral terms in business correspondence to avoid offending the recipient. Careful proofreading prevents the embarrassment of discovering a spelling or punctuation error in the letter's text or a misspelling of the recipient's name after the original letter has left the office. Medical correspondence deals primarily with routine matters, and letters of two or three paragraphs cover most subjects.

Introduction, Body, and Closing

The first paragraph of a letter should be positive in tone and deal immediately with the subject matter in a friendly and courteous manner. It should include a personal comment and an expression of interest in the patient or his or her health problem. Thoughts are presented in logical order in the body of the letter with sentences averaging no more than 20 words. A concise and courteous closing statement includes some reference to an action to be taken by the recipient. Thanks are expressed if a service has been rendered or a response expected; otherwise, the assistant waits until the request has been fulfilled before following up with an acknowledgment.

Characteristics of a Letter

All correspondence should be answered promptly—within 24 hours if possible. If there is a delay, the letter, when it is written, should include a tactful explanation. A well-written letter has the following characteristics:

1. It creates a favorable impression by arousing the reader's interest with the first sentence.

2. It appeals to the reader's point of view and avoids the use of the pronoun "I."

3. It is correct in every grammatical detail.

4. It is courteous, friendly, and sincere—promoting goodwill.

5. It is accurate, clear, concise, and complete.

6. It flows smoothly from paragraph to paragraph and concludes by telling the reader how to respond.

7. It avoids jargon and stilted phrases such as "please be advised," "as per," "enclosed please find," "in re," "under separate cover," and "attached hereto." It also avoids sexism by deleting the role use of "he" or "she."

8. It concludes on a positive note, emphasizing a pleasant closing thought.

Sample Letters

Sample letters for common situations are presented in Examples 11-15 through 11-20. See Chapter 3 for a "Letter of Withdrawal From a Case," "Letter to Confirm Discharge by Patient," and "Letter to Patient who Fails to Keep Appointment." See Chapter 13 for examples of collection letters.

Types of Letters

Basic types of letters used in medical offices include multipage letters, form letters, and interoffice memorandums.

Multipage Letter

When more than one page is needed for written correspondence, a simplified heading is placed at the top of each continuation sheet, using a horizontal or ver-

tical format (see Example 11-21). Continuation pages are keyed on plain bond paper or preprinted second sheets. The heading for all continuation sheets begins on line seven, which leaves a one-inch top margin. The letter is continued on the third line space after the heading. It is best to conclude a paragraph at the bottom of each page, but if this is not possible, at least

---

EXAMPLE 11-15

Outlining Office Visit Fees

Dear Mrs. Chai:

In response to your request for information on fees charged for office visits, Dr. Practon has asked me to send you a range of the customary charges. Fees vary according to the level of history, medical examination, and decision-making process performed by the physician. They are:

Office visit, new patient from $33.25 to $132.28

Office visit, established patient from $16.07 to $96.00

If you have any questions, do not hesitate to call our office for additional information.

EXAMPLE 11-16

Canceling an Appointment

Dear Miss Wooley:

Dr. Practon has asked me to cancel all of her scheduled appointments for the week of Monday, July 3, through Friday, July 7, because of a family emergency necessitating a trip to New Orleans. Therefore, I have canceled your appointment for Wednesday, July 5, at 2:00 p.m. I have been unsuccessful in my attempts to reach you by telephone, so would you please contact this office as soon as possible to schedule another appointment. Dr. Practon regrets any inconvenience this change may have caused you.

EXAMPLE 11-17

Response to a Referral

Dear Dr. Ames:

Thank you for referring your patient, Mrs. Phyllis Green, for consultation. She was examined by me today, and there were no significant symptoms of pulmonary disease. Her episodic asthma seems to be exercise related and should improve with a continuous exercise program.

Her chest x-ray was normal, as were the results of the CBC, BUN, and spirometry. She has a short ejection systolic murmur that does not vary with maneuvers.

My recommendation is that Mrs. Green continue the medication and diet you recommended and that she enroll in a daily supervised exercise program. Please do not hesitate to contact me if you have further questions regarding my findings.

EXAMPLE 11-18

Transferring Care to Another Physician

Dear Dr. Bailey:

This letter confirms my April 7 telephone referral of Marjorie Lowe transferring her to your care.

Mrs. Lowe has been my patient for five years and has experienced increased complaints of coughing and shortness of breath. I am referring Mrs. Lowe to you after a routine office exam and pulmonary function test indicated the possibility of emphysema. I appreciate your receiving Mrs. Lowe as a new patient for this condition, and I will continue to care for her other medical problems.

Her address and telephone number are 12135 Arbor Circle, Kearney, Nebraska 68845, Tel. 555/236-4068.

EXAMPLE 11-19

Letter About a Delinquent Account

Dear Miss Norton:

Two months ago on June 14, you visited our office for a complete physical examination. We have received no payment in response to our billing statements.

We are anxious to hear from you concerning the $250 balance. Please contact this office as soon as possible so we can set up a satisfactory payment plan. Your cooperation in this matter is appreciated.

EXAMPLE 11-20

Request for Information

Dear Sir or Madam:

In your Spring catalog on page 85, you advertised a designer-styled, steel stool with an adjustable seat. Dr. Davis would like to place an order; however, he first would like to know what type of padding is used in the construction of the seat and whether the stool is available with a washable cover.

Your prompt reply to this inquiry is appreciated.

EXAMPLE 11-21

Multipage Letter Headings

A. Leonard J. Warren, MD 2 May 1, 20XX
    (addressee)

B. RE: Lorraine Gonzaga (patient)
        Page 2
        November 19, 20XX

two lines of a paragraph are carried to the continuation sheet. Never use a second page to key only the complimentary close. The last word on a page is never divided, and there must be at least a one-inch bottom margin.

When using a computer, always look at the document in print preview before printing. Check to be sure that the page-two markings appear where they were intended. If transcribing a document that will be printed at another site with no opportunity for you to review the final printout, be sure someone verifies the printer setup and checks the document.

Form Letters

Form letters, also known as *repetitive letters*, are often used when the physician communicates repetitious information, such as notifying the health department of an individual who has contracted a contagious disease or notifying the Department of Motor Vehicles that an individual has developed epilepsy. Additionally, form letters are mailed to patients who fail to keep appointments, who do not follow the medical advice given them, or who need to be advised, with written documentation, of the physician's withdrawal from a case. Contents for some of these are shown in Chapter 3. The assistant must always be aware of the legal implications for the physician inherent in writing any such letter and never diagnose or make any unethical statements about a patient's illness or the prognosis for recovery.

Letters that provide instructions and details of an upcoming hospital stay, that appeal a denied health insurance claim, or that deal with routine collections are also typical instances in which form letters might be used. It is sometimes necessary to follow up a delinquent account with a series of collection letters before turning the matter over to a collection agency: these notices are often form letters. (See Chapter 13).

To save time and to reflect the physician's personality in writing form letters for his or her signature, model form letters should be kept in the reference folder along with frequently used paragraphs or phrases. A preprinted form letter that has been duplicated by a copy process can be personalized by adding a date line, an inside address, and a salutation that includes the patient's name. To make it appear to be an original copy, the medical assistant must use the same font (typestyle). Proper alignment and spacing are important when variable information is inserted into open areas within the body of the letter.

COMPLIANCE

Confidential matters should never be written in memos, because those messages are circulated throughout the office and may be part of permanent or temporary records.

When form letters are done via computer, they can be stored on disks. These letters can be merged with address, salutation, and date information. This is called mail merge. Top-quality form letters can be prepared in a few minutes.

Interoffice Memorandums

Preprinted **interoffice memorandums** (memos), in which no text placement decisions are required, are used by offices, clinics, and hospitals. Memos facilitate the exchange of ideas among individuals and departments within the organization in situations when informal written communication is appropriate. The message, which is casual in tone, should communicate instructions or other messages in a concise, impersonal manner so the reader can easily absorb the information.

Types of memos include the (1) *informative*, which provides facts with explanations; (2) *directive*, which gives brief instructions; and (3) *administrative*, which states policy or judgment on a specific topic.

A special memo format with appropriate guide words used as headings and followed by a colon may be printed on the computer or the headings may be keyed on plain bond paper (Figure 11-10). Some memos are printed on letterhead, but usually the title "Interoffice Memo" or simply "Memo" is sufficient as the heading. Four basic headings for memos are shown in Figure 11-10. When preprinted forms are not available, use either a vertical or horizontal format to type the main heading (Example 11-22).

The vertical style format is popular, easier to set up, and more appropriate when the subject line is lengthy. In the horizontal format, the two headings "TO" and "FROM" are double-spaced flush with the left margin; the "DATE" and "SUBJECT" lines would be placed to the right of the center of the page.

Margins are set at the point where the preprinted guide words begin or at a point two or three spaces after the longest guide word in the left column of the printed headings. Typist's initials, enclosures, and copy notations are single- or double-spaced at the

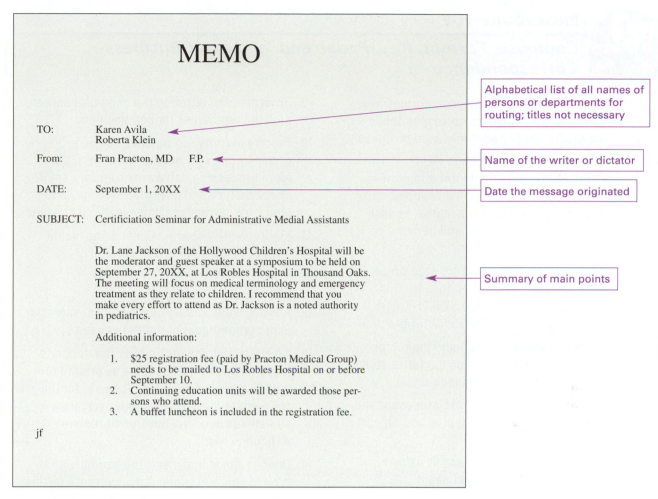

MEMO

TO: Karen Avila
             Roberta Klein

From: Fran Practon, MD   F.P.

DATE: September 1, 20XX

SUBJECT: Certificiation Seminar for Administrative Medial Assistants

             Dr. Lane Jackson of the Hollywood Children's Hospital will be
             the moderator and guest speaker at a symposium to be held on
             September 27, 20XX, at Los Robles Hospital in Thousand Oaks.
             The meeting will focus on medical terminology and emergency
             treatment as they relate to children. I recommend that you
             make every effort to attend as Dr. Jackson is a noted authority
             in pediatrics.

             Additional information:

             1. $25 registration fee (paid by Practon Medical Group)
                 needs to be mailed to Los Robles Hospital on or before
                 September 10.
             2. Continuing education units will be awarded those per-
                 sons who attend.
             3. A buffet luncheon is included in the registration fee.

jf

Callout boxes:
- Alphabetical list of all names of persons or departments for routing; titles not necessary
- Name of the writer or dictator
- Date the message originated
- Summary of main points

Figure 11-10. Preprinted headings on an interoffice memo to medical office personnel

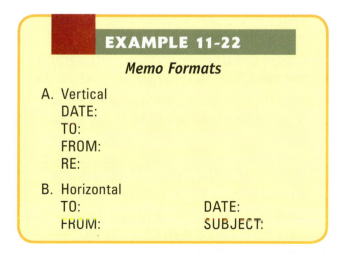

EXAMPLE 11-22

Memo Formats

A. Vertical
   DATE:
   TO:
   FROM:
   RE:

B. Horizontal
   TO: DATE:
   FROM: SUBJECT:

conclusion of the message, just as in any letter. Keying the writer's initials is not required, but it would be done if it is the custom determined by the medical office.

A keyed signature line is typically not used, nor does the author or dictator sign the memo. However, if the writer of the memo prefers to end the memo with a handwritten signature, then key the writer's name or initials on the fourth line below the last line of the message. Or, the writer's initials may be typed at the end of the memo and initialed by the author. If the writer inserts handwritten initials at the end of the memo or next to the typed name in the heading, as in Figure 11-10, omit the signature line altogether. Even if the memo is not signed by the author, it should always be submitted to him or her for approval before being distributed.

When a memo is to be read by several persons (copy routing), the names are listed either in alphabetic order or in order of seniority, with each person initialing his or her name after reading the information. If the memo continues to an additional page or pages, begin one inch from the top of the continuation page and key in headings vertically or horizontally:

PROCEDURE 11-2

Compose, Format, Key, Proofread, and Print Business Correspondence

Objective: To compose, format, key, proofread, and print business correspondence following guidelines of commonly used business-letter style.

Equipment/Supplies: Computer and printer or typewriter; letterhead paper, envelope, attachments (if necessary), thesaurus, English dictionary, medical dictionary, and pen or pencil.

Directions: Follow these step-by-step procedures, which include rationales, to learn this skill, which is presented in Job Skill 11-4, 11-5, 11-6, 11-7 and 11-10 of the *Workbook* for practice.

1. Assemble materials, determine the recipient's address, and decide on the letter style or format (modified or full block style).

2. Turn on the computer or word processor and select the word processing program. Open a blank document.

3. Create and key the letterhead. If using a typewriter insert letterhead paper.

4. Key the *date line* beginning at least three lines below the letterhead, making sure it is in the proper location for the chosen style.

5. Double-space down and insert the *inside address,* making sure it is in the proper location for the chosen style. Select a style to insert an attention line if necessary.

6. Double-space and key the *salutation,* using either open or mixed punctuation. A business letter is more formal than personal correspondence, so the salutation should include a title and the person's last name.

7. Double-space and enter the *reference line* ("Re:" or "Subject:") in the location for the chosen letter style. This helps the recipient identify the contents of the letter before thoroughly reading it.

8. Double-space and key the *body* (content) of the letter in single-space, making sure the paragraph style is proper for the format chosen. Double-space between paragraphs. Save your work to write computer hard drive every 15 minutes.

9. Proofread the letter on the computer screen, or in the typewriter for composition.

10. Proofread for typographical, spelling, grammatical, and mechanical errors. Use the word processing software program's spell-check feature and any reference books to check for correct spelling, meaning, or usage.

11. Key/type the *second page heading* (name, page number, and date) in vertical or horizontal format if a second page is necessary (see Example 11-20).

12. Key a *complimentary close,* making sure it is in the proper location for the chosen style.

13. Go down four spaces and key the *sender's name and title* or credentials as printed on the letterhead. This makes it easier for the recipient to identify the sender, because sometimes handwritten signatures are difficult to read.

14. Double-space and insert the sender's and typist's *reference initials* in lowercase letters, separating the two sets of initials with a colon or slash.

15. Single- or double-space to insert copy ("CC"), *enclosure* ("Enclosure" or "Enc"), or attachment notations.

16. Double-space to insert a *postscript* ("P.S."), if necessary.

17. Save the file before printing a hard copy, and proofread the letter again. Make corrections, if necessary.

18. Print the final copy to be sent, and proofread. Make a copy to be retained in the files so if questions arise, a copy of the letter can be referred to.

19. Save the file to a diskette, Zip disk, CD, or flash drive to be stored for future reference.

20. Prepare an envelope, using the format for optical scanning. If sending the correspondence registered or certified, be sure to place special mailing instructions on the envelope.

21. Clip any attachments to the letter and give to the physician for review and signature.

name of addressee, date, and page number. Triple-space and continue with the body of the memo.

When many memos are to be distributed by the office staff, it might save time to prepare a macro on the computer that can be recalled anytime it is necessary to compose or transcribe information. A *macro* is a group of keystrokes that have been combined, recorded, and assigned a brief name or key combination. By keying the macro, the word, phrase, or sentence automatically appears on the screen.

When electronic mail (e-mail) is used to send memos it is only necessary to insert the names of the recipients with their e-mail addresses and the subject because the date and name will appear as a regular part of the e-mail heading.

Ordinarily, interoffice memorandums delivered by mailroom personnel or office staff are not placed in envelopes. If, however, documents are to be enclosed, a large manila interoffice envelope may be used. It may be addressed using the receiver's name and department with "Internal Mail" keyed in the upper right corner. When interoffice envelopes are used, the sender crosses out the previous name, writes the name of the recipient and date, inserts the memo or items, and then fastens the envelope (without sealing, allowing for reuse).

CORRECTIONS IN BUSINESS CORRESPONDENCE

Corrections occur in business correspondence in spelling, word division, spacing, punctuation, capitalization, grammar, use of figures and symbols, and data input (typographical errors). While keying data, it is common to transpose and alter the sequence of letters and numbers, which changes the spelling of a word or the numeric order. When some type of correction, alteration, or refinement is necessary, these changes are referred to as **edits.** Any editing done to medical records should not change the content or meaning of the physician's dictated report. If questions arise, ask the physician prior to making changes.

Text-Editing Features

Word processing software has the capability to convert partial words to complete words. However, when this occurs, the word should always be checked for correctness. Certain codes or symbols may also be converted to complete words, phrases, sentences,

or paragraphs, expediting the input process. Electronic word processors and computer word processing software have special text-editing features, which include:

- Directional keys, which move the cursor up, down, left, and right

- Function keys, which perform tabulation, delete, and search operations

- Memory functions, which store spelling word lists and frequently used phrases

- Tool features, which flag misspelled words and misused phrases during the keying or scanning of a document; also provide word corrections and synonyms

- Edit features, which search for a page number or a word or phrase in the text and allow optional replacement

- Printing feature, which prints multiple copies of a standard letter and can merge letters with a list of names and addresses

- Format functions, which direct the placement of information in the document (indentation, centering, right and left margin justification); alignment of columns; use of boldface, italicize, and underline; cut and paste feature; insert and remove punctuation; and hyphenate words that go beyond the right margin

Automatic format features may also indicate a certain style, setup, or format. Inadvertent use of the above-mentioned features may result in a printout containing an incorrect format or an inappropriate word, phrase, or entire paragraph.

Proofreading

Proofreading may be done on-screen or while the paper is still in the typewriter and also on hard copy after printing. Careful **proofreading** and correcting of all copy prevents the embarrassment of errors in information presented to patients and associates. Proofreading on-screen is more difficult than scanning the printed page because errors can be easily overlooked. Errors that are not corrected might seriously affect a medical case or research information, so take extra care to find and correct errors when they appear on-screen. Reread final documents because in the process of making corrections using computer software, words may be lost, phrases may be duplicated, new paragraphs may be inserted, or old paragraphs may not be deleted.

Spelling and Grammar Check

Spell check, grammar check, and medical dictionary software programs are available, or may be packaged with a word processing program. These are great assets because these programs can find many types of mistakes. In addition, medical words may be looked up for their definitions or added to the dictionary to personalize it to a medical specialty. Separate software programs may be purchased for medical terms, pharmacology words, laboratory terminology, and so forth. Many of these programs use a marker system to point to problem words. Corrections can be made as the document is being keyed or after it is finished, using the search and replace function to locate words marked automatically (i.e., wavy line) by the software program.

Some grammar checkers allow a choice of six types of writing styles: general, business, technical, fiction, informal, and custom. This gives the operator a tremendous amount of flexibility, so such a program is very useful. It is not perfect, however; one needs to know basic grammar in order to make decisions about proper usage of words. Never rely on a spell or grammar checker to correct the overall document; stop if doubts occur about words and phrases and look them up. Researching these later is *not* a good idea, because they may not be picked up during the spell check and thus be overlooked or forgotten. Software that checks spelling offers tips for improvement, but the corrective action is still the proofreader's responsibility. Remember that spell checkers do not check for correct *use* of a word, so it is imperative that the proofreader be competent in the use of language. Sometimes the spell-check feature may indicate that words or sentences are wrong when they are actually correct. Therefore, do not accept suggested corrections without question. Other times a document may be run through the spell checker and no errors found. However, when manually proofing it, you may find a typographical error (e.g., *do* instead of *to*). Refer to Resources at the end of this chapter for online spelling and grammar help via the Internet.

Cut and Paste Features

Cut and paste features allow the operator to remove words or sections of text and rearrange by putting the removed (cut) item in another place. When using this editing feature it is easy to make mistakes while inserting or rearranging words or paragraphs. For example, you can end up with a missing subject or verb, or have a paragraph or word appear in the wrong place. Particular care must be taken whenever these procedures are performed.

Print Preview

When proofreading on the computer screen, the display can be deceptive as to how the format of a report may appear when printed. Most software programs offer a "view document" option (i.e., print preview) allowing the proofreader to view the document on the screen as it will appear when printed. Always view the document using "print preview" and proofread work on-screen and train eyes to spot the smallest of errors. Then print out and proofread the document again to see if anything slipped by unnoticed. This skill will improve with experience.

ENVELOPE ENCLOSURES

A letter's first impression is made by the envelope in which it is enclosed; much the same way that the first impression of a book is determined by its cover. The envelope should always have a professional appearance and follow accepted business style. See Chapter 12 for envelope guidelines.

When a letter goes to the physician to be signed, it is paper-clipped under the flap of the envelope so the physician sees both together (Figure 11-11). The envelope size depends on the type of communication and the number of enclosures. Attachments are stapled to the back of the letter. When the letter has been signed and is ready to mail, it is folded and inserted into the envelope so that it will be in reading position when it is removed.

Folding Enclosures

When folding a letter for a large (No. 10) envelope, the letter is placed flat on the desk in reading position. First fold from the bottom to a point a little less than

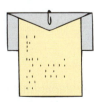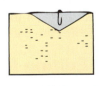

Figure 11-11. Two examples of paper-clipping a letter for signature to the underside flap of an envelope

PROCEDURE 11-3

Proofread a Business Document

Objective: To proofread a business document on screen and in hard copy to correct spelling, typographical, mechanical, grammar, and other errors.

Equipment/Supplies: Computer, document with errors (on screen and hard copy), and pen or pencil.

Directions: Follow these step-by-step procedures, which include rationales. Several job skills are presented in the *Workbook* for practice after keying a letter.

1. Proofread the document as you key in data using the word processing software program. You might turn off the automatic spell checker to force yourself to read the completed document carefully and look for spelling errors and use of wrong or incomplete words.

2. Slowly read the material aloud, if you can, to keep from skimming over material too quickly. Increasing the size of the font may make it easier to spot errors. However, be sure to reduce the font to the proper size and check the format before printing and sending.

3. Check for typographical and mechanical errors. Then review the document for style, spelling, grammar, and meaning. If you find one error, look carefully nearby for others.

4. Check punctuation. Watch for doubled periods, missing part of paired punctuation such as parentheses and quotation marks, missing comma, missing semicolon, putting in a comma instead of a semicolon, and so forth.

5. Check capitalization and lowercase letters for drug names, names of places, and medical specialty abbreviations.

6. Read titles and first lines carefully. Check that titles in headers or footers match those in the text.

7. Check consistency of headings and subheadings (same font, size, alignment, capitalization).

8. Check numbered and alphabetically ordered lists for correct sequence. Look for repeated, missing, or out-of-order numbers or letters.

9. Use the spell-check feature only for obvious errors since it cannot select words out of context (e.g., *injection* for *infection*, *palpation* for *palpitation*, *tick douloureux* for *tic douloureux*) or correctly spelled homonyms, (e.g., *their* for *there*, *callus* for *callous*, *vesical* for *vesicle*).

10. Load a medical dictionary or update the dictionary in the software program to include terms or acronyms unique to the medical practice's specialty.

11. Review a revised (cut and paste) document carefully. Words can be omitted or rekeyed, a new paragraph inserted without deleting the old, or a paragraph moved without deleting it at its original position. This can be verified with the search and find feature. Check immediately before and after cut-and-paste revisions.

12. Correct errors and reread the on-screen copy that comes immediately before and after revisions.

13. Read it a second time, word for word, letter by letter, watching for errors in spelling, punctuation, and grammar and for accuracy of facts.

14. Print a hard copy of the document.

15. Use a plastic ruler to remain on the correct line and proofread the hardcopy.

16. Read each line backward, a word at a time for long, complicated documents. This method will help you catch spelling and other errors that sometimes get overlooked during the conventional reading.

17. Divide the document into convenient viewing sections for proofreading, i.e., paragraph by paragraph or 10 to 12 lines at a time.

18. Look at the copy upside down to check spacing.

19. Check carefully for placement, appearance, and format.

20. Always strive for a perfect first printing of the final copy and do not send a document with errors.

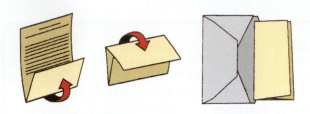

Figure 11-12. Folding a letter for insertion into a large (No. 10) envelope

one-third of the page and crease. Next fold downward from the top to within one-half inch of the first fold and crease. The last crease is inserted into the envelope first so that the top of the letter is at the top of the envelope (Figure 11-12).

For a small (No. 6¾) envelope, the letter is placed flat on the desk in reading position. First, fold from the bottom up to within one half-inch of the top and crease. Next, fold from the right a third of the way over to the left and crease; then fold from the left over to about one-half inch of the previous crease on the right. The last creased edge is inserted into the envelope first (Figure 11-13).

MEDICAL TRANSCRIPTION

A physician's transcription needs vary according to medical specialty, size of practice, amount of consultation work, involvement in medical and community affairs, and whether a mobile device, speech recognition, or template systems are used.

The medical **transcriptionist** (MT) may be a certified medical assistant (CMA), registered medical assistant (RMA), certified medical transcriptionist (CMT), or other health care professional. MTs may work in the physician's office or health care facility, at home, off site, or in another city, state, or country. As transcription technology advances, the profession becomes more specialized.

A transcriptionist should have an educational background in medical terminology and basic skills of business English, vocabulary, grammar, spelling, punctuation, and capitalization. These skills become paramount when a speech recognition system is used,

because the transcriptionist is acting as an editor. A superior transcriptionist can transcribe 10,000 characters an hour, but this degree of proficiency comes only after much practice and each organization has its own standards. Accuracy is more important than speed. With practice, the transcriptionist can learn to listen to a new group of words while still keying a previous group. Typically, a new transcriptionist is allowed a three- to six-month period to increase production to the expected level.

Transcription Procedures and Equipment

If the administrative medical assistant's position requires transcription, it is important to understand the equipment and methods of operating the system skillfully (Figure 11-14). Before using any transcription equipment, the assistant can read the basic operating instructions in the manual, discuss procedures with a coworker who has used the machine, or call the

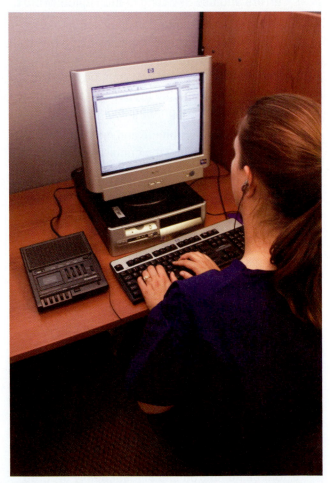

Figure 11-14. Medical transcriptionist operating a dictation-transcription machine, keying in data via computer

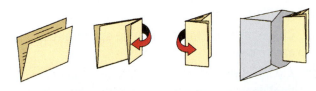

Figure 11-13. Folding a letter for insertion into a small (No. 6¾) envelope

sales representative for a demonstration. Transcription systems range from the small portable dictation unit hand-carried by the busy physician, to combination dictation and transcription desktop models that use standard micro- or mini-cassettes or magnetic tapes called *media*. The physician dictates into the machine, which records the message on the media. The assistant then activates the media by using a foot pedal or by hand and listens to the dictated information through a headset or earpiece, while simultaneously typing data on medical report forms or letterhead paper. Most machine dictation is transcribed using word processing software. All machines are equipped with a backspacing mechanism and can fast-forward to the next report. It is possible to select forward or reverse to listen to the prerecorded material. Tone, volume, and speed can be adjusted to each person's keying capabilities.

Sometimes the medical assistant is asked to transcribe from handwritten copy or edit a document. If handwritten copy is difficult to read, all the typist can do is try to figure out what the writer has in mind. In these instances, he or she should not key for speed but for accuracy.

If some letters are unclear, look for comparable letters elsewhere, and chances are difficult areas can be figured out. Sometimes a word can be deciphered if the typist understands the context of the sentence. However, if there are still problems, do not guess, ask the writer (dictator) to clarify confusing words, and never change any wording without informing him or her.

When the assistant can't make sense of a word or a phrase, he or she should leave a blank space and write the physician a note indicating the page number and the line of the missing or indistinct information. This is known as "flagging" and can also be easily indicated by using repositionable adhesive tape flags or tabs.

Every physician has a unique dictation style, with which the transcriptionist becomes familiar. Most physicians prefer to dictate patient information into the machine at the end of the day or at quiet periods during office hours when the medical assistant may be working on other projects. At the convenience of the assistant, material may be transcribed later.

Templates

A *template* can be a sequence of basic headings for content that needs to be included for a specific letter or report. To help with creation of a document, the writer uses the template as a guide for the report ele-

COMPLIANCE

The Health Insurance Portability and Accountability Act privacy rule does not prohibit the use of tapes for dictation, nor outsourcing of transcription. However, it requires that specific language addressing confidentiality be inserted in contracts with business associates (outside vendors).

ments that are needed. A template can be used in the dictation process, for electronically captured information, or in handwritten notes. In a computer system it is a keystroke saver and speeds generating a document.

A template in a paper-based system consists of a form that is checked off by the writer (physician). The form is then scanned to input the template-generated language into the computer system specific for the patient's complaints and symptoms or for the business letter that is to be generated.

Speech Recognition

Some physicians have begun using speech recognition software to generate documents. While the dictator uses a microphone and speaks, the dialogue appears on the computer monitor. The dictator is able to verbally order the record to be electronically signed when it is completed. It can be printed in hard copy, become part of the patient's electronic medical record, or both. However, all speech engines must be initially trained and the dictator must practice speaking into the machine so that his or her voice, style, syntax (way in which words are put together), and vocabulary allow the software to work at its optimum. Dictation must be distinct, clear, and unhurried. It is time-consuming because physicians are used to dictating rapidly.

If punctuation, paragraphing, and capitalization are not vocalized, the transcriptionist or editor must carefully edit the document at a later time. Onscreen editing may also include inserting figures as numbers instead of as words. As the transcriptionist edits and corrects the document using sound equipment, the incorrect phrase or word is highlighted so he or she can teach the program the correct word. One hundred percent accuracy is not realistic with voice recognition software; however, it can be significantly faster than keyboard entry.

STEP 1 2 3

PROCEDURE 11-4

Transcribe a Dictated Document

Objective: Transcribe a dictated letter or report without errors into hard copy using a computer or typewriter.

Equipment/Supplies: Letterhead stationery, transcription equipment (headset, earphones, foot control, media containing dictation), English and medical dictionaries, drug book, computer and printer or typewriter.

Directions: Follow these step-by-step procedures, which include rationales, to learn this skill.

1. Gather all necessary information and materials at the desk, including reference books.

2. Make sure the headset, earphones (or amplifier), and foot control are attached to the unit and comfortably positioned.

3. Verify that the unit is plugged in, turned on, and operating properly.

4. Insert the medium (tape). Priority (STAT) reports are transcribed immediately. Then the oldest dictation is transcribed and the most recent dictation keyed last.

5. Scan electronically to estimate the length of the report or letter, and listen for special instructions or comments before beginning to transcribe.

6. Adjust the volume, tone, and speed controls.

7. Set the margins and tabulator stops.

8. Select the paper and note how many copies are required.

9. Finally, begin transcribing after activating the voice on tape; listen and remember a phrase,

stop the voice, key the material, and repeat the process. Try to avoid rewinding and listening to the same material twice. Listen for pauses to indicate punctuation or the end of a sentence.

10. Look up the meaning of English and medical homonyms to end confusion and help you decide how to spell them, such as *mucus* (noun) or *mucous* (adjective), *ileum* or *ilium*. Homonyms sound the same but have different meanings.

11. Proofread the document on screen for content; typographical, spelling, grammar, style, and mechanical errors; and overall appearance.

12. Save the file to the hard drive before printing a hard copy, and proofread the document again. Make corrections, if necessary.

13. Print two copies, one to be sent and one to be retained in the files. If questions arise, a copy of the document can be referred to.

14. Save the file to a floppy disk, Zip disk, or CD-ROM to be stored for future reference.

15. Prepare an envelope using the format for optical scanning (presented in Chapter 12). If sending the correspondence by registered or certified mail, be sure to insert these special instructions on the envelope.

16. Clip any attachments to the document, and give to the physician for review and signature.

17. Turn off the transcription equipment.

Mobile Devices

As mentioned earlier, mobile devices such as personal digital assistants (PDAs) save physicians time and offer access to clinical information. PDAs now have technology that allows the recording of dictation in real time over a secure and wireless network. Voice files are transmitted wirelessly to the server and do not take up space on the portable device. Their reliability is still being tested, but with more than 40 percent of physicians owning mobile devices, adoption of PDA-based dictation software is expected to increase.

PHOTOCOPYING PROCEDURES

The term **photocopy** means any process using light or photography to reproduce multiple copies of original (graphic) material; also known as reprograph-

STEP 1 2 3

PROCEDURE 11-5

Prepare Documents for Photocopying

Objective: To prepare documents with multiple pages for photocopying.

Equipment/Supplies: Photocopy machine, paper, equipment instruction book, document(s) to be photocopied, stapler with staples, and staple remover.

Directions: Follow these step-by-step procedures, which include rationales, to practice this skill.

1. Warm up the photocopy machine if it has been turned off.

2. Assemble all pages of the document.

3. Check the original to see it is free of smudges and stains before making a copy.

4. Remove paper clips and staples, and assemble documents to be copied before taking them to the copier. Staples or paper clips may damage the photocopy equipment.

5. Copy only the portion of the medical record that is requested and that the patient has authorized. If the document is from a patient's medical record, verify that there is a signed authorization to release the information.

6. Use correction tape when lines, smudges, or phrases of a master copy need to be corrected. To avoid photocopy "lines" appearing where the tape is attached to the master, paint edges of tape with correction fluid or place adhesive tape over the correction tape.

7. Place the original(s) in the machine according to the instructions for the photocopy equipment. If single-sheet copying, place each document facedown on the glass. If the machine accepts the entire document, load them (facedown or faceup) into the feeder according to directions.

8. Select the correct format for size (e.g., letter or legal size paper, size of copy) and set the machine for the number of copies desired. Make at least one file copy of all documents.

9. Press the settings so copies will be collated, stapled, or both, if the equipment has these features.

10. Regulate for light or dark copy if the machine does not automatically adjust for this. Careful preparation will save time and money by preventing running the job again.

11. Always make copies with the copier lid closed, because the drum picks up toner to cover the entire glass opening. An open lid wastes toner and may lead to more service calls, and intense light can be a health hazard.

12. Press the "start" or "print" button.

13. Arrange the document pages in the correct sequence, and staple if the equipment does not have the stapling feature.

14. Verify the number of document pages. If the patient or an attorney has requested copies, then submit the number of pages to the person responsible for billing.

15. Avoid lengthy exposure to sunlight or room light, which may damage the developing roller, if toner cartridges are used.

16. Notify the office manager if copy paper and supplies are at the reorder point.

17. Be sure to take all originals and photocopies from the trays before the next person copies a document.

18. Refill paper trays, unless another person has been assigned this duty.

19. Make sure the copier is turned off at the end of the day.

ics. Medical offices are experiencing the need to make more copies of patient records, medical reports, correspondence, insurance claim forms, bills, memos, and other documents. A computer printer can be programmed to produce multiple copies, and the fax machine may also have reproduction capabilities; however, the most popular machine to reproduce documents is the photocopier.

When high-quality copies are needed quickly in limited quantities, the **photocopy machine** is one of the most important pieces of equipment in the medical office. Documents can be reproduced on ordinary paper stock, specially coated paper, copying paper, letterhead, preprinted forms, and colored stock. The copies resemble the original, the equipment is easy to operate, and paper and toner are the only supplies necessary. Some models can reduce or enlarge copy size, collate, and staple multiple documents. Although the cost of making one copy is small, employees should be discouraged from duplicating items unnecessarily.

A reply to a letter may be duplicated directly on the back of the letter being answered, to save paper and to eliminate bulky medical records and misplaced correspondence. Both sides of an insurance card can be copied using the same piece of paper and running it through a second time. Caution should be taken because certain copyrighted material cannot be legally copied without permission.

Multifunction Devices

A multifunction device (MFD) is linked to a computer system and provides a printer, scanner, copier, and often a fax in a single unit. It comes in small sizes, just larger than a printer, which saves desktop space, and in large sizes that offer all the functions of a deluxe photocopy machine.

Photocopy Machine

In most offices, the copier is a busy machine (Figure 11-15). Always place the machine away from file cabinets or walls to prevent overheating. Keep the area surrounding the machine neat and clean, and recycle used photocopy paper. Schedule lengthy copy projects for times when the machine is least busy. Study the operating manual for specific instructions and place it a prominent place for reference.

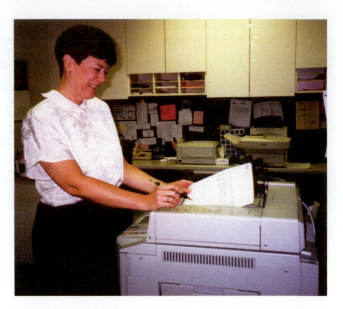

Figure 11-15. Medical assistant preparing to copy a medical document on a photocopy machine

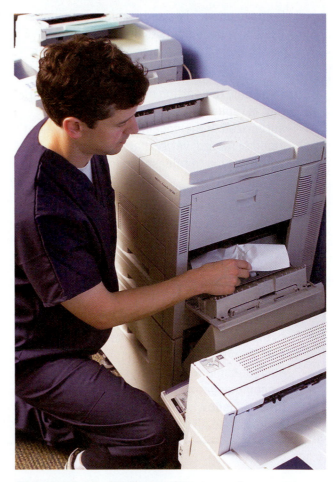

Figure 11-16. Medical assistant opening a copy machine to remove a paper jam

To make a photocopy, the original material is either fed into the machine or placed facedown on the platen glass. After machine adjustments are made according to size, darkness, and quantity, copies may be produced in seconds from paper stored in cassettes. The "print" button is pressed to activate the copy machine.

Common Photocopy Machine Problems

Table 11-2 offers suggestions for troubleshooting some of the most common photocopy machine problems.

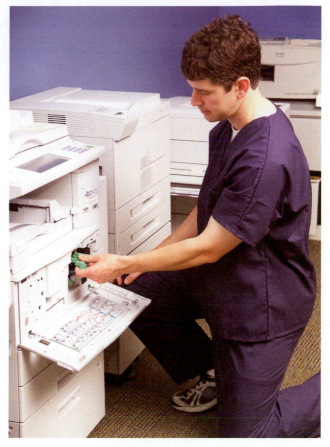

Figure 11-17. Medical assistant opening a copy machine to remove or install an ink cartridge

Table 11-2. Copier Problems with Possible Causes and Solutions

Difficulty	Possible Cause	Solution
Feeding problems	Letterhead or heavy-stock paper may cause static buildup	Substitute lighter-weight paper (20 lb. is standard)
Misfeeding	Uneven edges or curl; may be caused by mixing weights of paper in the same tray or cassette	Open another ream of paper or turn the existing paper over; fan to allow air to circulate between sheets
Jamming in the bins or sheets sticking together	Excessive curl of paper; moisture or low humidity may be the cause	Turn the paper over; check storage conditions; ask maintenance or supplier to check static eliminator
Wrinkling	High moisture due to damp storage, or paper has remained in copy machine too long	Check storage conditions; substitute another ream of copy paper
Smoking or making strange noise	Cause unknown	Turn machine off immediately; contact person in charge of maintenance

STOP AND THINK CASE SCENARIO

Edit a Thank-You Letter for Final Copy

Scenario: Dr. Fran Practon gives you a rough draft of a letter that she wants you to put into final copy to send to the patient, Jason Chieu. It reads as follows:

Dear Mr. Chieu, I wanted to express my thank-you due to the fact that you referred your friend, Cherry Hotta, to our medical practice. I recognize that this referral indicates that I provided good medical care for you and your family. I'm grateful for both your confidence and consideration. My staff and I are committed to deliver the same quality care that you have come to expect from me. Again thanks for your kindness in referring your friend to me. Sincerely,

Critical Thinking: What should you do? Respond to each choice and list the changes you would make if you selected response 1, 2, or 3.

1. Rewrite it to give it a conversational tone?

_____

_____

_____

2. Rewrite it to make it more concise and clear?

_____

_____

_____

3. Rewrite it to give it a formal tone?

_____

_____

_____

4. Send it as written?

_____

_____

_____

_____

STOP AND THINK CASE SCENARIO

Edit a Transcribed Medical Report

Scenario: Dr. Gerald Practon dictated a medical report on Charlotte Greenwich, who came in with a right inguinal hernia. You transcribed the report, but certain sections are unclear and you have had to leave several blanks.

Critical Thinking: What should you do? Respond to each choice stating whether you would or would not proceed in that manner and give the reasons behind your decision.

1. Look at the patient's medical record and try to obtain the data to insert.

_____

_____

2. Pull a medical record of another patient who had the same complaints and try to fill in the data by reading through that chart.

_____

_____

_____

3. Mark the hard copy of the medical report with notes to the physician asking for clarification.

_____

_____

_____

4. Other (please state).

_____

_____

_____

STOP AND THINK CASE SCENARIO

Select the Correct Homonyms in a Medical Report

Scenario: Dr. Fran Practon dictated a medical report, and some sentences contained homonyms. You want to put it into final copy. A section reads as follows:

"Mrs. Frye has completed one (coarse, course) of radiation therapy after her mastectomy. There was (mucous, mucus) draining from the site of treatment. She complained that the prescribed medication for her nausea had the (effect, affect) of making her drowsy. She cannot (bare, bear) to be lethargic."

Critical Thinking: Look at each set of homonyms and decide how you would determine the correct word, then circle it. Respond to each choice below expressing why you would or would not proceed in the manner stated.

1. Look in the patient's medical record for any notes to decide which word is more appropriate.

   _____

2. Look up each of the words in the medical dictionary and decide from the meaning which one suits the context of the sentence.

   _____

3. Flag the section of the report and ask the dictator which words are the correct ones.

   _____

FOCUS ON CERTIFICATION*

CMA Content Summary
- Medical terminology
- Spelling, correspondence, letters, memos
- Data entry; keyboard fundamentals
- Letter and memo formats
- Envelopes
- Computer and printer usage
- Computer storage devices
- Word processing
- Databases

RMA Content Summary
- Medical terminology
- Spelling

- Written communication skills
- Compose correspondence
- Transcription and dictation
- Word processing computer applications

CMAS Content Summary
- Spell medical terms
- Written communication
- Format business documents
- Basic computer operations
- Fundamental knowledge of a PC-based environment
- Word processing and databases
- Medical office software applications

*This textbook and the accompanying Workbook meet the entry-level administrative and general competencies for the CMA outlined by the AAMA Examination Content Outline and Role Delineation Study and for the RMA and CMAS outlined by the AMT Competencies and Examination Specifications (see Competency Grid in Appendix B).

REVIEW   EXAM-STYLE QUESTIONS

1. Computer software is programmed to permanently store data on the hard drive, which can be duplicated and transferred to other data-storing media such as:

   a. floppy disks

   b. Zip disks

   c. CDs

   d. flash drives

   e. all the above

2. Working at a computer in one position hour after hour performing the same movements over and over can cause injuries referred to as:

   a. repetitive trauma disorders

   b. cumulative stress injuries

   c. repetitive stress injuries

   d. ergonomic injuries

   e. movement disorders

3. Select the correct description for pica and elite type.

   a. pica 12 characters per inch, elite 14 characters per inch

   b. pica 10 characters per inch, elite 12 characters per inch

   c. pica 12 characters per inch, elite 10 characters per inch

   d. pica 14 characters per inch, elite 12 characters per inch

   e. pica 8 characters per inch, elite 10 characters per inch

4. Select the correctly spelled word.

   a. indespensable

   b. indispinsable

   c. indispinseble

   d. indispensable

   e. indespinsable

5. What determines the letter style used in a physician's office?

   a. equipment used

   b. physician's preference

   c. type of letter being sent

   d. office manager's preference

   e. personal choice of staff member

6. When a colon or comma is used after the complimentary close, it is referred to as:

   a. full punctuation

   b. open punctuation

   c. mixed punctuation

   d. internal punctuation

   e. closed punctuation

7. To *justify* means to:

   a. start all lines flush with the left margin

   b. space words so that the ends of lines are flush at right and left margins

   c. align text flush with the right margin

   d. center text

   e. indent when starting a new paragraph

8. The date line is typically placed:

   a. 1 double space below the letterhead

   b. 1 space below the letterhead

   c. 2 spaces below the letterhead

   d. 3 spaces below the letterhead

   e. 4 spaces below the letterhead

9. Select the correct statement regarding the *salutation.*

   a. There is no punctuation after the salutation in *open punctuation.*

   b. There is a colon following the salutation in *open punctuation.*

   c. "Ms." is never used in the salutation.

   d. When a woman's title is not known, the salutation should read: "To whom this may concern."

   e. When it is not known whether the addressee is a man or woman, the salutation should read: "To whom this may concern."

10. A thesaurus lists:

    a. synonyms

    b. antonyms

    c. definitions

    d. synonyms and antonyms

    e. all the above

11. The informal exchange of ideas among individuals and departments within an organization or business are written on:

    a. form letters

    b. formal letters

    c. multipage letters

    d. repetitive letters

    e. interoffice memorandums

12. When moving sections of text in a letter using word processing software, the following text-editing feature should be used:

    a. format feature

    b. directional keys

    c. cut and paste feature

    d. spell check

    e. search feature

13. The job of a medical transcriptionist:

    a. is no longer needed with modern technology

    b. has become more specialized as technology advances

    c. is only found in large medical practices and hospitals

    d. is not needed with the use of templates

    e. is not needed with speech recognition software

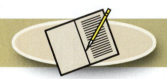

WORKBOOK ASSIGNMENT

To develop competency-based job skills, refer to the *Workbook* and complete the:

- Abbreviation and Spelling Review
- Review Questions

- Critical Thinking Exercises
- Job Skill activities, which are outlined at the beginning of this chapter under "Performance Objectives in the *Workbook*."

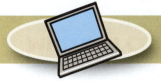

COMPUTER ASSIGNMENT

To review the concepts you have learned in this chapter, insert the *Student Practice* CD-ROM into a computer and work through the *StudyWARE* activities and games. Answer review questions in the practice mode and read the feedback, studying the questions you have missed. Take the chapter quiz until you achieve a minimum score of 90 percent. Successfully completing the *Critical Thinking Challenge* at the end of this course will help you think through scenarios and develop problem solving skills.

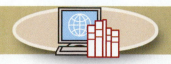

RESOURCES

Books

Achieving the Competitive Edge through Office Ergonomics
Quill Corporation
100 Schelter Road
Lincolnshire, IL 60069-3621
(800) 789-1331
Web site: http://www.quill.com
Web site: http://www.randomhouse.com

Complete Office Handbook
International Association of Administrative Professionals
10502 N W Ambassador
Kansas City, MO 64153
(816) 891-6600
Web site: http://www.iaap-hq.org

The Gregg Reference Manual
William A. Sabin
Glencoe/McGraw-Hill
PO Box 543
Blacklick, OH 43004
(800) 334-7334

Medical Keyboarding and Transcribing Techniques and Procedures
M. O. Diehl and M. T. Fordney
W. B. Saunders/Mosby/Elsevier Science
11830 Westline Industrial Drive
St. Louis, MO 63146
(800) 545-2522
Web site: http://www.us.elsevierhealth.com

Medical Transcription Guide, Do's and Don'ts
Marilyn T. Fordney and Marcy O. Diehl
W.B. Saunders Company/Elsevier Science
11830 Westline Industrial Drive
St. Louis, MO 63146
(800) 545-2522

Internet

Association for Healthcare Documentation Integrity (AHDI)
Formerly the American Association for Medical Transcription
Web site: http://www.aamt.org

Big Dog Grammar
Web site: http://aliscot.com/bigdog

The Blue Book of Grammar and Punctuation
Web site: http://www.grammarbook.com

Common Errors in English—Type "Brians errors" in the search window and then click the Site button. From the list of possible sites, choose Common Errors in English.
Web site: http://www.wsu.edu

Directory of Professional Translation Services
Web site: http://www.proz.com

The Elements of Style—Click on Reference, select English, then click on Elements of Style
Web site: http://www.bartleby.com

Health Professions Institute—Click Transcription Zone
Web site: http://www.hpisum.com

Medical Dictionaries, Resources, Glossaries, Databases, and Encyclopedias
Web site: http://www.useekufind.com/medres.htm

Medicine Net.Inc
Medical dictionaries
Web site: http://www.medicinenet.com

MT Desk (medical word glossary and medical terminology links)
Web site: http://www.mtdesk.com

The Online English Grammar
Web site: http://www.edufind.com

PDA Resources for Health Professionals—Click Library then PDAs and Medicine
Web site: http//www.medicalpocketpc.com
Web site: http://www.healthypalmpilot.com

Pocket PC Magazine
Web site: http://pocketpcmag.com

CHAPTER 12

Processing Mail and Telecommunications

OBJECTIVES

After reading this chapter and learning step-by-step procedures to gain job skills,* you should be able to:

Learning Objectives

▍ Select appropriate mail equipment and stationery supplies.

▍ Describe various options for purchasing postage and postal supplies.

▍ State the characteristics of suspicious mail.

▍ Explain how incoming mail is handled and sorted.

▍ Define methods for annotating incoming mail.

▍ Coordinate distribution of mail when the physician is on vacation.

▍ Determine the most economical classification for various mailings.

▍ Choose the safest service for mailing valuable items and important papers.

▍ State the envelope address format following preferred United States Postal Service regulations.

▍ Explain electronic mail etiquette and format.

▍ Determine the advantages of an electronic communication system for a medical practice.

▍ Cite etiquette, guidelines, and operating procedures for fax transmission.

Performance Objectives (Procedures) in This Textbook

▍ Operate a postage meter (Procedure 12-1).

▍ Open, sort, and annotate mail (Procedure 12-2).

▍ Prepare outgoing mail (Procedure 12-3).

▍ Complete U.S. Postal Service forms to send a letter by certified mail (Procedure 12-4).

*This textbook and the accompanying Workbook meet the educational components for entry-level administrative and general competencies outlined by CAAHEP and ABHES.

▌ Address a business envelope using U.S. Postal Service regulations (Procedure 12-5).

▌ Compose an e-mail message (Procedure 12-6).

▌ Prepare a fax cover sheet and send a fax (Procedure 12-7).

Performance Objectives (Job Skills) in the *Workbook*

▌ Process incoming mail (Job Skill 12-1).

▌ Annotate mail (Job Skill 12-2).

▌ Classify outgoing mail (Job Skill 12-3).

▌ Address envelopes for OCR scanning (Job Skill 12-4).

▌ Complete a mail-order form for postal supplies (Job Skill 12-5).

▌ Compose a letter and prepare an envelope for certified mail (Job Skill 12-6).

▌ Prepare a cover sheet for fax transmission (Job Skill 12-7).

▌ Key and fold an original letter; address a small envelope for certified mail, return-receipt-requested (Job Skill 12-8).

▌ Key and fold an original letter; address a large envelope for certified mail, return-receipt-requested (Job Skill 12-9).

OUTLINE WITH LECTURE NOTES

United States Postal Service

_____
_____
_____
_____

Stamp Services

_____
_____
_____
_____

Supplies and Equipment
Postal Scale

_____
_____
_____
_____

Postage Meter

_____
_____
_____
_____

Handling Incoming Mail
Mail Security

_____
_____
_____
_____

Opening Mail

_____
_____
_____
_____

Annotating Mail

E-Mail Usage

Handling Mail When the Physician is Away

E-Mail Etiquette

Handling Outgoing Mail

Mail Classifications

E-Mail Format

Special Services

Basic Guidelines for Using E-Mail

Other Delivery Services

Facsimile (Fax) Communication

Addressing Envelopes for Computerized Mail

Fax Etiquette

Envelope Guidelines

Fax Machine Features

Fax Operating Guidelines

Managing Office Mail

Faxing Confidential Records

Electronic Mail

KEY TERMS

annotate
bar code sorter (BCS)
Certified Mail
DHL WorldWide Express
domestic mail
electronic mail
enclosure (enc)
facsimile (fax) communication

Federal Express (FedEx)
mail classifications
optical character recognition (OCR)
Registered Mail
service endorsement
United Parcel Service (UPS)
United States Postal Service (USPS)
zone improvement plan (ZIP + 4)

HEART OF THE HEALTH CARE PROFESSIONAL

Service

Processing mail is a "behind the scenes" job and not thought of as very important. However, when not done efficiently and in a timely manner, the entire office can grind to a stop and a variety of responsibilities that addresses patients' needs may not be met.

UNITED STATES POSTAL SERVICE

The volume of incoming and outgoing mail in the physician's practice is a major factor in determining mail procedures. The medical assistant's goal is to take appropriate steps to sort and distribute incoming mail and to choose the service that speeds the delivery of outgoing mail at minimum cost. With the advent of the Internet, sending First-Class letters and other documents using standard mail delivery has diminished. Sending documents by fax and electronic mail (e-mail) has replaced that system because of the ease and speed in sending and receiving a communication as well as the reduced cost by eliminating postage. The Internet also offers options in purchasing postage and metering outgoing mail.

The **United States Postal Service (USPS)** is used by the majority of citizens in the United States to deliver both domestic and international mail. To obtain quick and up-to-date information on regulations and take advantage of many online services, access the USPS Web site (see Resources at the end of the chapter). There you can obtain **domestic mail** zone (United States, Canada, and Mexico) and international mail postage rates, locate ZIP codes, register change of address, find abbreviations for city names that exceed 13 characters, calculate postage according to the weight of the item, purchase stamps, print postage onto envelopes or labels, obtain forms, create cards, and more. If a medical practice does not have access to the Internet, use the White Pages of the local telephone directory to obtain the toll-free 800 number.

A nine-digit **zone improvement plan (ZIP + 4)** code on the envelope expedites sorting and delivery because mail can be processed by computerized equipment. The United States is divided into 10 large areas. Each area is assigned a number between 0 and 9, which represents the first digit in a ZIP code. Key post offices in each area are designated sectional centers represented by the next two digits. Each sectional center serves a series of associated post offices represented by the last two digits. The four-digit add-on number identifies a specific delivery segment such as a city block, floor of a building, department within a company, or group of post office boxes. A hyphen appears after the five-digit ZIP code and before the four-digit add-on code. If the ZIP + 4 code is known, it should be used.

Using the ZIP + 4 code, particularly for business mail, reduces the number of handlings, decreases the potential for human error, reduces the possibility of misdelivery, and leads to better control of postal costs. Automated mail equipment can read the nine-digit code. It reads the first-class letters and cards by **optical character recognition (OCR)**, and then the **bar code sorter (BCS)** imprints a bar code on the lower right corner of the envelope. Local ZIP codes can usually be found in telephone directories in addition to the USPS Web site.

SUPPLIES AND EQUIPMENT

In a small-volume mail operation, some or all of the following supplies will be useful: letter opener, postal scale, postage meter, stapler, rubber stamps, labels, adhesive tape, stickers, and postage stamps.

Postal Scale

The postal scale, used to determine the weight of mail, is available in spring, beam, pendulum, and electronic models. A postal scale can be checked for accuracy by weighing nine pennies on it; they should weigh 1 ounce. If they do not, an adjustment needs to be made. If the office has a pediatric scale, it can be used as a postal scale.

Postage Meter

Postage meters are used to print prepaid postage directly on envelopes or onto a meter tape that is affixed to large envelopes or packages (Figure 12-1). The imprint, or meter stamp, serves as postage payment, postmark, and cancellation mark. Because metered mail does not have to be cancelled at the post office, mail handling is expedited. The meter may be used for all classes of mail except periodicals and for any amount of postage. Envelopes that contain bulky items should be stamped by hand *before* placing contents inside. Write "Hand Stamp" in large letters on the envelope under or to the left of the stamp.

Postage meters may be purchased or leased and rental fees are based on the amount of usage. The medical assistant should keep a daily record to make sure the office is not being over charged for minimum usage. Models vary in design, from a lightweight, hand-operated machine to a computer-controlled meter that can fold, stuff, and weigh mail items.

The USPS offers three ways to fund postage meters, which can also be used to reset postage.

- Automated Clearing House (ACH) Debit—provides postage instantaneously after a debit account has been set up. It can be accessed by telephone or via computer.
- Automated Clearing House (ACH) Credit—provides automatic payment, upon request

from the office bank account for large volume mailings.
- Federal Wire—allows transfer of funds from the office bank account but is typically used when purchasing over $25,000 in postage.

After the model has been selected from a list of manufacturers authorized by the USPS, an application for postage meter license is submitted to the post office where the metered mail is to be deposited. A one-time fee permits an imprint account. There is no separate fee for bulk mailing; however, an annual fee must be paid. All metered mail must be deposited at the post office where the permit was issued. Bulk mail drop offs are recommended early in the day, early in the week, and early in the month. Manual postage meters have been retired, all are now set remotely. It is illegal to possess a postage meter without paying for postage.

Stamp Services

There are several ways to order postage without having to make a special trip to the post office. Ordering by mail, over the telephone, and via the Internet are three common ways.

Stamps by Mail

Stamps by Mail can be purchased by filling out Form 3227 provided by the U.S. Postal Service and mailing it to the local post office. Within five days, postage stamps will be mailed to the medical office at no extra charge. Stamps by Mail order forms may be kept on hand for use at any time. After indicating on the form the items needed and the cost, a check or money order for the total amount is inserted in a self-addressed attached envelope. Any order totaling $200 or more is returned by Certified Mail and a signature is required upon delivery.

Stamps by Telephone

Stamps by Telephone involves a call to the toll-free number (800-STAMP-24) anytime 24 hours a day, 7 days a week. Stamps are delivered within five business days and may be charged to an office credit card. There is no minimum order, but there is a service charge based on the total price of the order.

PROCEDURE 12-1

Operate a Postage Meter

Objective: To set up a postage meter and apply postage to an envelope or package for mailing, according to U.S. Postal Service guidelines.

Equipment/Supplies: Postage meter, addressed envelope or package, and manual or electronic postal scale.

Directions: Although postage meters differ in size and function, the following step-by-step procedures, which include rationales, are basic to learning this skill.

1. Purchase or lease a postage meter and contact the USPS to buy a license for metered mail.

2. Contact the meter company and set up an account to pay so the meter can be put into the function mode.

3. Find the location where the meter registers the date. Change the date daily and check the meter to verify that it is correct. U.S. Postal Service guidelines state that the day an envelope or package is mailed must be the date that appears on the postage label, or postage may be forfeited.

4. Verify that contents and enclosures are included in the envelope or package.

5. Weigh the envelope or package (unless the machine does this automatically) to determine if it is over 1 ounce, using a postage scale.

6. Seal the envelope or package (unless the meter seals it).

7. Key in the amount of postage on the meter and press the Enter button. Proofread the amount. If postage is deficient, the article will be returned by the U.S. Postal Service.

8. Process the mail and packages:

   a. *Envelopes:* Apply postage to the envelope by holding it flat with the right side up so the address can be read. Locate where to slide the envelope through near the bottom

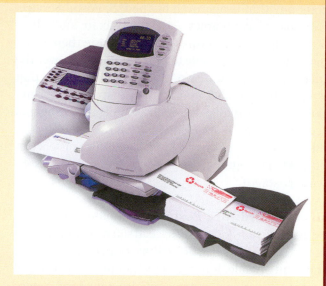

Figure 12-1. Postage meter and scale. (Courtesy of Pitney Bowes, Inc., Stamford, CT.)

of the meter. Place the envelope to the left side and push toward the right. Make certain the postage is printed in the upper right corner of the envelope.

   b. *Packages:* Weigh the package to determine postage. Create a postage label to affix to the package by following the same procedure as making a postmarked label for an envelope. Affix the postmarked label on the package in the upper right corner.

9. Check the postmarked label to verify the printed date and the amount and to see if it is legible.

10. Reset the meter to zero when all mail has been metered.

11. Save all unused and spoiled postage-metered tapes and envelopes and apply for a refund within the year. Request a refund (up to 90 percent of postage value) if an error is made by the meter (poor ink or incorrect postage amount), and do not imprint further postage until the problem has been corrected.

12. Reorder postage by telephone or via computer depending on how the account was set up.

Online Postage

Exact postage can be purchased and printed from a personal computer (PC) by using an online software company that is approved by the U.S. Postal Service. Example of companies are Stamps.com and Click-Stamp Plus (Pitney Bowes product). Using these products, customers are able to purchase postage over the Internet and print a two-dimensional bar code that is digitally encoded and contains various information about the mail piece, such as mail processing and security-related data elements (Figure 12-2). It also allows for mail piece tracking. Two types of services offer PC postage: offline hardware and online software postage.

Offline Hardware Postage—An offline hardware postage system consists of special software and a small postal security device (PSD) that connects to the PC at the printer cable. It may or may not have an attached postal scale. Some systems require a postage meter–like device or tiny printer. After obtaining this special hardware, the medical assistant must go to the company's Internet site, buy postage (e.g., $500) using a credit card or bank fund transfer, download it into the PSD, and log off the Internet. Postage may be printed anytime. A fee is charged for obtaining postage via the Internet and a per month charge is applied. Postal regulations require that the mail piece be mailed on the date that appears on the postage label.

Online Software Postage—Online software postage is a software-based product (e.g., Stamps.com) in which the amount of postage purchased by a customer is stored on the company's Internet site. No special hardware (PSD) is required. Some companies offer free software that interfaces with address books and other business software programs. To obtain online software postage, the customer goes to the Internet site and remains online to print the address and postage. If using labels rather than envelopes, some companies require that the customer purchase proprietary labels for addressing. Some systems verify addresses by matching the address with an existing database and will not print the address unless it matches. The postage amount is deducted from the customer's prepaid account, and a fee is charged for drawing postage off the Internet.

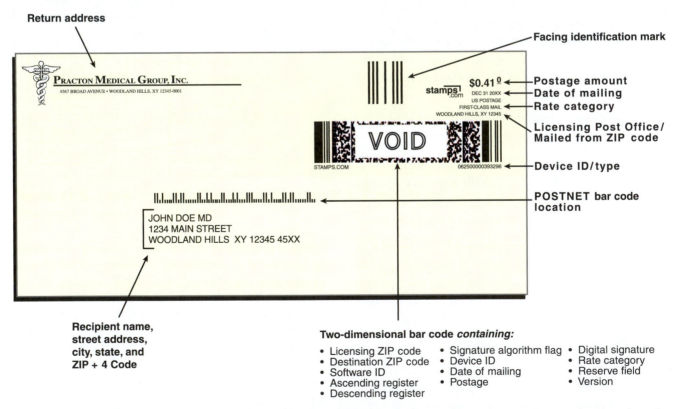

Figure 12-2. Example of an information-based indicia (IBI) bar coded envelope shown addressed, printed, and electronically stamped using online postage

HANDLING INCOMING MAIL

Incoming mail should be opened and processed expediently while keeping confidentiality and security in mind.

Mail Security

It is vital to know how to handle suspicious mail safely since the increase of terrorist activity in the United States. During alerts, it is wise to wear rubber gloves to handle incoming mail, especially if a cut or abrasion is present on hands or fingers. Suspicious characteristics are any mail that is:

- Unexpected or from someone you do not know
- Addressed to someone no longer at your address
- Postmarked with a city that does not match the return address
- Handwritten or poorly typed with no return address or bearing one that you cannot confirm is legitimate on the mail piece
- Showing misspelled common words
- Incorrectly titled
- Oddly sealed or has excessively taped-over areas on the mailed piece
- Stamped with excessive postage
- Excessive in weight
- Marked with restrictive endorsements ("Personal" or "Confidential")
- Exhibiting signs of leakage of liquid (residue of a brown or sandy-brown powdery substance on the exterior, oily stains, or discolorations)
- Lopsided or lumpy, containing an unknown item
- Protruding wires or aluminum foil
- Visually distracting or contains ticking sounds

The USPS caution and commonsense guidelines for those handling a large volume of mail are:

1. Wash your hands thoroughly with soap and water before and after handling any suspicious piece of mail.

2. Do not eat or drink around mail.

3. Do not handle a letter or package that you suspect is contaminated.

4. Stay calm. Do not panic. Do not open, empty, shake, bump, or sniff the contents of any suspicious envelope or package.

5. If you have open cuts or skin lesions on your hands, put on disposable latex gloves.

If a suspicious piece of mail is opened, follow these guidelines:

1. Isolate the specific area of the workplace so that no one disturbs the item, and put the suspicious mail item into a plastic bag or other container.

2. Leave the room and close the door.

3. Keep others away from the area.

4. Wash your hands with warm water and soap for at least 1 minute. Have anyone who has touched the envelope or package do the same.

5. Do not allow anyone who might have touched the envelope to leave. List all people in the room and give the list to the local public health authorities or law enforcement officials.

6. Do not clean up spilled powder. Cover with plastic, paper, or a trash can and leave the room.

7. Remove contaminated clothing, place in a plastic bag, and give it to emergency responders. Shower with soap and water. Do not use bleach or disinfectant on your skin.

8. Turn off fans and ventilation units if there is a question of room contamination by aerosolization. Leave the area immediately, close the door, seal off the area, and shut down the air handling system in the building.

9. Notify your supervisor and local law enforcement authorities immediately.

Opening Mail

The medical assistant should set aside a regular time each day to open the physician's mail as soon as possible after delivery (Figure 12-3). Typically, the assistant handles the mail that deals with statements, payments, insurance, invoices, laboratory test reports, samples, and magazines for the reception room.

Unless the physician has stated otherwise, letters marked "Personal" or "Confidential" are not opened by the assistant. However, if a personal letter is opened by mistake, it should be resealed with transparent tape, labeled "Opened by mistake," and initialed. The

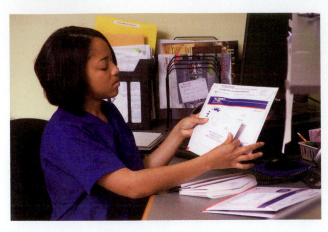

Figure 12-3. Medical assistant opening a physician's mail

letter may then be placed with other personal mail on the physician's desk.

The medical assistant might choose to have readily available for opening the mail a hand or portable automatic letter opener, a stapler, paper clips, transparent tape, a date stamp, and an ink pad (stored upside down to allow the ink to soak into the top).

Date all incoming correspondence with a rubber stamp or a handwritten entry in an upper corner. The date may have legal significance in fixing responsibility for any delay in delivery or response.

When correspondence requests patient data or requires background information, the medical assis-

tant should pull the medical record from the file to place with the letter on the physician's desk. If a letter refers to previous correspondence, gather information from the file folder and fasten it to the back of the letter, perhaps with "See attached" written in the margin.

If an **enclosure (enc)** is mentioned in the letter or noted on the enclosure line but nothing has been inserted, the assistant writes "No enclosure" opposite the notation at the bottom of the letter and contacts the correspondent for the missing material. Enclosures are usually attached to the upper left corner of the letter. A single small enclosure may be stapled to the front of the letter, but a large attachment is usually fastened to the back. X-ray films and photographs must be protected from marks or mutilation by placing a small piece of paper over the material before attaching a paper clip. Cash, checks, and money orders are routed to the bookkeeper according to established procedures. After the medical assistant has opened all the mail, it is then stacked and distributed according to distribution guidelines listed in Table 12-1.

After opening packages, the assistant checks the contents to determine that nothing is missing or broken. All newspapers, booklets, and catalogs are flattened and new catalogs are filed and outdated ones discarded. Advertising items should not be allowed to accumulate to be opened later because they clut-

Table 12-1. Daily Mail to a Physician's Office and Its Distribution

Mail	Distributed to...
Faxes, certified or registered letters, Express and Priority Mail, Telegrams and Mailgrams	Physician
Personal letters, e-mail, and letters from other professionals	Physician
Checks from patients, insurance forms, invoices, letters about accounts	Medical assistant
Letters soliciting contributions	Medical assistant, who annotates
Radiology and laboratory reports; other test results	Medical assistant, who pulls patients' medical records and gives them and test results to physician
Announcements of meetings, medical society bulletins, professional materials	Physician
Journal reprints, medical journals, newspapers	Physician
Magazines for the office	Medical assistant
Advertisements, catalogs, and equipment and supplies information	Medical assistant
Drug samples	Medical assistant, who stores in cabinet

ter the office and could conceal a letter or card among them. Several sheets of advertising that arrive in one envelope should be stapled together unless the physician has given instructions to discard them. If there is an accumulation of periodicals while the physician has been on vacation, photocopy the table of contents of each and store the magazines in a predetermined cabinet. The physician can then scan the photocopied sheets to determine which magazines need to be pulled from storage for study without having to take the time to read them all.

Annotating Mail

The physician may request that you **annotate** all business correspondence. This means to read the correspondence and either underline or highlight important words and phrases or make explanatory notes in the margins so action can be taken. Annotating should be done sparingly because it loses its value if it is overdone. When there is doubt about underlining a word or phrase, it is best not to do so. The assistant should approach each letter looking for the answers to who, what, why, when, and where. Colored pencils will differentiate notes written by the assistant from those written by the physician, and different colors may be used to distinguish general information from items that require particular attention.

A simple "yes" or "no" written by the physician in the margin of a letter will often indicate to the assistant the written response or action to be taken. In, out, and hold baskets or trays on the physician's desk will keep both incoming and outgoing correspondence organized and prevent loss.

Handling Mail When the Physician is Away

Before the physician leaves the office for an extended time, the assistant should discuss procedures for handling the mail in his or her absence. Some questions to pose might be:

1. Should all personal mail be forwarded unopened, can it be opened at the office and a photocopy forwarded, or should it be held?

2. May the assistant decide which mail to forward after opening it?

3. Should any correspondence be answered?

4. Does the physician want all correspondence held until his or her return?

5. Should the assistant prioritize the mail into various piles with the most important on top (see Procedure 12-2)?

If the medical assistant is instructed to forward personal correspondence at different times to different addresses listed on the itinerary, numbering the envelopes consecutively will permit the physician to determine if all communications have been received. Items not forwarded could remain in a "Correspondence to Be Read" folder for action on the physician's return, or they might be sorted into a four-pocket folder set up with sections headed:

- Correspondence Requiring Immediate Action
- Correspondence to Be Read
- Correspondence Awaiting the Physician's Signature
- Miscellaneous Items

Trays could be labeled:

- Urgent
- Not So Urgent
- Junk Mail
- Acknowledged Items (including business and personal mail)

Another system for managing the physician's mail in an absence is to set up a correspondence digest that summarizes in chronological order in outline or tabular form the text and details of each piece of mail. If a communication arrives requiring an immediate response from the physician, the assistant should write a note to the correspondent or send an e-mail or fax to explain that the physician will reply promptly on his or her return.

When the entire office closes for vacation, arrangements must be made with the post office to hold the mail or forward it to a specific address.

HANDLING OUTGOING MAIL

The medical assistant has numerous responsibilities when processing outgoing mail for the office. In order to choose the least expensive and most efficient system for mailing items, a knowledge of **mail classifications** and the steps to take before mailing documents is necessary.

STEP 1 2 3

PROCEDURE 12-2

Open, Sort, and Annotate Mail

Objective: To open, sort, annotate and process incoming mail using a standard procedure.

Equipment/Supplies: Letter opener or portable automatic letter opener, date and time stamp (manual or electronic), ink pad, stapler, paper clips, transparent tape, and adhesive notes.

Directions: Follow these step-by-step procedures, which include rationales, to learn this skill, which is presented in the *Workbook* (Job Skill 12-1 and 12-3) for practice.

1. Tap the lower edges of a stack of envelopes on the desk to settle the contents so no item will be accidentally cut as the envelope is opened. Any item cut by mistake should be immediately mended by tape.

2. Check the address on each letter or package to verify it has been delivered to the correct location.

3. Set aside all letters marked "Personal" or "Confidential" unless you have permission to open them.

4. Arrange all envelopes with the flaps facing up and away from you. Place the first envelope to be opened with its flap to the right if you are right handed. Holding the envelope with the left hand, slip the opener under the flap, and with one stroke, cut the edge open.

5. Open all envelopes.

6. Remove and flatten the contents of each envelope, then hold the emptied envelope up to the light to make certain nothing remains inside.

7. Attach each envelope to every check received so when the payment is posted, the patient's return address on the envelope can be compared with the account ledger and verified.

8. Attach all envelopes to the back of letters that do not have complete return addresses or lack a signature to identify a sender.

9. Verify the enclosure notation on the letter with the actual enclosures. Contact the sender if anything is missing. Clip together each letter with its enclosures.

10. Check the date of the letter with the postmark. If a delay is shown, keep the envelope because this may be needed for reference in legal matters or cases of collection. If dates correspond, discard the envelope.

11. Date stamp and time stamp, if required, each piece of correspondence in the upper right corner.

12. Sort and prioritize mail as follows:

    First priority—Items sent by overnight delivery, registered mail, certified mail, and special delivery. In addition, faxes, e-mail messages, telegrams, and Mailgrams are given first priority.

    Second priority—Personal or confidential mail.

    Third priority—First-Class Mail, airmail, Express Mail, and Priority Mail. Separate according to payments received, insurance forms, reports, and other correspondence. Stamp bank checks with a restrictive endorsement, "For Deposit Only."

    Fourth priority—Packages (e.g., drug samples).

    Fifth priority—Magazines, medical journals, and newspapers.

    Sixth priority—Advertisements, catalogs, equipment and supply information, and junk mail (unsolicited or inapplicable advertisements).

13. Annotate letters by underlining or highlighting important words and phrases, and write notes or questions on the front or back of the correspondence that require action.

Mail Classifications

Mail is classified by size, contents, weight, frequency of mailings, destination, and speed of delivery. Types of mail classifications have changed over the years and obsolete but familiar titles have been included in parentheses to increase understanding.

First Class

First-class mail includes letters, cards, flats, bills, statements of account, small parcels, and all matter sealed or otherwise closed to inspection. It is the fastest and most economic service because mail goes by air when air service is available without an added fee and it includes forwarding and return services. All sealed, most up to and including 13 ounces in weight fall into this category.

Postcards are also included; however, first-class mail that weighs one ounce or less may be subject to a nonmachinable surcharge. A *surcharge* is an additional amount added to the usual postage fee.

Following are minimum and maximum requirements for standard types of first-class mail:

- Postcard—minimum length and height: 5 × 3½ inches; maximum length and height: 6 × 4¼ inches
- Letter—minimum length and height: 5 × 3½ inches; maximum length and height: 11½ × 6⅛ inches

- Large Envelope—minimum length and height: 11½ × 6⅛ inches
- Package—length and girth (distance around thickest part of package) cannot exceed 130 inches; weight cannot exceed 70 pounds

First-class mail to Mexico and Canada requires more postage than the rate within the United States.

Priority Mail

Priority mail is the designation for first-class mail that weighs more than 13 ounces and up to and including 70 pounds. The cost is based on distance and weight if over one pound. First-class mail is typically used to send documents and merchandise in large or thick envelopes, tubes, and packages. It is the fastest way to get heavier mail to its destination within one to three days. Using the free USPS Priority Mail envelopes, boxes, and tubes for this class of mail ensures first-class handling.

Periodicals (Second Class)

Periodicals, formerly called second-class mail includes newspapers and periodicals that must be regularly issued at least four times a year, at which time the rate for mailing is computed. This class of mail is forwarded.

STEP 1 2 3

PROCEDURE 12-3

Prepare Outgoing Mail

Objective: To prepare outgoing mail for delivery.

Equipment/Supplies: Manual or electronic postal scale, postage meter or PC stamps, envelope or package for mailing.

Directions: Follow these step-by-step procedures, which include rationales, to learn this skill, which is presented in the *Workbook* (Job Skill 12-2) for practice.

1. Sort all pieces of mail according to postal class for processing; bundled mail is processed faster.

2. Weigh the item to be mailed with the use of a manual or electronic postal scale.

3. Compute the amount of postage needed to ensure fast delivery service.

4. Affix the correct postage to the item for mailing. Delivery is expedited by using online postage and postmarked labels applied by postal meters because this type of postage does not have to be canceled or postmarked at the post office.

5. Place the mail in the office designated outgoing mail area or take the mail to the post office. Establishing a central location for outgoing mail ensures quick pickup and delivery.

Media Mail (Third Class)

Media Mail, formerly called third class, and sometimes referred to as "Book rate," is a special classification for mailing books, manuscripts, film, sound recordings, videotapes, and computer media (such as CDs, DVDs, and diskettes), and other printed matter that weighs less than 16 ounces and not more than 70 pounds. All pieces of media mail mailed at the single-piece rate, whether sealed or not, must carry the proper endorsement, "Media Mail," written under the postage. Bulk rates are available for multiple mailings of identical matter with special requirements, including a permit obtained from the post office. Nothing may be written on these items but the date and address, and no personal correspondence can be included. Media mail is not forwarded unless it contains a special endorsement.

Parcel Post (Fourth Class)

Parcel post, formerly known as fourth-class mail, includes thick envelopes, tubes, and packages containing gifts and merchandise weighing 1 to 70 pounds and mailed within the continental United States. The combined length and girth must not exceed 130 inches. Postage depends on the weight and the destination.

For purposes of airline security, the U.S. Postal Service recommends packages weighing more than a pound be mailed in person at the post office. When a package is to be sealed with tape, glass-reinforced waterproof strapping that will not split is recommended. Masking tape is not advisable. Address labels should be readable from a distance of 30 inches. All parcel post mail is forwarded unless the sender specifically says it is not to be forwarded. If a piece of mail is forwarded, the recipient can keep it and pay the forwarding charges or refuse the article. If the recipient refuses the article, it is returned to the sender who pays the forwarding and return charges.

Bound Printed Matter (Special Fourth Class)

Bound printed matter, formerly called special fourth class, is a rate applied to promotional material (advertising), directories, or educational material. All items must consist of 90 percent printed material (other than typewritten or handwritten) and be securely bound by permanent fastenings such as staples, spiral binding, glue, or stitching. No personal correspon-

dence is allowed. Barcode discounts are available and bulk rates are available for a minimum of 300 pieces.

Mixed Class

Mixed class, or *combination mailing,* may be used when a letter must be sent with a parcel. If it is sent parcel post, first-class postage is required on the letter, which either may be attached to the outside of the package or placed inside. When x-rays are mailed with a letter by a medical office, this classification is often used.

Express Mail

Express mail is the fastest and most reliable delivery service offered by the USPS. It includes tracking and insurance up to $100 and guarantees overnight delivery of letters and packages to most major metropolitan areas. The charge is based on weight, and the item must be 70 pounds or less. Express Mail next day service offers four types of service:

1. *Post office to post office.* Ensures that mail deposited by 5 p.m. at a designated post office or in any express mail box will be available for customer pickup in the receiving post office by 10 a.m. the next business day.

2. *Post office to addressee.* Requires that the mail be deposited into any express mail box or at a designated post office by 5 p.m. for it to be delivered to the addressee by 3 p.m. the next day.

3. *Custom-designed service.*

4. *Same day airport service.*

If a letter or package fails to arrive at its destination by the following day, there is an immediate refund of postal charges; delivery is made on Saturdays, Sundays, and the holidays with no extra charge. The local post office furnishes a network directory of cities served by express mail as well as labels and various sizes of envelopes and boxes.

International Mail

There are many delivery options for *international mail,* and each offers specific features, including volume mailing services. Delivery time and cost vary. Standard services include:

- Global Airmail—Mail can be sent anywhere in the world; delivery within four to seven days with return receipt.

- Global Economy—Worldwide mail delivered within four to six days with return receipt featuring bargain prices starting at $2.85 for one pound.

Expedited services include:

- Global Express Guaranteed® (GXG)—Guarantees delivery to more than 200 countries. Offers tracking, insurance, online discounts, and prints shipping labels.

- Global Express Mail® (GEM)—Fast and economical delivery to more than 190 countries. Offers tracking, insurance, return receipt, online discounts, and prints shipping labels.

- Global Priority Mail® (GPM)—Economical way to send mail four pounds and under to 51 major countries. Offers priority handling and prints shipping labels.

Instructions for package preparation, shipping, international forms, addressing mail, postage payment options, and an international rate fee calculator can be found on the USPS Web site. Restrictions and rates can also be checked at any post office in the *Directory of International Mail*.

Special Services

The USPS offers *special services* to track mail, provide proof of mailing, and ensure delivery. The level of tracking desired will determine which service to use.

Registered Mail

Registered Mail is first-class mail of a declared value such as mail containing checks, money, or valuable merchandise. A trip to the post office is required to complete the forms, which include proof of mailing and delivery (date and time). A delivery receipt, signed by the addressee may be purchased for an additional fee; no other person can accept delivery. Insurance coverage based on declared value of the item (up to $25,000) can be added. Both documents and packages can be registered. First-class or Priority mail postage is required on domestic Registered mail.

STEP 1 2 3

PROCEDURE 12-4

Complete U.S. Postal Forms to Send a Letter by Certified Mail

Objectives: To complete a Certified Mail Receipt and delivery confirmation to accompany a letter.

Equipment/Supplies: U.S. Postal Service Certified Mail Receipt PS Form 3800, Domestic Return Receipt PS Form 3811, and pen or pencil.

Directions: Follow these step-by-step procedures, which include rationales, to learn this skill, which is presented in the *Workbook* (Job Skill 12-4) for practice.

1. Handwrite and print legibly the addressee's name, street address, city, state, and ZIP + 4 code in the bottom right corner of the Certified Mail Receipt form. When processing this at the U.S. post office, the mail clerk will tear off and adhere part of the receipt with the receipt number to the mail piece.

2. Handwrite and print legibly the sender's name, street address, city, state, and ZIP + 4

code on the front side of the domestic return receipt form.

3. Handwrite and print legibly the addressee's name, street address, city, state, and ZIP + 4 code in the number 1 block on the reverse side in the bottom left corner of the domestic return receipt form.

4. Handwrite and print legibly the 20-digit number obtained from the front side of the Certified Mail receipt form and place it in the number 2 block of the domestic return receipt form.

5. Insert a check mark in the number 3 block, indicating the appropriate service type (Certified Mail).

6. Attach this card to the back of the mail piece, or on the front if space permits.

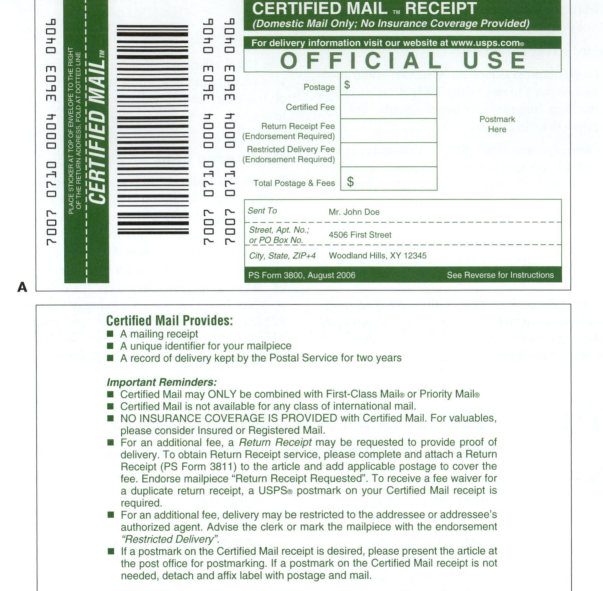

Figure 12-4 A and B. (A) Front of a completed Certified Mail receipt, U.S. Postal Service Form 3800. (B) Back of receipt listing important provisions and instructions.

Certificate of Mailing

Certificate of mailing is a form to be filled out by the assistant indicating the name and address of the office and of the addressee to show proof that a special communication was sent by a deadline. The form is initialed and postmarked at the post office and returned to the assistant for office file records. Because the post office does not keep a record of the mailing, this certificate costs less than certified mail.

Certified Mail

Certified Mail is used when it is necessary to prove that a piece of mail has been mailed and delivered at a certain time and date. This type of mail service is used often by medical offices for collection purposes and for important letters (e.g., notification of practice relocation, closure, or dismissal of a patient). The sender is provided with a receipt of mailing and the receiver must sign a receipt of delivery when it arrives. The

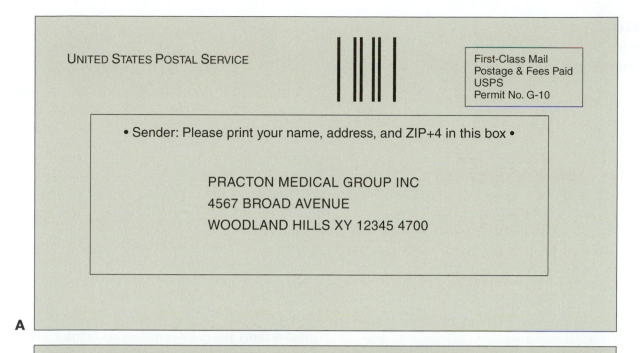

Figure 12-5 A and B. (A) Front of domestic return receipt, U.S. Postal Service Form 3811, addressed with sender's information. (B) Back of receipt addressed with recipient's information and indicating tracking number and type of service (Certified Mail).

record of delivery remains on file at the receiver's post office for two years.

Checks, bankbooks, money orders, legal papers, and income tax forms are usually mailed under this classification. Certified Mail forms may be kept in the office to eliminate special trips to the post office (Figure 12-4 A and B).

Delivery Confirmation

For a small additional fee, a return receipt can be requested for both Registered and Certified mail. A postcard with the addressee's signature is sent to the sender that provides the date and time of delivery or attempted delivery (Figure 12-5 A and B).

Restricted Delivery

Restricted delivery is available for Certified Mail, Insured Mail, or Registered Mail and assures that only a specified person will receive a piece of mail. The signature of the person who signed for the item, along with the date and time of delivery or attempted delivery is included.

Other Delivery Services

Many private carriers compete with the U.S. Postal Service to provide shipment of letters and packages. Some of the most popular are **United Parcel Service (UPS)**, **Federal Express (FedEx)**, and **DHL World-Wide Express** (formerly Airborne Express). The USPS may contract with an outside service for the transportation and delivery of mail, such as the alliance they have with FedEx for delivering Global Express Guaranteed (GXG) mail items.

Most delivery services offer next-day service, second-day service, and regular shipping service. Delivery times and costs vary according to the size of the package and the distance involved. The assistant may want to be familiar with the range of services and delivery schedules provided by these carriers and to be aware of special packaging and labeling requirements. Arrangements can be made to have letters and packages picked up at the medical office. The Yellow Pages of the telephone directory provides names of other private shipping and courier companies listed with toll-free numbers under "Shipping Services."

ADDRESSING ENVELOPES FOR COMPUTERIZED MAIL

There are two popular envelope sizes used in the medical office. The small, personal size (number 6¾) is 6½ inches long and 3⅝ inches wide. The larger business size (number 10) is 9½ inches long and 4⅛ iches wide. The upper left corner of the envelope is reserved for the name and address of the sender. If not preprinted, this is placed on line three about one-half inch from the left edge of the envelope. The name and address of the person who is to receive the communication should be keyed as they appear in the inside address and should be placed within the reading zone determined by the U.S. Postal Service for OCR electronic scanning.

Optical character recognition (OCR) is a fully computerized system that processes the mail by the complete address at a speed of 36,000 pieces an hour or 10 pieces every second. Specific typing and address-

EXAMPLE 12-1
Bar Code

ing standards must be adhered to when preparing an envelope for OCR processing. At the bottom right-hand corner of the envelope is a space reserved as a bar code read area. After the OCR scanner has read the mailing address printed on the envelope, it prints a bar code of minute vertical lines representing the nine-digit ZIP code in the bar code read area (see Example 12-1). This reserved area, which is about 4½ inches wide and no more than ⅝ inch from the bottom of the envelope, must remain free of extraneous markings, such as printing and colored borders. Although the U.S. Postal Service accepts any color combination of ink and paper, black printing on white paper is the easiest to read.

Word processing software programs include a feature that addresses envelopes in the OCR format and inserts the bar code. These programs also have mail merge capabilities so an address book can be accessed and names and addresses can be easily inserted into documents.

All major U.S. cities employ computerized mail processing; therefore, medical assistants should adopt the required envelope format (Figure 12-6) to avoid rejection by an OCR. The electronic "reader" scans envelopes with two "eyes." One scans upward from the lower edge, and the other scans inward from the left edge, covering together a zone that measures 2¾ inches from the bottom and 8 inches from the left. In processing mail for delivery, both postal employees and sorting equipment ignore everything but the address in the line immediately above the city name. The last line must always contain the city, state, and ZIP code. Nothing may be typed below the last line of the address because the computer will consider it an error and redirect the envelope for hand processing.

Envelope Guidelines

The following guidelines are used to address business mail according to U.S. Postal Service OCR processing.

1. Key and machine print all address lines using a block format (four to six lines maximum), that is, single-spaced, at least 10-point type, in all capital letters with no characters touching. Table 12-2 shows names and address formats for

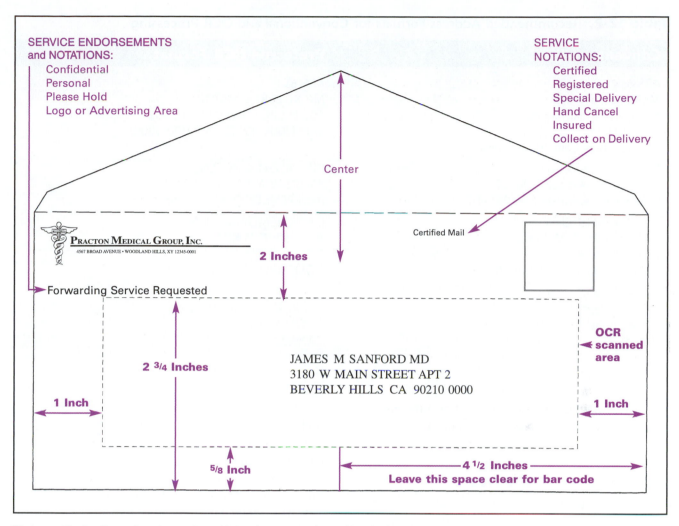

Figure 12-6. Completed number 10 business envelope (9½ inches by 4⅛ inches) using optical character recognition (OCR) format for placement of recipient's address, sender's return address, and special service endorsements. (Envelope is not shown to scale.)

conventional OCR processing. The U.S. Postal Service prefers all capital letters, but this is no longer required with the newer equipment.

2. Use standardized address abbreviations (see Table 12-3 at end of chapter).

3. Use standardized state abbreviations (see Table 12-4 at end of chapter).

4. If a city in an address exceeds 13 digits, refer to the "Address Abbreviation" section of the *National ZIP Code Directory*, published annually by the U.S. Postal Service, to find the accepted abbreviation. The computer is programmed to read only those cities listed in the directory.

5. Key an attention line (when one is necessary) on the second line of the mailing address (see Example 12-2).

EXAMPLE 12-2

Envelope Address Attention Line

PRACTON MEDICAL GROUP INC
ATTN FRAN PRACTON MD
4567 BROAD AVENUE
WOODLAND HILLS XY 12345 4700

or

PRACTON MEDICAL GROUP INC
ATTN FRAN PRACTON MD
4567 BROAD AVENUE
WOODLAND HILLS XY
12345 4700

Table 12-2. Recommended Address Formats for Conventional and OCR Processing

Conventional	Preferred OCR Format
ARS 654 Mr. Robert L. Major 608 North Broadway Place Suite 402 San Francisco, Calif. 91400-0000	ARS 654 MR ROBERT L MAJOR 608 N BROADWAY PL STE 402 SAN FRANCISCO CA 94100 0000
Mrs. Alison McKenzie 35 102 West Avenue K, Rm. 21 Independence, Missouri 64055-4178	MRS ALISON MCKENZIE 35 102 W AVE K RM 21 INDEPENDENCE MO 64055 4178
Lane Memorial Clinic Attention: Dr. C. M. Kim 770 12th Street E Columbus, Ohio 43202-0000	LANE MEMORIAL CLINIC ATTN DR C M KIM 770 12 ST E COLUMBUS OH 43202 0000
Monsieur John Kaput 120 Rue Nepean, Apt 8 Ottawa (Ontario) K2P0B6 Canada	MONSIEUR JOHN KAPUT 120 RUE NEPEAN APT 8 OTTAWA ON K2P0B6 CANADA

6. Mail destined for a foreign country must have that country's full name on the last line of the address typed in capital letters.

Two Delivery Addresses

When mail that has two delivery addresses, a post office box (POB) number and street address, the mail is delivered to the address that appears directly above the city–state–ZIP code line (Example 12-3). If the two addresses have different ZIP codes, the ZIP must be the one that serves the address of actual delivery.

EXAMPLE 12-3

Two Addresses

MIDWAY PHARMACY
2221 W MAPLE STREET
PO BOX 54 [mail would be delivered here]
NEW YORK NY 10017 0000

MIDWAY PHARMACY
PO BOX 64
2221W MAPLE STREET [mail would be delivered here]
NEW YORK NY 10017 0000

To speed mail delivery when a mailing address includes both street and POB number, always address the correspondence to the POB number. Recipients can pick up mail addressed to a POB as early as 8 or 9 a.m., whereas mail addressed to a street address may not be delivered until the afternoon of the same day. Also, when a medical office moves to a new location, the POB number usually remains the same. Consequently, the process of forwarding to a new street address can delay delivery of mail for one or two days when it could have been delivered promptly if it had been addressed to a POB.

Standard U.S. Postal Service procedure requires that mail addressed to an old street address be forwarded to a new street address, even if the addressee has a POB. This has been a source of frustration to POB holders who happen to move, but there is no way to avoid it apart from consistently using the POB number rather than the street address on all mailings.

Service Endorsements and Notations

Service endorsements are used to request a new address and to provide the USPS with instructions on how to handle undeliverable mail (Figure 12-6). The endorsements must appear in 8-point type or larger and should stand out clearly with a ¼ inch clear space on all sides. It cannot interfere with the return address or the mailing address that appears within the OCR-read area. Endorsements may appear in one of the following areas:

- Below the return address (line 9, flush with the left edge of the return address)
- Below the postage area (clear of all stamp markings)
- To the left of the postage area (clear of all stamp markings)
- Above the delivery address (not interfering with the OCR-read area)

A medical practice may request one of the endorsement types listed below. When the office is notified of a new address, be sure to update the patient's personal information in the computer database as well as their medical and financial records.

1. *Address Service Requested*—Mail is forwarded for 12 months at no charge and notice of new address provided; address correction fee ($0.50)

is charged. Mail will be returned after 12 months; action depends on length of time and type of mail.

2. *Return Service Requested*—Mail returned with new address and reason for nondelivery; may be a nominal charge for certain classes of mail.

3. *Change Service Requested*—Mail disposed of and a separate notice of new address or reason for nondelivery provided; address correction fee charged.

4. *Forward Service Requested*—Mail forwarded to new address for 12 months at no charge; this is the same with no endorsement appearing. Between 13 and 18 months the mail piece is returned with new address; may be minimal charge. After 18 months or if undeliverable, mail is returned with reason; may be minimal charge.

Other notations, such as "confidential" typically appear below the return address and *special service*

PROCEDURE 12-5

Address a Business Envelope Using United States Postal Service Regulations

Objective: To address business envelopes according to United States Postal Service regulations for accurate and timely delivery.

Equipment/Supplies: Computer and printer with envelope tray, or word processor or typewriter.

Directions: Follow these step-by-step procedures, which include rationales, to learn this skill, which is presented in the *Workbook* (Job Skill 12-7) for practice.

1. Refer to Figure 12-6 for visual guidance in preparing envelopes.

2. Choose the envelope format using a computer or word processor software program or insert each envelope in the typewriter. An option is generating labels using a software program.

3. Key the sender's name, street address, city, state, and ZIP + 4 code in upper- and lowercase letters in the upper left corner

of the envelope. If the letter needs to be returned to the sender for additional postage or address correction, a return address will ensure prompt return.

4. Start to the left of the center and at least 2 inches from the top of the envelope, key the receiver's mailing address in uppercase letters, maintaining a uniform left margin for each line. The U.S. Postal Service prefers this format. Eliminate punctuation in the address except the hyphen in the ZIP + 4 code. Leave a minimum of one space between the city name and the two-character state abbreviation and the ZIP + 4 code (see Table 12-3).

5. Key any notation for special services as noted in Figure 12-5.

6. Proofread the envelope and make corrections before printing from a computer program or prior to removing it from the typewriter. Accurate address information and placement of date will ensure fast and correct delivery to the recipient.

notations such as "certified" typically appear to the left or below the stamp, but cannot interfere with the OCR-scanned area for the address (Figure 12-6).

Window Envelopes

Window envelopes are popular because their use eliminates the need to type an address twice. They also reduce the possibility of a letter being placed in the wrong envelope. They are often used for mailing patient statements. Correspondence with address inserts for window envelopes must follow post office specifications. That is, they must be on white or very light-colored paper of a size that matches the opening to allow a clear view of the entire address. One-fourth inch of clear space must be visible between the address and all edges of the window; the only information that may show through the window is the name, address, and any key number used by the sender. If any part of the address is hidden, the OCR will reject the envelope.

When folding a letter for a window envelope, the letter is placed flat on the desk in the reading position. First, fold from the bottom third up, and then fold the top third *backward*. The last crease goes in the envelope first, with the envelope window-side up (Figure 12-7). Be sure to check the placement of the address when using a window envelope.

MANAGING OFFICE MAIL

Tight control of office mail procedures will expedite collections, save postage expense, and leave the staff time for other duties. Letters and packages that need to be rushed should be taken directly to the post office. Some guidelines when managing office mail are:

1. Check each outgoing letter for a written signature and for enclosures before sealing the envelope.

2. Avoid surcharges by keeping envelopes and cards within size limitations because nonstandard mail costs more.

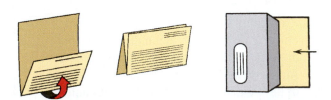

Figure 12-7. Folding a letter for insertion into a window envelope

3. Use window envelopes only if an address has four or fewer lines.

4. Indicate the proper mailing class to avoid being charged at the First-Class rate.

5. Use a service endorsement on the outside of envelopes that instructs the post office to forward mail to the patient at a new address if the patient moves. This procedure ensures that patients will receive their bills with minimum delay.

6. Print the bar code on the envelope if the office has a computer.

7. Use lightweight paper when sending international mail because rates are measured in half-ounce increments.

8. Purchase a postage scale and keep it accurately adjusted or keep a supply of Postage by Mail forms on hand to save a trip to the post office if mail is not metered.

9. Prepare computer disks for mailing by placing them in cardboard or heavy plastic before inserting them into a box or padded envelope.

10. Include a letter with any computer disks to identify the contents and the sender.

11. Place filament tape over the fastened clasp of an envelope to avoid damaged mail caught in automated equipment. If staples or paper clips must be used, fold the material so the fasteners are on the inner part of the documents. Write "Non-Automation Compatible Mail," "Do Not Run on Automation Equipment," "Please Hand Stamp," "Do Not Bend," or "Disk Enclosed" prominently on the envelope if the envelope is thick or contains disks, x-rays, or delicate objects.

12. Include APO (Army/Air Force Post Office) or FPO (Fleet Post Office) initials followed by a designated city and ZIP code on military mail envelopes.

13. Encourage patients to pay fees at the time of their office visit or personally hand them their statement with a return envelope.

14. Send several health insurance claim forms to the same carrier in one large manila envelope.

The medical assistant may want to use one of the many automated mailing stations and information centers that provide words, pictures, and videos to

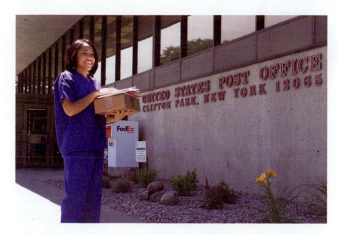

Figure 12-8. Medical assistant taking mail and packages to the United States Post Office

give postal information and help determine the type of service desired. The USPS Web site (http://www.usps .com) also has the information needed to mail everything from a letter to a 70 pound package. A "decision tree" is available; you choose the type of mail, size, weight, and then indicate how many pieces you have and whether you want it sorted, and it will automatically give you the best option for mailing. Postage and labels for special services are dispensed and receipts are provided.

ELECTRONIC MAIL

Electronic mail (e-mail) is a type of mail service that electronically sends, receives, stores, and forwards messages in digital form over telecommunication lines. E-mail saves time, is flexible, and encourages a rapid response. Instead of having to make contact by mail or telephone, the sender can leave a message in the electronic mail box of a distant computer where it can be retrieved by the receiver at a convenient time. If a response is required, it can be returned using the same system.

E-mail can improve patient satisfaction, increase accessibility to information, and enable patients to be more involved in their care. For physicians, e-mail can create self-documenting medical records, improve time management, and enrich the provider–patient relationship.

E-Mail Usage

Physicians have found multiple uses for e-mail, and many medical practices have an active electronic mail (e-mail) address. E-mail can greatly reduce tele-

phone calls, eliminate phone tag, speed up services to the patient, allow the patient communication with office staff, and allow the physician to respond to the patient at a convenient time, and it is an efficient tool for referrals. The physician can easily access e-mail from home, office, hospital, and distant locations when traveling. Errors are reduced through the elimination of verbal and handwritten data. Uses in a medical practice include:

- *Prescription requests and refills:* Pharmacy refill requests can be made via e-mail. The medical assistant pulls the patient's chart, routes it to the responsible physician for review, and sends an e-mail to the pharmacy.

- *Test results:* Laboratory and radiology reports may be e-mailed to the requesting physician to review. After printing a hard copy, the reports would be filed in the patient's chart or, if the office has an electronic medical record (EMR) system, transferred to the patient's EMR. The physician may e-mail the normal findings with any comments to the patient's private nonshared or monitored e-mail address. Abnormal findings would warrant a telephone call to the patient.

- *Transfer of patient records:* If medical records are stored electronically in the physician's computer system, selected portions of the medical record or the entire record can be e-mailed to a consulting physician. In return, the consulting physician can e-mail comments about the patient to the referring physician. This can be printed in hard copy and filed in the patient's chart or transferred to the patient's EMR.

- *Insurance processing:* E-mail has multiple uses for the insurance department. It may be used

PATIENT EDUCATION

E-mail communication to patients can consist of data about the medical practice and the staff, for example, office hours, satellite locations, and announcements, such as when flu vaccines have arrived and are available or times for walk-in blood pressure checks. Patients need to be informed when a medical practice uses e-mail and what they can use it for.

to verify the patient's eligibility; substantiate the deductible amount and status; obtain authorization for referral, service, or procedure; follow up on outstanding claims; and appeal denied or downcoded claims.

- *Appointment scheduling:* Patients may request appointments online by entering dates and times they prefer. A return e-mail message confirms the appointment.

- *Health news and information:* Notices can be sent out regarding new health information or screening tests (e.g., blood pressure checks, cholesterol tests). Links to Web sites that offer patient education can be provided.

- *In-office communication:* E-mail messages often work better than forgotten verbal messages. E-mail is able to facilitate faster, more efficient business communications (announcements and reminders) with colleagues and among coworkers who do not need an immediate response. When computers are in a network, electronic mail can substitute for an interoffice memo. The office assistant composes the memorandum on the computer screen to be transmitted to other areas of a medical facility. Large medical facilities may have an in-house Web site for employees that may have links to the Internet; this is called an *Intranet*. This network provides a way of disseminating information internally and cannot be accessed by the general public.

COMPLIANCE

Health care providers may not use or disclose protected health information without a valid authorization. The patient must sign an e-mail consent form to communicate electronically. In the form, the patient should acknowledge that he or she understands the risks of e-mailing information (Figure 12-9).

Subscription Services

It is possible to subscribe to an online computer information service via the Internet (e.g., America Online, CompuServe, Yahoo) or a local service (cable or telephone company) and communicate with any other

COMPLIANCE

Data transmission security must be ensured. The Health Insurance Portability and Accountability Act (HIPAA) requires the use of password protection, encryption, and authentication in transmission of patient information on an open network to ensure confidentiality.

person who has an e-mail address around the world. Medical assistants, medical billing services, and others subscribe to these services to network information with each other. These services also feature "bulletin boards" (electronic method of exchanging information publicly).

Transmission and Receiving E-Mail

To use e-mail, the computer needs to be connected to a modem that is serviced by a long distance telephone carrier or cable company for transmission of information across its lines. When sending a message, an online service is accessed by designating the mailbox code of the recipient and then keying in the message on the word processor (see Example 12-4). When opening unsolicited or unknown e-mail, there is a risk of exposing the computer system to viruses, so it is important to follow office guidelines in this regard.

When receiving a message, the user accesses an e-mail service on the computer and enters the password for the appropriate "mailbox." Any message stored can be brought up on a screen and saved to a disk or printed. In some electronic mail systems, a printed copy of the message is sent if the electronic

EXAMPLE 12-4

Electronic Mail (E-Mail) Address

Dbrown@aol.com

Dbrown	Individual user (David Brown)
@	at
aol	site (America Online, an on-line service provider)
com	type of site (commercial business)

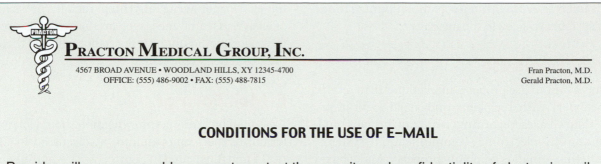

PRACTON MEDICAL GROUP, INC.

4567 BROAD AVENUE • WOODLAND HILLS, XY 12345-4700
OFFICE: (555) 486-9002 • FAX: (555) 488-7815

Fran Practon, M.D.
Gerald Practon, M.D.

CONDITIONS FOR THE USE OF E-MAIL

Provider will use reasonable means to protect the security and confidentiality of electronic mail (e-mail) information sent and received. Provider cannot guarantee the security and confidentiality of e-mail communication, and will not be liable for improper disclosure of confidential information that is not caused by provider's intentional misconduct. Therefore, patients must consent to the use of e-mail for patient information. Consent to the use of e-mail includes agreement with the following conditions:

1. All e-mail messages to or from the patient concerning diagnosis or treatment will be printed and made part of the patient's medical record. Because they are a part of the medical record, other individuals authorized to access the medical record, such as staff and billing personnel, will have access to those e-mail messages.
2. Provider will not forward e-mail messages to independent third parties without the patient's prior written consent, except as authorized or required by law.
3. Provider cannot guarantee that any particular e-mail message will be read and responded to within any particular period of time. The patient shall not use e-mail for medical emergencies or other time-sensitive matters.
4. It is the patient's responsibility to follow up and/or schedule an appointment if warranted.

ACKNOWLEDGMENT AND AGREEMENT

I acknowledge that I have read and fully understand the risks associated with the communication of e-mail between the provider and me, and consent to the conditions outlined herein. I agree to the instructions outlined herein and any other instructions that the provider may impose to communicate with patients by e-mail. Any questions I may have had were answered.

_____   _____

Patient's Signature   Date

_____

Patient name:

_____

Patient address:

_____

Patient e-mail address:

Figure 12-9. E-mail consent form that can be adapted to a medical practice

form is not retrieved within a certain amount of time. Other systems will delete the message.

E-Mail Etiquette

It is important to use proper e-mail etiquette to retain good rapport with recipients and avoid legal problems. Court cases regarding issues of privacy and ownership in electronic communication systems indicate that e-mail is company property. Make business e-mail businesslike and do not write personal e-mails on company time. Do not send messages of a sensitive nature, such as termination or a legal issue, via e-mail. E-mail messages may not be confidential and should not contain any data that could prove embarrassing to the sender, the business, or other people. Compose the e-mail, then reread it with this in mind.

Users need to be careful about expressing emotion in a message. Choose words carefully and eliminate humor, sarcasm, and anger. These can be misinterpreted easily because the receiver cannot see a grin or hear a chuckle. If you get emotional after receiving an e-mail message, write a reply and put it aside until the next day. Emotional responses to messages should not be made immediately. Before sending the message, reread and rewrite it to make it sound less harsh. Do not write anything racially or sexually offensive. Assume messages are forever. Misdirected messages should not be ignored but followed through to the intended recipient.

E-Mail Format

An e-mail business communication should follow the format of the memorandum, as discussed in Chapter 11 and illustrated in Figure 11-10. Anything more formal should justify using a letter format, which can be attached to the e-mail or sent instantly by fax. Use a font that is clean-cut and professional looking, such as Times New Roman, 12 point, black, and minimize the use of color and design (Figure 12-10).

Use a brief, meaningful, and specific subject line, such as "request for a meeting" or "insurance announcement" instead of one that is vague in nature. If there is a date or location involved, include this in the subject line.

Salutations may be formal; however, because the sender, recipient, and subject are identified in the heading, they may be informal and require no more than a name or an initial and a dash (see Example 12-5).

Left justify the message because this makes it easier to read.

Electronic Mail (E-mail) Message

Subj: **Appointment reminder**
Date: April 19, 20XX
To: Mary Avery

Reminder: Your next appointment with Dr. Gerald Practon is on Thursday, April 20, 20XX, at 2:00 p.m.

Connie Wheeler
Secretary to Gerald Practon, MD
General Practitioner
4567 Broad Street
Woodland Hills, XY 12345-0001
Phone: (555) 486-9002
Fax: (555) 488-7815
E-mail: gpractonmd@doctor.com

NOTE: THE INFORMATION CONTAINED IN THIS E-MAIL TRANSMISSION IS INTENDED TO BE SENT ONLY TO THE STATED RECIPIENT OF THE TRANSMISSION. IF THE READER OF THIS MESSAGE IS NOT THE INTENDED RECIPIENT OR THE INTENDED RECIPIENT'S AGENT, YOU ARE HEREBY NOTIFIED THAT WE DO NOT INTEND TO WAIVE ANY PRIVILEGE THAT MIGHT ORDINARILY ATTACH TO THIS COMMUNICATION AND THAT ANY DISSEMINATION, DISTRIBUTION, OR COPYING OF THE INFORMATION CONTAINED IN THIS E-MAIL IS THEREFORE PROHIBITED. YOU ARE FURTHER ASKED TO NOTIFY US OF ANY SUCH ERROR IN TRANSMISSION AS SOON AS POSSIBLE AND TO RETURN THE E-MAIL TO US. THANK YOU FOR YOUR COOPERATION.

Figure 12-10. E-mail message reminding a patient about an upcoming appointment

> ### EXAMPLE 12-5
> #### E-Mail Salutations
>
> Dear Mrs. Smith: (formal)
>
> Hi Joe, (informal)
>
> Greetings or Good morning/afternoon- (informal)

The message communicated in the body of the letter needs to be brief and to the point. *Pronouns may be omitted* if the interpretation is not lost in the reading of the message (see Example 12-6).

> ### EXAMPLE 12-6
> #### E-Mail Grammar
>
> A. Received lab report so please call for the results. (no pronouns)
>
>   *We* received *your* lab report so please call *us* for the results.
>
> B. Sent x-ray films to Dr. Stevens on March 18. (no pronouns)
>
>   *I* sent *your* x-ray films to Dr. Stevens on March 18.

Use correct grammar, word usage, and spelling along with standard capitalization and punctuation rules. Do not write in all capital letters; this is referred to as shouting. The way you produce an e-mail message reflects your professionalism and the importance of the message.

Do not use "emoticons," such as smiley faces ☺ and frowns ☹ in business e-mail. Use these only in personal communications with people you know well. Use only well-known acronyms and abbreviations. Limit messages to a maximum of two screens.

If responding to a long e-mail message, print out the letter and refer to it as you respond to ensure all items have been addressed accurately. Do not paraphrase from the message, but use quotes for the exact words when necessary. Create several paragraphs instead of one long body of text. Use numbered lists, when appropriate, to increase comprehension and speed reading. However, be careful when using for-

matting features such as bullets, underline, italics, and boldface because they may not translate correctly.

Tell the recipient what you want him or her to do and when you want action taken. Indicate to the recipient if you want a confirmation upon reception of e-mail. Proofread your e-mail before sending it and always check your spelling.

A complimentary close may be used for a formal closing and may or may not be used informally (see Example 12-7).

> ### EXAMPLE 12-7
> #### E-Mail Complimentary Closings
>
> Very truly yours, (formal)
>
> Sincerely, (formal)
>
> Bye. (informal)
>
> Regards to Jennifer (informal)

Most e-mail programs append signature lines automatically to the end of each message you send. A standard may be required by the medical practice for employees' signature lines, such as employee's name, business address, and telephone number. A maximum of six lines is recommended (see Example 12-8).

> ### EXAMPLE 12-8
> #### E-Mail Signature Lines
>
> A. (Ms.) Charlotte Evans
>   Insurance Billing Specialist
>   Practon Medical Group, Inc.
>   4567 Broad Avenue
>   Woodland Hills, XY 12345-4700
>
> B. Maria Valdez
>   Office Manager for Drs. Fran and Gerald Practon

Answering E-Mail

Some e-mail tools automatically save and include the text that you are answering. After going back and forth a few times, this history can get unwieldy, so use judgment in cutting off the bottom of the message. Leave enough of the message to establish context because an individual may not remember the message. Update the subject line when you receive or send a reply. Otherwise, the receiver may think that he or she has read the message and may accidentally delete it.

Use the "reply all" function with discretion. If four people received the message and you select "reply all," then all four people will receive your reply. Instead reply to the original sender unless the situation requires a "response to everyone."

Forwarding E-Mail

Never forward chain letters and beware when forwarding a message. To protect against viruses, the message may be copied and posted to a new message to be sent. Clean it up if the message has been forwarded several times. Erase all the "forwarded from" information and anything else that is irrelevant. By doing this, your recipient will not have to scroll through screens of routing information to find the one paragraph to read.

E-Mail Attachments

Limit the use of attachments, and if sending one, explain what it is about. Attachments are useful for sending large, formatted documents but not as a substitute for the regular text of an e-mail. Make sure the person you are sending an attachment to knows how to open it. Do not open attachments from someone you do not know because they may contain a virus that could infect your computer.

Basic Guidelines for Using E-Mail

Office policies should be instituted to regulate e-mail use for personal correspondence. There should also be an employer's policy on inspection of messages. Make sure employees understand office policies regarding when telephone calls or face-to-face communication is preferred. Following are some basic guidelines:

- Develop an office e-mail policy.
- Use strong encryption and password protection.
- Have the patient sign an informed consent form. If a patient refuses, do not accept e-mail from him or her.
- Do not provide any patient identifiers or personal health information in the body or subject field.
- Identify office staff who have permission to read and receive the physician's e-mail.

- Check your e-mail at designated times during each workday so you will not miss time-sensitive messages or let e-mail build up. Some e-mail software will make a beeping sound when e-mail arrives; that is, if the software is up and running and the speakers are turned on. Limit how often you check your e-mail inbox so it does not interrupt your work focus.
- Indicate appropriate times to send messages.
- Print e-mail if it contains important information or if there is need for a paper record. Append it to the patient chart when necessary.
- Answer messages promptly. If you cannot give an immediate response, let the sender know you will reply within a specified time, for example, within 24 hours.
- If you plan to be away from the office for an extended period of time, create an automatic reply function to let people know when you will return so the sender will not be waiting for an immediate response.

E-Mail Policies and Security

A number of professional organizations have established policies relating to e-mail, including the American Medical Association, the American Medical Informatics Association, and HealthyE-Mail, a non-profit physician outreach program. Protection of patient confidentiality, provision of quality health care, and physician liability should be three considerations when establishing office policies for e-mail transmission.

E-mail communication, like all forms of communication may present a threat to the patient's confidentiality and privacy. If strict guidelines are not established, patients may attempt to use e-mail for urgent needs, resulting in potential harm to themselves and liability for the physician. Post an informed consent document outlining the office policies and security capabilities and an authorization to use e-mail forms on the medical practice's Web site. Make sure the function is designed so that the consent must be read and signed prior to sending and receiving messages. Statements about who has access to patient e-mails, where patient e-mails go after they are read and printed, expected response times, various ways patients can use e-mail, and what topics are appropriate for e-mail usage should be included.

PROCEDURE 12-6

Compose an E-Mail Message

Objective: To compose and prepare e-mail messages for transmission via the Internet.

Equipment/Supplies: Computer with Internet connection.

Directions: Follow these step-by-step procedures, which include rationales, to learn this skill.

1. Use Times New Roman font, 12 or 14 point, black ink.

2. Insert the recipient's e-mail address.

3. Insert a descriptive subject line.

4. Insert a salutation.

5. Compose a single-spaced, left-justified message in the body of the letter.

6. Append closing signature line(s) at the end of the message.

7. Proof message and check for spelling errors.

8. Click "Send" and wait for an on-screen message to indicate the mail has been sent.

9. Mail that has been returned as undeliverable will appear in your mailbox. Verify the address and read carefully the reason for nondelivery.

Use a secure messaging service that allows the sending and receiving of encrypted messages. When using such a service, messages are picked up and delivered through the Internet or the medical practice's Web site, which is linked to the vendor's Web server. The server is protected by a firewall. A secure messaging service also allows the physician to limit staff access to specific categories of messages, restrict forwarding messages to standard e-mail systems, and permit patient communication for only those patients who have signed an informed consent and authorization document.

Each workstation should have a password to ensure unauthorized persons cannot access patient information. Patients' e-mail addresses must not be used for marketing purposes and written consent must be obtained before sending patient-identifiable information to a third party, even another physician.

COMPLIANCE

E-mail between patients and physicians involves protected health information (PHI) in electronic form. Therefore, even though HIPAA does not directly address e-mail in any of its standards, both the privacy and security rules apply.

Managing E-Mail

An e-mail management system should be developed so that you do not get overwhelmed with e-mail communication. Following are management tools that can be applied:

- Check and empty your e-mail box regularly

- When opening a message, be prepared to act on it; this eliminates the need to open and read messages multiple times

- Organize your mailbox into several categories or folders where messages can be stored

- Include a "miscellaneous" e-mail folder for messages that do not fit into basic folders

- Include a "temporary" e-mail folder for messages that do not need to be kept permanently

- Include a prompt when closing or deleting all e-mail messages that says, "Do you want to make this a part of the health care business record?" This allows one last time to decide if the mail should be kept or deleted

- Set up and use distribution lists that include names to which you can legally send e-mail messages to

- Set time limits for retaining and deleting messages; a retention policy will alleviate confusion and help ensure appropriate messages are kept

- Save all e-mail responses that contain PHI

FACSIMILE (FAX) COMMUNICATION

Facsimile (fax) communication, more commonly called *fax transmission* is an important communications tool for sending and receiving printed copies of information over telephone lines because the transmission is instant, reliable, and inexpensive. Although faxes are typically used less frequently than e-mail in today's business world, when used properly they can add a useful dimension when forms or documents need to be sent quickly.

To determine whether a document should be faxed, decide whether a telephone call would be more appropriate, particularly if only a short reply is required. Physicians use fax machines to transmit prescriptions to pharmacies, resubmit unpaid insurance claims, obtain preauthorization for services or procedures, network with other medical assistants, and send medical documents such as laboratory, pathology, x-ray, and biopsy reports (Figure 12-11).

To use fax transmission, each office needs a fax machine or a computer with fax capabilities, a printer, and a telephone line. Fax transmission saves time because messages can be sent in seconds to anyplace in the world. It saves money because the sender pays only the price of a telephone call each time a single or multipage document is sent. It prevents errors because it is an exact copy of the original document, whether it is typewritten, handwritten with a pen, or a graphic illustration. Fax transmission is a fast—3 seconds to 6 minutes per page—and an inexpensive alternative to using courier services or internal messengers in a large medical facility.

Fax Etiquette

It is inappropriate to send some documents by fax. Do not fax letters of appreciation, apology, or condolence or messages containing negative information, such as news of impending layoffs. Do not send insulting or sloppy messages or chain letters. Avoid sending a fax and asking the recipient to make and distribute copies. Do not send advertisements for wide distribution, and avoid using the fax machine for sending messages of a personal nature.

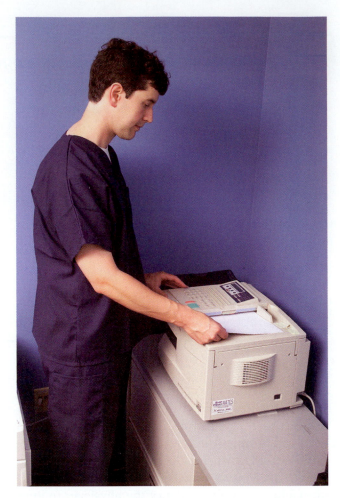

Figure 12-11. Medical assistant faxing a document

Cover Sheet

A cover sheet is mandatory to ensure protection and verify reception. It may consist of either a separate small half-sheet or a full-sheet letter, a small self-adhesive form attached to the top of the first page or a stamp on page one. The transmittal sheet or form may be handwritten or typed (Figure 12-12).

Fax Machine Features

Special features offered on fax machines are:

- Automatic document feeder (ADF), which saves time because handfeeding originals is eliminated.
- Coded mailboxes, which keep fax messages confidential. The sender punches in a code indicating the individual to whom the fax is addressed; that person then must punch in his or her own code to activate the printer.

PRACTON MEDICAL GROUP, INC.

4567 BROAD AVENUE • WOODLAND HILLS, XY 12345-4700
OFFICE: (555) 486-9002 • FAX: (555) 488-7815

Fran Practon, M.D.
Gerald Practon, M.D.

FAX TRANSMITTAL SHEET

To: *College Hospital*

Date *April 5, 20XX*

Fax Number: *555-487-6790*

Time *10:30 a.m.*

Telephone No. *487-6789*

From: *Gerald Practon, MD*

Telephone No. *555-486-9002*

Number of pages (including this one): *1* Fax No. *555-488-7815*

Note: This transmittal is intended only for the use of the individual or entity to which it is addressed, and may contain information that is privileged, confidential, and exempt from disclosure under applicable law. If you are not the intended recipient, any dissemination, distribution, or photocopying of this communication is strictly prohibited. If you have received this communication in error, please notify this office immediately by telephone and return the original FAX to us at the address below by U.S. Postal Service. Thank you.

Remarks: *Please send immediately the lab and x-ray reports on patient, Irene Snell.*

If you cannot read this FAX or if pages are missing, please contact:
PRACTON MEDICAL GROUP, INC.

INSTRUCTIONS TO THE AUTHORIZED RECEIVER: PLEASE COMPLETE THIS STATEMENT OF RECEIPT AND RETURN TO SENDER VIA THE ABOVE FAX NUMBER.

I, *Mary Smith* , verify that I have received *1*

(no. of pages including cover sheet)

from *Gerald Practon, MD*
(sending facility's name)

Figure 12-12. Example of a completed fax cover sheet for medical document transmission

- Automatic page cutting and collating for incoming documents.
- Store-and-forward (broadcasting) features, which schedule specific times for transmission, resulting in reduced telephone costs, automatic image reduction, activity reporting, voice request, delayed transmission, memory, remote control, and polling.

Transmit faxes only to and from machines located in secure or restricted access areas to protect the patient's confidentiality.

Fax Operating Guidelines

When a document is placed in the fax machine, it is scanned and the text is converted to electronic impulses that are transmitted over telephone lines. The impulses are then converted back to text by the receiving fax machine. The medical assistant should be aware of certain general operating procedures when using a fax machine:

- Plug fax equipment into a special fax power surge suppressor, preferably one with an uninterruptible power supply (UPS) to prevent damage. In addition, the entire office should be protected by a surge suppressor installed near the electric circuit breaker panel. This device is called an all-office or whole-office surge suppressor.
- Study the owner's manual for explicit information on the machine's care and use.
- Designate one or two staff members to monitor the fax machine.
- Keep the machine clean to avoid poorly reproduced copies.
- Write fax numbers in red and telephone numbers in black for easy identification.
- Avoid using correction fluid or tape on documents; remove staples and paper clips to prevent damage to the fax rollers.
- Wait for the signal that indicates receiving transmission has ended before trying to remove any document from the machine.
- Press the stop button to interrupt transmittal of a document; do not pull the paper out by hand.

- Try to transmit at times of the day when telephone rates are least expensive.
- Never leave the machine until the transmission is complete because noise or interference from telephone lines can be severe enough to garble a fax message.
- Place the machine away from direct sunlight or heat of any kind to avoid damage to documents.
- Turn the machine off when paper is replaced; failure to do so may cause incorrect sensor readings.
- Avoid sending documents that contain dark areas because they reproduce poorly. Lighten documents using photocopy machine settings prior to transmission.
- Reduce clerical time by maintaining a list of addresses and fax telephone numbers. Make copies of fax transmission sheets for frequently faxed numbers.
- Use faxes in rural areas to transmit test reports to expedite the diagnostic process and to save time and money.
- Send legal-sized documents only if the target fax machine can handle them.
- Enlarge a standard telephone message slip on a photocopier and forward the message by fax to the intended person if there is a problem reaching the person by telephone.
- Keep fax transmission short, not more than 10 pages.
- Telephone the recipient and ask when it is a good time to transmit a lengthy fax (20 pages or more). A message may be lost if the recipient's machine runs out of paper, toner, or both.
- It is not advisable to use a thermal paper fax; the edges of thermal paper roll and documents fade. If a thermal fax is used, photocopy all documents received prior to filing them.

Faxing Confidential Records

When handling faxed records, the assistant should be aware of specific legal and confidential requirements. They are:

1. Fax health information only when it is absolutely necessary to save time critical to the patient's welfare, not for convenience.

COMPLIANCE

The American Health Information Management Association (AHIMA) recommends that fax machines not be used for *routine* transmission of patient information and should be used only when (1) hand or mail delivery will not meet the needs of immediate patient care, or (2) a third party requires it for ongoing certification of payment for a hospitalized patient.

2. Do not fax personal documents, psychiatric records except for emergency requests, or records containing information on sexually transmitted diseases, drug or alcohol treatment, or AIDS or human immunodeficiency virus (HIV) status.

3. Never fax a patient's financial data. In court, faxing medical information can be justified on the basis of medical necessity, but faxing financial information cannot be justified.

4. Fax only to machines located in physician offices, nursing stations, or other secure areas. Do not fax to machines in mail rooms, office lobbies, or other open areas unless someone is standing by to receive the fax or they are secured with passwords.

5. Before faxing medical records, remember that issues of patient confidentiality, physician liability, invasion of privacy, and potential breach of the patient-physician privileged relationship are serious concerns.

6. Prior to the release of confidential medical information, have the patient sign a properly

COMPLIANCE

For Medicare patients, wording on the release of information form must meet government requirements for confidentiality.

completed authorization form. Edit your release of records authorization form to allow for fax transmission.

7. Ask the receiving party for a patient reference number (e.g., the patient's medical record number). Blank out the patient's name and write in the reference number on the document before faxing it. Ask other senders to fax records by reference number rather than by patient name.

8. Prepare a properly completed transmittal sheet with each transmission including a statement similar to that in Example 12-9.

EXAMPLE 12-9

Facsimile Confidentiality Statement

Unauthorized interception of this telephonic communication could be a violation of federal or state laws. The documents attached to this transmittal contain confidential information. They belong to the sender and are legally privileged. The information contained here is intended for use only by the authorized receiver named above. It cannot be redisclosed or used by any other party. If the assistant is not the authorized receiver, he or she will be notified that any disclosure, copying distribution, or taking any action on the information contained here is prohibited. If the assistant has received this document in error, notify the sender immediately by telephone or arrange for the return of the original documents to sender or to receive instructions for their destruction.

9. For confidential information, verify the telephone number and make arrangements with the recipient for a scheduled time of transmission or send it to a coded mailbox; otherwise, do not fax it. Coded mailboxes require the sender to punch in a code indicating the individual to whom the fax is addressed and the receiver to then punch in his or her own code to activate the printer. Place a telephone

call to the recipient about 15 minutes after faxing patient records to verify receipt. Or request that the authorized receiver sign and return an attached receipt form at the bottom of the cover sheet on receipt of the faxed information.

10. If a fax document gets misdirected, note the incident along with the misdialed number in the patient's medical record. Program frequently used numbers into the fax machine to avoid misdirecting faxed communications.

11. Keep a fax report of all transmissions, indicating the date, time, and destination telephone number.

12. Monitor incoming faxes frequently to maintain confidentiality.

Legal Document Requirements

The Federal Rules of Evidence (Rule 803) of the Uniform Rules of Evidence (URE) affects duplication of documents. More than half of the states have adopted rules based on the URE, which states, "a duplicate is admissible to the same extent as an original unless (1) a genuine question is raised as to the authenticity or continuing effectiveness of the original, or (2) in the circumstances it would be unfair to admit the duplicate in lieu of the original."

A number of states have adopted the Uniform Photographic Copies of Business and Public Records Act. This authorizes the admissibility of reproductions in legal cases that are made in the regular course of business without need to account for the original.

The Bureau of Policy Development of the Centers for Medicare and Medicaid Services (CMS) stated in June 1990 that the use of fax to transmit physicians'

STEP 1 2 3

PROCEDURE 12-7

Prepare a Fax Cover Sheet and Send a Fax

Objective: To prepare a cover sheet and send information quickly and accurately by fax.

Equipment/Supplies: Document to fax, fax machine, and telephone line.

Directions: Follow these step-by-step procedures, which include rationales, to learn this skill, which is presented in the *Workbook* (Job Skill 12-6) for practice.

1. Prepare a cover sheet for the document to be faxed containing:
   - Date
   - Time fax was sent
   - Name of the recipient
   - Fax number of recipient
   - Telephone number of recipient
   - Name of sender
   - Telephone number of sender (in case of a transmittal problem; e.g., lost page or dropped line)

   - Statement that it is personal, privileged, and confidential medical information intended for the named recipient only (see Figure 12-12).
   - Total number of pages, including the cover sheet

2. Place the document face down in the fax machine to align it for transmission.

3. Dial the fax number of the recipient. Preprogram all commonly used fax numbers to prevent misdialing errors. If the fax machine has a digital display that shows the fax number dialed, verify it for accuracy.

4. Press start when you hear the fax tone.

5. After the document has processed through the fax machine, press the button requesting a receipt if the machine does not automatically generate a report.

6. Remove the documents from the machine. If necessary, call the recipient to be sure the fax was received.

orders to health care facilities is permissible. When fax is used, it is not necessary for the prescribing practitioner to countersign the order at a later date. However, a legible copy of the physician's order must be retained as long as the medical record is retained. Thus, if thermal paper is used, photocopy it for preservation purposes. Some hospitals may not accept faxed physician orders, or they may limit transmission during certain times and require verifications of signature. The assistant should check with local hospitals or clinics about their fax policies.

Consult an attorney in your state to make sure documents (e.g., contracts, proposals, outlines, charts, graphs, plans, artwork composites, or photographs) requiring signatures are legal if faxed. Follow these guidelines to maximize a document's legal validity:

- Have the cover page of the fax refer specifically to what is being sent.

- Transmit the entire document, front and back, to be signed and not only the page to be signed so the receiver has full disclosure of the agreement.

- Obtain confirmation that the receiver is in receipt of all pages sent, because an incomplete document may be invalid and unsupportable in court.

- Insert a clause in the contract stating that faxed signatures will be treated as originals; for example, "Facsimile signatures shall be sufficient unless originals are required by a third party."

- Ask the recipient to obtain the signature of a witness while signing the document.

- Follow up and obtain the original signature in hard copy form as soon as possible by mail.

Table 12-3. Common Address Abbreviations

Alley	ALY	Center	CTR	Lake	LK	President	PRES	Street	ST
Annex	ANX	Circle	CIR	Lakes	LKS	Ranch	RNCH	Suite	STE
Apartment	APT	Cliffs	CLFS	Lane	LN	Rapids	RPDS	Summit	SMT
Arcade	ARC	Club	CLB	Mall	MALL	Ridge	RDG	Terrace	TER
Association	ASSN	Court	CT	Manager	MGR	River	RIV	Track	TRAK
Avenue	AVE	Drive	DR	Manor	MNR	Road	RD	Trail	TRL
Bayou	BYU	East	E	Mount	MT	Room	RM	Tunnel	TUNL
Beach	BCH	Estates	ESTS	Mountain	MTN	Route	RT	Turnpike	TPKE
Bend	BND	Expressway	EXPY	North	N	Row	ROW	Union	UN
Bluff	BLF	Extension	EXT	Northeast	NE	Run	RUN	Valley	VLY
Bottom	BTM	Freeway	FWY	Northwest	NW	Rural	R	Viaduct	VIA
Boulevard	BLVD	Grove	GRV	Orchard	ORCH	Secretary	SECY	Vice President	VP
Branch	BR	Harbor	HBR	Palms	PLMS	Shoal	SHL	View	VW
Bridge	BRG	Heights	HTS	Park	PK	Shore	SH	Village	VLG
Brook	BRK	Hill	HL	Parkway	PKWY	South	S	Ville	VL
Burg	BG	Hospital	HOSP	Place	PL	Southeast	SE	Vista	VIS
Bypass	BYP	Institute	INST	Plaza	PLZ	Southwest	SW	Walk	WALK
Camp	CP	Isle	ISLE	Point	PT	Spring	SPG	Way	WAY
Canyon	CYN	Island	IS	Port	PRT	Square	SQ	Wells	WLS
Cape	CPE	Junction	JCT	Prairie	PR	Station	STA	West	W
Causeway	CSWY								

Table 12-4. Two-Letter Abbreviations for the United States and Territories and Canadian Provinces

United States and Territories

Alabama	AL	Kentucky	KY	Ohio	OH
Alaska	AK	Louisiana	LA	Oklahoma	OK
Amer. Samoa	AS	Maine	ME	Oregon	OR
Arizona	AZ	Marshall Islands	MH	Palau	PW
Arkansas	AR	Maryland	MD	Pennsylvania	PA
California	CA	Massachusetts	MA	Puerto Rico	PR
Colorado	CO	Michigan	MI	Rhode Island	RI
Connecticut	CT	Minnesota	MN	South Carolina	SC
Delaware	DE	Mississippi	MS	South Dakota	SD
District of Columbia	DC	Missouri	MO	Tennessee	TN
Federated States of Micronesia	FM	Montana	MT	Texas	TX
Florida	FL	Nebraska	NE	Utah	UT
Georgia	GA	Nevada	NV	Vermont	VT
Guam	GU	New Hampshire	NH	Virginia	VA
Hawaii	HI	New Jersey	NJ	Virgin Islands, U.S.	VI
Idaho	ID	New Mexico	NM	Washington	WA
Illinois	IL	New York	NY	West Virginia	WV
Indiana	IN	North Carolina	NC	Wisconsin	WI
Iowa	IA	North Dakota	ND	Wyoming	WY
Kansas	KS	No. Mariana Islands	MP		

Canadian Provinces

Alberta	AB	Northwest Territories	NT	Quebec	QC
British Columbia	BC	Nova Scotia	NS	Saskatchewan	SK
Manitoba	MB	Nunavut	NU	Yukon Territory	YT
New Brunswick	NB	Ontario	ON		
Newfoundland and Labrador	NL	Prince Edward Island	PE		

STOP AND THINK CASE SCENARIO

Practice Mail Security

Scenario: You are opening mail for Practon Medical Group, Inc., and come across a piece of mail that looks like it has been opened and resealed with tape.

Critical Thinking: How would you proceed? List several things that you might do to verify the safety of the mail.

1. _____
   _____

2. _____
   _____

3. _____
   _____

STOP AND THINK CASE SCENARIO

Classify Outgoing Mail

Scenario: You are preparing outgoing mail and need to classify each piece.

Critical Thinking: Refer to the guidelines for mail classifications under "Handling Outgoing Mail" and use critical thinking skills to determine the mail classification for the following items:

1. Medical supply catalogue issued in the Spring, Summer, Fall, and Winter

   _____

2. Unsealed letter from Practon Medical Group, Inc., with one page advertisement for free blood pressure testing

   _____

3. Diagnostic codebook (package, 9 inches long, 6 inches wide, 2¼ inches thick, 3 pounds)

   _____

4. Consultation letter (envelope, 9½ inches long, 4⅛ inches wide, 6 ounces)

   _____

5. Referral letter that must be received the following day (envelope, 9½ inches long, 4⅛ inches wide)

   _____

6. Medical reports in a sealed envelope (9½ inches long, 4⅛ inches wide, 16 ounces)

   _____

7. Postcards (standard size), sent with a "Happy Birthday" wish to patients whose birthdays are this month

   _____

8. Package (18 inches long, 10 inches wide, and 10 inches high; weighs 50 pounds)

   _____

STOP AND THINK CASE SCENARIO

Select the Best Communication Method

Scenario: Following are several situations where communication is necessary.

Critical Thinking: Determine what the best form of communication is for the following scenarios and indicate by writing one of the following:

Letter   Memo   Telephone   Fax   E-Mail

1. The physician wants to send a note of condolence to a patient.

   _____

2. The insurance billing specialist wants to send a copy of a claim form that was already submitted to the insurance company.

   _____

3. The office manager wants to notify all office staff of an emergency meeting that will take place tomorrow morning.

   _____

4. The office manager wants to notify all office staff of a local medical society meeting that will take place next month.

   _____

5. Drs. Fran and Gerald Practon want to ask another physician group in the community whether they will be on call while the Practons go on vacation.

   _____

FOCUS ON CERTIFICATION*

CMA Content Summary

- Medical terminology and abbreviations
- Receive, organize, prioritize, and transmit information
- Format envelopes
- Operate photocopy machine
- Operate fax machine
- Send electronic mail

*This textbook and the accompanying Workbook meet the entry-level administrative and general competencies for the CMA outlined by the AAMA Examination Content Outline and Role Delineation Study and for the RMA and CMAS outlined by the AMT Competencies and Examination Specifications (see Competency Grid in Appendix B).

- Security/password
- Screen and process incoming and outgoing mail
- Classify mail
- OCR guidelines
- Postal meter

RMA Content Summary

- Medical terminology
- Common abbreviations
- Written communication
- Encryption and personal passwords

- Understand firewall software
- Compose correspondence

CMAS Content Summary

- Medical terminology
- Written communication
- Process incoming and outgoing mail
- Confidentiality
- Ensure confidentiality of computer-stored information
- Software and e-mail applications
- Manage office mailing and shipping services

REVIEW   EXAM-STYLE QUESTIONS

1. In the ZIP + 4 code, the four-digit add-on number is important because it identifies:
   a. a particular city block
   b. the floor of a building
   c. a department within a company
   d. a group of post offices boxes
   e. all the above

2. To verify the accuracy of a postage scale, weigh the following item(s), which equals one ounce.
   a. glass thermometer
   b. 9 pennies
   c. 6 pennies
   d. 1 nickel
   e. 1 dime

3. Metered mail must be deposited:
   a. at the nearest post office to the office address
   b. at any post office
   c. at the post office where the permit was issued
   d. on Mondays only
   e. anywhere regular mail is accepted

4. If mail to the physician marked "Personal and Confidential" is opened by mistake, how should it be handled?
   a. put it on the physician's desk by itself
   b. reseal with transparent tape
   c. personally hand it to the office manager
   d. reseal with transparent tape and label it "opened by mistake"
   e. ignore the error and place it with the other mail

5. When the medical assistant reads correspondence and either underlines or highlights important words and phrases or makes explanatory notes in the margin, this is referred to as:
   a. proofreading
   b. editing
   c. annotating
   d. commenting
   e. paraphrasing

6. Letters, cards, flats, bills, statements, and small parcels are typically sent by:
   a. first-class mail
   b. second-class mail
   c. third-class mail
   d. priority mail
   e. express mail

7. Priority mail usually reaches its destination in:

   a. 1 day

   b. 2 days

   c. 1 to 3 days

   d. 1 to 5 days

   e. 24 hours

8. Domestic registered mail can be insured for a value up to:

   a. $1,000

   b. $10,000

   c. $15,000

   d. $25,000

   e. $35,000

9. When the medical office sends an important letter notifying patients of the pending office relocation and wants to ensure its arrival, which USPS special service would be used?

   a. certified mail

   b. certificate of mailing

   c. registered mail

   d. express mail

   e. priority mail

10. Select the correct statement regarding mail addressed to a post office box *and* to a street address.

   a. Mail is delivered to the address appearing directly below the name.

   b. Mail is delivered to the address that appears directly above the city-state-ZIP code line.

   c. Mail is always delivered to the post office box.

   d. Mail is always delivered to the street address.

   e. Mail cannot be delivered if two addresses appear.

11. Select the correct statement regarding e-mail and the Health Insurance Portability and Accountability Act.

   a. HIPAA does not directly address e-mail in their standards; therefore, no rules apply.

   b. Only HIPAA security rules apply to e-mail.

   c. Only HIPAA privacy rules apply to e-mail.

   d. If e-mail involves PHI, privacy and security rules apply.

   e. none of the above

12. Select the correct statement regarding the fax machine.

   a. Fax machines are typically used less frequently than e-mail.

   b. Fax machines are typically used more frequently than e-mail.

   c. Fax machines send electronic messages more quickly than e-mail.

   d. Fax machines are no longer needed since the development of e-mail.

   e. Fax machines are useful for sending letters of appreciation, apology, or condolence.

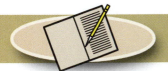

WORKBOOK ASSIGNMENT

To develop competency-based job skills, refer to the *Workbook* and complete the:

- Abbreviation and Spelling Review
- Review Questions

- Critical Thinking Exercises
- Job Skill activities, which are outlined at the beginning of this chapter under "Performance Objectives in the *Workbook*."

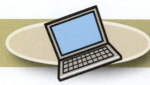

COMPUTER ASSIGNMENT

To review the concepts you have learned in this chapter, insert the *Student Practice* CD-ROM into a computer and work through the *StudyWARE* activities and games. Answer review questions in the practice mode and read the feedback, studying the questions you have missed. Take the chapter quiz until you achieve a minimum score of 90 percent. Successfully completing the *Critical Thinking Challenge* at the end of this course will help you think through scenarios and develop problem solving skills.

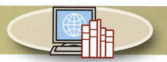

RESOURCES

Internet

To obtain answers to questions and get up-to-date information on mailing and shipping regulations, go to the following Internet Web sites.

DHL World Wide Express
    Web site: http://www.dhl-usa.com
Federal Express
    Web site: http://www.fedex.com

The Postal Store
    Web site: http://www.stampsonline.com
United Parcel Service
    Web site: http://www.ups.com
United States Postal Service
    Web site: http://www.usps.com

UNIT 5

Financial Administration

CHAPTER 13

Fees, Credit, and Collection

OBJECTIVES

After reading this chapter and learning step-by-step procedures to gain job skills,* you should be able to:

Learning Objectives

▎ Define credit and collection terminology and use collection abbreviations.

▎ Explain fee schedules and fee discounts.

▎ Discuss fees with patients and communicate fee policies.

▎ Understand billing methods.

▎ Report how billing services are used in the medical office.

▎ Describe credit laws.

▎ List the services of a credit bureau.

▎ State the importance of aging accounts and dun messages.

▎ Pursue telephone debt collection tactfully.

▎ Determine when to seek and how to select a collection agency.

▎ Decide when to use small claims court.

▎ Explain federal bankruptcy and garnishment laws.

▎ Trace a debtor who has moved and left no forwarding address.

Performance Objectives (Procedures) in This Textbook

▎ Explain professional fees in an itemized billing statement (Procedure 13-1).

▎ Perform mathematical functions using a calculator (Procedure 13-2).

▎ Prepare and post to a patient's ledger card (Procedure 13-3).

---

*This textbook and the accompanying Workbook *meet the educational components for entry-level administrative and general competencies outlined by CAAHEP and ABHES.*

- Prepare monthly itemized billing statements (Procedure 13-4).

- Establish a financial agreement with a patient (Procedure 13-5).

- Perform debt collecting using a telephone (Procedure 13-6).

- Take collection action, write off an uncollectable account, then post money from a collection agency (Procedure 13-7).

- File an uncollectable account in small claims court (Procedure 13-8).

- Trace a skip (Procedure 13-9).

Performance Objectives (Job Skills) in the *Workbook*

- Role-play collection scenarios (Job Skill 13-1).

- Use a calculator (Job Skill 13-2).

- Complete and post on a ledger card: charges, payments, a returned check and a check from a collection agency (Job Skill 13-3).

- Complete cash reciepts (Job Skill 13-4).

- Compose a collection letter, prepare an envelope and ledger: post transactions (Job Skill 13-5).

- Complete a credit card authorization form (Job Skill 13-6).

- Complete a financial agreement (Job Skill 13-7).

OUTLINE   WITH LECTURE NOTES

History of Credit
Credit and Collection Information

_____

_____

_____

_____

Fee Schedules
Medicare Fees

_____

_____

_____

_____

Changes in Fees and Discounts

_____

_____

_____

_____

Discussing Fees

_____

_____

_____

_____

Billing
Payment at Time of Service

_____

_____

_____

_____

Multipurpose Billing Form

_____

_____

_____

_____

Monthly Itemized Statement

_____
_____
_____
_____

Cycle Billing

_____
_____
_____
_____

Credit Card Billing

_____
_____
_____
_____

Debit Cards

_____
_____
_____
_____

Individual Responsibility Program

_____
_____
_____
_____

Billing Services

_____
_____
_____
_____

Credit and Collection Laws

Fair Debt Collection Practices Act (FDCPA)

_____
_____
_____
_____

Equal Credit Opportunity Act

_____
_____
_____
_____

Federal Truth in Lending Act

_____
_____
_____
_____

Truth in Lending Consumer Credit Cost Disclosure

_____
_____
_____
_____

Fair Credit Billing Act

_____
_____
_____
_____

Fair Credit Reporting Act (FCRA)

_____
_____
_____
_____

Collections

Aging Accounts

_____
_____
_____
_____

Office Collection Problem Solving

_____
_____
_____
_____

Telephone Collections

_____
_____
_____
_____

Collection Letters

_____
_____
_____
_____

Collection Agencies

_____

_____

_____

Small Claims Court

_____

_____

_____

Estate Claims

_____

_____

_____

Bankruptcy

_____

_____

_____

Tracing a Skip

_____

_____

_____

KEY TERMS

account receivable (A/R)
aging accounts
bankruptcy
bill
calculator
charge
collection ratio
credit
cycle billing
debit card
dun

fee-for-service
fee schedule
garnishment
ledger card
multipurpose billing form
open accounts
professional courtesy
quantum merit
receipt
skip

HISTORY OF CREDIT

The physician's primary aim is to provide health care for those who require it; however, it would be unrealistic to ignore another reason for practicing medicine, that is, to provide a livelihood for the physician and the physician's family. This livelihood depends on the good **credit** of those the physician serves. The word "credit" comes from the Latin, *credere*, which means "to believe" or "to trust." In today's world it simply means a trust in a person's integrity and in his or her financial ability to meet all obligations when they come due.

Credit for medical services and credit cards grew out of the Depression of the 1930s. Through

HEART OF THE HEALTH CARE PROFESSIONAL

Service

Communicating fees tactfully during a first encounter establishes patient responsibility. Answering questions and explaining fees is a courtesy to the patient. Offering payment options and arranging monthly payments may be of great assistance to the patient who is having financial difficulties.

the Depression years and before, when a patient was unable to pay cash, the doctor was paid in chickens, vegetables, or other material or by an exchange of labor. In Western society, it is the custom to pay the physician after services have been rendered. In other societies, such as ancient China, the doctor regularly visited the patient every three to six months in order to keep the patient healthy and was paid when the patient was well, payment was suspended when the patient became ill, until the patient was cured or much improved.

Times have changed; payment is now expected at the time of service unless an insurance contract is in place. It is not uncommon for patients to use some type of debit or credit card. In large clinics or a hospital setting, patients may use a patient record card that when passed through an electronic terminal will give a printout of their medical history, insurance coverage, and financial information. Patients may authorize via the card the billing of the insurance company or their credit card, so the doctor receives payment quickly.

Credit and Collection Information

The first important step in credit and collection is to obtain a complete and accurate registration of the patient at the time of the first visit, securing enough personal and financial history to be able to effectively collect on an account or trace a patient who moves (See Procedure 5-2). Figure 5-5 in Chapter 5 is an example of a patient registration record, which covers in detail the information that should be obtained from a patient. A comprehensive registration form lays the groundwork for a good flow of information that will help in sending statements, billing the insurance company, and collecting. Be sure the registration form includes spaces for a street address in addition to a PO Box, apartment number, business telephone number with extension, and a statement regarding interest charged on account. If a patient invokes the privacy laws and refuses to divulge any information, it should be policy to require payment for services at the time care is rendered.

It is important to update this form regularly so data is current. This can be done by having the patient review a copy of his or her original registration form and inserting changes in red ink. This will be vital when follow-up on a delinquent account is necessary.

FEE SCHEDULES

Each physician establishes fees depending on what other physicians in the same specialty receive for various services, the physician's education and experience, the geographic location of the practice, and the overhead for maintaining the practice (i.e., rent, utilities, salaries, equipment, supplies, insurance, telephone, laundry, office maintenance, taxes, Social Security, and so forth). **Quantum merit**, which means "as much as he deserves," is a common-law principle on which fees are based. Literally this term simply translates as the promise by the patient to pay the doctor as much as he or she deserves for labor.

A **fee schedule** is then determined, which is a typed list of the most common services the physician offers, including procedure code numbers, with a description of each service and its price. This must be available to all patients and under federal regulations, a sign to this effect must be posted in the office. This schedule can be used to quote prices to patients either before or after treatment is rendered. Practices may have more than one fee schedule except in those states with fair pricing laws that allow only one schedule stating standard fees for each service. For states that allow multiple schedules, there may be separate fee schedules for workers' compensation, managed care contracts, Medicare, and private pay patients depending on the specialty of the practice and the type and number of signed contractual insurance and managed care plan agreements.

Sometimes a physician charges a fee for a service that is not on the fee schedule, such as telephone calls to another physician for medical consultation, an uncanceled "no show" appointment, completion of insurance forms, a narrative of medical reports to other facilities requested by the patient, interest charges for delinquent accounts, or annual summary sheets of the patient's account for income tax purposes. It is wise and tactful to inform a patient verbally or in writing before billing for any such services; otherwise the patient-physician relationship may be adversely affected.

Medicare Fees

The Medicare fee schedule involves three columns. A *participating* fee is the amount paid to physicians who have contracts with Medicare. A *nonparticipating* fee is

---

EXAMPLE 13-1

2007 Medicare Fee Schedule for Southern California

Procedure Code	Participating Fee	Nonparticipating Fee	Limiting Charge
99211	$8.81	$8.37	$9.63
62270	$176.35	$167.53	$192.66

---

the amount paid to physicians who do not have contracts, and a *limiting charge* is the highest amount a nonparticipating physician can charge a Medicare patient (see Example 13-1). Additional information on this topic is presented in the Medicare section of Chapter 16, Health Insurance Systems.

Changes in Fees and Discounts

Some doctors give discounts for cash payment. Such discounts must be offered to *all* patients, posted in the office, and outlined in a patient brochure. If fees are raised, a message to patients explaining the increase should accompany the monthly billing, and the assistant should post a notice in the reception room.

Hardship Discounts

Discounts may be granted dependent on income level. Patients should be asked to verify their level of need by filling out an asset disclosure form or by bringing in their income tax returns. Document the reason (i.e., hardship discount) for the fee reduction in the patient's financial record.

Hill-Burton Act—Occasionally a patient seeking medical care has no way to pay for services and is ineligible for state aid. Most metropolitan areas have certain hospitals that have received federal construction grants to enlarge their facilities, in exchange for which they must care for indigents needing medical care. This obligation falls under the Hill-Burton Act of 1946. By contacting the local department of health, the assistant can obtain the names of hospitals participating in this service and send patients to these outpatient departments. Generally, the patients must complete financial applications to determine eligibility. Application forms and criteria vary from hospital to hospital.

Professional Courtesy

The term **professional courtesy** is a euphemism for a discount or a no-charge exemption extended to certain people by the physician. The medical assistant must know the physician's policy so as not to bill in error. Computerized systems allow accounts to be coded so no statements are sent to the patient.

When a bill is requested by the spouse of a physician who has a reciprocal treatment agreement, the phrase "by request" is typed on the billing statement. Currently the trend among physicians is toward billing their colleagues; psychiatrists bill all patients including fellow doctors.

Hospitals and many surgeons have largely given up the practice of free care, especially inasmuch as most physicians have health insurance coverage for medical expenses. If one physician does not bill another for services rendered, a result is that a third-party payer is relieved of its contractual obligation; this may fall under the False Claims Act.

COMPLIANCE

The Office of the Inspector General's compliance program guidelines state that professional courtesy arrangements may violate fraud and abuse laws, but this depends on two factors:

1. How the recipients of the professional courtesy are selected
2. How the professional courtesy is extended

If recipients are selected in a manner that directly or indirectly affects referrals, it may implicate the antikickback statute. An insurance claim submitted as a result of such a professional courtesy may also be affected by the False Claims Act.

Copayment Waiver

In the past to reduce the cost of medical care for some patients, a physician who accepted assignment (payment directly from the insurance company) might waive the copayment amount. However, the physician could be accused of not treating everyone with the same insurance coverage equally.

In most situations, both private insurers and the federal government ban waiving the copayment. It is, therefore, not recommended. There is one exception to this rule, Medicare recognizes a credit adjustment for this purpose on a doctor-to-doctor basis.

Discussing Fees

Physicians generally prefer not to discuss financial matters (e.g., insurance deductibles, unpaid bills) with their patients. The job of discussing and collecting fees is the responsibility of the medical assistant.

If the physician is charging **fee-for-service**, that is, set dollar amounts for professional services, it is important to tell patients when they call for appointments that the office policy is to collect the fee at the time services are given. This type of practice increases collections and decreases the number of billing statements sent. It has been shown that a policy of stating fee-for-services also improves public relations and reduces patient complaints, business-office turnover, accounts receivable, and write-off amounts. The percentage of patients who pay their bills and return the next time they need health care will increase.

The medical assistant may state fees and answer any questions about charges when making appointments by telephone. If the patient is a member of a managed care plan, he or she should be advised that the copayment will be collected at the time of the visit. In some instances (e.g., elective surgery) and in some types of specialty practices, the policy may be

COMPLIANCE

Because financial matters are personal, it is important that any conversation regarding fees be private so discussion of patients' accounts are not overheard by others and patients feel free to talk about any financial problems. A mature, courteous, tactful, firm, and businesslike approach is vital.

EXAMPLE 13-2

Obstetric Fees

An obstetrician-gynecologist may collect at each prenatal visit a portion of the charge for delivering a baby so that the entire patient responsibility for the obstetric bill is paid before the child is born. This eliminates having to ask the patient to pay a lump sum after delivery or after the insurance company has paid its portion.

to collect for services as they are rendered while also requiring payment of a small amount toward the performance of future services. Obstetric fees are a case in point (Example 13-2).

There is a right time and a wrong time for everything, including the discussion of medical fees. Most patients who come to the office seeking medical care are more concerned with their health problem than with the expense incurred by their office visit. The assistant begins by listening to the patient's medical problem but is prepared to discuss the expense, should the patient inquire about costs. After the patient explains his or her medical problem, the assistant should tactfully ask whether the patient has health insurance coverage. Generally a patient who has insurance will have coverage that will offset a portion of the office and hospital expense.

It is wise to ask, "Would you like to know something about the expense?" because occasionally a patient is emotionally unable to handle a discussion of fees. If a patient is elderly and someone in the family is responsible for the bill, the fee discussion should take place with both the guarantor (paying party) and the patient.

Never assume anything about a patient's financial status, and do not judge by outward appearance. Even if someone appears poorly dressed, or conveys the impression that they cannot afford to pay, the medical assistant must refrain from asking embarrassing questions. Tact is called for in all inquiries, whether dealing with credit (the ability to pay) or with the choice of a room at the hospital. "What type of room would you like to reserve?" is preferable to, "You'll want a private room, of course." To eliminate psychologically misleading statements about "credit," it is best to use the terminology "patient accounts department" when referring to the credit department

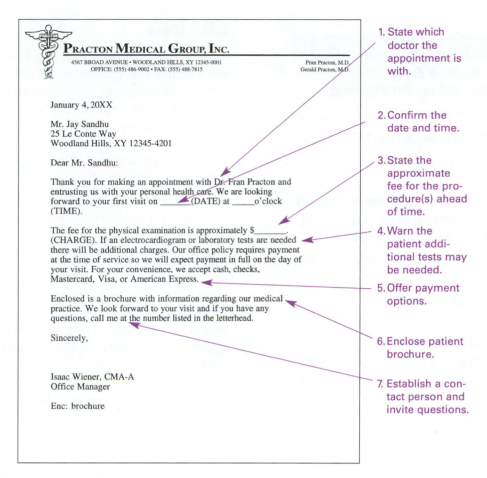

Figure 13-1. New patient confirmation letter

Guidelines for Communicating Fees

Fees for medical service should be stated clearly and accurately. A misquoted cost may make a patient angry. The medical assistant should neither hesitate when stating the approximate amount nor apologize for the fee. Use an approach that makes it easier for the patient to pay than to avoid payment (see Example 13-3). If the patient cannot pay at the time of service, do not reward such behavior by letting him or her leave quickly.

If a patient is having financial difficulties, this may come out during the initial interview. Then the assistant can discuss a payment plan, or a discount if it is warranted. Physicians expect patients to make acceptable monthly payments on their accounts regardless of pending payments by insurance companies.

In some instances, the physician is the person to handle the financial discussion, particularly when surgery is recommended. The examination room, however, is not the place to discuss fees. Fee discussion should wait until the patient has dressed and is in the privacy of the physician's office. The physician should communicate directly with the patient by asking if there are any questions about the cost of the operation and, if so, review the surgical fees involved. Surgical costs should be quoted after the insurance

verbally or in correspondence. "Our payment policy" is preferable to "our credit policy." Terms that project a positive tone, such as "fee" instead of "**charge**," will be reflected in patients' attitudes.

PATIENT EDUCATION

Patients must be made aware that payment is expected. Exhibit a sign on the front desk or in the waiting room stating the payment policy. Send a brochure, patient information pamphlet, or confirmation letter to new patients welcoming them to the practice (Figure 13-1) and informing them of the approximate cost.

EXAMPLE 13-3

Positive Expressions When Asking for Payment

1. When a patient calls for an appointment:

   "Copayment is expected at the time of service."

   or

   "The office visit will be approximately $_____. We accept cash, checks, and credit cards for your convenience."

2. When the patient checks in at the front desk:

   "Your copayment will be $_____ today."

3. When the patient checks out:

   "The office visit is $_____. Would you like to pay by cash, check, or credit card?"

   or

   "I see your deductible has been met and your insurance pays 80%. Your portion of the bill comes to $_____."

BILLING

Each office has its own policy for fee collection based on whether the patient is insured and a fee-for-service contract is in place, enrolled in a managed care plan with copayment requirements, or not insured. Collection of fees may also depend on the specialty of the physician, the amount of the average bill, and the patient load. The following section covers popular collection methods.

Payment at Time of Service

Collection for office visits when the service is rendered is an opportunity not to be missed. The medical practice may introduce a "pay now" policy by sending a letter to patients indicating the need for such a policy (Figure 13-2). Attractive features include increase of cash flow, reduction of collection costs (in both postage and administrative time), reduced billing chores, settlement by insurance companies directly to the patient, quick identification of nonpayers (see Example 13-4) and increase in the **collection ratio**, i.e., the proportion of money owed compared to money collected on the accounts receivable. Offering patient payment options and a reason to pay will increase collections.

company has given information on how much the policy pays on a specific procedure. If the preoperative examination and postoperative care are included in a surgical fee, this should be stated so the patient knows in advance what to anticipate. Hospital costs should be quoted only if current room rates and extra fees are known. Otherwise, direct the patient to the financial department of the hospital.

A deadbeat (one who evades paying bills) may be spotted in advance, so payment may be requested at the time of service. Some signals to watch for are:

1. Questionable employment record
2. No business or home telephone
3. Many moves of residence
4. A motel address
5. A record of doctor hopping
6. No referral
7. No insurance
8. Many unfilled blanks on the patient registration form

EXAMPLE 13-4

Incentives to Discuss with Patients to Receive Payment at Time of Service

1. Accepting cash, check, or credit/debit card offers patient convenience

2. Paying at time of service helps the practice avoid further billing costs, which contribute to rising health care costs

3. Paying insurance deductibles and copayment fees at time of service allows the insurance company to take care of the entire balance after billing

4. Owing money and receiving bills is reduced

5. Paying in monthly installments to a credit card company eases monthly debt

6. Avoiding collection agencies decreases bad credit reports

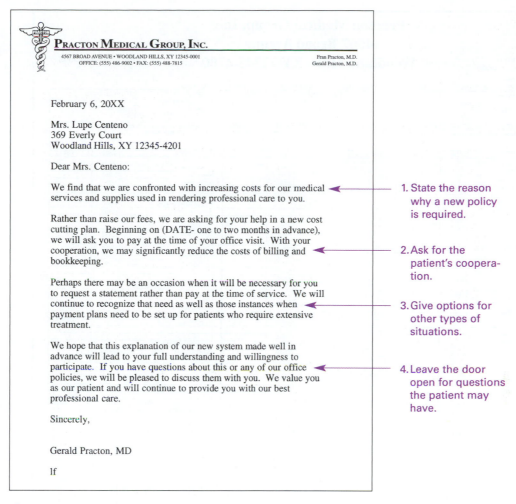

Figure 13-2. Pay now policy letter

A common excuse for nonpayment is the forgotten checkbook; a remedy is to keep *early-pay envelopes*, stamped and self-addressed, within easy reach to give to patients with requests to mail a check on arrival at home. Also, provide payment options such as credit or debit card payment.

Meeting with the Patient

Meeting face to face with the patient at the time of service regarding outstanding balances is often more successful than telephoning or sending statements. The day before the visit, the patient appointment schedule can be printed from the computer or copied from the appointment book. Each patient's account balance is reviewed and balances over 60 days are flagged. When the patient arrives, he or she is courteously escorted into a private room to discuss the bill. The patient can see how committed the assistant is in regard to solving the collection problem and the chance of a mutually satisfactory resolution is greatly improved. Although the physician does not per-

form credit and collection work, he or she can make patients aware of their outstanding debt. The realization that the physician is aware of the delinquency is often effective in encouraging payment.

Multipurpose Billing Form

The **multipurpose billing form** is a combination bill, insurance form, and routing document, which may be given to the patient at the time of the office visit (Figure 13-3). It is also referred to as a *charge slip, communicator, encounter form, fee ticket, patient service slip, routing form, superbill,* and *transaction slip.* The form (two or three parts) can be used in a manual (pegboard charge-slip system) or computerized office bookkeeping system (Chapter 15). It contains the patient's name, date, services rendered, procedure codes, diagnostic codes, the physician's identifying data, and a section to indicate the patient's next appointment. It may also include an assignment of benefits, other insurance requirements, and a section for the

Practon Medical Group, Inc.
4567 Broad Avenue
Woodland Hills, XY 12345-4700

Phone: 555-486-9002

STATE LIC. # C1503X
SOC. SEC. # 000-11-0000
PIN # _____

1. Physician's identifying data

☐ PRIVATE	☐ BLUECROSS	☐ IND.	☐ MEDICARE	☐ MEDI-CAL	☐ HMO	☒ PPO	

PATIENT'S LAST NAME	FIRST	ACCOUNT #	BIRTHDATE	SEX ☐ MALE	TODAY'S DATE
Chang	Kim	2936	10 / 05 / 41	☑ FEMALE	03 / 05 / XX

INSURANCE COMPANY	SUBSCRIBER	PLAN #	SUB. #	GROUP
Aetna	self		463-XX-3699	

2. Patient and insurance data

ASSIGNMENT: I hereby assign my insurance benefits to be paid directly to the undersigned physician. I am financially responsible for non-covered services.
SIGNED: (Patient, or Parent, if Minor) _____ DATE: / /

RELEASE: I hereby authorize the physician to release to my insurance carriers any information required to process this claim.
SIGNED: (Patient, or Parent, if Minor) _____ DATE: / /

3. Assignment of benefits and authorization to release information

✓	DESCRIPTION	CODE	FEE	✓	DESCRIPTION	CODE	FEE	✓	DESCRIPTION	CODE	FEE
	OFFICE VISITS	NEW	EST.		IMMUNIZATIONS				MAJOR SURGERY		
	Blood Pressure Check		99211		Allergy Inj. X1	95115			Circumcision	54150	
	Level II	99202	99212		Allergy Inj. X2	95117			Vasectomy	55250	
✓	Level III	99203	99213	70.92	Trigger Pt. Inj.	20550			Mole Removal	* 17100	
	Level IV	99204	99214		Therapeutic Inj.	90799			Flat Warts	* 17110	
	Level V	99205	99215			Drug			Biopsy, 1 Lesion	11100	
	SUPPLEMENTAL VISITS					Dose			Biopsy, Addt'l. Lesions	11101	
	HPR Meet Dr.		90001						Endometrial Bx	58100	
	HPR GYN		90089		VACCINATIONS						
	Post-Op N/C		99024		DPT	90701			SURGERY		
	PREVENTIVE EXAM	NEW	EST.		DT	90702			Skin Tags to 15	* 11200	
	Intermediate	99385	99395		Tetanus	90703			Each Addt'l. 10	11201	
	Age 12 - 17	99384	99394		MMR	90707			Elec. Skin Tags to 15	* 17200	
	Age 5 - 11	99383	99393		OPV	90712			Each Addt'l. 10	17201	
	Age 1 - 4	99382	99392		Polio Inj.	90713			I & D Abscess	* 10060	
	Infant	99381	99391		Flu	90724					
	Newborn Ofc		99432		Rabies	90726					
	OB / NEWBORN CARE				Hepatitis B Vac	90731			SUPPLIES / MISCELLANEOUS		
	OB Package		59400		Pneumovax	90732			Surgical Tray	99070	
	Post-Partum Visit N/C				HIB Vaccine	90737			Trays S L		
	LAB PROCEDURES								Casting Supplies		
	Urine Dip		81000		OFFICE PROCEDURES				Type:		
✓	UA Only		81005	15.00	Anoscopy	46600			Splints/Slings		
	Pregnancy Urine		81025		Diaphragm Fitting	57170					
	Wet Mount		87210		Ear Lavage	69210					
	KOH Prep		87220		IUD Insert/Removal	58300	58301		SPECIAL SERVICES		
	Occult Blood		82270		Spirometry	94160			Special Report	99080	
	Venipuncture		36415		Nebulizer Rx	94664			Handling Charge	99000	
	Strep Screen		86403		Splint Site						
	TB Skin Test		86585		Casting Site Removal						
	Hematocrit		85013								
	Glucose Finger Stick		82947								

4. Codes for professional services

DIAGNOSIS   ICD-9

CARDIOLOGY:
__ Angina 413.9
__ Atrial Fibrillation 427.31
__ Cardiopulmonary Dis. .429.2
__ CHF 428.0
__ CVA/Old 437.1
__ Heart Murmur 785.2
__ Irregular Heart Beat ..427.9
__ Mitral Valve Disease ..356.9
__ PVD 443.9
__ Tachycardia/Unsp. ...785.0
__ TIA 435.9

ENT:
__ Allergic Rhinitis 477.9
__ Cerumen Impacted ...380.4
__ Labyrinthitis 386.30
__ Otitis Externa 381.23
__ Otitis Media 381.01
__ Otitis Media/Sanguinous 381.03
__ Pharyngitis 462
__ Pharyngitis/Strep 034.0
__ Rhinitis/Chronic 472.0
__ Sinusitis/Acute 461.9
__ Sinusitis/Chronic 473.9
__ Thrush 112.0
__ Tinnitus 388.30
__ Tonsillitis 463

__ Tympanum/Rupture ..384.20
__ Viral Syndrome 079.99

EYE:
__ Blepharitis 373.00
__ Conjunctivitis, Acute .372.00
__ Conjunctivitis, Bi-Lat. .372.30
__ Conjunctivitis, Pink-Eye 372.03

FEMALE / OB-GYN:
__ Amenorrhea 626.0
__ Bleeding/Uterine ...626.9
__ Breast Mass 611.72
__ Cervical Dysplasia ..622.1
__ DUB 626.8
__ Dysmenorrhea 625.3
__ Fibrocystic Breast ..610.1
__ Menopausal Synd. ..627.2
__ Menorrhagia 626.2
__ Ovarian Cyst 620.2
__ Pelvic Mass 789.3
__ PID 614.9
__ Premenstrual Tension .625.4
__ Uterine Fibroid 218.9
__ Vulvovaginitis 616.10
__ Vulvovaginitis/Monilia .112.1
__ Vulvovaginitis/Trich. ..131.01

MEDICINE:
__ Arthritis/Inflammatory .714.9
__ Arthritis/Rheumatoid ..714.0

__ Chronic Pain Sys., Myalgia 729.1
__ Condyloma 078.10
__ Constipation 564.0
__ Cuarts-Common 078.10
__ Cuarts-Venereal 078.19
__ Cystitis/Acute 595.0
__ Diabetes/Type I 250.01
__ Diabetes/Type II ...250.00
__ Diverticulitis 562.11
__ Diverticulosis 562.10
__ Gastritis 535.50
__ Gout 274.9
__ Headache/Tension ..307.81
__ Headache/Vascular ..784.0
__ Hemorrhoids 455.6
__ Herpes 054.9
__ Hypercholesterol ...272.0
__ Hypertension 401.9
__ Hypothyroidism 244.9
__ Irritable Bowel Syndr. .564.1
__ Kidney Stone 592.0
__ Migraine 346.90
__ Peptic Ulcer Disease .533.30
__ Plantar Fasoitis 728.71
__ Pyelonephritis 590.10
__ Rectal Bleeding 569.3
__ Renal Colic 788.0
__ Skin Tag 709.1

✓ UTI 599.0
__ Warts-Common 078.10
__ Warts-Venereal 078.19

PAIN:
__ Abdom/Epigastric ..789.06
__ Abdom/Generalized .789.02
__ Abdom/LLQ 789.04
__ Abdom/LUQ 789.02
__ Abdom/Periumbilic .789.05
__ Abdom/RLQ 789.03
__ Abdom/RUQ 789.01
__ Abdom/UNSP 789.00
__ Anal/Rectal 569.42
__ Ankle/Foot 719.47
__ Back 724.5
__ Breast 611.71
__ Chest 786.50
__ Ear 388.70
__ Generalized/Chills ..780.9
__ Hip 719.45
__ Limb 729.5
__ Low Back/Lumbago .724.2
__ Neck 723.1
__ Pelvic 625.9
__ Shoulder 719.41
__ Upper Arm 719.42

RESPIRATORY:
__ Apnea/Sleep 780.57

__ Asthma/Allergic 493.00
__ Asthma/Bronchial ...493.90
__ Bronchitis/Acute 466.0
__ Bronchitis/Chronic ..491.9
__ COPD 496
__ Croup 464.4
__ Emphysema 492.8
__ Pneumonia 486
__ Shortness of Breath ..786.09
__ URI 465.9

V-CODES
__ Cntrcpt./Pres/IUD. ...V45.51
__ Cntrcpt./Pres/Norplant .V45.52
__ Cntrcpt. Surv. & Exam .V25.40
__ Desens. to Allergens .V07.1
__ Eating/Inap Diet/Habits .V69.1
__ Exercise/Lack of Phys. .V69.0
__ Fam. Hx/Breast Malig ..V16.3
__ Fam. Hx of Diab. Mellitus .V18.0
__ Family Planning V25.09
__ Gynecological Exam ..V72.3
__ Health Check/Adult ..V70.0
__ Hlth. Check/Auto Accid. V71.4
__ Health Check/Child ..V20.2
__ Hx Tobacco Use V15.82
__ Laboratory Examination V72.6
__ Personal Hx/Brst. Malig V10.3
__ Pp/Imm Aft Del/Unc. ..V24.0

__ Pregnant State V22.2
__ Routine or Ritual Circum. V50.2
__ STD/Exposus V01.6
__ TB Skin Test V74.1
__ Tet. Tox./Vacc V03.7
__ Vaccination/DTP V06.1
__ Vacc./Inoculation/Influ. .V04.8
__ Vacc./Meas/Mumps/Rub V06.4
__ Vacc./Poliomyelitis ...V04.0
__ Vacc./Proph/Hem.Type B V03.81
__ Vacc./Prop/Oth Sp Bact.V03.89
__ Vacc./Proph/Stre./Pneu V03.82

SYMPTOMS
__ Abn. Blood Chemistry .790.6
__ Abnormal Bld. Pressure 796.4
__ Abnormal Pap 795.0
__ Anemia 280.9
__ Anxiety 300.00
__ Diaper Rash 691.0
__ Drug Abuse 305.9
__ Drug Dependency ..304.90
__ Edema 782.3
__ Insomnia 708.52
__ Pyrexia 780.6
__ Rash, Unspecified ..782.1
__ Seizure Disorder ...780.3
__ Weakness 780.7

5. Diagnostic code

6. Additional diagnoses

Injury Diagnosis	C Spine	T Spine	L Spine	Pelvis	Clavicle	Shoulder	Scapula	Humerus	Elbow	Forearm	Wrist	Hand	Finger	Hip	Femur	Patella	Leg	Ankle	Foot	Toe
SPRAIN/STRAIN	847.0	847.1	847.2	848.5	840.0	840.9	840.9	840.9	841.9	841.9	842.00	842.10	842.12	843.9	843.9	844.9	844.9	845.00	845.10	845.1
TENDINITIS/BURSITIS	—	—	—	—	—	726.11	—	—	726.33	—	726.4	726.4	726.8	726.5	—	726.60	—	726.71	726.7	—

DIAGNOSIS:	DOCTOR'S SIGNATURE / DATE

_____ Sliding Scale

7. Appointment information

RETURN APPOINTMENT INFORMATION:	-WITH WHOM	SELF/OTHER	REC'D. BY:	TOTAL TODAY'S FEE	85.92
DAYS ____ WKS. 2 MOS. ____			☐ CASH ☐ CHECK # ____	AMOUNT REC'D. TODAY	0

PLEASE REMEMBER THAT PAYMENT IS YOUR OBLIGATION, REGARDLESS OF INSURANCE OR OTHER THIRD PARTY INVOLVEMENT.

8. Total charges and payments received

INSUR-A-BILL ® BIBBERO SYSTEMS, INC. • PETALUMA, CA • © 7/90 (BIBB ST SB SAMP)   (REV. 1/97)

Figure 13-3. Multipurpose billing form; procedure codes for professional services are taken from the *Current Procedural Terminology (CPT)* codebook and diagnostic codes are taken from the *International Classification of Diseases, 9th revision, Clinical Modification (ICD-9-CM)* codebook. (Courtesy of Bibbero Systems, Inc., Petaluma, CA. Telephone: (800) 242-9330; Web site: http://www.bibbero.com.)

patient to complete. This form is clipped to the front of patients' charts on their arrival at the office. The physician checks off procedures that are performed during the office visit and all applicable diagnoses, and, at the bottom of the slip indicates if the patient should return for an appointment. The transaction slip is routed back to the medical assistant to be totaled for payment. It is designed to provide insurance billing information, eliminate paperwork, encourage payment immediately after services have been rendered, and change the patients' habits by making them financially responsible for themselves. In some states private insurance programs accept a multipurpose billing form from the patient and in some cases the insurance benefits can be assigned to the physician directly, which means the insurance company will mail the check to the physician instead of the patient. The physician's signature is not necessarily required. It may be given as a **receipt** if the patient paid for services at the time they were rendered.

This form is, in some respects, an attending physician's statement. It is an important document that should be prenumbered, filed in numeric and chrono-logical order with the most recent first, and used for audit control. A multipurpose form should be annually reviewed and updated to include new or revised procedure and diagnostic codes and any other changes in the practice. All fees and payments should be posted daily to the patient's account or ledger and daysheet.

Monthly Itemized Statement

A **ledger card** is a record showing charges, payments, adjustments, and balance owed and is created for each patient when he or she first receives medical services (Figure 13-4). Some offices copy these as a monthly itemized statement. Other practices generate a computerized **bill**, which uses the same information found on the ledger, to be sent to the patient stating the fees owed (Figure 13-5). When compared to payment at the time of service, this increases collection costs and delays cash flow.

In a computerized system, the computer can be directed to search the database and print financial account records for patients who have outstand-

PROCEDURE 13-1

Explain Professional Fees in an Itemized Billing Statement

Objective: To explain professional fees in a private setting so the patient's right of privacy is observed and he or she understands financial obligations.

Equipment/Supplies: Fee schedule for the medical practice, patient's monthly statement, and quiet private room.

Directions: Follow these step-by-step procedures, which include rationales, to learn this skill.

1. Obtain a copy of the patient's itemized monthly billing statement to review amounts owed (see Figure 13-5).

2. Refer to the medical practice's fee schedule for the services and procedures rendered (see Part IV of the *Workbook*).

3. Examine the billing statement for any errors.

4. Correct any error that may have occurred prior to discussing the bill with the patient.

5. Invite the patient into a quiet private room to discuss financial matters, observing the patient's right to privacy.

6. Explain the itemized billing statement for each date of service, type of procedure, and fee(s) charged if there are no errors. This will verify with the patient the extent of the services rendered and the fees.

7. Correct and apologize for any error, clearly explaining the new revised billing statement.

8. Show a willingness to answer questions politely.

9. Find out if the patient has specific concerns regarding ability to pay, in case special financial arrangements need to be instituted.

10. Arrange for a discussion between the accounts manager, office manager, or physician and patient if additional explanation is necessary to resolve the problem.

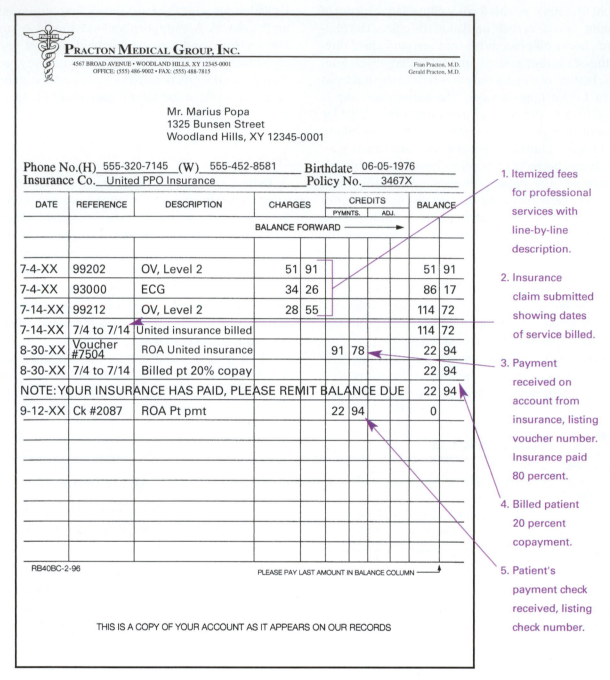

Figure 13-4. Ledger card illustrating posting of professional service descriptions, fees, payments, and balance due

ing balances. An individual or an entire family can be listed on the statement, which shows fees, payments, credit adjustments, balance due, and whether an insurance claim has been submitted. The statement usually shows a breakdown of the amounts that are due or delinquent, and how many days they are delinquent (e.g., 30, 60, 90, 120 days). This informa-tion is called *aging analysis* and is a feature usually not found in a manual bookkeeping system (See Aging Accounts, page 434).

In the event an insurance company sends a check and the patient has already paid, a credit balance will appear indicating an overpayment on the account and the patient should be sent a statement showing

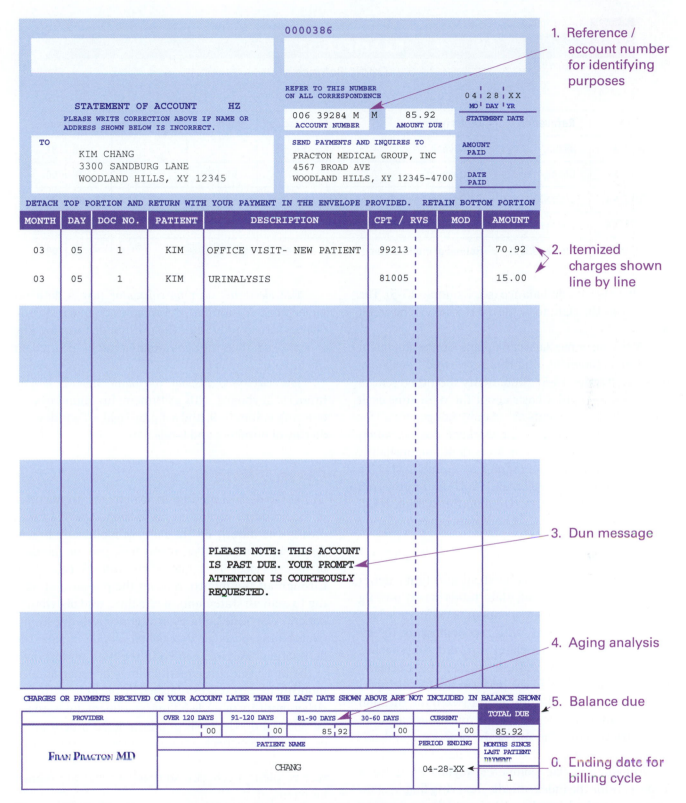

1. Reference / account number for identifying purposes

2. Itemized charges shown line by line

3. Dun message

4. Aging analysis

5. Balance due

6. Ending date for billing cycle

Figure 13-5. Computer-generated monthly itemized billing statement showing a dun message

EXAMPLE 13-5
Credit Balance

Date	Reference	Description	Charges	Payments	Adjustments	Balance
				Credits		
3/12/XX	99202	OV, level 2	51 91			51 91
3/12/XX	Check #189	Pt payment		51 91		0 00
3/13/XX	3/12/XX	ABC Insurance billed				0 00
4/15/XX	Check #8954	ABC Insurance payment 80%		41 53		<41 53>
5/1/XX	Check #2389	Refund pt credit balance		<41 53>		0 00

that there is a credit balance (see Example 13-5). The patient has the right to request a refund for the credit amount.

A phrase or message can appear on the statement to promote payment, and this is referred to as a *dun* message (Figure 13-5). Statements should be sent to patients on a regular basis about the same time each month. Such statements are usually not generated for patients on the Medicaid or workers' compensation programs, because there is no patient responsibility. If a patient belongs to a managed care plan, such as health maintenance organization (HMO) or preferred provider organization (PPO), different billing, bookkeeping, and reporting methods may be required.

Office Calculator

One of the administrative medical assistant's duties will be to accurately calculate totals when posting charges and payments to a patient account or ledger, preparing bank deposits with reconciliations, inserting fees on an insurance claim form, ordering supplies, and verifying invoices. Desk **calculators** (formerly known as *adding machines*) perform arithmetic operations—addition (+), subtraction (−), multiplication (×), and division (÷)—and some machines can store and retrieve data. The size of the practice will determine the type of calculator that is best for the office.

Calculators, like computer keyboards, have a home row for the index, middle, and ring fingers. Fingers rest on the home keys (4, 5, and 6). Each of the fingers moves independently from its home row to a position above or below. For example, the index finger moves up to reach the 7 key and down to reach the 1 key. Practice in keying numbers will develop touch operation so your eyes can stay fixed to the input copy, similar to touch typing.

The *electronic printing calculator* prints data on paper tape. A number is entered and shown on the display screen only until the arithmetic function key is depressed; then the accumulated total is printed on the tape.

The *electronic display calculator* has a 10-key numeric keyboard with arithmetic function keys for entering values 0–9, and a digital readout window for display of numbers and totals.

Cycle Billing

Cycle billing is a method in which certain portions of the accounts receivable are billed at specific times during the month on the basis of alphabetic breakdown, account number, insurance type, or the date of first service. This allows continuous cash flow throughout the month, relieves the pressure of having to mail all statements at one time, and distributes patient telephone calls regarding account questions. Cycle billing, based on date of first service, enables the first patient statement to be in the mail within days of the first visit; subsequent billings are then mailed monthly in the cycle established by the first billing. In either monthly or cycle billing, statement dates might be selected on the basis of a local government office or business paycheck-issuing pattern with the goal of having the patients' bills in their hands before they receive their paychecks, so they can allocate money for payment.

Credit Card Billing

Credit card transactions are often used in group practices and in specialties that entail major expenditures such as dental care, eye care, and plastic surgery procedures. Figure 13-6 (see page 427) illustrates how

PROCEDURE 13-2

Perform Mathematical Functions Using a Calculator

Objectives: To accurately calculate and verify mathematical totals using an electronic display calculator with or without tape.

Equipment/Supplies: Calculator, numeric list (invoice or ledger card), and pen or pencil.

Directions: Follow these step-by-step procedures, which include rationales, to learn this skill, which is presented in the *Workbook* (Job Skill 13-4) for practice.

1. Turn on the calculator machine.

2. Clear the calculator machine's total by pressing the clear (C) button. Verify that it is clear by viewing the digital display window or producing a printed tape. It should indicate 0.

3. Enter all figures or fees from the numeric list (invoice, account, or ledger) together with the arithmetic function (+, −, ×, ÷). Add all charges (+) and subtract all payments or adjustments (−).

4. Indicate the total on a sheet of paper.

5. Double-check the math by repeating steps 2 and 3 and enter all numbers a second time.

6. Print the tape and compare the second total with the total already written on the sheet of paper in step 4.

7. If the two totals are the same, the total is correct. If the totals are different, look for an error and repeat steps 2 and 3 until the totals are identical. Then transfer the numbers to the appropriate form.

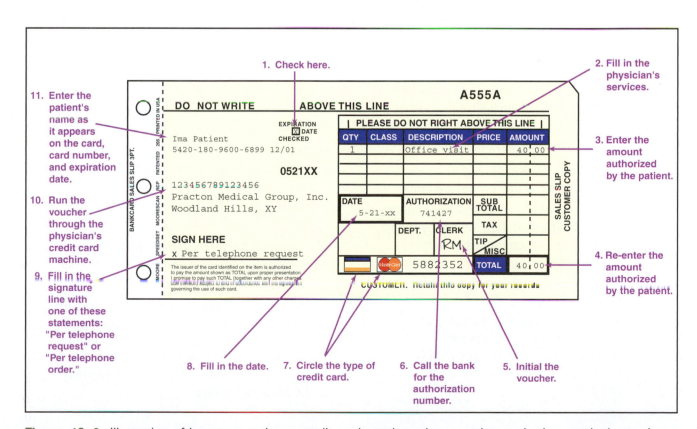

Figure 13-6. Illustration of how to complete a credit card voucher when a patient authorizes a telephone charge

PROCEDURE 13-3

STEP 1 2 3

Prepare and Post to a Patient's Ledger Card

Objectives: To prepare, insert descriptions on, and post fees, payments, credit adjustments, and balances due to a patient's ledger card.

Equipment/Supplies: Computer or typewriter, patient accounts or ledger cards, and calculator.

Directions: Follow these step-by-step procedures, which include rationales, to learn this skill, which is presented in the *Workbook* (Job Skill 13-3) for practice.

1. **Personal data:** Insert the patient's name and address on the ledger card. Note: Some practices may use a ledger that requires additional personal data, which may appear either on the front or back side of the card, such as home and work telephone numbers; birth date; Social Security number; driver's license number; spouse's and or dependents' names; name, address and telephone number of nearest relative; insurance company's name with policy and group numbers.

2. **Date:** In the first column on the first available line, post the current date (date transaction is recorded), which is usually the same as the date of service (DOS). If the DOS differs from the posting date, list the DOS in the reference column. This date column should never be left blank.

3. **Reference:** Write a reference to the transaction being posted.
   a. *Charges:* List the *CPT* procedure code.
   b. *Payments:* List the type of payment (cash, check, debit/credit card, or money order) and check or voucher number (e.g., voucher #543).
   c. *Adjustments:* List the date of service the adjustment is being made on.
   d. *Billing Comments:* List the dates of service(s) billed. Note: the balance at the end of the line may not coincide with the amount being billed to the insurance company.

4. **Description:** Write a brief description of the transaction that is being posted.
   a. *Charges:* Use a key at the bottom of the ledger or standard abbreviations to indicate charges posted (e.g., OV [office visit], HV [hospital visit]. Indicate the Evaluation and Management service levels (1 through 5) using the last digit of the E/M code (e.g., 99205 = Level 5). Abbreviate the name of other services or surgical procedures (e.g., ECG, vaccination, tonsillectomy).
   b. *Payments:* Indicate ROA (received on account), and who made the payment (e.g., pt [patient] or name of insurance company).
   c. *Adjustments:* Indicate the type of adjustment (e.g., insurance plan adj., contract adj., courtesy adj.).
   d. *Billing Comments:* Indicate the name of the insurance company billed or that a patient statement was sent and amount due if different from the current balance (e.g., patient billed $50.00 balance after insurance payment).
   e. *Other Comments:* Indicate other comments that pertain directly to the account (e.g., account sent to XYZ Collection Agency, account scheduled for small claims court).

5. **Charges:** Refer to the fee schedule (Part IV of *Workbook*) and post each fee (charge) on a separate line in the "charge" column. Charges are debited (subtracted) from the account balance.

6. **Payments:** Enter the amount paid in the "payment" column. Payments are credited (added) to the account balance.

7. **Adjustments:** Enter the amount adjusted off the account in the "adjustment" column. If the ledger card does not have an adjustment column, enter the amount in the payment column. Adjustments are credited (added) to the account balance.

PROCEDURE 13-3 *continued*

8. **Current Balance:** Line by line, add (credit) and subtract (debit) postings to the running balance to determine the amount for the "current balance" column. If a line is used to indicate a date an action was taken (e.g., insurance company or patient billed, account sent to collection), bring down the *running balance* from the previous line. This column must always contain an amount and should never be left blank.

9. **Credit Balances:** If an overpayment or double payment is received, the dollar amount of credit left on an account is enclosed with a symbol (e.g., <20.00> means twenty dollars credit); some offices post these in red ink. When a refund is made on a credit balance, the amount of the check that is written by the medical practice is listed either in the "Payment" or "Adjustment" column as a negative <> number and the amount is added back into the balance (see Example 13-5).

10. **Account Sent to Collection:** When an account is sent to a collection agency, write off the entire balance of the account in the adjustment column and indicate a zero balance. When the collection agency collects and sends a check, post the monies back onto the account as a payment and a reverse adjustment (e.g., 50.00 in the payment column and <50.00> in the adjustment column); the balance remains zero.

11. **Returned Checks:** When a check is returned, post the NSF charge in the charge column (which will be added to the balance) and reverse the amount of payment by check in the payment column (e.g., <37.00>), which will also be added to the balance. When the patient pays for the returned check by cash, credit card, or money order, post the amount in the payment column (which should include the check charge) with a clear description.

STEP 1 2 3

PROCEDURE 13-4

Prepare Monthly Itemized Billing Statements

Objective: To prepare monthly itemized billing statements.

Equipment/Supplies: Typewriter or computer, patient accounts, and billing statement forms (ledger cards).

Directions: Follow these step-by-step procedures, which include rationales, to learn this skill.

1. Gather all patient accounts or ledger cards with outstanding balances.

2. Separate the accounts or ledgers that have been marked as delinquent.

3. Prepare the itemized billing statements for the monthly billing, verifying the following information:

a. Date of the billing statement

b. Name and address of the person responsible for payment

c. Name of the patient if different from the person responsible for payment

d. Itemized dates of procedures and services, and charges

e. Unpaid balance carried forward and due

4. Determine action to take on delinquent accounts (dun messages, telephone calls, collection letters, assignment to collection agency, or small claims court).

5. Document on each account or ledger the action taken, in case further follow-up is necessary.

to complete a credit card voucher. After completion, mail the patient a copy of the charge slip. A charge is put on the patient's credit card and the physician receives payment directly from the credit card company. The patient can authorize for the entire balance to be paid or for a partial payment. A phone authorization must be made each month if a partial amount is authorized. The patient makes a payment directly to the credit card company. The original voucher is deposited to a bank credit card account. Always check with the credit card company for specific procedures and written instructions for completing telephone transactions. Credit card companies (e.g., Visa, MasterCard, Discover) charge a minimum monthly fee per location as well as a percentage based on the charges submitted. This method reduces office overhead and collection costs. However, under certain circumstances banks may hold participating merchants or professionals liable for the collection of credit card accounts. For instance, if the bank previously circulated a list of card numbers that should not be honored and if the physician accepted one, the physician could be responsible for the amount charged.

A record of the credit card number should always be kept with the patient's financial records and may be useful if the patient needs to be traced or if collection action is necessary. If the patient is reluctant to charge a large amount to a credit card, a payment plan may be instituted, which allows monthly payments via credit card (Figure 13-7).

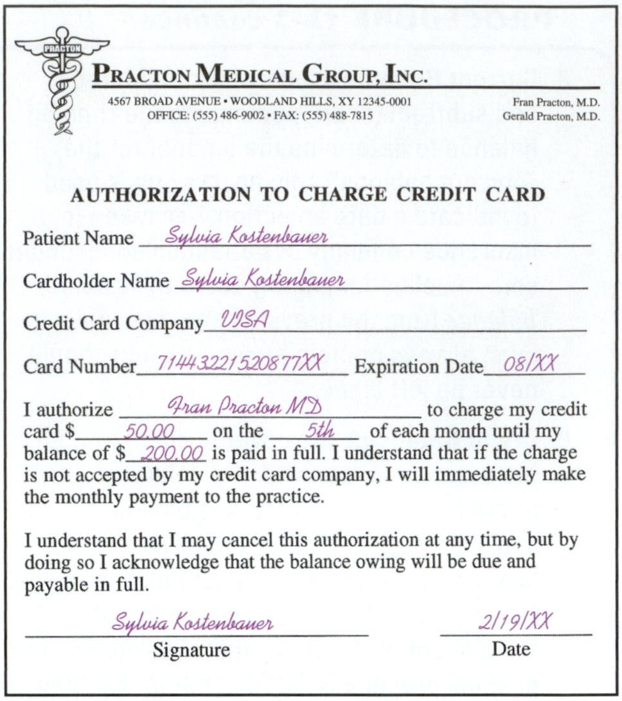

PRACTON MEDICAL GROUP, INC.
4567 BROAD AVENUE • WOODLAND HILLS, XY 12345-0001
OFFICE: (555) 486-9002 • FAX: (555) 488-7815
Fran Practon, M.D.
Gerald Practon, M.D.

AUTHORIZATION TO CHARGE CREDIT CARD

Patient Name Sylvia Kostenbauer

Cardholder Name Sylvia Kostenbauer

Credit Card Company VISA

Card Number 71443221520877XX Expiration Date 08/XX

I authorize Fran Practon MD to charge my credit card $ 50.00 on the 5th of each month until my balance of $ 200.00 is paid in full. I understand that if the charge is not accepted by my credit card company, I will immediately make the monthly payment to the practice.

I understand that I may cancel this authorization at any time, but by doing so I acknowledge that the balance owing will be due and payable in full.

Sylvia Kostenbauer — Signature
2/19/XX — Date

Figure 13-7. Authorization to charge credit card form

Debit Cards

A **debit card** also known as a *check card* is used by bank customers to either withdraw cash from any affiliated automated teller machine (ATM) or make electronic transfers of cash from a customer's bank account to a merchant's account. A small fee may be charged to the customer's checking account when the card is used; however, this fee is usually applied once a month regardless of how many times the card is used during the month. Since these cards accompany checking accounts and are easy to use, more patients will have these. Cards are issued either by banks or through credit card companies (e.g., Visa debit card, MasterDebit card).

There are two types of debit cards: off-line and on-line. Off-line debit cards do not require personal identification numbers (PIN) and generate an electronic check that is debited in about one to three days against the bank account like a handwritten check. On-line debit cards require PIN numbers and withdraw money immediately from the holder's account (e.g., VISA Check card or MasterCard's MasterMoney card).

If the office processes credit cards electronically, then it can usually use the same electronic credit card machine to swipe the debit card for verification and approval. The bank that issued the debit card is responsible for paying the funds that were approved, so there are no checks returned for nonsufficient funds.

Individual Responsibility Program

In some states, a program has been established whereby physicians accept all patients but refuse to accept reimbursement from any third party, private, or government programs. They bill the patient directly, and the patient then applies to the carrier or program for reimbursement. This is called an individual responsibility program (IRP).

Billing Services

Some medical practices employ billing services to prepare and mail patient bills. These services have a number of advantages over billing done by office personnel, on office time, using office equipment and supplies:

1. Patient understanding of statements is improved because all charges and payments are shown.

2. Prompt billing is ensured, because sending out statements is the business of the service; the medical practice is free of office disruptions while billing.

3. Billing services save the medical office money because expensive billing equipment is not required and valuable space need not be allocated for billing supplies.

4. Collection calls to patients do not disrupt the practice, because they are handled by the billing service.

Most billing services use professional computerized monthly statements generated with dun messages, if required. These billing services either pick up copies of multipurpose forms or receive account information via modem transmission to produce statements and complete insurance claims.

CREDIT AND COLLECTION LAWS

Credit laws govern the way fees are collected. There are federal laws regulating the entire nation, and state laws that vary among states. To keep well informed, the assistant needs to be aware of federal laws and should obtain information about state laws from the state attorney general's office.

Fair Debt Collection Practices Act (FDCPA)

Although the act is not designed to govern most medical collection activities, it does affect anyone who collects a debt in the same manner as a collection agency. The following guidelines will help avoid negative patient relations and enhance collections:

1. Debtors may be contacted only once a day.

2. Calls may be placed after 8 a.m. and before 9 p.m.

3. Debtors may not be contacted on a Sunday or a day the debtor recognizes as the Sabbath.

4. Contact the debtor at work only if attempts to contact the debtor elsewhere have failed; if the employer disapproves, no contact should be made.

5. Collectors must identify themselves and the medical practice they represent; they must not mislead the patient.

6. The physician or representative may not contact the debtor except to convey the message that there will be no further contact if the debtor states in writing that the physician is not to contact him or her.

7. An action must be taken, such as turning the patient over to a collection agency, if the physician or representative states that a certain action will be taken.

8. All contact must be made through the attorney if an attorney represents the debtor.

9. The medical assistant may contact other people for tracing purposes only; the nature of the call should not be disclosed to another party.

10. Postcards are not allowed for collection purposes.

11. Collectors should not threaten or use obscene language.

12. Collectors are obligated to send the patient written verification of the name of the creditor and the amount of the debt within five days of the initial contact.

Equal Credit Opportunity Act

Under the Federal Equal Credit Opportunity Act, which became law in 1975, if the physician agrees to extend credit to one patient, the same financial arrangement must be extended to all patients who request it. Refusal can be based only on ability or inability to pay, and the physician either must tell the patient the reason for a credit refusal or give the patient notice that no credit will be granted. The patient then has 60 days to request the reason in writing why credit was denied. Once the physician has granted credit, the Equal Credit law coverage applies.

Federal Truth in Lending Act

The Federal Truth in Lending Act, which became law on July 1, 1960, governs anyone who charges interest or agrees to more than four payments for a given service. If the physician charges interest rates, the rates

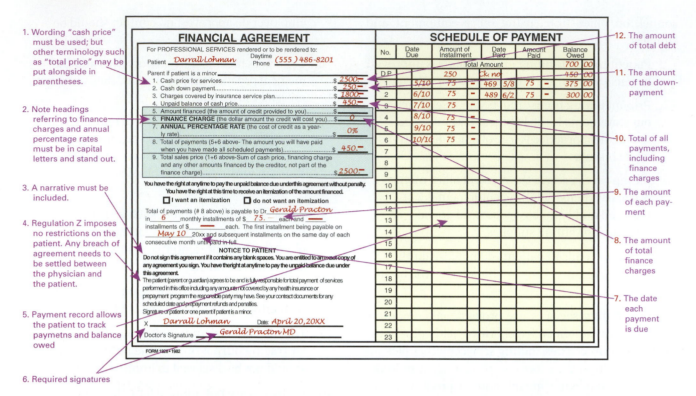

Figure 13-8. Truth in Lending Disclosure Form or Financial Agreement Form. By completing this form, the physician provides all information on full disclosure required by the Truth in Lending Act Regulation Z. (Reprinted with permission from Delux Small Business Sales, Inc. Form 21826 available from Sycom Healthcare Products & Services. Telephone: (800) 356-8141; Web site: http://www.sycom.com.)

may be governed by state laws; therefore, it is important to check with the appropriate agency before beginning such charges.

Regulation Z requires that a disclosure form (Figure 13-8) be completed and signed when a payment plan is instituted; one copy going to the patient and one to the office files (see Procedure 13-5). According to the Federal Trade Commission (FTC), the Truth in Lending Act does not apply and no disclosures are required if a patient offers to pay in installments or whenever convenient. In discussing an installment plan with a patient, the assistant would cover the amount of the total debt, the down payment, amount and date of each installment, and the date of final payment. However, if a patient has a delinquent account, the courts have said that continued medical care implies an extension of credit, even if the old account remains unpaid. Therefore, the physician and the medical assistant should consider referring such patients elsewhere for their care. When the patient has paid the overdue amount, he or she can be taken back with the understanding that payment will be required at the time of service.

Truth in Lending Consumer Credit Cost Disclosure

The Truth in Lending Consumer Credit Cost Disclosure is similar to the Federal Truth in Lending Act. It requires that providers disclose *all* costs including interest, late charges, and so on, *prior* to the time of service. If interest is charged on monthly billing, the amount of each payment, due date, unpaid balance at the beginning of the billing period, finance charge, and date balance due must be included on each statement.

Fair Credit Billing Act

The Fair Credit Billing Act states that patients have 60 days from the date the statement is mailed to complain about an error. The complaint must be acknowledged and documented within 30 days of receiving it. The provider has two billing cycles (maximum of 90 days) to correct the error if an actual error occurred; otherwise the accuracy of the bill should be explained to the patient.

PROCEDURE 13-5

STEP 1 2 3

Establish a Financial Agreement with a Patient

Objective: To assist the patient in making credit arrangements by completing and signing a Truth in Lending form.

Equipment/Supplies: Patient's account or ledger, calendar, Truth in Lending form, typewriter or computer, calculator, and quiet private room.

Directions: Follow these step-by-step procedures, which include rationales, to learn this skill, which is presented in the *Workbook* (Job Skill 13-7) for practice.

1. Discuss the patient's balance due and answer questions about credit.

2. Inform the patient of the office policy about extending credit payments.

3. Discuss an installment plan, including the amount of the total debt, the down payment, amount and date of each installment, and the date of final payment.

4. Subtract the down payment from the total debt. Divide the remaining amount by the number of months the debt is being carried to determine the monthly installment amounts and date of final payment.

5. Complete a Truth in Lending form after mutually agreeing on the terms if the payments require more than four installments. This procedure complies with Regulation Z.

6. Review the completed Truth in Lending form with the patient.

7. Ask the patient to sign the Truth in Lending form.

8. Make a photocopy of the form for the patient to retain.

9. File the original Truth in Lending form in the patient's financial files in the office.

When making a collection call and the patient has a complaint, always address the complaint seriously. Listen with an open mind, and note specifically what the complaint is and what the person wants to do. Do not sidestep the issue, because it will only add fuel to the fire. Apologize whether the patient is right or wrong. Be sincere and do not try to interject humor. Decide on a resolution, and let the patient know specifically what action will be taken.

Fair Credit Reporting Act (FCRA)

The Fair Credit Reporting Act became law in 1971 and was amended in the Budget Bill of 1996. Consumer reporting agencies (CRAs) gather and assemble information on private individuals to evaluate and determine the credit standing and credit capacity of consumers; they sell consumer reports that detail the information for future creditors, employers, insurers, and other businesses. The FCRA, enforced by the Federal Trade Commission is designed to promote accuracy and ensure the privacy of the information used in consumer reports.

Credit Bureaus

The most common type of consumer reporting agency is the Credit Bureau. The industry is divided into two branches. The first branch consists of companies that issue noninvestigative consumer credit reports when someone applies for credit.

The second branch consists of companies that issue consumer investigative reports requested by insurance companies, employers, prospective employers, credit grantors, and others who show a legitimate business need. Some also operate a collection department, receiving delinquent accounts from participating businesses.

As a member of a credit bureau service, a physician may obtain information about a consumer over the telephone. The information may consist of the patient's residence or previous residence (which will show if the patient is transient), the patient's employment verification, approximate salary, number of dependents, how the patient pays on other merchant accounts, and derogatory information, such as bankruptcy, use of an alias, and so forth.

The Fair Credit Reporting Act permits a person to check the credit report for mistakes, outdated information, disputed information, and negative credit information from earlier years. If there are inaccuracies, the consumer can have them corrected. If a physician joins a credit bureau and uses its services, the medical assistant may be designated to check new patients for information on their credit history.

If a credit refusal is based in whole or in part on a report from a credit bureau or similar agency, then the medical assistant must provide the patient with the name and address of the agency, although the exact nature of the information obtained does not have to be revealed. If a patient does not ask for the name and address of the credit bureau, the medical assistant must volunteer it because failure to do so can result in legal action. The procedure is to send a letter courteously informing the patient that the credit has been denied because credit requirements have not been met. The name and address of the bureau that supplies credit information should be given and a copy of the letter should go in the files.

COLLECTIONS

There is a statute of limitations, which varies from state to state, establishing the maximum time during which a legal collection suit on a delinquent account may be rendered against a debtor. Table 13-1 lists the time limits for collections in the various states. The statutes also vary according to oral and written contracts; there are three kinds of accounts:

1. *Open-book account*—(also called **open accounts**) record of business transactions on the books that represents an unsecured account receivable where credit has been extended without a formal written contract; payment is expected by a specific period. The physician's patient accounts are usually of this type.

2. *Written-contract account*—agreement a patient signs to pay the bill in more than four installments under the Truth in Lending provisions.

3. *Single-entry account*—account with only one charge listed and generally for a small amount.

Aging Accounts

To follow up on accounts in a timely manner, it is important to know when an account begins to become delinquent. A system is used called **aging accounts**, which is an analysis of accounts receivable indicating a breakdown of the length of time (30, 60, 90, and 120 days) the account is overdue.

In a manual accounting system, some offices use colored tabs or clips that fit onto patients' ledger cards to indicate the age of accounts that are delinquent. This system has the disadvantage of clips having to be removed when each ledger is photocopied for billing and of becoming entangled with other ledger cards. Removable, self-adhesive, color-coded labels may also be used to indicate delinquent accounts. They are inexpensive, allow quick identification, and can be used several times.

A method of keeping track of aging accounts is to establish an accounts receivable log (see Example 13-6). This helps keep track of the accounts so follow-up action can be instituted. Notations about telephone calls, dun messages, and collection letters can also be made on the back of the patient's ledger card.

In practices employing a computer system, accounts are entered with the patient's name, date of service, charge, and payment. The balance is automatically calculated and aged by the computer. Insurance payments are applied to specific charges and patient payments are applied to the oldest unpaid charge unless specifically directed to a particular date of service. Computerized collection reports are a valuable tool used to monitor patient and insurance payments and to evaluate the staff on their collection

---

EXAMPLE 13-6

Accounts Receivable Log

Date	Patient's Name	Old Balance	New Balance	Age of Account 30 60 75 90 120	Action Taken	Patient Response
10/1/XX	West, Brian	$150	$150	X	telephone call	Promise to pay $50 10/7/XX

Table 13-1. Individual State Time Limits (Statute of Limitations on Civil Actions) for Collection of Open Accounts and Oral/Written Contracts. (Abstracted from *Summary of Collection Laws.* Reprinted with permission of the American Collectors Association, Inc., 2006. All rights reserved.)

Statute of Limitations (in Years)

State	Open Accounts	Contracts: Written/Oral	State	Open Accounts	Contracts: Written/Oral
Alabama	6	6	Montana	5	8
Alaska	10	10	Nebraska	4	5
Arizona	3	6	Nevada	4	6
Arkansas	3	5	New Hampshire	3	3
California	2	4	New Jersey	6	6
Colorado	6	6	New Mexico	4	6
Connecticut	3	6	New York	6	6
Delaware	3	6	North Carolina	3	3
D.C.	3	3	North Dakota	6	6
Florida	4	5	Ohio	6	15
Georgia	4	6	Oklahoma	3	5
Guam	3	4	Oregon	6	6
Hawaii	6	6	Pennsylvania	4	4
Idaho	4	5	Puerto Rico	3	15
Illinois	5	10	Rhode Island	10	10
Indiana	6	6	South Carolina	3	3
Iowa	5	10	South Dakota	6	6
Kansas	3	5	Tennessee	6	6
Kentucky	5	15	Texas	4	4
Louisiana	3	3	Utah	4	6
Maine	6	6	Vermont	6	6
Maryland	3	3	Virgin Islands	4	6
Massachusetts	6	6	Virginia	3	5
Michigan	6	6	Washington	3	6
Minnesota	6	6	West Virginia	5	10
Mississippi	3	3	Wisconsin	6	6
Missouri	5	10	Wyoming	8	10

Note: Most open accounts fall under the "oral contract" time limit. Contracts under seal may have an extended time limit.

efficiency. Regardless of the system used the key to success is working the accounts receivable regularly, keeping accurate records on aging accounts, and updating notes consistently. See Chapter 15 for further information about financial management using a computer.

Office Collection Problem Solving

A patient under the physician's care may fall deep into debt and find it impossible to pay bills. In a discussion to find the cause of the problem, the patient may ask the administrative assistant to suggest a solution.

Credit Counseling

Patients with financial problems may be directed to a consumer credit counseling service that can be found in most communities; it is a nonprofit agency that assists people in paying off their debts. Or the debtor may contact his or her own bank or labor union, either of which may provide counseling at no charge. If these suggestions do not help, then a budget consultant might be the solution. A budget consultant is a financial planner who recommends solutions for a debt by itemizing income and expenses for a projected time period. Commercial debt consolidators charge high fees and should be sought only as a final resort. The assistant must be careful to give only legitimate recommendations and referrals, because if the patient is dissatisfied, the medical assistant or the physician may be blamed.

Verifying Checks

A *check* is a written order to pay a sum of money, the most common form of money exchange other than actual cash. When accepting checks, always ask to see two sources of identification. Call to verify checks drawn on out-of-state bank accounts. Examine the check to be sure it is made out to the correct party, it is for the correct amount, and the signature matches other identification. Verify the address and telephone number on the check with the patient's account.

Nonsufficient Funds—When notice is received from a bank indicating a check was not honored because of nonsufficient funds (NSF), call the bank and patient to see if they suggest redepositing it. If it is not worthwhile or if a second NSF notice is received, call the person who wrote the check and tell him or her to bring in payment to the office immediately. Accept only cash, a certified check, money order, or in certain cases a credit or debit card. Be courteous but straight to the point. If restitution is not received within three days, notify the patient in writing to start the legal process. An NSF demand letter (Figure 13-9) would include the following:

1. Check date
2. Check number
3. Bank the check is drawn on
4. To whom check was payable
5. Check amount

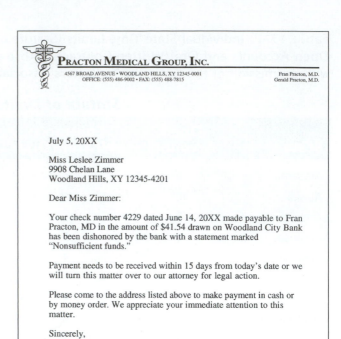

Figure 13-9. Nonsufficient funds (NSF) demand letter

6. Any allowable service fee
7. Total amount due
8. Number of days the check writer has to take action
9. Send certified mail with return receipt requested

In most states if the debtor has not responded within 30 days, a claim may be filed in small claims court (see page 442). It may be possible to collect an additional $100 in damages, and in some states the person can be sued for three times the amount of the check. Section 1719 of the State Civil Code addresses penal sanctions for individuals who pass checks on nonsufficient funds. The district attorney, district justice, state attorney, or other government official may also help with the collection of a bad check.

The patient must also be informed that the medical facility will no longer be able to accept checks as a payment on future services. Future payments need to be in the form of cash, money order, cashier's check, or debit or credit card if office policy permits. See Procedure 13-3 for step-by-step directions on posting returned checks.

Bad Check Preventive Measures—Larger medical facilities may want to consider a check authorization system. This type of system involves a company that supplies a terminal that will give an approval number for each check and guarantees payment on those that are authorized. To help discourage bad checks, charge a penalty for returned checks. This information should be detailed in the new patient brochures and posted in the office for all patients to see.

Use of debit cards will also eliminate bad checks. Additional information on payment disputes regarding NSF, misdated checks, incorrect payee's name on check, missing payer's signature, variable amounts, payment-in-full checks, third-party checks, and forged checks appear in Chapter 14, Banking.

Dun Messages

If a payment has not been made after obtaining personal and financial data from the patient and rendering professional services, then an itemized billing statement is sent every 30 days. The statement should be simple and to the point. Patients should be able to open a statement, peruse it, and understand the date of service, service rendered, amount owed, and how long past due the account is, that is, 30, 60, 90, or 120 days (see Figure 13-5). At the time of the second

---

EXAMPLE 13-7

Dun Message

"The balance above is due and payable. Please remit immediately. Unless we receive payment within 10 days, it will be necessary to take further action."

---

billing, a reminder in the form of a written note (dun message) on a statement is appropriate.

Dun comes from the Old English word *dunnen*, which means "to make a loud noise." A *dun message* is a phrase used to remind a delinquent patient about payment (see Figure 13-5 and Example 13-7). Brightly colored self-adhesive collection labels are also available for this purpose. If a patient speaks a foreign language, a dun message should be written in suitable language.

A notation indicating the type of dun message sent should go on the back of the patient's ledger card, on the accounts receivable log, or on the computer comment area, such as "N1" or "N2" (see Table 13-2), along with the date the notice was mailed. When a payment is received, post it immediately. Patients who

---

Table 13-2. Collection Abbreviations

B	bankrupt	NSF	not sufficient funds (check)
BLG	belligerent	NSN	no such number
EOM	end of month	OOT	out of town
EOW	end of week	OOW	out of work
FN	final notice	Ph/Dsc	phone disconnected
H	he or husband	POW	payment on way
HHCO	have husband call office	PP	promise to pay
HTO	he telephoned office	S	she or wife
L1, L2	letter one, letter two (sent)	SEP	Separated
LB	line busy	SK	Skip or skipped
LD	long distance	SOS	same old story
LMCO	left message, call office	STO	she telephoned office
LMVM	left message voice mail	T	telephoned
N1, N2	note one, note two (sent)	TB	telephoned business
NA	no answer	TR	telephoned residence
NF/A	no forwarding address	U/Emp	unemployed
NI	not in	UTC	unable to contact
NLE	no longer employed	Vfd/E	verified employment
NR	no record	Vfd/I	verified insurance

send a check and subsequently receive a bill with a stern dun message may decide to look elsewhere for care.

Telephone Collections

Generally if an account remains delinquent for over 60 days, it is important to make personal contact by telephone. First, arrange the accounts according to aging parameters (e.g., 30, 60, 90, 120 days) and select all accounts in the 60-day range. Next prioritize the calls that need to be made according to the amounts owed; take action on accounts that may be difficult to collect first. It is best to prepare thoroughly for the call by outlining what is going to be said. A telephone that allows privacy should be used and the call should be made at a time when there will be no interruptions. According to surveys, the best times to phone are between 5:30 and 8:30 p.m., Tuesdays and Thursdays, and between 9:00 a.m. and 1 p.m. on Saturdays. It may be prudent to add one evening per week to the practice schedule for collection purposes or offer the medical assistant a flexible schedule to make collection calls during these hours.

The longer an account remains delinquent, the harder it will be to collect. Although the assistant may hear the same excuses over and over, it is important to convey an understanding of the circumstances. When a patient is talking nonstop, use a "bridge" in the conversation such as "Yes, I understand that, and we do need to talk, but . . . the collection agency picks up our accounts on Friday," or "Our accountant won't allow a payment plan over 90 days, so you probably need to take out a loan," or "In order to keep your account current, we need to have your check in the office this week," and so forth.

Insurance Check Sent to Patient

If the "assignment of benefits" has been signed and the insurance check has gone to the patient, it is the insurance company's responsibility to generate a new check to the physician and collect the amount of the check directly from the patient. Follow up immediately in such situations.

Solutions for Payment Excuses

The following are some patient tactics used for stalling payment and solutions the medical assistant may use:

1. *Situation:* Saying the check is in the mail.
   Solution/Response: Get a check number, amount, and mail date. Call in three days if not received.

2. *Situation:* Experiencing a broken promise.
   Solution/Response: Follow up within 48 hours. Determine the reason for the broken promise. Get immediate payment.

3. *Situation:* Sending unsigned checks that must be returned.
   Solution/Response: Have patient come to the office to sign.

4. *Situation:* Paying an incorrect amount.
   Solution/Response: Have patient come to the office and exchange a new check for the one made out in error.

5. *Situation:* Saying, "I never received your bill."
   Solution/Response: Verify name, address, and resend the bill the same day. Call in three days to see if the patient received it.

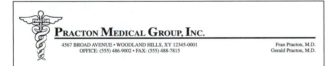

September 22, 20XX

Mr. Richard Urasali
1990 Corvalis Court
Woodland Hills, XY 12345-4201

Dear Mr. Urasali:

This is a reminder of the agreement we made in our phone conversation on September 21, 20XX, regarding your past due account in the amount of $200. We will expect a payment of $50 on your account on or before September 28, 20XX.

We have enclosed a return envelope for your convenience.

Sincerely,

Karen Bringham

Karen Bringham, CMA
Collection Department

Encl: envelope

Figure 13-10. Collection letter following a telephone agreement

PROCEDURE 13-6

Perform Debt Collection Using a Telephone

Objective: To make a telephone call to request payment from a patient who has a delinquent account balance.

Equipment/Supplies: Telephone, patient's account or ledger, and pen or pencil.

Directions: Follow these step-by-step procedures, which include rationales, to learn this skill.

1. From the point that the patient incurs a debt, be clear about how and when payment is expected.

2. Telephone patients who are slow payers shortly before their scheduled appointments. Remind them of the date and time of their appointment, and at the same time, ask them to bring in their payment or suggest they use their debit/credit card.

3. Follow the Fair Debt Collection Practices Act when making a telephone call.

4. State the name of the caller, the practice represented, and identify the patient.

5. Verify the patient's address and any telephone numbers listed.

6. Ask for full payment, stating the total amount owed when speaking to a patient about an overdue amount. Ask for payment courteously but firmly, conveying a sense of urgency and requesting that the patient keep payments prompt.

7. Speak slowly in a low voice; staying calm and polite prevents quarreling.

8. Elicit grievances, answer questions, ask why there has not been a payment, give the patient a choice of action, and then set immediate deadlines for payment.

9. Pause for effect and do not assume that if the patient does not respond immediately it is a "no." Some questions to ask include "How much are you short?" "When do you get paid?" and "Do you have a checking account?" Asking for a postdated check is another option if allowed per office policy.

10. Make positive instead of negative statements such as "We will NOT send your account to our collection agency as long as we receive payment by (date)" instead of "if we do not receive payment by (date), we WILL send your account to our collection agency."

11. Treat patients who owe money as you would want to be treated in the same situation. Be assertive and empathetic instead of aggressive.

12. Tune in to the feelings and concerns of patients, showing patience and openness. Respond to patients instead of reacting to them.

13. Ask the patient to write down the payment agreement when an agreement is reached, and read it back to be sure there has been no misunderstanding.

14. Write a short note outlining the conversation and the agreement that was made as a follow-up to the telephone call (Figure 13-10).

15. Make abbreviated notations (see Table 13-2 for abbreviations) on the back of the patient's ledger card, on the accounts receivable log, or in the computer system and also indicate the date any telephone calls were made. It is vital to be consistent in follow-up procedures and policies.

Collection Letters

If regular statements have been sent, two or three months have elapsed since the service, and the patient cannot be reached by telephone or a promised payment has not been received, then it is time to send a collection letter. There are a number of letter formats to consider, such as a form letter (Figure 13-11), a letter with a checklist (Figure 13-12), or a personally composed and typed letter. The letter in the chosen format may be sent either in a plain envelope or a brightly colored one to attract attention. A debtor

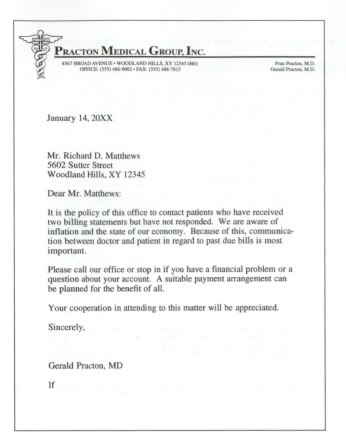

Figure 13-11. Form collection letter

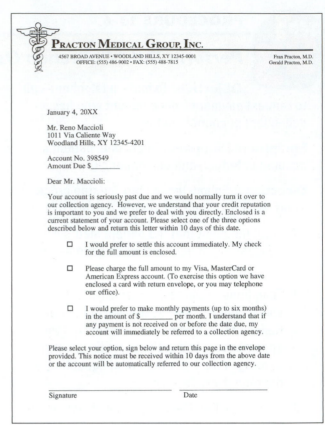

Figure 13-12. Multipurpose form collection letter with checklist

is more likely to open the envelope and read the contents if it does not look like a bill. If the patient has moved and left a forwarding address, the post office will forward the letter. For a small fee, the post office will also supply a card indicating the new address if "Address Service Requested" or "Forwarding Service Requested" is printed on the envelope as described in Chapter 12 and illustrated in Figure 12-6.

A collection letter should be brief and direct. It should mention how much is owed for a specific service; what the patient should do about the delinquency; when, where, and why the patient should remit; and how the patient can facilitate payment. Enclosing a self-addressed, stamped envelope may help obtain a response. A letter written over the physician's signature rather than the medical assistant's may be more successful in prompting a payment. Collection letters may also be purchased for a small price, such as those sold by Telecredit, and the collection follow-up is left in the medical assistant's hands.

When mailing a collection letter in November or December before the end of the income tax year, it might be helpful to remind the patient that medical expenses, if large enough, could qualify as an income tax deduction if the account is settled before the year-end deadline. A message, such as "The medical expense listed on this statement may be used as a deduction on your 20__ income tax, provided it is paid by December 31, 20__," could be used as an incentive.

Patients can also be encouraged to pay their debts with income tax refunds. Arrangements can be made for patients to make small payments January through March and a large payment when they get their refund in April. Suggest that patients file their income tax returns electronically to expedite the refund. Whenever a letter is sent, it should be noted on the back of the ledger card, on the accounts receivable log, or in the computer comment area as L1, L2, and so on, with the date on which it was mailed.

Depending on the policy of the office, when the account has aged 120 days, a decision needs to be made whether to (1) send another bill with a dun message, (2) turn the account over to a collection service, or (3) file in small claims court. After a certain amount of time, some physicians prefer to write off a small debt (e.g., $25) rather than to increase administrative collection costs. From a medicolegal standpoint, a consideration regarding a small claims suit would be not to file until a counterclaim by the patient alleging negligence is barred by the statute of limitations.

Collection Agencies

Before seeking the services of a collection agency, the medical assistant needs to determine the type of agency that best meets the office needs. The agency typically takes a percentage of the bill owed, which can be as much as 50 percent, and the physician's office is no longer permitted to communicate with or bill the patient. National agencies that have local and regional branches have advantages when tracking an individual with a debt who moves and leaves no forwarding address. The agency should be licensed and bonded. Following are guidelines for the medical assistant seeking to employ an agency.

1. Check with physicians who have used the agency for over two years to determine the agency's rate of accomplishment. A collection rate of 30 to 60 percent of the accounts assigned to it would be considered successful.

2. Look for an agency that charges on a sliding scale, usually between 33 and 50 percent, with the higher rate applied to older and smaller accounts.

3. Find out if there is a minimum fee charged if nothing is collected.

4. Make sure the agency does not hold partial payments until the account is collected in full.

5. Ask the agency to provide the form letters sent to patients so the physician can approve or disapprove of their tone.

6. Keep a record of the money that the agency actually collects. If it is more than 25 to 30 percent of what is owed, the assistant's own collection procedures need strengthening.

7. Ask whether accounts are forwarded to another collection office if a debtor moves and whether there are penalties for withdrawing an account.

8. Find out if the agency is covered by errors and omissions insurance that would protect both the agency and physician in the event of a lawsuit.

9. Check the agency's policy for a hold harmless clause, which protects the physician from being sued if the agency is accused of harassing a debtor.

Do not hold onto an account too long before turning it over to a collection agency. For best collection results, agencies like to get the delinquent accounts at a maximum of five or six months after the debt has

---

EXAMPLE 13-8

Write Off an Uncollectable Account; Post Monies from a Collection Agency

Date	Reference	Description	Charges	Credits Payments	Credits Adjustments	Balance
6/13/XX	30520	Septoplasty	660 88			660 88
7/15/XX	6/13/XX	Billed pt				660 88
8/15/XX	6/13/XX	Billed pt				660 88
9/15/XX	6/13/XX	Billed pt				660 88
10/1/XX 10/2/XX 10/5/XX		Telephoned pt re: collections—UTC X 3				660 88
10/15/XX	6/13/XX	Sent collection notice				660 88
11/1/XX	6/13/XX	Sent acct to XYZ Collection Agency			660 88	0 00
12/15/XX	Ck # 8970	XYZ Collection Agency pd		250 00	<250 00>	0 00

PROCEDURE 13-7

Take Collection Action, Write Off an Uncollectable Account, Then Post Money from a Collection Agency

Objective: Post an adjustment on a ledger card for an uncollectible account that is being sent to collection, then post monies received from the collection agency.

Equipment/Supplies: Ledger card or patient account with applicable data; pen.

Directions: Follow these step-by-step procedures, which include rationales, to learn this skill.

1. Send statements for at least three billing cycles (90 days). It is important for the patient to receive consistent statements itemizing the amount owed.

2. Contact the patient by telephone. Several attempts should be made by telephone to try to find out why the patient has not paid and/ or get a promise to pay.

3. Send a collection notice if unable to reach the patient or if the patient is not interested in paying the debt. The notice should state clearly when the account will be turned over to a collection agency if payment is not received (e.g., 10 days).

4. Send the account to the collection agency and post on the account/ledger as follows:

   a. *Date:* Post on the date mentioned in the collection notice.

   b. *Reference:* Date(s) of service for amounts owed.

   c. *Description:* Record "Sent account to collection agency," naming the agency.

   d. *Adjustments:* Post the amount owed in the adjustment column and subtract it from the balance.

   e. *Balance:* The entire amount should have been written off leaving a zero balance.

5. Flag the patient's medical record (chart) and financial record (ledger) so that all staff members know that the account has gone to collection. A bright colored piece of paper with "COLLECTION" written on it, placed in the front of the chart alerts all employees; write "COLLECTION" across the front of the ledger. Make note in computerized accounts in the comment sections of the financial statement, medical record, and appointment schedule.

6. Post monies received from the collection agency as follows:

   a. *Date:* Date received.

   b. *Reference:* Check or voucher number.

   c. *Description:* Pd by (name of collection agency).

   d. *Payment:* Post the amount of the check.

   e. *Adjustments:* Post the amount of the payment as a "reverse adjustment" thereby adding it back onto the account (e.g., <250.00>).

occurred. When an account has been turned over to a collection agency, the patient's financial record should be removed from the regular file and marked with the date and name of the agency. It is illegal for the physician's office to send a bill to a patient after the account has been turned over to a collection agency. If payment should come to the physician's office instead of the agency after the account has been turned over, the assistant must notify the agency immediately, because a percentage of this payment may be due the agency.

When an account is assigned, it is suggested that the doctor send the patient a letter of discharge by certified mail for liability protection. Refer to Chapter 3 for sample letters of discharge or withdrawal from a case.

A record of the total monies owed to the medical practice is referred to as the **accounts receivable (A/R)**. Management consultants recommend that the patient's account balance be written off the A/R when an account is turned over to a collection agency. When money is received, the charged amount is reposted (debited) to equal the payment received (see Example 13-8).

Small Claims Court

A physician may decide to file a claim for a delinquent bill in small claims court rather than turn it over to a collection agency. Small claims court proceedings are an inexpensive collection method; but after the

PROCEDURE 13-8

File an Uncollectible Account in Small Claims Court

Objective: To file a delinquent or uncollectible account in small claims court.

Equipment/Supplies: Small claims court filing form and instructional booklet, check for filing fee, and photocopies of financial records for cases to be presented.

Directions: Follow these step-by-step procedures, which include rationales, to learn this skill.

1. Obtain a form from the clerk's office located at the municipal or justice court; there are booklets and material to help guide the claimant through the process.

2. File the initiating papers.

3. Pay the filing fee. Filing fees vary by state, by county within some states, and by the amount of the claim.

4. Make arrangements to serve the defendant. If the summons is served on the patient by a sheriff or court-appointed office, a fee plus mileage for the officer who serves it is necessary. There must be a street address where the patient can be found. The person serving the defendant completes the proof of service form.

5. After being served, a patient has one of four options:

   a. *Pay the claim*—to the court clerk. This will be forwarded to the physician, but the filing fee or service charge will not be refunded.

   b. *Ignore the claim*—the physician will win by default. In some states a judgment may be requested in writing, but in other states the physician or the medical assistant must appear on a specified date. If the patient does not appear, the judgment is granted in the physician's favor and usually court costs are included in the judgment.

   c. *Request a small claims hearing*—the court clerk will let both parties know when to appear. The patient may file a counterclaim against the physician at this time.

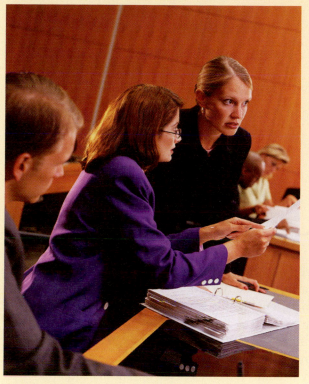

Figure 13-13. Medical assistant in a courtroom presenting a small claims case

   d. *Demand a jury trial*—the case will be taken out of small claims court. The physician will be notified by the court clerk to file a formal complaint in a higher court, and an attorney must represent the physician.

6. Appear in court (physician or the medical assistant) on the specified date, or claim will be dismissed and cannot be refiled.

7. Basic information required by the court is:

   a. Physician's name, address, and telephone number

   b. Patient's name and address

   c. Delinquent amount

   d. Summary of the claim including the date the physician's bill was due, date of the last visit, date of the last payment, unpaid amount, and all records of telephone contacts and letters sent

(continues)

PROCEDURE 13-8 *continued*

8. Determine what the judge needs to hear to decide a favorable case. Good preparation for the trial can make the difference between success or failure.

9. Organize all the exhibits in a notebook, in chronological order. A timeline showing the sequence of events can be useful.

10. Take a businesslike professional approach at the hearing, giving concise and accurate answers to the judge's questions, and speaking slowly and clearly. The physician or assistant must bring any witnesses, statements, receipts, contracts, notes, dishonored checks, or other evidence to

court. The judge will question the medical assistant or physician and the patient, review the evidence, and then make a ruling.

11. Put a lien on the debtor's wages, automobile, bank or personal assets, or real property if the judgment, which is usually effective for many years, is in the physician's favor. This is the physician's legal right. The small claims office will show the medical assistant or physician how to execute a judgment.

12. Pay a small fee if the physician decides to execute against the patient's assets. It is recoverable from the patient.

judgment is made, the physician is still the one who has to pursue the money. Sometimes that is not easy. To be eligible for small claims court, the bill must be within the limit the state has set on the amount. This figure varies from $300 to $25,000 state to state and, in some instances, within the state. The majority of states have increased maximum amounts from $2,000–3,000 to $5,000–10,000. There also may be limits on the number of claims over specific dollar amounts per year, and other dollar limits regarding claims filed against a guarantor of a debt. In many states, lawyers are not permitted to represent litigants; however, an incorporated physician must usually be represented by an attorney. For large balances when small claims court is no longer a viable choice, collection attorneys are the second highest choice in alternative enforcement.

If the account has been turned over to a collection agency, the debt cannot be filed in small claims court. Such agencies have different filing protocols.

Federal Wage Garnishment Law

Title III of the Consumer Credit Protection Act, which became effective on July 1, 1970, set down the legislation affecting garnishment. **Garnishment** means attaching a debtor's property and wage by court order so monies can be obtained to pay debts. Personal earn-ings include wages, salary, tips, commissions, bonuses, and income from pensions or retirement programs. Enforcement is carried out by the compliance offices of the Wage and Hour Office, U.S. Department of Labor, whose offices are located across the United States. Two basic provisions of the garnishment law are:

1. It limits the amount of employee earnings withheld for garnishment in a workweek or pay period.

2. It protects the employee from being dismissed if his or her pay is garnished regardless of the number of levies included in the garnishment.

The garnishment law is a continuous garnishment judgment. In other words, if the debt is not paid within 90 days, the garnishment can be continued for another 90 days. The garnishment law does not apply to federal government employees, court-ordered support of any person, court orders in personal bankruptcy cases, or state or federal tax levies. The amount of wages subject to garnishment is based on the patient's disposable earnings. This is the amount left after deductions for federal, state, and local taxes and Social Security. Union dues, health and life insurance, assignment of wages, and savings bonds are not considered in disposable earnings. Garnishment is limited to the lesser of 25 percent of disposable earnings in any workweek or the amount by which disposable earnings for that week exceed 30 times the highest current federal minimum wage. Special restrictions apply to court orders for child support and alimony.

When state garnishment laws conflict with federal laws, the statute resulting in the smaller garnishment applies. For further information, the assistant can contact the local Wage and Hour Office listed in most telephone directories under U.S. Government, Department of Labor, Employment Standards Administration.

Estate Claims

There are various state time limits and statutes governing the filing of a claim against an estate. First, an itemized billing statement (or in some states, a special form) is completed for the collection of a deceased patient's account. This is mailed in duplicate to the estate administrator by certified mail with return receipt requested. The name of the estate administrator can be obtained by calling the probate department of the superior court, county recorder's office. The administrator of the estate will either accept or reject the claim. If accepted, an acknowledgment of the debt will be sent to the physician. If rejected, the physician should file a claim against the administrator within a time specified by state law.

Bankruptcy

Bankruptcy laws are federal laws, and a patient who files for **bankruptcy** becomes a ward of the federal court and is thereby protected by the court. If a patient writes or telephones stating bankruptcy has been declared, under the law the medical assistant must not send monthly statements or make an attempt to collect; a creditor can be fined for contempt of court for failing to follow the law. If the account has been turned over to a collection agency and the agency has been notified of the bankruptcy, it is the same as if the physician has been notified.

Bankruptcy laws are organized in sections called *chapters*. The chapters applicable to patients' debts in a medical practice are as follows:

- Chapter 7, *straight petition in bankruptcy*, allows a person, family, or small business to liquidate all debts and to be able to restart with a clean financial slate. First the patient declares bankruptcy to those to whom money is owed. If the physician is listed, since there is no collateral, he or she will be the last person paid. If the physician is not listed and the patient wishes to make payments, then this is allowed. In this bankruptcy process, a court-appointed trustee takes charge of the patient's assets, subject to certain exemptions, and then sells them and distributes the collected money among the creditors. If the court determines

there are assets to be distributed, the physician will be notified to file a creditor's claim.

If a patient files a straight petition in bankruptcy, the physician should file a proof-of-claim form available from an attorney, county clerk's office, or local stationery store. Copies of the patient's outstanding bill are attached to the form and it is mailed to the bankruptcy court. Physician debts are "unsecured" and often go unpaid in bankruptcy cases. However, the physician will never be paid if a claim is not filed. Once a patient has declared bankruptcy, he or she cannot do so again for six years. The only exception to this is a Chapter 13, or wage earner's bankruptcy.

- Chapter 13, *wage-earner's bankruptcy*, a milder proceeding in which a federal district court acts as a consumer counseling service. The object is to protect wage earners from bill collectors and to make arrangements for the wage earner to pay bills over time. The court fixes a monthly amount that the debtor can pay, collects that sum, and parcels it out among the creditors according to an extended repayment plan that may take as long as five years. The plan often includes a reduced repayment of debts. To be paid, the physician must file a claim as directed by the debtor's attorney.

Tracing a Skip

A patient who owes a balance and moves, leaving the physician's office no forwarding address, is called a **skip**. A skip is discovered when a statement goes out and is returned unopened and marked by the post office "Returned to Sender, Addressee Unknown." This problem can often be avoided by having envelopes printed with "Address Service Requested" or "Forwarding Service Requested" below the physician's return address as discussed in Chapter 12 (Figure 12-6). If the address is a rural delivery box number, go to the post office and fill out a Freedom of Information Act Form, pay a nominal search fee, and the United States Postal Service will give the physical location of the person's residence.

It is important to begin tracing a skip as soon as possible. Move quickly in these efforts to locate the patient. If unable to trace and contact the patient, turn the skip over to a collection agency *immediately*. Time is an important factor. Some agencies offer customized skip tracing. Various levels of tracing are offered

PROCEDURE 13-9

Trace a Skip

Objective: To use search techniques to trace a debtor who has moved leaving no forwarding address and owes a balance on his or her account.

Equipment/Supplies: Telephone, patient's account ledger card, and pen or pencil.

Directions: Follow these step-by-step procedures, which include rationales, to learn this skill.

1. Check the address on the returned statement against the patient's registration form, account or ledger, to make sure all match and it was mailed correctly.

2. Check the ZIP code directory to see if the ZIP code corresponds with the patient's street address or post office box.

3. Telephone the patient's nearest relative, neighbor, or references given on the patient information record, using utmost discretion.

4. File a request with the local post office to try and get a new or corrected address.

5. Look in the local telephone directory or call information, and check for a new or current listing or for the same name. Telephone and ask for the patient by name if the patient has an unusual last name; the person who answers might be a relative. If directory assistance says the number is unpublished, the patient could still be in town.

6. Telephone the primary care physician for updated information when investigating for a physician specialist or any referring practice.

7. Call the patient's employer without disclosing to coworkers the reason for the call. If the patient is no longer employed, ask to speak to the personnel department to inquire if they have a lead.

8. Find out if the Department of Motor Vehicles has been notified of a change of address, if the driver's license number is available.

9. Look in the street directories, city directories, and cross-index directories (available at the public library or via the Internet), and locate a neighbor, relative, or landlord to inquire what happened to the patient.

10. Call the bank and ask if the account was transferred or is still open, if the patient information record contains information about the patient's bank.

11. Call the local hospital's inpatient admission office to see if they have a forwarding address, if the patient was hospitalized.

12. Look in the patient's medical record for referrals or reports from other physicians or laboratory, radiology, or physical therapy reports, and call other facilities.

13. Search other sources of information, such as tax records, voter registration records, court records, death and probate records, credit bureau reports, other creditors, marriage licenses, hunting and fishing licenses, moving companies, police department, school district, or utility company.

14. Obtain the services of a local credit bureau to check reports and notify you if the patient's Social Security number appears under a different name or the party is listed at a new address.

for specific dollar amounts. As each level increases, more time is spent trying various tactics to locate the patient. The more time spent, the more money the agency charges. When using such a service, the medical assistant should choose a specific level for each account depending on what dollar amount is owed.

Determine how much to spend tracing each debtor. Depending on the amount owed and the time estimated to locate the patient, there may be a decision to write off the balance.

Also, on-line information services can be used for skip tracing via the Internet. A search is made of the database that contains millions of records. If a match is made with the given data, helpful information may be discovered.

To make locating a skip easier, remember to keep records updated and verify information each time the patient visits the office.

Search via Computer

When using the Internet for a search, it is important to remember that information is not secure and the patient's right to privacy must never be violated. Some excellent methods of skip tracing using electronic databases or on-line services to locate a debtor are:

Surname scan—Searches (locally, regionally, or nationally) based on data that have been compiled from public source documents.

Address search—Gives property search and any change of address from all suppliers of data to the database, including the U.S. Postal Service; names of other adults in the household, who may have the debtor's telephone number listed under their name, may also be included.

Electronic directory—Gives access to the regional telephone operating company's screen of information.

Credit holder search—Used to discover occupation.

Phone number search—Allows access to the names of other adults in the same household who have a telephone number.

Neighbor search—Shows names, addresses, and telephone numbers of the debtor's former neighbors.

ZIP code search—Provides names, addresses, and telephone numbers of everyone within that ZIP code who has the same last name as the debtor.

City search—Finds everyone with the same last and first name within a given city, as well as all people who live in that city.

State search—Locates all individuals with the same last name or same last and first name within the state, and lists their addresses and telephone numbers.

National search—Operates the same way as the state search; use for people with unusual last names.

Business search—Lists the names of businesses in the neighborhood of the patient's last known residence; may help find where the patient has relocated or will help verify the patient's place of employment.

Refer to the Resource section at the end of this chapter for Web sites used in skip tracing.

STOP AND THINK CASE SCENARIO

Tackle Payment Obstacles

Scenario: An established patient, Martha Gay, is leaving the office after her appointment and stops by your desk. You state today's fee and she says, "Oh, I forgot my checkbook."

Critical Thinking: Determine what your response should be.

_____

_____

_____

_____

_____

STOP AND THINK CASE SCENARIO

Handle Collection Problems

Scenario: Harold Benger's account has become delinquent. You telephone the patient and he says, "I sent in the payment."

Critical Thinking: Formulate questions to ask the patient and state what action you will take.

_____
_____
_____
_____
_____
_____
_____
_____

FOCUS ON CERTIFICATION*

CMA Content Summary
- Medical abbreviations
- Telephone technique
- Ledgers
- Charges, payments, adjustments
- Collecting and updating demographic data
- Itemized and cycle billing
- Aging accounts receivable
- Collection procedures

RMA Content Summary
- Medical terminology and abbreviations
- Payments and write-off amounts
- Aging reports
- Fee schedules
- Calculate and post payments

- Ledgers and accounts
- Truth in Lending Statements
- Itemized statements and billing methods
- Skip tracing
- Fair Debt Collection Practices Act
- Bankruptcy and small claims procedures
- Collection procedures

CMAS Content Summary
- Spell medical terms
- Accounts receivable
- Fee structure
- Credit arrangements
- Patient accounts/ledgers
- Billing methods
- Collections

*This textbook and the accompanying Workbook meet the entry-level administrative and general competencies for the CMA outlined by the AAMA Examination Content Outline and Role Delineation Study and for the RMA and CMAS outlined by the AMT Competencies and Examination Specifications (see Competency Grid in Appendix B).

REVIEW   EXAM-STYLE QUESTIONS

1. When establishing fees, the following are taken into consideration:

   a. fees of physicians in the same specialty

   b. the physician's education and experience

   c. geographic location of the practice

   d. overhead for maintaining the practice

   e. all of the above

2. Select the correct statement regarding physician's giving cash discounts.

   a. The physician has the right to determine who he or she can offer cash discounts to.

   b. Discounts can only be offered to patients with insurance coverage.

   c. If cash discounts are offered, they must be offered to all patients.

   d. Cash discounts can only be offered to patients without insurance coverage.

   e. Cash discounts should never be offered in a medical practice.

3. Certain hospitals have received federal construction grants to enlarge their facilities in exchange for caring for indigent patients, this obligation falls under the:

   a. Medicare program

   b. federal Medicaid program

   c. state Medicaid program

   d. Hill-Burton Act

   e. Indigent-Care Act of 1946

4. The most important collection practice to increase collections, improve public relations, and reduce patient complaints, business-office turnover, accounts receivable, and write-off amounts is:

   a. stating fee-for-service and collecting fees at the time services are given

   b. sending timely billing statements every 30 days

   c. utilizing a collection agency early in the collection process

   d. sending friendly collection letters

   e. telephoning patients who have overdue accounts

5. Cycle billing:

   a. allows billing at certain times of the month based on alphabetic breakdown, account number, insurance type, or date of first service

   b. allows continuous cash flow, relieves mailing statements all at once, and distributes billing telephone calls

   c. distributes statements during the month based on dollar amounts; those with the highest amount due are billed first

   d. is not recommended for the medical office

   e. both a and b

6. The credit law that states, "Collectors must identify themselves and the medical practice they represent; they must not mislead the patient," is:

   a. Equal Credit Opportunity Act

   b. Fair Debt Collection Practices Act

   c. Federal Truth in Lending Act

   d. Truth in Lending consumer Credit Cost Disclosure

   e. Fair Credit Billing Act

7. If a physician denies credit to a patient, according to the Equal Credit Opportunity Act, how many days does the patient have to request the reason in writing?

   a. 10 days

   b. 30 days

   c. 60 days

   d. 90 days

   e. 120 days

8. Regulation Z of the Federal Truth in Lending Act applies to:

   a. patients who decide to pay (on their own) their debt in more than four installments

   b. patients who do not pay all of their debt in one payment, but spread it out over time

   c. patients who offer to pay in installments

   d. patients who agree to pay in more than four installments

   e. all of the above

9. Breaking down accounts into lengths of time that money is owed is called:

   a. account divisions

   b. separating accounts

   c. aging accounts

   d. analyzing accounts

   e. maturation of accounts

10. Select the correct statement regarding collections.

    a. Use a public telephone to make collection calls.

    b. Be flexible about interruptions when making collection calls.

    c. The best times to make collection calls is prior to and after regular working hours.

    d. Collection letters to obtain payment are better than telephone calls.

    e. The longer an account remains delinquent, the harder it will be to collect.

11. When interviewing a collection agency, what collection rate would be considered good?

    a. 25 to 45%

    b. 30 to 60%

    c. 50 to 75%

    d. 60 to 80%

    e. 75% or above

12. After a judgment is made in favor of the medical practice in small claims court:

    a. the physician still has to pursue the money

    b. the money is always exchanged in the court room and turned over to the physician

    c. the court follows up to make sure payment is made

    d. a court order is sent to the patient mandating payment

    e. a court representative follows up to make sure payment is made

13. Garnishment is:

    a. limited to 10% of disposable earnings in any workweek

    b. limited to 15% of disposable earnings in any workweek

    c. limited to 25% of disposable earnings in any workweek

    d. limited to 30% of disposable earnings in any workweek

    e. there is no limit on the amount that can be garnished

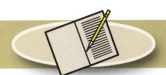

WORKBOOK ASSIGNMENT

To develop competency-based job skills, refer to the *workbook* and complete the:

- Abbreviation and Spelling Review
- Review Questions

- Critical Thinking Exercises
- Job Skill activities, which are outlined at the beginning of this chapter under "Performance Objectives in the *Workbook*."

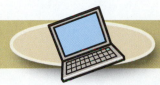

COMPUTER ASSIGNMENT

To review the concepts you have learned in this chapter, insert the *Student Practice* CD-ROM into a computer and work through the *StudyWARE* activities and games. Answer review questions in the practice mode and read the feedback, studying the questions you have missed. Take the chapter quiz until you achieve a minimum score of 90 percent. Successfully completing the *Critical Thinking Challenge* at the end of this course will help you think through scenarios and develop problem solving skills.

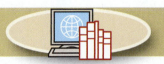

RESOURCES

Collection Resources

American Medical Billing Association
   Online billing seminars, billing conferences, and billing resources
   Web site: http://www.ambanet.net/AMBA.htm
Insurance Companies
   Search for an insurance company (e.g., Blue Cross Blue Shield [www.bcbs.com]) for frequently asked billing questions (FAQ)

Credit Bureaus

Equifax
   PO Box 740241
   Atlanta, GA 30374
   (800) 685-1111
   Web site: http://www.equifax.com
Experian
   PO Box 2002
   Allen, TX 75013
   (888) 397-3742
   Web site: http://www.experian.com
TransUnion
   PO Box 1000
   Chester, PA 19022
    (800) 888-4213
   Web site: http://www.transunion.com

Internet Skip Tracing

Anywho	http://www.anywho.com
Bigfoot	http://www.bigfoot.com
InfoSpace	http://www.infospace.com
InfoUSA	http://www.infousa.com (bankruptcy)
SearchBug	http://www.searchbug.com
WhoWhere?	http://www.whowhere.com (Free: address, phone, and reverse search)
Yahoo People Search	http://www.yahoo.com (people search)
411Locate	http://www.411locate.com

Newsletters

The Doctor's Office
   HCPro
   PO Box 1168
   Marblehead, MA 01945-5168
   (800) 331-5196
The Health Care Collector
   Aspen Publications, Inc.
   PO Box 990
   Frederick, MD 21705-9727
   (800) 638-8437
   Web site: http://www. aspenpublishers.com

CHAPTER 14

Banking

OBJECTIVES

After reading this chapter and learning step-by-step procedures to gain job skills,* you should be able to:

Learning Objectives

- Define common banking terms.
- List different types of checking accounts.
- Name several types of checks.
- Explain the difference between a blank, a restrictive, and a full endorsement.
- Describe various methods of paying bills.
- Discuss reasons to make prompt bank deposits.
- State precautions when using an automated teller machine.
- Understand the steps used in reconciling a bank statement.

Performance Objectives (Procedures) in This Textbook

- Prepare a bank deposit (Procedure 14-1).
- Write a check using proper format (Procedure 14-2).
- Reconcile a bank statement (Procedure 14-3).

Performance Objectives (Job Skills) in the *Workbook*

- Prepare a bank deposit (Job Skill 14-1).
- Write checks (Job Skill 14-2).
- Endorse a check (Job Skill 14-3).
- Inspect a check (Job Skill 14-4).

*This textbook and the accompanying Workbook meet the educational components for entry-level administrative and general competencies outlined by CAAHEP and ABHES.

■ Post payment to a ledger (Job Skill 14-5).

■ Post entries to ledger cards and calculate balances (Job Skill 14-6).

■ Reconcile a bank statement (Job Skill 14-7).

OUTLINE WITH LECTURE NOTES

Financial Institutions

_____

_____

_____

_____

Accounts
Savings Account

_____

_____

_____

_____

Checking Account

_____

_____

_____

_____

Checks
Types of Checks

_____

_____

_____

_____

Check Fraud Prevention

_____

_____

_____

_____

Check Endorsements

_____

_____

_____

_____

Bank Deposits
Banking by Mail

_____

_____

_____

_____

Direct Deposit Program

_____

_____

_____

After-Hours Deposits

_____

_____

_____

_____

Automated Teller Machines
Basic Rules of Precaution

_____

_____

_____

_____

Checkbook Management
Check Writer Machine

_____

_____

_____

_____

Banking Online

_____

_____

_____

_____

Payment Disputes and Check-Writing Errors

_____

_____

_____

_____

Bank Statements
Bank Statement Reconciliation

_____

_____

Balance Differences

_____

_____

_____

KEY TERMS

ABA number
automated teller machine (ATM)
automatic transfer of funds
bank by mail
bank statement
bearer
check (CK)
checking account
credit
currency
debit
deposit record
deposit slip
deposits
direct deposit service
electronic funds transfer system (EFTS)
endorsement
forgery

money order
negotiable instrument
nonsufficient funds (NSF)
notes
overdraft
payee
payer
postdated check
reconciliation
savings account
service charges
signature card
stale check
stop payment orders
voucher
warrant
withdrawal

HEART OF THE HEALTH CARE PROFESSIONAL

Service

A medical assistant who is knowledgeable about financial transactions can assist the patient when payments are made for professional medical services.

FINANCIAL INSTITUTIONS

Banks are financial institutions that receive deposits into accounts, lend money, and render other services. It is important to select a financial institution that offers services that can be tailored to the particular needs of a medical practice. Such services as free online banking and 24-hour telephone banking, access to ATM banking, a variety of interest-bearing accounts; specialized services such as courier, direct deposit, safe deposit boxes, and high-volume checking accounts; lines of credit that include business debit and credit cards, a wide variety of loans and credit lines, equipment financing, and face-to-face interaction with decision-makers are all important considerations when choosing a financial institution.

Similar services are offered by credit unions, savings and loan associations, and other financial institutions. By comparing these services and making the most effective use of them for the medical practice, a knowledgeable medical assistant can be a financial asset to an employer.

Every financial transaction between a medical practice and a bank concerns some form of money (e.g., cash, checks, money orders). Therefore, the medical assistant must understand fundamental banking procedures and common banking terms.

ACCOUNTS

Premier accounts, money market accounts, and both personal and business accounts are offered at financial institutions. The most common types of accounts are savings and checking accounts.

Savings Account

A **savings account** is an interest-bearing account into and from which deposits and withdrawals may be made; there is no stated maturity date. Savings accounts typically do not offer check-writing capabilities; however, some may offer limited check-writing (e.g., three checks per month). A physician's office may have a savings account into which regular deposits are made, then money may be transferred into the checking account monthly or as the need arises for practice expenses and payroll.

Checking Account

A **checking account** may or may not be interest bearing; it is subject to withdrawal of funds on deposit by check.

Types of Checking Accounts

The medical assistant may be responsible for opening a checking account, making deposits and withdrawals, and reconciling the bank statement at the end of each month. There are various types of checking accounts, but the most common are the individual or joint checking accounts and the business or commercial checking accounts.

- *Individual or joint checking account*—The depositor purchases a supply of checks and places money in the checking account to cover the amount of checks written. A joint checking account is owned by two or more people and requires signatures either singly or jointly for withdrawals or check writing, depending on how the account is set up. The bank keeps a signature card on file for each account, showing those authorized to sign or endorse and cash checks. There may be no fee with a specified minimum balance, a flat monthly fee, or a per-check charge.

- *Business or commercial checking account*—A large amount of checks are purchased or furnished by the bank to the depositor. Typically, if the account has a minimum balance, there is no charge, but if the balance of the account falls below the minimum amount (e.g., $10,000), a service charge may be levied.

Electronic Funds Transfer System—A system by which preauthorized automatic transfers are made from savings to checking accounts is called an **electronic funds transfer system (EFTS)**. The physician can arrange with the bank to have money automatically transferred from an interest-paying savings account into a noninterest-paying checking account whenever money is needed. Mortgage, utilities, insurance premiums, and payroll can be handled with this system. Employees' paychecks may be deposited directly into their bank accounts by magnetic tape.

Pay-by-Phone System—*Pay-by-phone* is a system that is a substitute for check writing whereby the medical assistant telephones the bank or savings and loan association to initiate payments. A bank

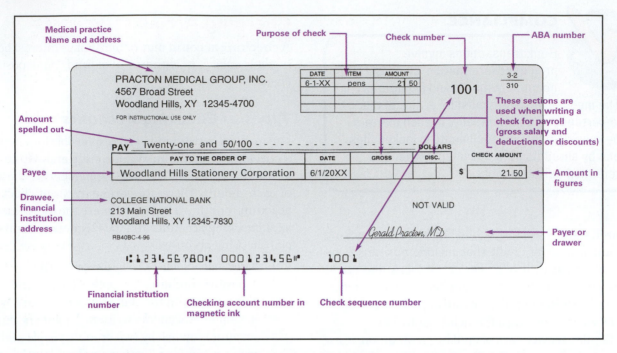

Figure 14-1. Completed check with its various parts identified. In the ABA number (3-2/310), numbers 1 through 49 before the hyphen designate the cities where Federal Reserve banks are located or other key cities, and numbers 50 through 99 designate the states or territories. The number after the hyphen is the bank's assigned number. The denominator (310) is the number of the Federal Reserve district where the bank is located.

can only transfer between accounts they hold called **automatic transfer of funds**. There may be a nominal fee for the service, which is usually less than the postage to mail a check; some financial institutions provide this as a free service if a minimum balance is maintained.

Automatic Bill Paying—Automatic bill paying is another substitute for writing a check. The bank is given permission by the account holder to transfer funds monthly for bill paying. This service is used most commonly for monthly bills such as mortgage payments, loan payments, insurance premiums, utilities, and so forth. Often there is no charge for this service, and there may even be a reduction in the loan interest rate or monthly payment but, generally, only for those bills on a preferred list.

Point-of-Sale Banking System—Point-of-sale banking (POS) is a system that brings banking to the business location. It allows instant transfer of funds from a patient's bank account at the time services are received. The system uses a plastic debit card plus an identification number, which is known only to the owner, and an electronic terminal.

CHECKS

A large percentage of the money received in a physician's office are payments made by checks. A **check (CK)** is a written order to a bank to pay money on demand (Figure 14-1). Each check is numbered in the top right corner. The check sequence number is also imprinted by the bank at the bottom, along with the first series of numbers identifying the financial institution and a second series of numbers identifying the checking account number. The American Bankers Association code number, called the **ABA number**, appears as a fraction and is located on the face of the check in the top right area. The name and address of the owner of the checking account appears in the top left portion of the check. The blank areas to be completed include the date, name you are writing the check to (payee), amount of the check (written in figures and spelled out), and signature of payer. It concerns three parties:

1. The *drawer*/**payer** (or depositor) who orders the bank to pay

2. The *drawee* (or financial institution) where the money is deposited in a checking account

3. The **payee** (or person) who is directed to receive the money

A check is negotiable, that is, legally transferable, to another person by endorsement when it meets the following requirements. It must be:

1. Written

2. Signed by the drawer, or *maker*

3. An unconditional order to pay a specific amount of money

4. Payable to the order of the bearer

5. Payable on demand or on a definite date

6. Written to the payee

The payee endorses the check, thereby transferring the right to receive the money.

Types of Checks

Various types of checks may be presented in a medical practice. Always inspect a check to be sure it is properly completed. Obtain a state driver's license number and a second form of identification and check them against existing records before accepting a check for payment. Call the bank to verify all out-of-state or suspicious checks. The medical assistant can call the bank to see if checks that have a carbon strip through the center can be used, such as those provided in a pegboard bookkeeping system (discussed in Chapter 15). A check authorization system or private company that offers a check verification service may be worthwhile in a large medical practice or clinic setting.

Checks containing dates that are over six months old will not be accepted by the bank. If the numerical and written amounts do not agree, the payee receives the amount that is written out.

Cashier's Check

A *cashier's check* is drawn by the bank, made payable out of the payee's bank account, and signed by an authorized bank official. No stop payments are allowed so this type of check is considered as good as cash.

Certified Check

A customer's check may be presented to the bank for authentication and guarantee, making it a *certified check*. The bank makes note of the details, with-draws the funds specified, sets the funds aside until the check is presented for payment, stamps "certified" on the check face, and has the check signed by an authorized bank official. This check is not used very often.

Counter Check

A *counter check* is one available at the bank for the depositor to draw funds from his or her own account. The wording on the check, "Pay to the Order of Myself Only," makes the counter check nonnegotiable. A counter check can also be a blank check used to transact payment when a person does not have checks with him or her. The name of the bank must be written in as well as other standard information. A counter check might be needed if a physician goes to the bank to withdraw money from the account but forgets the checkbook.

Electronic Check

An *electronic check* is a check created from digital images of the original. The 21st Century Act, known as "Check 21," is a federal law granting the usage of electronic checks that went into effect October 28, 2004. Instead of the bank transporting checks physically, they can now transport them electronically to other banks in the check collection process. The reproductions are called *substitute checks*. Both the front and back of the check are copied and a legend that states, "this is a legal copy of your check" appears; the substitute check serves all uses of the original check and may be returned with the bank statement.

Some companies will take a paper check that has been sent by the medical office and convert it into an electronic transaction that is processed via the automated clearinghouse (ACH) system. The paper check is not forwarded to the bank for payment and, therefore, is not returned to the medical practice. Also, regular billers, such as telephone and utility companies, may convert check payments into electronic ACH transactions that are sent to the bank for payment. The original check is destroyed by the biller and is also not returned.

A retailer may convert a paper check into an electronic ACH payment at the time of purchase (point of purchase [POP]). The cashier captures the information on the check electronically and hands back the physical check.

Limited Check

A *limited check* is one bearing a statement that indicates the check is void if written over a certain amount. Such checks are used for payroll or may be received as payment of insurance claims. A limited check also specifies a time limit during which it is negotiable, for example, "Void twelve months from issue date." If the time limit has passed, the check is referred to as a **stale check**.

Money Order

A **money order** is an instrument similar to a check purchased for face value plus a fee. It is signed by and issued according to the purchaser's instructions. The seller sets aside funds until payment of the money order is made. Money orders are issued by banks, financial institutions, money order companies, and the post office.

Traveler's Check

Traveler's checks were developed to use while traveling and in situations where personal checks may not be accepted or carrying large amounts of cash is not desirable. They are printed in denominations of $10, $20, $50, and $100. The checks, purchased from banks or traveler's clubs, are signed on their face in the presence of a bank witness at the time of purchase. Then, when cashing a check for a purchase, the owner fills in the name of the payee and signs his or her name again on the face of the check. The second signature must be done in the presence of the person cashing the check, who can then compare the two signatures for authenticity. This provides protection against loss or theft. When a bank deposit slip is completed, traveler's checks are listed as checks, not cash.

Voucher Check

A *voucher check* is a check that is available in a variety of styles. Some medical offices order the style that is bound with three checks to a page. A perforation divides the actual check from that portion that outlines written details of the payment. Another style is unbound checks in assembled packs, and a copy is retained as a record of the transaction.

Warrant

A check that is not considered negotiable but can be converted into a **negotiable instrument**, that is, a written order promising to pay a specific sum, or cash is called a **warrant**. A warrant shows that a debt is due because services have been rendered, entitling the bearer to payment. Government and civic agencies may issue warrants. An insurance adjuster issues drafts, known also as warrants, that order the insurance company to pay a claim. Warrants do not have ABA numbers (see "Bank Deposits"). To receive payment on a warrant, it must be submitted to the bank that has the funds for collection and final payment. A warrant can be subjected to lengthy delay before funds are available in the source bank.

Check Fraud Prevention

A check written with the knowledge that there is not sufficient money in the account to cover the check is considered an *intent to defraud* and is unlawful. Businesses are more vulnerable during the following times:

- Friday afternoons
- Evenings
- Weekends
- Holidays

Be cautious when receiving checks. Do not give out bank or credit card information over the telephone, and ask the bank about fraud prevention features when checks are ordered.

Check Endorsements

Checks and money orders must be endorsed on the back by the payee (the person or company the check is made out to) exactly as written. If the endorser's name is incorrect on the face of the check, it should be endorsed twice—first as it appears on the face of the check and then as it appears on the account **signature card**. If a check is made out to "**bearer**" or "cash," it is considered a negotiable instrument and requires no endorsement, although banks may require a signature as evidence of who received the money.

To endorse a check, the payee or the payee's authorized agent writes, types, or stamps his or her name and other pertinent matter on the back of the check within the specified area, 1½ inches from the *trailing edge*. The trailing edge is the left end of the check that has the payee's name and address printed on it. Going over the 1½ inch limit can result in collection delays and possible Federal Reserve Board fines against the medical practice. An authorized agent may be the physician, office manager, bookkeeper, or administrative medical assistant in charge of bank deposits. After the check is properly endorsed, it may then be deposited in a bank or cashed.

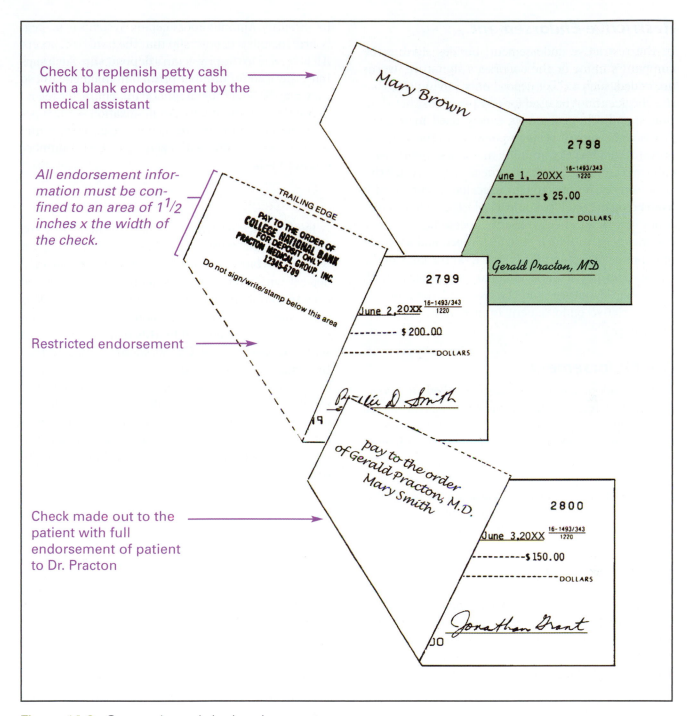

Check to replenish petty cash with a blank endorsement by the medical assistant

All endorsement information must be confined to an area of $1^1/2$ inches x the width of the check.

Restricted endorsement

Check made out to the patient with full endorsement of patient to Dr. Practon

Figure 14-2. Commonly used check endorsements

The most commonly used **endorsements** in a physician's practice are *blank*, *restrictive*, and *full endorsements* (Figure 14-2).

Blank Endorsement

The blank endorsement is the most common way of endorsing a check. The payee simply signs his or her name on the back of the check near the left end.

A check so endorsed should be cashed or deposited immediately. The medical assistant is most likely to use a blank endorsement when cashing a check made out to replenish petty cash. The physician's office manager or bookkeeper writes a check to "cash" or "petty cash," and the assistant endorses the check when receiving the cash from the bank, thereby verifying who received payment.

Restrictive Endorsement

In the restrictive endorsement, besides signing the company's name or the endorser's signature, words are added, such as "For deposit only," to indicate that the check cannot be used for any purpose other than that stated. This custom is widely used in medical practices because it protects payment to the payee by preventing a **forgery** (fraudulent endorsement). Use a rubber stamp and stamp the check with a restrictive endorsement immediately on receipt to safeguard it from being negotiable should it be lost or stolen. Sometimes insurance checks require a personal signature endorsement, in which case a stamped endorsement may not be accepted; this is stated on the back of the check. The payee must endorse such checks with his or her signature, and the assistant then stamps the restrictive endorsement immediately below the signature.

Full Endorsement

A full endorsement, sometimes called a *special endorsement,* is used when a check is to be transferred to another person or company. This is referred to as a third-party check, mentioned later in this chapter. The bearer to which the check is made out to writes "Pay to the order of," followed by the name of a specified person or company and signs his or her name, further protecting the check from improper use. Only the new payee can endorse it for further processing.

BANK DEPOSITS

Preparing daily bank **deposits** is one of the routine chores usually handled by the administration medical assistant. Deposits of checks and **currency** (paper money) should be made promptly to prevent payments being lost, misplaced, or stolen. Timely deposits also reduce the possibility of a check being returned due to insufficient funds. It is an act of courtesy to cash checks promptly so payers' bank statements can be more easily reconciled at the end of the month.

Checks received for payments numbered anywhere from 101 to 300 or 1001 to 1050 are usually an indication of a newly established checking account. It is particularly important to deposit such checks immediately because it has been established that kiting (writing a check not backed by funds in the bank) occurs more frequently in such new accounts.

Some computerized financial software programs create a daily deposit slip when payments are posted to accounts. Manual bookkeeping systems (e.g., pegboard) include a deposit slip that the bank will accept if it is stapled to the physician's **deposit slip**. Such slips have the account number printed in magnetic ink so they may be "read" by magnetic ink character recognition (MICR) equipment. An itemization of the types of money included in the deposit (e.g., checks and cash) are listed along with each check's ABA number (Figure 14-3).

Banking by Mail

A bank service whereby deposits are mailed by the customer to the bank for credit to his or her account is known as **bank by mail**. Banks provide special mail deposit slips and envelopes with either preprinted account numbers or with space to record them. This saves the medical assistant considerable time, but cash cannot be deposited by this method unless it is sent by registered mail. Checks should include restrictive endorsements, "For deposit only" or "For deposit and credit to the account of John Doe, MD; account number 12 34 56." The bank will send the depositor a receipt along with another envelope and deposit slip, or some banks use a duplicate deposit slip system, whereby the depositor keeps the duplicate as the receipt.

Direct Deposit Program

A **direct deposit service** is the automatic deposit of wages or benefits (e.g., Social Security check, payroll check) into a customer's bank account. This expedites the deposit of a check and the availability of funds. It also eliminates mailing expenses or going to the bank to accomplish the transaction.

In a physician's practice, payroll may be deposited directly into an employee's bank account or arrangements can be made for regular insurance payments (e.g., Medicare) to be deposited into the physician's bank account.

After-Hours Deposits

If the physician's office closes after banking hours, a depositor may use the after-hours depository service of a bank. The deposit is placed in an envelope and dropped through a slot located on the outside of the bank. The deposit is processed by the bank the following morning or held unopened until the depositor can get to the bank personally to make the deposit; then during banking hours it is necessary to obtain a

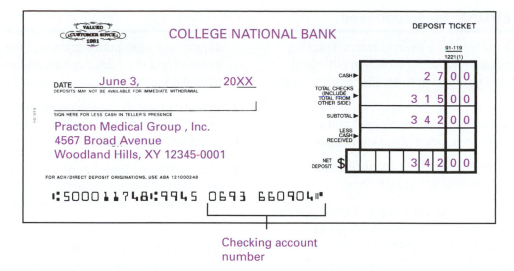

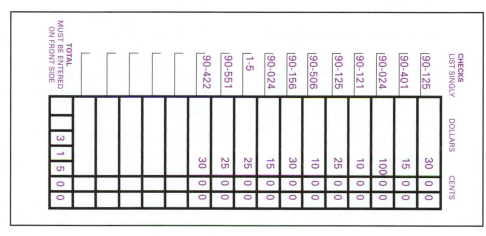

Figure 14-3. Both sides of a completed deposit slip, showing boxed areas where itemized checks and totals are entered

PROCEDURE 14-1

Prepare a Bank Deposit

Objective: To prepare a bank deposit slip for the day's receipts (cash and checks), complete financial records related to the deposit, and deposit the day's receipts into a bank account.

Equipment/Supplies: Items for deposit—currency, money orders, checks, bank deposit slip—endorsement stamp (optional), computer or typewriter, envelope, and pen.

Directions: Follow these step-by-step procedures, which include rationales, to learn this skill, which is presented in the *Workbook* (Job Skill

14-1) for practice. Refer to Figure 14-4 for a visual example.

1. Type or handwrite the name and address of the physician on the deposit slip if it is not preprinted; list the date of the deposit. Never use pencil or erasable ink.

2. Insert the checking account number if it is not preprinted on the deposit slip.

3. Organize the receipts by dividing the bills, coins, checks, and money orders into separate piles.

(continues)

PROCEDURE 14-1 *continued*

4. Sort the currency by denomination, stacking bills face up in the same direction with larger bills on top graduating to smaller ones or vice versa.

5. Total the currency (paper money) and write this amount on a piece of scratch paper.

6. Total the amount of coins and write this amount on a piece of scratch paper.

7. Total the amount of currency and coins, verify it against the total of the day's accounts receivable on the computer, daysheet, or general ledger, and enter the amount on the deposit slip under "cash."

8. Place the currency and coins in an envelope. If there are a large number of bills, paper clip or wrap them according to denomination. Banks provide special paper bands for wrapping bills. If there are a large number of coins roll them in coin wrappers supplied by the bank with the physician's name and account number written or stamped on each wrapper.

9. Verify that a restrictive endorsement has been placed on the back of all the checks and money orders.

10. Examine each check to be deposited to ensure it is properly drawn. Watch for **postdated checks** (dated for sometime in the future) and discrepancies between written amounts and figures. If a check is written improperly, the payer must be contacted.

11. List each check separately on the deposit slip, including the top portion of the ABA number (see Figure 14-1) and the amount. Deposit slips may appear with some screened or shaded areas; write all numbers inside the amount boxes and do not use fractions or dashes. Avoid numbers touching each other. Keep other writing away from amount boxes. Some deposit slips may not have preprinted decimal points, and others may appear printed. Follow the bank's directions as to whether decimal points should be inserted.

12. Total all checks and verify the amount with the total listed in the computer or on the daysheet or general ledger. When using a pegboard system, checks are arranged in the order received and amounts are written on the deposit slip listing the names of the patients' account and the ABA transit numbers. This is helpful if future reference is required.

13. Enter the total of checks deposited on the reverse side of the deposit slip, or in an area listed as "total checks."

14. Clip the checks together or put them in an envelope or in bank wrappers. The account number should be written on each envelope wrapper.

15. List other items of currency after the checks, for example, money orders, traveler's checks, share drafts (checks from credit unions), and promissory notes.

16. Subtotal the amount of cash and currency and verify this amount with the amount listed in the computer or on the daysheet or general ledger.

17. Recalculate the "net deposit total" for verification (total amount of currency, coins, and checks) and enter this on the deposit slip. Banks accept a date-stamped adding machine tape indicating the amounts of the checks, cash, and change. The tape should be duplicated and the original stapled to the deposit slip; the duplicate should be stapled to the duplicate deposit slip or daysheet or general ledger.

18. Make a photocopy of the deposit slip, if needed, to retain in the office.

19. Enter the amount of the deposit (preferably with red ink so deposits can be quickly located) in the checkbook register and add it to the current balance, indicating the new balance.

20. Place coins, currency, checks, and the deposit slip in a large envelope or bank deposit bag to transport it to the bank in person. Or if mailing the deposit, put them in a bank-by-mail envelope and send by registered mail.

21. Obtain a **deposit record** or receipt from the bank at the conclusion of the transaction for deposits made in person. File it for later reference when reconciling the monthly bank statement.

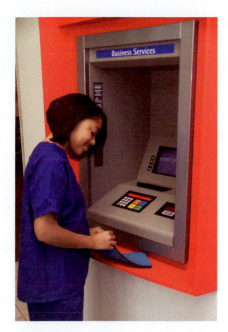

Figure 14-4. Medical assistant depositing money in an automated teller machine

replacement envelope and a deposit receipt. A double-locked security bag is available from banks for a small fee for this purpose. Always double-check that the deposit bag has gone into the evening deposit drawer properly by reopening the drawer.

AUTOMATED TELLER MACHINES

An **automated teller machine (ATM)** is a computerized terminal that enables a customer to make a deposit, withdraw cash, transfer funds, or obtain other bank services (Figure 14-4). Automated teller machines are accessible 24 hours a day, 7 days a week, and are installed in the outer wall of a bank. Additional terminals can be found in airports, train stations, shopping centers, college campuses, and supermarkets. Depositors are given a debit card and select a personal identification number (PIN) that gives them access to their own computerized bank accounts. If cash is needed and the bank is not open or located in a convenient area, a debit card allows **withdrawal** (removal of funds) at an ATM. The card may also be used at other locations (e.g., restaurants, stores) to make cashless purchases from funds on deposit without incurring revolving finance charges for credit. Do not keep a copy of the checking account number and ATM personal identification number in the same place; if found together, these numbers

make it easy for a thief to steal from an account even without a check.

Basic Rules of Precaution

ATM "skimming" has led to billions of dollars in yearly losses. Thieves have used portable card reading devices that fit over the card slot to record data on a card's magnetic strip. They have also used tiny cameras that videotape customers entering their PINs into the machine, or a transparent sheet placed over the ATM keyboard that can record PINs, and even a framed laptop computer that has been placed on top of the ATM screen with a look-alike screen featuring the bank logo and instructions for transactions has been used to duplicate debit cards with PINs written on the back and later sold on the black market.

Because ATMs dispense cash, it is wise to use the machines with caution and awareness. Some guidelines are:

- Complete the deposit envelope ahead of time to speed up the transaction.

- Park close and in a well-lighted area near a walk-up ATM and look for suspicious individuals or activity near the ATM. If you begin a transaction and you notice something unusual, cancel and leave the area.

- Pull close to the machine when using a drive-up ATM and be sure your vehicle doors are locked and all windows are closed except when it is necessary to lower the driver's window to conduct your transaction.

- Select a PIN that does not have numbers that appear in birthdates, addresses, phone numbers, and Social Security numbers, or numbers that appear on anything that is carried in a wallet.

- Never disclose your PIN to anyone, including merchants, bank employees, government officials, or police officers.

- Protect the PIN secret code when accessing the account. Do not write it down; memorize it. Use your hand or body as a shield to prevent others from seeing the code input. Stand directly in front of the panel containing the push buttons. If someone is using the ATM ahead of you, allow that person room for privacy by remaining a few steps back.

- Avoid ATMs with new equipment protruding from or near the card slot or signs noting new equipment.

- Retain the transaction receipt or ATM statement to keep the account information confidential. Do not leave it at the machine or throw it into a nearby trash receptacle. Receipts should be checked against the monthly bank statement.

- For night use, it is preferable to use an ATM that is indoors at a market or shopping mall or to locate a well-lit ATM. If using an enclosed ATM, close the vestibule entry door completely after entering the ATM and do not open the vestibule door to any unknown person(s) at any time.

- Never count or display money at the ATM. Put it away immediately and count it later, in a safe place.

- Never accept offers of help from anyone not associated with the bank.

- Put away your cash, card, and receipt and leave immediately upon completion of your transaction. Look around as you prepare to leave the ATM.

- Ask your bank what the ATM withdrawal limit is on your account and lower it if it is too high.

- Keep track of your account balance and report any discrepancies to the bank immediately.

- Call 911 if emergency assistance due to criminal activity or medical emergency is needed.

CHECKBOOK MANAGEMENT

At the time a check is handwritten, the assistant should take the precaution of completing the **voucher** or stub attached to the check or designated area in the checkbook register (Figure 14-5). This routine reduces the possibility of forgetting to record information and prevents incorrect calculations. Computer software programs that generate checks electronically are available. The bank balance should be

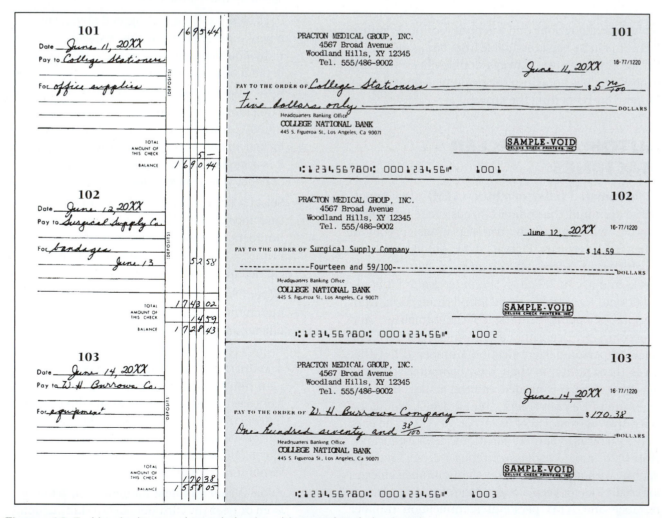

Figure 14-5. Handwritten and typed checks with completed check stubs

known at all times so a check is not written for an amount greater than the balance, causing an **overdraft**. A continuous record of the bank balance is kept on the stub or posted in a check register. Deposits are **credited**, or added, to the balance (preferably in red ink) and checks issued are **debited**, or subtracted, to compute the new balance. Bank service charges must also be subtracted to keep the balance accurate. Other bank charges for collecting **notes** and drafts, for writing drafts or cashier's checks, or for handling checks returned by the bank for insufficient funds must be subtracted or debited in the check register. A note is a document indicating an obligation to pay funds, such as promissory notes, collateral notes, and installment notes. If a check is not written properly (see Procedure 14-2) financial responsibility for any loss is borne by the drawer.

Check Writer Machine

Some offices use a check writer that imprints the figures on a check so that they cannot be changed. First, the date, the name of the payee, and the amount (in figures) are typed on the check. Then the check is inserted into the check writer machine. Next the dollar and cent amounts of the check are set on the machine, and a lever is pressed down. In one operation, the check is imprinted and embossed with the dollar amount. Some machines also imprint over the payee's name so it cannot be altered. Always double-check the figures before imprinting the check; incorrect checks must be voided. The check should be signed by the physician.

Banking Online

An optional banking method, called online banking or Internet banking, that benefits both bank and client is offered by credit unions, savings and loan associations, and other financial institutions. The physician must have a computer with a modem using a telephone or cable line and must subscribe to an Internet service provider with a browser (e.g., Netscape Navigator, Microsoft Internet Explorer). Each of the accounts at the financial institution is governed by the Deposit Account Agreement and Disclosure, Funds Availability Act Disclosure, Electronic Funds Transfer Act Disclosure, and related account agreements. To access, you have to have an eligible account (e.g., checking, savings, certificates of deposit, loans), a user identification number, and an online bank password. Usually there is no monthly fee for accessing accounts,

but fees may apply to services ordered online. Access is available 24 hours a day, 7 days a week. Features that are available with this type of communication include viewing account balances; reviewing transaction history; viewing the front and back of a paid item; transferring money between accounts; printing a statement; searching for specific transactions by date, check number, or amount; placing a stop payment on a check; and many other benefits. It is possible to send electronic mail messages to the financial institution and obtain a response.

Payment Disputes and Check-Writing Errors

A normal check endorsement constitutes acceptance. If a patient writes on a statement "paid in full," but the check amount is for less than the balance due, do not return the check to the patient. For legal protection, do not cross out "payment in full"; instead write the words "without prejudice," "under protest," "received as payment on account," "endorsement disputes payment in full," or "endorsed under protest as per UCC 1-207; payment not in full." Write "balance due" and the amount above your endorsement and make a copy of this endorsement to be kept in the files for future reference. Send a copy to the patient along with a request for payment in full, or telephone the patient to discuss the fee before sending a bill for the balance. The check may be deposited if bank policy allows acceptance of a conditional endorsement—in this way any disputed balance may be collected. If not resolved, you might consider referring this account to a professional collector.

Correction notices or **stop payment orders** are sent from the bank because of bookkeeping errors, if a deposit did not include as much money as shown on the deposit slip, or for reporting uncashable checks of several categories. They are:

1. *Nonsufficient funds (NSF).* This occurs because the payer did not have sufficient money in the account to cover the check. First, call the patient and then call the bank to verify the balances, or ask the patient to pay in cash, money order, or credit card. Keep a record of patients who habitually write such checks. Accept only cash, money order, or credit or debit cards for future payments.

2. *Misdated checks.* If a bank clerk spots a post-dated check or an old check dated three to six months before the day of deposit, it is usually

PROCEDURE 14-2

Write a Check Using Proper Format

Objective: To write a check, record it in the checkbook, and calculate a new balance.

Equipment/Supplies: Blank check, checkbook, and pen.

Directions: Follow these step-by-step procedures, which include rationales, to learn this skill, which is presented in the *Workbook* (Job Skill 14-2) for practice.

1. Balance the checkbook so it is up-to-date and be sure there are sufficient funds to cover the check to be written.

2. Number the checks consecutively unless prenumbered by the bank, making sure the stub number agrees with the corresponding check.

3. Complete the stub showing the date the check is being written, the payee's name, the amount of the check, and the purpose for which payment is being made.

4. Subtract the amount of the check from the running balance and list the new balance.

5. Carry the new balance forward to the next stub.

6. Handwrite the information on the check in ink; do not use an erasable ballpoint pen. If a check is typed and an error is made, you can do either one of the following:

   a. Correct the error and initial it.

   b. Draw a diagonal line across the face of the check and write "void." Write "void" on the stub, and then file the voided check with the canceled checks.

7. Use a check-printing device to prevent tampering, that indents the paper when dollar amounts are inserted, or apply tape or fixative spray over the dollar amount. Checks can be altered by a skilled crook if nonindelible ink is used, or correctable carbon ribbons.

8. Enter the current date, including the month, day, and year (checks may be dated on Sundays and holidays). A postdated check can be issued only with permission from the person accepting the check, because this practice may result in an overdraft, embarrassing the physician and reflecting poorly on the financial soundness of the medical practice.

9. Enter the payee's full name without title (e.g., Ms., Mr., Dr., or Mrs.); begin writing to the extreme left and, following the name, draw a line from the name to the dollar sign at the right to protect the check against alteration. Use abbreviations only when instructed to do so or when space is limited. If the payee is an officer of an organization, the check should be written as "John Doe, Treasurer."

10. Write the amount of the check in figures, placing them close to the dollar sign and close to each other. If typing, use the hyphen or asterisk key to fill in all blank spaces; if handwriting, draw a line in any remaining spaces. The amount should agree with the check stub or register. Use commas if the amount of the check is over four figures; for example, $4,500.50.

11. Write the amount of the check in words on the line, which typically appears below the payee's name; begin at the extreme left of the line so no additional words can be inserted to increase the amount, and draw a line from the end of the written amount to the printed word "Dollars." Separate the cents amount from the dollar amount by writing the word "and," and write the cents as a fraction; for example, 50/100. If there are no cents, write the word "no" as the numerator or the word "only" in place of the fraction (see Example 14-1). If there are no dollars, only cents, the figures following the dollar sign should be circled; for example: $ .75; the printed word "Dollars" should be crossed out (see Example 14-2).

PROCEDURE 14-2 *continued*

EXAMPLE 14-1

Check with Dollar Amount and No Cents

Ten dollars only

Ten dollars and no/100

Ten dollars and no cents

EXAMPLE 14-2

Written Amounts on Checks

Only seventy-five cents ———— Dollars

No and 75/100 ———————— Dollars

Note: The written words on a check always represent the correct amount no matter what is expressed in figures.

12. Write the purpose of the check on the face of the check on a memo line (if included).

13. Obtain the physician's or other authorized person's signature on each check.

14. Keep the checkbook in a secure place out of the reach and sight of unauthorized persons.

---

not honored—"bounced" by the bank. Look at the date of every check you receive. Federal collection law states that if a check dated more than 5 days in advance is accepted, the patient must be notified no more than 10 days and no less than 3 days before the check is deposited. State laws vary, and some states add regulations in addition to those mandated by federal law. When a check bounces, both the check writer and the person to whom the check is written are usually charged a fee.

3. *Incorrect payee's name.* If the physician's name or practice's name on a check is incorrect, many banks will refuse to accept the check. For accuracy and to save time, offer the patient a rubber stamp containing the account name. If the name is written incorrectly, correct it and have the patient initial by the correction.

4. *Missing payer's signature.* Glance over each check to be sure it is signed. If you receive an unsigned check from a patient, first try to obtain a signature by asking the patient to come to the office and sign the check or send a new one. If unable to reach the patient or if there is a transportation or time limitation problem, type "over" on the check where the customer normally signs, then type "lack of signature guaranteed," your physician's name, and your name and title on the back of the check, leaving space above your name. Then sign your name in the space above the typed version. When the

check is deposited, your bank is assured that if the patient's bank does not honor the check, you will take it back as a charge against your account. This is the normal procedure for a dishonored check. Some banks will process the check if funds are available in the customer's account but other banks will process only if there is a written authorization on file. However, a debtor can protest a check that is deposited without a signature.

5. *Variable amounts.* If the numerical amount and the written-out amount are different, the bank will credit only the written-out amount. Make sure the two amounts agree before accepting the check.

6. *Third-party checks.* These include paychecks, government checks, and insurance checks made out to one party (e.g., the patient) and fully endorsed over to the physician. Acceptance of a third-party check made out in an amount over that which is being collected may entail handing out so much cash that the cash drawer is depleted. Good office policy is to inform patients that third-party checks cannot be accepted.

7. *Forged checks.* Accept checks only from patients who are known or, if from an unfamiliar person, obtain two forms of identification such as a driver's license, bank and employee identification cards, or a U.S. passport. Forgers are more likely to have national cards, for example, MasterCard, Visa, and American

Express. Identifications that are insufficient are Social Security cards, library cards, voter registration cards, and unfamiliar credit cards.

PATIENT EDUCATION

Educate patients about different types of payment accepted by the medical practice. If patients are aware that the office accepts debit and credit cards, the problem of returned checks will be minimized.

BANK STATEMENTS

Every month, banks mail each depositor a statement of his or her checking account. Canceled checks or substitute checks that have been debited from the account during the month are also included (Figure 14-6). The **bank statement** lists the date and amount of each deposit and of each withdrawal by date presented for payment, not the date written. The statement also lists electronic transfers of money to the checking account, payments made via electronic banking (debit cards), and deposits made by mail. **Service charges**, interest, credit, and corrections are also listed, and check numbers are shown. The state-

ment should be compared with the checkbook register immediately to determine the cause of any disparity in figures. The balance on the statement and the balance on the checkbook stub or register may not agree due to outstanding checks, so each month the two balances must be reconciled.

Bank Statement Reconciliation

As soon as a bank statement is received, the process of **reconciliation** should be performed (see Example 14-3). A form on the reverse side of the bank statement can be used for this purpose (Figure 14-7).

Balance Differences

If the checkbook balance and bank statement balance do not agree, all details must be rechecked to locate the error, which may result from:

1. Omission of a written check, or one or more outstanding checks, which may have been written without recording the information on a stub or register. This could occur if the physician wrote a check without the medical assistant's knowledge.

2. Omission of a deposit in the checkbook stub or register

3. Unrecorded deposit sent by mail or left in a night depository

---

EXAMPLE 14-3

Reconciliation Formula

Checkbook				Statement
Checkbook ending balance	$_____		$_____	Ending balance from bank
Subtract service charge and any other charges shown on bank statement; also enter these in your check register	−		+	Add any deposits made after the date of the bank statement
Subtotal	$_____		$_____	Subtotal
Add interest earned; also enter in your check register	+		−	Subtract total of outstanding checks and withdrawals listed above
	$_____		$_____	
Adjusted checkbook balance	$_____		$_____	Bank account balance

These two should agree.

College National Bank
700 West Main Street
Woodland Hills, XY 12345

(800) 540-5060

COLLEGE NATIONAL BANK
ACCOUNT ACTIVITY

STATEMENT PERIOD: May 17, THROUGH
June 16, 20XX

PRACTON MEDICAL GROUP, INC   140
4567 BROAD AVENUE
WOODLAND HILLS XY   12345

ACCOUNT
12345-6789
ACCESS# 0082

PAGE   1

ITEM COUNT   30

CHECKING		ACCOUNT 12345-6789	

SUMMARY

BEGINNING STATE BALANCE ON 5-127-20XX.................................... $ 633.87

TOTAL OF   4 DEPOSITS/OTHER CREDITS 1414.75

TOTAL OF   25 CHECKS PAID...   271.53
             5 WITHDRAWALS/OTHER CHARGES.................................   73.00

ENDING STATEMENT BALANCE ON   6-16-20XX...............................   1704.09

CHECKS/
WITHDRAWALS/
OTHER CHARGES

CHECKS:

NUMBER	DATE	AMOUNT	NUMBER	DATE	AMOUNT
0317	06-08	17.40	0328	06-10	29.90
1319	05-25	30.00	0329	05-26	32.05
0320	05-30	7.59	0330	06-02	2.75
0321	05-27	9.00	0331	06-02	30.79
0322	05-24	1.00	0332	06-02	11.47
0323	06-03	6.13			
0324	05-30	1.78			
0325	06-02	67.50			
0326	05-25	21.92			
0327	06-03	2.25			

TOTAL OF 25 CHECKS PAID $271.53

WITHDRAWALS/OTHER CHARGES:

DATE	TRANSACTION DESCRIPTION	AMOUNT
06-10	SURGICAL SUPPLY PAYMENT AT ELECTRONIC BANKING	34.30
06-07	STAR FREE PRESS PAYMENT AT ELECTRONIC BANKING	2.00
06-07	MARINER'S MAIL PAYMENT AT ELECTRONIC BANKING	1.00
06-07	CELLULAR ONE PAYMENT AT ELECTRONIC BANKING	16.00
06-03	CLINT PHARMACY PAYMENT AT ELECTRONIC BANKING	19.70

DEPOSITS/
OTHER CREDITS

DEPOSITS:

DATE	TRANSACTION DESCRIPTION	AMOUNT
06-07	BRANCH DEPOSIT	250.24
06-09	BRANCH DEPOSIT	1000.00
06-15	BRANCH DEPOSIT	156.69
06-16	CHECK DEPOSIT AT BANK BY MAIL	7.82

DAILY BALANCES

DATE	BALANCE	DATE	BALANCE	DATE	BALANCE
05-24	632.87	06-02	418.02	06-09	1605.78
05-25	580.95	06-03	389.94	06-10	1573.88
05-26	548.90	06-07	623.18	06-15	1730.57
05-27	539.90	06-08	605.78	06-16	1704.09
05-30	530.53				

Figure 14-6. Bank statement illustrating date and amount of each deposit and withdrawal, service charges, interest, credits, corrections, check numbers, electronic transfers of money, payments made via electronic banking, and deposits made by mail

FOUR EASY STEPS TO HELP YOU BALANCE YOUR CHECKBOOK

1. UPDATE YOUR CHECKBOOK
   - Compare and check-off each transaction recorded in your check register with those listed on this statement.
     These include checks, direct deposits, direct debits, deposits, ATM transactions, etc.
   - Add interest and subtract service charges.

2. DETERMINE OUTSTANDING ITEMS
   - Use the charts below to list transactions shown in your check register but not included on this statement.
   - Include any from previous months.

OUTSTANDING CHECKS OR OTHER WITHDRAWALS					DEPOSITS NOT CREDITED		
CHECK NO.	AMOUNT		CHECK NO.	AMOUNT	DATE	AMOUNT	
	$			$		$	
248	2	50					
318	14	59					
337	5	00					
338	6	15					
339	170	38					
340	5	00					
			TOTAL	$ 203.62	TOTAL	$	

3. BALANCE YOUR ACCOUNT
   - Enter Ending Statement Balance shown on this statement. $ 1704.09
   - Add deposits listed in your register and not shown on this statement.   +   52.58
   - Subtract outstanding checks/withdrawals.   -   203.62
   - **ADJUSTED TOTAL** (should agree with your checkbook balance). $ 1553.05

4. IF THE BALANCE IN YOUR CHECKBOOK DOES NOT AGREE WITH THE ADJUSTED TOTAL, THEN
   - Check all addition and subtraction.
   - Make sure all outstanding checks, withdrawals and deposits have been listed in the appropriate chart above.
   - Compare the amount of each check, withdrawal and deposit in your checkbook with the amounts on this statement.
   - Review the figures on last month's statement.

IN CASE OF ERRORS OR QUESTIONS ABOUT YOUR ELECTRONIC TRANSFERS, telephone us at the telephone number shown on this statement, or write us at: P.O. Box 30987, City of Industry, CA 91896-7987 as soon as you can if you think your statement or receipt is wrong or if you need more information about a transfer on the statement or receipt. We must hear from you no later than 60 days after we sent you the FIRST statement on which the error or problem appeared. Tell us your name and account number, and describe the error or the transfer you are unsure about. Please explain as clearly as you can why you believe there is an error or why you need more information. You must also tell us the exact dollar amount of the suspected error. If you tell us orally, we require that you send us your complaint or question in writing within 10 business days. If you do not put your complaint or questions in writing or we do not receive it within 10 business days, we may not recredit your account. If we decide that there was no error, we will send you a written explanation within 3 business days after we finish our investigation. You may ask for copies of the documents that we used in our investigation. For purposes of error resolution, our business days are Monday through Friday, 8:30 a.m. to 5:00 p.m., Pacific Time. We are closed Saturdays, Sundays and federal holidays.

All Non-POS, MasterMoney™ or Foreign Transactions
We will tell you the results of our investigation within 10 business days after we receive your written complaint and will correct any error promptly. If we need more time, however, we may take up to 45 days to investigate your complaint or questions. If we decide we need additional time, we will recredit your account within 10 business days for the amount you think is in error, so that you will have the use of the money during the time it takes us to complete our investigation.

POS, MasterMoney™ and Foreign Transactions
If the transfer results from a point-of-sale transaction, MasterMoney™ transaction or a transfer initiated outside the United States, we will still correct any error promptly. However, we may take up to 20 business days after we receive your written complaint to tell you the results of our investigation. If we need more time, we may use an additional 90 days. Should we take this additional time, we will recredit your account within 20 business days for the amount you think is in error. This will allow you to have the use of this money while we complete our investigation.

CF 5299F (5/96)

Figure 14-7. Reverse side of a bank statement showing account reconciliation form

4. Check drawn for a different sum than that recorded on the stub or register

5. Check that has cleared for a different amount than what is shown on the transaction register or checkbook stub

6. Addition or subtraction error(s) in the bank statement or stub or register while carrying figures forward

7. Transposition of figures on the stub or register (divide the amount by nine to pinpoint a transposition error)

8. Canceled check not returned by the bank or omitted on the bank statement in error

If an error is found, mark the stub or register where the error occurred with a reference to the stub or register number where the correction is made. Enter the correction after the last entry, together with a cross-reference to the stub or register number where the error occurred. After the last entry on the stub register, write "Reconciliation" and the date.

PROCEDURE 14-3

Reconcile a Bank Statement

Objective: To verify that all bank deposits and withdrawals agree with the medical practice's financial records of deposits and withdrawals.

Equipment/Supplies: Ending balance of previous bank statement, current bank statement, reconciliation worksheet, deposit receipts, red pencil, check stubs or checkbook register, canceled or returned checks, calculator, and pen or pencil.

Directions: Follow these step-by-step procedures, which include rationales, to learn this skill. Exercises are available in the *Workbook* to practice this job skill.

1. Compare the opening balance on the current bank statement with the previous month's ending balance. They should agree.

2. Organize the cancelled checks in numeric order and compare the entries of the checks on the bank statement with the returned checks to make sure the number and amounts are correct. Verify that all checks are from the medical office and are for the statement period.

3. Compare the deposits listed on the bank statement with the amounts of the deposits listed on the check stubs or check register.

4. Beginning in numeric order, compare the bank imprinted dollar amount on the bank statement of the canceled checks with the amount listed on the checkbook transaction register or checkbook stubs; place a red check mark next to the amount of each returned check as it is verified.

5. List the outstanding checks not returned with the statement on the bank reconciliation form. Certified checks are not listed as outstanding because the amount has already been deducted from the account. If a check has been outstanding for an unusual length of time (e.g., for two monthly statements), it may be lost. Call the payee to see if it has been received.

6. Total all outstanding checks and record the figure in the proper area, "balance your account."

7. List all deposits in transit, that is, those that were made since the last entry on the bank statement.

8. Total all deposits made and not included on the statement and record this amount in the proper area, "balance your account."

9. Record the ending statement balance and add the total amount of deposit in transit and subtract the total amount of outstanding checks from the ending statement balance. The result is the adjusted bank statement balance.

10. Enter on the check stubs or register and subtract from the checkbook balance any

(continues)

PROCEDURE 14-3 *continued*

fees appearing on the bank statement, such as service charges, automatic withdrawals, or payments. The result is the adjusted checkbook balance.

11. The two adjusted balances should agree. If not in agreement, recheck each step to locate the error. The most common errors are missing an outstanding check and mathematical calculations.

STOP AND THINK CASE SCENARIO

Determine What Type of Checks to Write

Scenario A: The physician has asked you to send away to the American Medical Association for very expensive continuing education video series. The physician left on vacation, and you do not have access to a business credit card. You are completing the order form and note that it states that "personal checks" are not accepted. You have check signing authority on the business account.

Scenario B: The physician is purchasing a used automobile from a private party for his eldest son to drive back and forth to college. The seller wishes to meet with the physician and deliver the car to the office tomorrow afternoon at which time payment will be required.

Critical Thinking: Study the differences in cashier's checks, certified checks, counter checks, electronic checks, limited checks, money orders, traveler's checks, voucher checks, and warrants and determine the type of check you should obtain for payment for each scenario; state the reasons for your choice.

A. _____

_____

_____

B. _____

_____

_____

_____

STOP AND THINK CASE SCENARIO

Determine Accepting Payment

Scenario: Dr. Practon's patient, Walter Knott, wants to pay an outstanding account ($100) at the end of an office visit. He hands you a check in the amount of $200 that is made out to him and signed by someone unknown to you.

Critical Thinking: Respond to the situation stating what type of check this is, how you would proceed, and the reason for your answer.

_____

_____

_____

_____

_____

_____

FOCUS ON CERTIFICATION*

CMA Content Summary
- Medical abbreviations
- Banking procedures
- Process accounts receivable
- Preparing bank deposit
- Electronic banking
- Reconciling bank statement
- Maintaining financial records

RMA Content Summary
- Medical terminology and abbreviations
- Collect and post payments
- Patient ledgers and accounts
- Bank deposits

- Checking accounts
- Reconcile bank statements
- Understand check processing procedures
- Process payables and maintain disbursement records
- Perform account calculations

CMAS Content Summary
- Spell medical terms
- Financial computations
- Accounts payable
- Accounts receivable
- Patient accounts/ledgers
- Banking services and procedures

REVIEW EXAM-STYLE QUESTIONS

1. A joint checking account requires:
   a. the signature of both parties
   b. the signature of only one party
   c. the signature of a bank employee and the owner of the account
   d. the signature of one or both parties depending on how the account is set up
   e. the signature of a bank employee only

2. A system by which preauthorized automatic transfers are made from savings to checking accounts is known by the abbreviation:
   a. EFT
   b. EFTS
   c. AFT
   d. AFTS
   e. PAT

3. The "drawee" is:
   a. the person who orders the bank to pay
   b. the person who is directed to receive the money
   c. the financial institution where the money is deposited in a checking account
   d. the maker of the check
   e. the bearer to whom the check is written

4. If the numerical and written amounts of a check do not agree:
   a. the bank will not accept it
   b. the bank will hold it until the writer of the check verifies the correct amount
   c. the payee receives the amount that is spelled out
   d. the payee receives the numerical amount
   e. the check will be returned unpaid

*This textbook and the accompanying Workbook meet the entry-level administrative and general competencies for the CMA outlined by the AAMA Examination Content Outline and Role Delineation Study and for the RMA and CMAS outlined by the AMT Competencies and Examination Specifications (see Competency Grid in Appendix B).

5. If the endorser's name is written incorrectly on the face of a check:

   a. the incorrect name should be used to endorse the check

   b. the correct name should be used to endorse the check

   c. the incorrect and correct name should both be used to endorse the check

   d. the bank will always refuse the check

   e. the check should be voided

6. All checks received in a medical office should:

   a. be stamped with a restrictive endorsement upon receipt

   b. include a blank endorsement

   c. include a full endorsement

   d. be placed in a safe until they are deposited

   e. be turned over to the physician for safe keeping

7. Select the correct statement about bank deposits.

   a. Bank deposits are routinely prepared by the administrative medical assistant.

   b. Bank deposits should be made promptly to prevent payment from being lost, misplaced, or stolen.

   c. Timely deposits reduce the possibility of a check being returned due to insufficient funds.

   d. It is an act of courtesy to cash checks promptly so payers' bank statements can be more easily reconciled.

   e. all of the above

8. ATM pin numbers:

   a. should include either telephone numbers, address numbers, birthdates, or Social Security numbers so that they can be easily memorized

   b. should be shared confidentially with bank employees in case you forget them

   c. should not be disclosed to anyone except police officers in the case of an investigation

   d. should be written down and kept in a secret place for easy access

   e. should be memorized and shared with no one

9. If a check is not written properly, financial responsibility for any loss is borne by the:

   a. drawee

   b. drawer

   c. payee

   d. depositor

   e. financial institution

10. When reconciling a bank statement:

    a. first start with the beginning balance from the bank statement

    b. subtract all deposits made after the date of the bank statement

    c. add the total of outstanding checks and withdrawals

    d. subtract the total of outstanding checks and withdrawals

    e. add the service charge to the checkbook

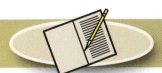

WORKBOOK ASSIGNMENT

To develop competency-based job skills, refer to the *Workbook* and complete the:

- Abbreviation and Spelling Review
- Review Questions

- Critical Thinking Exercises
- Job Skill activities, which arc outlined at the beginning of this chapter under "Performance Objectives in the *Workbook*."

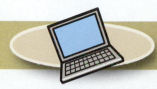

COMPUTER ASSIGNMENT

To review the concepts you have learned in this chapter, insert the *Student Practice* CD-ROM into a computer and work through the *StudyWARE* activities and games. Answer review questions in the practice mode and read the feedback, studying the questions you have missed. Take the chapter quiz until you achieve a minimum score of 90 percent. Successfully completing the *Critical Thinking Challenge* at the end of this course will help you think through scenarios and develop problem solving skills.

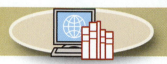

RESOURCES

Internet

ATM Machines
    Search: ATM
    Select from table of contents:
    • Introduction to How ATM Works
    • How Do ATMs Work
    • ATM Card Versus Check Cards
    • Parts of the ATM Machine
    • ATM Security
    Web site: http://www.howstuffworks.com

Bank News (Internet Banking Products)
    Web site: http://www.digitalinsight.com
National Check Fraud Center
    (843) 571-2143
    Web site: http://www.ckfraud.org
Safe Checks (Check Fraud Prevention Package)
    Web site: http://www.safepay123.com

CHAPTER 15

Bookkeeping

OBJECTIVES

After reading this chapter and learning step-by-step procedures to gain job skills,* you should be able to:

Learning Objectives

▎ Define bookkeeping terminology and use proper abbreviations.

▎ Name four bookkeeping systems and compare their differences and similarities.

▎ Determine ledger card components.

▎ State posting procedures on a ledger and on a computerized account.

▎ Explain daysheet posting procedures.

▎ Discuss several ways bookkeeping errors can be located.

▎ Describe accounts receivable control procedures.

▎ Explain two types of cash funds typically used in a medical office.

▎ Use a pegboard bookkeeping system.

Performance Objectives (Procedures) in This Textbook

▎ Prepare the pegboard; post charges, payments, and adjustments, and balance the daysheet (Procedure 15-1).

▎ Establish, record, balance, and replenish petty cash fund (Procedure 15-2).

Performance Objectives (Job Skills) in the *Workbook*

▎ Prepare ledger cards (Job Skill 15-1).

▎ Bookkeeping Day 1—Post to patient ledger cards and prepare cash receipts (Job Skill 15-2).

▎ Bookkeeping Day 1—Prepare daily journal (Job Skill 15-3).

This textbook and the accompanying Workbook meet the educational components for entry-level administrative and general competencies outlined by CAAHEP and ABHES.

- Bookkeeping Day 1—Post charges, payments, and adjustments using a daily journal (Job Skill 15-4).

- Bookkeeping Day 1—Balance daysheet (Job Skill 15-5).

- Bookkeeping Day 2—Prepare daily journal (Job Skill 15-6).

- Bookkeeping Day 2—Post charges, payments, and adjustments to patient ledger cards and to the daily journal; prepare cash receipts and bank deposit (Job Skill 15-7).

- Bookkeeping Day 2—Balance daysheet (Job Skill 15-8).

- Bookkeeping Day 3—Prepare daily journal (Job Skill 15-9).

- Bookkeeping Day 3—Post charges, payments, and adjustments to patient ledger cards and to the daily journal; prepare cash receipts and bank deposit (Job Skill 15-10).

- Bookkeeping Day 3—Balance daysheet (Job Skill 15-11).

- Set up daysheet for new month (Job Skill 15-12).

OUTLINE WITH LECTURE NOTES

Bookkeeping Process

_____

_____

_____

_____

Bookkeeping Systems

_____

_____

_____

_____

Patient Accounts

Ledger Card/Patient Account

_____

_____

_____

_____

Daysheet

_____

_____

_____

_____

Accounts Receivable Control

Computerized Reports

_____

_____

_____

_____

Locating Errors

_____

_____

_____

_____

_____

Cash Funds

Change Drawer

_____

_____

_____

_____

Petty Cash

_____

_____

_____

_____

KEY TERMS

account
accounts payable (A/P) ledger
accounts receivable (A/R) ledger
adjustment
assets
balance
bookkeeping
capital
cash
credits
daysheet
debits

double-entry accounting
extend
general ledger
ledger card
liabilities
open accounts
petty cash fund
post
proprietorship
single-entry accounting
voucher

HEART OF THE HEALTH CARE PROFESSIONAL

Service

Confidence is communicated and mistakes are minimized when the medical assistant is knowledgeable about financial matters and has competent bookkeeping skills. All charges, payments, and adjustments should be posted precisely and figures computed accurately. It is the medical assistant's responsibility to do so and to trace financial transactions should the patient have a question about a bill or payment. It is important to display a concerned attitude when handling financial accounts and trying to locate and correct an error.

BOOKKEEPING PROCESS

The main purpose of any **bookkeeping** system is to record the financial affairs of a business. Most medical practices rely on the medical assistant to manage bookkeeping transactions accurately so the physician has a clear daily picture of the income derived from patient accounts, detailed information on office expenditures, and the necessary figures for income tax purposes.

The combination of private patients and managed care patients who are insured under a variety of contracts makes accounting a complex and challenging task. Because managed care plans vary in their financial reimbursement structure, a variety of accounting procedures is required. Such plans can range from fee-for-service (using various fee schedules) to capitation (fixed amounts paid for each enrollee in the plan; usually monthly). Many contracts require either a fixed-dollar amount copayment or a percentage to be paid by the patient for each office visit. Some contracts have a *stop loss* section, which means that if the patient's services go over a certain amount, the physician can begin asking the patient to pay. In such cases, the patients' accounts or ledgers would need monitoring. Managed care contracts may also retain a portion of the monthly capitation payment called a *withhold* until the end of the year for incentive and to reduce overutilization.

This chapter begins with an explanation of basic bookkeeping guidelines. Chapter 18 gives additional information about financial responsibilities for managers (e.g., accounts payable and payroll). Although many medical practices are computerized, manual bookkeeping skills are explained and taught in this chapter to help increase understanding of the basic computations a computerized system automatically does, as well as the various steps needed to balance books.

Bookkeeping Systems

In a medical practice, one of four bookkeeping systems is usually chosen based on the complexity of the physician's practice, whether it is a group or single-physician office, and on elements of the physician's

Table 15-1. Explanation of Debits and Credits

Debit is anything that:	Examples	Credit is anything that:	Examples
Increases assets	Items of value owned by the practice: cash, money owed by patients (receivables), building, land, equipment, supplies, office furniture	Decreases assets	Sale of equipment, building furniture
Decreases liabilities	Payment of bills owed by the practice	Increases liabilities	Monies owed for business expenditures, mortgage, supplies, equipment, furniture
Decreases earnings	Money owed by patients	Increases earnings	Payment by patients for services rendered by physician

other personal income. Whichever system is chosen—single-entry, double-entry, pegboard, or computerized—it will include a record of daily income (receipts) and payments (disbursements), showing amounts owed to the physician by patients and amounts paid for expenses. When these transactions are recorded completely, the books will reflect where all money comes from and where it goes.

The terms *debit* and *credit* are basic bookkeeping terms used in all accounting systems (see Table 15-1).

Increases in assets are termed **debits**. Decreases in assets are called **credits**.

Single-Entry Accounting

Single-entry accounting is relatively easy to learn and use and is acceptable to both federal and state authorities as a basis for filing tax returns. In this system, records include:

1. The **general ledger** or journal, called a daysheet, daily log, daybook, or charge journal, in which all fees for services rendered and payments are recorded every day

2. An **accounts-receivable (A/R) ledger**, which consists of all of the patients' accounts showing the amounts owed for services rendered; should be insured against fire or flood damage

3. An **accounts payable (A/P) ledger** (check register or checkbook), which shows amounts paid out for the expenses of the business practice

4. The petty cash fund, which contains records showing monies that are available for minor office expenses and monies that have been disbursed

5. The payroll records, which indicate salaries and wages paid and deductions made

Single-entry accounting is neither self-balancing nor well formulated. It does not rely on equal debits or credits, therefore errors are not obvious in this system. Mistakes can be easily made because entries must be registered on one sheet and then transferred onto other journals and ledgers. The medical assistant handles these books of original entry. Many physicians hire accountants, who keep the general ledgers (books of final entry). The assistant gives the accountant the information from the books of original entry, which the accountant then turns into a double-entry system.

Double-Entry Accounting

Double-entry accounting is an exact science because the books must **balance**. Advanced accounting skills are necessary so most medical offices do not require the administrative assistant to use double-entry bookkeeping. However, it is advisable for the assistant to understand the basics of this system, including related terminology such as *assets*, *capital*, *liabilities*, and *prietorship*.

Assets are anything owned by the business, such as equipment, furniture, bank accounts, buildings, accounts receivable, and so on. The physician may own some of the assets outright and may have some that are not completely paid for. **Capital** is original investment money and other property of a corporation that is owned. **Liabilities** are monies that are owed for business expenditures (debts). **Proprietorship** is the owner's net worth or equity, which consists of the amount by which the fair market value of all assets exceeds liabilities.

EXAMPLE 15-1

Formulas Explaining Assets and Proprietorship

The following equations can help you remember:

Assets = Capital + Liabilities

or

Assets − Liabilities = Proprietorship (Owner's Equity)

For recording the transactions, a general ledger sheet is divided in half, with the assets on the left side and the liabilities and capital on the right side. These two sides should balance; that is, the totals of all columns would be the same if no errors occur. The bookkeeper **posts** (records) each transaction to the daily ledger, a book of original entry, and then records totals into this general ledger. For example, when you pay a debt, such as a mortgage on a building, your liability decreases, but so does the cash account. Thus, if you write a check for $1,000, the cash account (asset) would decrease by $1,000. To balance this transaction, the accounts payable (liability) would also decrease by $1,000. In other words, when posting, a debit entry on the left side of the ledger sheet becomes a credit on the right-hand side, and a credit on the right becomes a debit on the left.

Places of business that offer merchandise for sale keep accounts on an *accrual basis;* that is, income is considered earned when the merchandise is sold. Physicians' accounts are kept on what is called a *cash basis,* indicating only what happens to the money taken in. Earned money is not considered income until the patient pays, and purchases are not recorded as expenses until the physician actually pays the bills. Therefore, only two journals are required, one for cash receipts and one for cash disbursements.

A cash receipt journal page shows one month's transactions. Each day an entry is made in the general ledger, listing incoming receipts, bank deposit, and miscellaneous cash expenditures. A cash disbursement page is a record of every check drawn on the physician's checking account as well as bank service charges and fees for checks. As each check is written, the amount is carried over to a disbursement column indicating where the expenditure occurred. In a physician's practice, the columns have various headings depending on the needs of the medical practice (e.g., rent, utilities, insurance). Accounts payable is further discussed in Chapter 18. The accountant will balance the ledgers and produce a periodic profit-and-loss statement and an annual balance sheet.

Pegboard Accounting

Pegboard accounting has been a popular bookkeeping method used in physicians' offices for decades. Although most offices have computerized their medical practices, it is felt by many educators that learning the pegboard system makes the student aware of how all parts are related and gives a good basic foundation for bookkeeping. The principles of the pegboard system can be transferred easily when adapting to a computer system. The pegboard system is accurate, easy to learn, and uses a write-it-once process for recording daily office transactions. It minimizes errors and saves clerical writing time. The system uses a lightweight board with pegs on the left side and often on the top and right side too. Various forms (e.g., transaction slips, cash receipts, ledger, deposit slip) have holes to affix over the pegs, thus aligning them to post a transaction. Using this method, several forms may be layered, one on top of the other, and held in place on the board (Figure 15-1A and B). Usually the layered forms are printed on no-carbon-required (NCR) paper or card stock.

To begin the day's transactions, a new daysheet **(A)** is placed on the pegboard. Then a series of prenumbered, shingled perforated transaction slips, known by many names **(B)** are aligned so the posting line is directly over the first available line on the daysheet near the top. Use of these slips increases cash flow because they are presented to the patient at the time the service is rendered. Each slip acts as a receipt if payment is made, and a portion of the slip can be removed and given to the patient to show the next appointment date. If an error is made on the slip, it is voided and retained. Embezzlement is prevented because the slips are prenumbered and must be accounted for at the end of each day. This is called

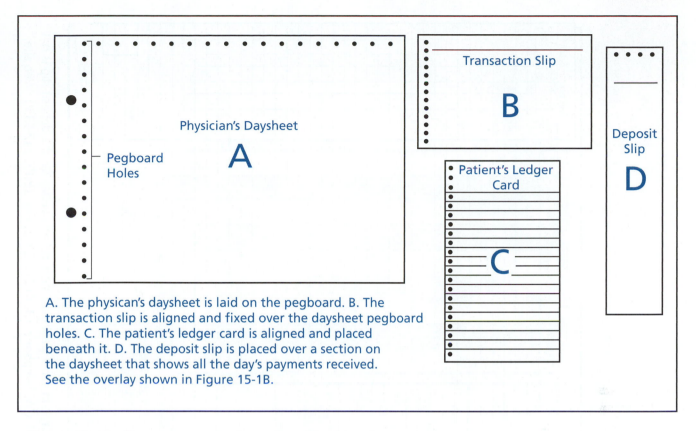

A. The physican's daysheet is laid on the pegboard. B. The transaction slip is aligned and fixed over the daysheet pegboard holes. C. The patient's ledger card is aligned and placed beneath it. D. The deposit slip is placed over a section on the daysheet that shows all the day's payments received. See the overlay shown in Figure 15-1B.

Figure 15-1A. Component parts of a pegboard bookkeeping system

an audit control. An example of a multipurpose billing form is shown in Chapter 13, Figure 13-3.

As each patient arrives, his or her ledger card, also referred to as an **account** (C), is slipped between the daysheet and the transaction slip. When an entry is written, it registers simultaneously on all three items—the daysheet, the patient's ledger card, and the transaction slip, thus decreasing posting errors. This slip acts as a charge slip, receipt for cash or check, statement of account showing prior and new balances, and an appointment reminder. The transaction slip acts as a billing statement and can be used to obtain insurance information for input into a computerized system or to file insurance claims in some states. After each patient has left the office, the ledger card is removed and the next patient's card is inserted.

All monies (cash and checks) are totaled and recorded on a bank deposit slip **(D)** at the same time that they are recorded on the daysheet, using overlapping forms in the same manner. A cash control log is usually included, which tracks beginning cash on hand, total daily receipts, cash paid out, bank deposit,

and closing cash on hand. Figure 15-2 is a visual presentation of the pegboard bookkeeping tasks performed by the administrative medical assistant.

At the end of the day, the journal sheet is balanced using a proof of posting area so if an error has been made it can be corrected the same day; this reduces the chance of an error being discovered at the end of the month. Daily totals are then added to the previous day's totals, providing month-to-date figures. An accounts receivable control and proof of accounts receivable are performed to ensure that the books are balanced.

Computerized Accounting

Computerized accounting is a method adopted by medical practices to expedite posting, reduce paper, increase accurate accounting, and incorporate electronic billing capabilities. Computer software and hardware are now affordable for both large and small offices. The computer automatically adds all credits, subtracts all debits, and computes a running balance. It also generates data that calculate overhead costs and

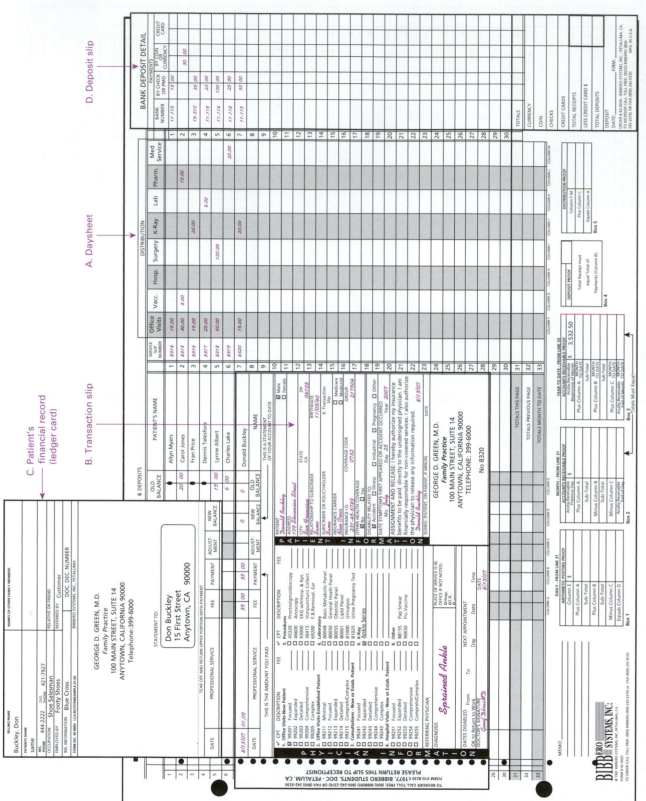

Figure 15-1B. Pegboard bookkeeping system complete with overlays. In some pegboard systems, an overlay for the deposit slip is not used. (Reprinted with permission of Bibbero Systems, Inc., Petaluma, CA. Telephone: (800) 242-2376; Fax: (800) 242-9330; Web site: http://www.bibbero.com.)

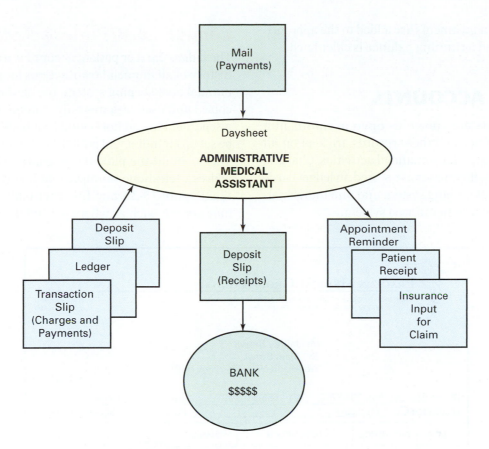

Control of Cash/Check Receipts in the Medical Office

1. Prepare daysheet.
2. Align transaction slip over daysheet.
3. Slip patient ledger card between transaction slip and daysheet.
4. Enter name and post daily charge.
5. Post cash/check payments.
6. Calculate account balance.
7. Stamp checks with restrictive endorsement.
8. Give patient transaction slip copy (receipt and appointment reminder).
9. Give insurance biller transaction slip copies to submit insurance claims.
10. Total cash/checks on daysheet and compare balances.
11. Prepare deposit slip.
12. Take deposit to bank.

Figure 15-2. Control of cash and check receipts in the medical office, showing the routing of components of the pegboard bookkeeping system

compare monthly billings, payments from insurance carriers, percentage of adjustments (amount written off), and percentage of accounts receivable assigned to each insurance carrier. The computer replaces all manual systems, such as pegboard bookkeeping, and has the capability of generating hard copies (paper printouts) of financial data. Basic computerized accounting elements are discussed in Chapter 18.

From Manual Accounting to Computerized Accounting—To understand how the components of a manual bookkeeping system compare to a computerized system is an easy transition. Instead of having to post on a separate account (ledger), daysheet (daily journal), cash receipt, and deposit slip, or having to layer each on a pegboard so they are posted simultaneously, you post charges and payments on each computerized patient account. As this is done, data is entered into the computer database and it becomes available (automatically posted) on the daily journal, cash receipt, and deposit slip as well as the patient's statement, accounts receivable, and various report forms. Calculations are automatically made so all charges, payments, and adjustments are added to the appropriate columns and a running balance is calculated.

PATIENT ACCOUNTS

Patient accounts are known as **open accounts** in a physician's practice and these records are kept on all individual patients' daily financial activities. Charges, payments, and adjustments are posted on ledger cards in a manual bookkeeping system and into individualized accounts in a computerized system.

Ledger Card/Patient Account

The **ledger card** or patient account is a chronological history of all financial transactions for a patient. In a manual bookkeeping system, the card may be photocopied and used as a monthly statement. It is kept in a separate file and not bound in a book. Ledgers may be set up for individual patients or for an entire family. They contain the patient's or guarantor's full name, address, telephone number, and insurance information (Figure 15-3A and B). Other billing information may appear, such as where to send the statement if it

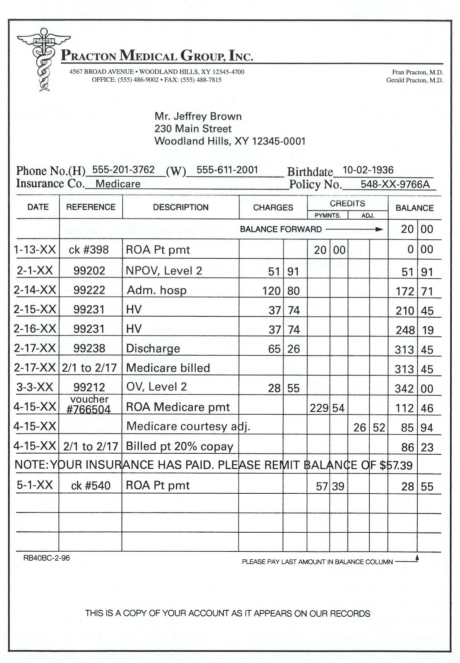

PRACTON MEDICAL GROUP, INC.

4567 BROAD AVENUE • WOODLAND HILLS, XY 12345-4700
OFFICE: (555) 486-9002 • FAX: (555) 488-7815

Fran Practon, M.D.
Gerald Practon, M.D.

Mr. Jeffrey Brown
230 Main Street
Woodland Hills, XY 12345-0001

Phone No.(H) 555-201-3762 (W) 555-611-2001 Birthdate 10-02-1936
Insurance Co. Medicare Policy No. 548-XX-9766A

DATE	REFERENCE	DESCRIPTION	CHARGES	CREDITS PYMNTS.	CREDITS ADJ.	BALANCE
		BALANCE FORWARD ⟶				20 00
1-13-XX	ck #398	ROA Pt pmt		20 00		0 00
2-1-XX	99202	NPOV, Level 2	51 91			51 91
2-14-XX	99222	Adm. hosp	120 80			172 71
2-15-XX	99231	HV	37 74			210 45
2-16-XX	99231	HV	37 74			248 19
2-17-XX	99238	Discharge	65 26			313 45
2-17-XX	2/1 to 2/17	Medicare billed				313 45
3-3-XX	99212	OV, Level 2	28 55			342 00
4-15-XX	voucher #766504	ROA Medicare pmt		229 54		112 46
4-15-XX		Medicare courtesy adj.			26 52	85 94
4-15-XX	2/1 to 2/17	Billed pt 20% copay				86 23
NOTE: YOUR INSURANCE HAS PAID. PLEASE REMIT BALANCE OF $57.39						
5-1-XX	ck #540	ROA Pt pmt		57 39		28 55

RB40BC-2-96

PLEASE PAY LAST AMOUNT IN BALANCE COLUMN ⟶

THIS IS A COPY OF YOUR ACCOUNT AS IT APPEARS ON OUR RECORDS

Figure 15-3A. Ledger card illustrating how charges, payments, and adjustments should be posted. Ledger cards may become statements, which are given to or sent to patients.

BROWN, JEFFREY

TELEPHONE	SPOUSE NAME	DATE OF BIRTH	SOC. SEC. NO.	DRIVERS LIC. NO.
555-739-0887	FRANCES	5-8-30	548-XX-9766	G0073459

EMPLOYER: CITY - STATE - PHONE	SPOUSE EMPLOYER: CITY - STATE - PHONE
Retired	Self-employed

NAME - ADDRESS - PHONE OF NEAREST RELATIVE	OTHER PROF. SERVICE USED: CITY - STATE - PHONE
Carl and Anne Brown (brother and sister-in-law) 555-257-0961	None

CREDIT/INSURANCE INFORMATION

Medicare

OWN
HOME ☒ RENT ☐

COMMENTS

USE LEAD PENCIL - FELT TIP MARKER - TYPEWRITER

Figure 15-3B. Top, back side of ledger card shown in Figure 15-3A

is not to be sent to the home address. Additional information may be found on the back of the card, as well as dates that document letters sent or telephone calls made to collect on an account.

In a computerized system, separate screens are used to input patient demographics (e.g., name and address), insurance information, and to post charges, payments, and adjustments. The demographic information is usually input at the time of the patient's first appointment and all entries are incorporated into the database. When a patient checks out after a visit, data are entered for professional services and amounts paid into an account screen, which acts as a *patient ledger.* The computer shares information from the database to print statements, receipts, or other financial data. Although the computer screen looks different from the ledger, the columns in which you post are the same, as are all mathematical computations. The computer's calculations will be error free; however, figures can still be input incorrectly, leading to account errors that may be hard to detect. Daily and end-of-month journal calculations are made automatically, saving time and offering more accurate records.

If a ledger becomes full using all lines on the card, it is necessary to bring the balance forward and **extend** the account. To do this, the first entry on the

reverse side or on a new card is called the balance forward amount. See the first posted entry of $20 to the ledger shown in Figure 15-3A.

Since ledger cards concern money they should be kept in a secure place, locked and fireproof. Cards may be divided into active accounts and inactive accounts, with the inactive accounts purged and kept in another location when the patient will not be returning. Color-coded tabs may be used to flag "collection agency accounts," "delinquent accounts," and so forth. The assistant should make it a point to keep every ledger card in its file unless it is set temporarily aside for posting or billing. Ledger cards should never be attached to medical records or correspondence; instead, the assistant can attach a photocopy to prevent ledger loss.

In some cases, two active accounts are needed for the same patient. If, for instance, an established private patient is injured on the job, the account becomes an industrial case, which requires a separate ledger card or account number. A private patient is one who is paying for medical care out of his or her own funds with or without insurance and is not on a state program for the medically needy. Patients who are private one month and on the Medicaid program another month may require two accounts to keep private and state records separate.

Charges

Fees are posted on the date of service, and at the same time, the transaction is recorded on the medical practice's daysheet in a manual system. In a computer system, it is posted to the patient's account and simultaneously recorded in a journal. The ledger or account should always be current and show the balance forward, date of posting, description of services, and charges incurred. Charges would include fees for office visits, surgery, house or hospital calls, laboratory tests and x-rays, medical supplies, and medication. The services are often abbreviated (e.g., office visit = OV, hospital visit = HV) to fit into the description area of the ledger card; they automatically populate the description area of the computerized screen when the procedure code is input (e.g., 99202 = office visit level 2). The level of office visit recorded corresponds with the last digit of the procedure code. For example, a new patient office visit coded 99202 would be recorded as: NP OV, Level 2. The diagnostic code may also be input at this time and later used on the computerized claim form. The account may be called up on the screen at any time if a patient makes an inquiry, or it can be printed as hard copy (Figure 15-4).

Payments

Payments at the time of service or payments received by mail must be recorded daily. Payments are posted on the date received to the patient's ledger card using the abbreviation "ROA," received on account. If the payment is received by the patient, the abbreviation "pt" is used, and if received by an insurance company the name of the company must be recorded. The method of payment is also listed as cash, check (ck), money order, and so forth along with the check number. Checks received from insurance companies are called **vouchers**. All payments are debited (subtracted) from the account balance.

Adjustments

An **adjustment** is made on an account when an amount must be written off the balance, such as when the contracted insurance payment plus the patient responsibility is less than the amount of the charge. The amount over the "allowed amount" is written off the books as a contract adjustment. When a contract adjustment is made it is recorded at the same time as the insurance payment, either balancing the account

COMPLIANCE

A statement on how patients' payments are posted should be written in the office policy manual. If audited, reviewers can examine this document to determine whether the medical assistant has complied. For example, the policy might say that in the absence of instructions from the patient, the payment should be applied to the portion of the balance that has remained on the books the longest. By applying the patient's payment to the oldest amount, the accounts receivables are reduced in the oldest aged categories (e.g., 90 days), which is considered good accounting practice.

to zero or indicating the amount the patient is responsible for. When billing Medicare cases, a "courtesy" adjustment is made after receiving the Medicare payment if the charged amount is over the allowed amount. The word "courtesy" implies that Medicare patients are treated well and is preferred to phrases like "not allowed" or "write off" (Figure 15-3A).

It may also be necessary to record the adjustment of a small amount on an uncollectible debt. Any adjustment to an account other than the known contractual write-off amounts should be authorized by the office manager before being posted (e.g., bad debt write-off, adjustment for an unhappy patient). Document the individual who authorizes the adjustment on the patient's account. Parentheses are used around an adjusting entry figure when it is posted to a charge column if there is no adjustment column.

If a ledger needs an adjustment entry, "adj" is noted; or if a patient is not to be charged, "NC" or "Professional Courtesy" should appear. All financial transactions should be recorded in bookkeeping codes as shown in Table 15-2.

DAYSHEET

In single-entry or pegboard bookkeeping, the **daysheet** is known by various names, such as a daily journal sheet, daily record sheet, or daybook, but all are basically the same (Figure 15-5). The daysheet is a cumulative listing of each patient seen in the office, services rendered, fees charged, payments made, and adjustments calculated on one day, with each patient's current daily balance indicated. As patients receive

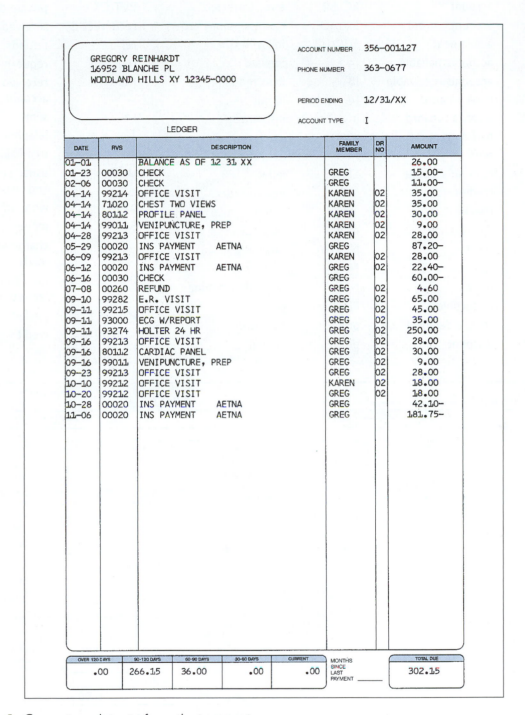

GREGORY REINHARDT
16952 BLANCHE PL
WOODLAND HILLS XY 12345-0000

ACCOUNT NUMBER   356-001127

PHONE NUMBER   363-0677

PERIOD ENDING   12/31/XX

ACCOUNT TYPE   I

LEDGER

DATE	RVS	DESCRIPTION	FAMILY MEMBER	DR NO	AMOUNT
01-01		BALANCE AS OF 12 31 XX			26.00
01-23	00030	CHECK	GREG		15.00-
02-06	00030	CHECK	GREG		11.00-
04-14	99214	OFFICE VISIT	KAREN	02	35.00
04-14	71020	CHEST TWO VIEWS	KAREN	02	35.00
04-14	80112	PROFILE PANEL	KAREN	02	30.00
04-14	99011	VENIPUNCTURE, PREP	KAREN	02	9.00
04-28	99213	OFFICE VISIT	KAREN	02	28.00
05-29	00020	INS PAYMENT AETNA	GREG		87.20-
06-09	99213	OFFICE VISIT	KAREN	02	28.00
06-12	00020	INS PAYMENT AETNA	GREG	02	22.40-
06-16	00030	CHECK	GREG		60.00-
07-08	00260	REFUND	GREG	02	4.60
09-10	99282	E.R. VISIT	GREG	02	65.00
09-11	99215	OFFICE VISIT	GREG	02	45.00
09-11	93000	ECG W/REPORT	GREG	02	35.00
09-11	93274	HOLTER 24 HR	GREG	02	250.00
09-16	99213	OFFICE VISIT	GREG	02	28.00
09-16	80112	CARDIAC PANEL	GREG	02	30.00
09-16	99011	VENIPUNCTURE, PREP	GREG	02	9.00
09-23	99213	OFFICE VISIT	GREG	02	28.00
10-10	99212	OFFICE VISIT	KAREN	02	18.00
10-20	99212	OFFICE VISIT	GREG	02	18.00
10-28	00020	INS PAYMENT AETNA	GREG		42.10-
11-06	00020	INS PAYMENT AETNA	GREG		181.75-

OVER 120 DAYS	90-120 DAYS	60-90 DAYS	30-60 DAYS	CURRENT	MONTHS SINCE LAST PAYMENT _____	TOTAL DUE
.00	266.15	36.00	.00	.00		302.15

Figure 15-4. Computer printout of a patient account

services, the assistant posts the fee to each patient's ledger and to the current daysheet, totaling the charges for each patient's account. Additional information for posting onto the daysheet comes from a number of sources: hospital visits, surgery, home visits, and nursing home visits; laboratory and x-ray fees; and any payments (cash or check) received in person or by mail. It is important for the assistant to check with the physician each morning in the event a hospital emergency call has been made after hours and to collect information on other services provided.

At the end of the day, all charges and receipts or adjustments are totaled along with the total of all previous and current balances. These final figures are recorded on a monthly summary of charges and receipts appearing at the bottom of the daysheet (proof

Table 15-2. Bookkeeping Abbreviations and Definitions

AC or acct	account	EC, ER	error corrected	PVT CK	private check
A/C	account current	Ex MO	express money order	recd, recv'd	received
adj	adjustment	FLW/UP	follow-up	ref	refund
A/P	accounts payable	fwd	forward	req	request
A/R	accounts receivable	IB	itemized bill	ROA	received on account
B/B	bank balance	I/f	in full		
Bal fwd, B/F	balance forward	ins, INS	insurance	snt	sent
BD	bad debt	inv	invoice	T	telephoned
BSY	busy	J/A	joint account	TB	trial balance
c/a, CS	cash on account	LTTR	letter	UCR	usual, customary, and reasonable
cc	credit card	MO	money order		
ck	check	mo	month	w/o	write off
COINS	coinsurance	msg	message	$	money/cash
Cr	credit	NC, N/C	no charge	–	charge already made
CXL	cancel	NF	no funds		
DB	debit	NSF	nonsufficient funds	0	no balance due (zero balance)
DED	deductible	PD	paid		
def	charge deferred	pmt	payment	✔	posted
disc, discnt	discount	pt	patient	<$0.00>	credit

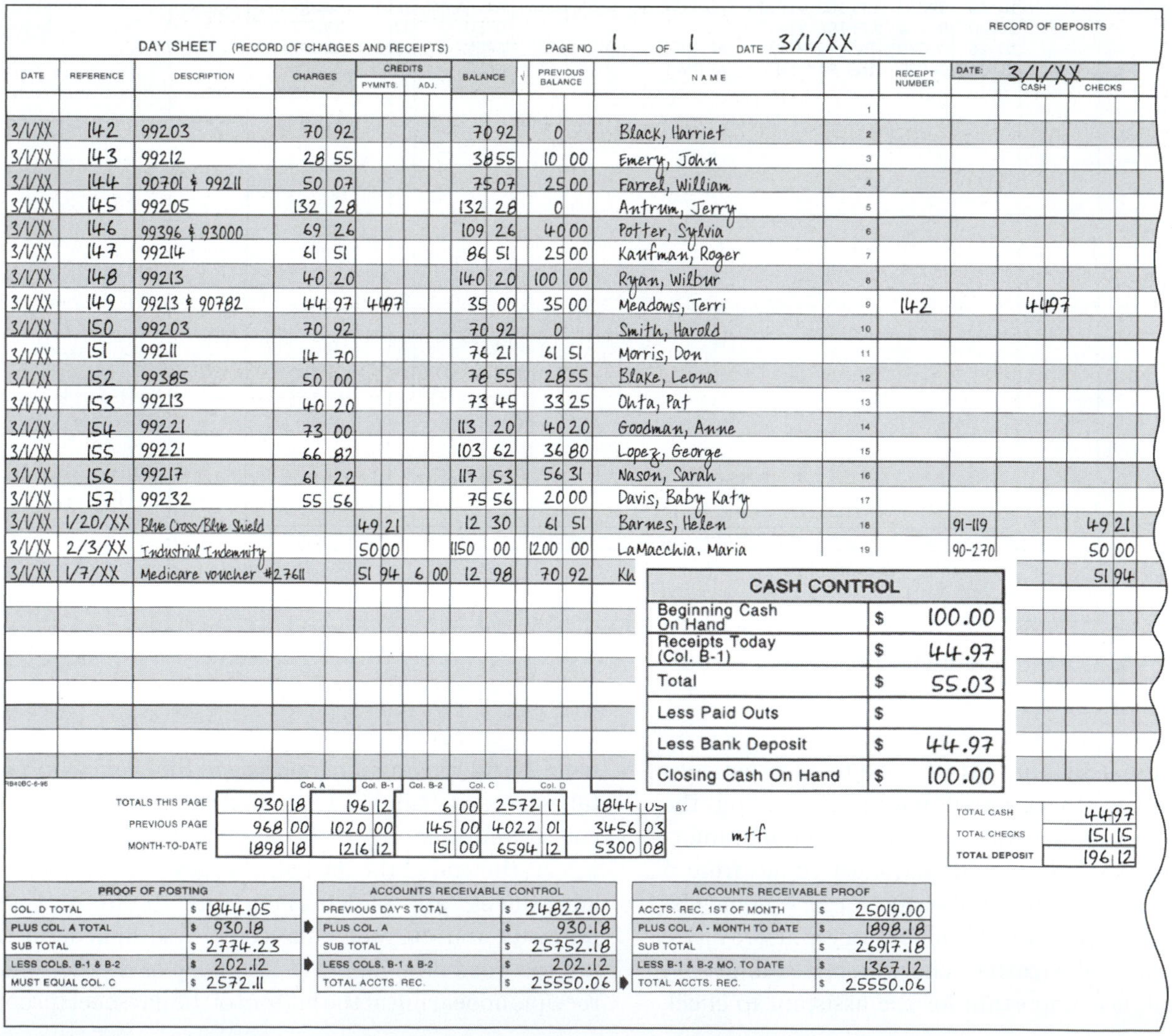

DAY SHEET (RECORD OF CHARGES AND RECEIPTS) PAGE NO 1 OF 1 DATE 3/1/XX

RECORD OF DEPOSITS DATE: 3/1/XX

DATE	REFERENCE	DESCRIPTION	CHARGES	CREDITS PYMNTS.	CREDITS ADJ.	BALANCE	√	PREVIOUS BALANCE	NAME		RECEIPT NUMBER		CASH	CHECKS
										1				
3/1/XX	142	99203	70 92			70 92		0	Black, Harriet	2				
3/1/XX	143	99212	28 55			38 55		10 00	Emery, John	3				
3/1/XX	144	90701 & 99211	50 07			75 07		25 00	Farrel, William	4				
3/1/XX	145	99205	132 28			132 28		0	Antrum, Jerry	5				
3/1/XX	146	99396 & 93000	69 26			109 26		40 00	Potter, Sylvia	6				
3/1/XX	147	99214	61 51			86 51		25 00	Kaufman, Roger	7				
3/1/XX	148	99213	40 20			140 20		100 00	Ryan, Wilbur	8				
3/1/XX	149	99213 & 90782	44 97	44 97		35 00		35 00	Meadows, Terri	9	142		44 97	
3/1/XX	150	99203	70 92			70 92		0	Smith, Harold	10				
3/1/XX	151	99211	14 70			76 21		61 51	Morris, Don	11				
3/1/XX	152	99385	50 00			78 55		28 55	Blake, Leona	12				
3/1/XX	153	99213	40 20			73 45		33 25	Ohta, Pat	13				
3/1/XX	154	99221	73 00			113 20		40 20	Goodman, Anne	14				
3/1/XX	155	99221	66 82			103 62		36 80	Lopez, George	15				
3/1/XX	156	99217	61 22			117 53		56 31	Nason, Sarah	16				
3/1/XX	157	99232	55 56			75 56		20 00	Davis, Baby Katy	17				
3/1/XX	1/20/XX	Blue Cross/Blue Shield		49 21		12 30		61 51	Barnes, Helen	18		91-119		49 21
3/1/XX	2/3/XX	Industrial Indemnity		50 00		1150 00		1200 00	LaMacchia, Maria	19		90-270		50 00
3/1/XX	1/7/XX	Medicare voucher #27611		51 94	6 00	12 98		70 92	Kh					51 94

RB40BC-6-96

	Col. A	Col. B-1	Col. B-2	Col. C	Col. D
TOTALS THIS PAGE	930 18	196 12	6 00	2572 11	1844 05
PREVIOUS PAGE	968 00	1020 00	145 00	4022 01	3456 03
MONTH-TO-DATE	1898 18	1216 12	151 00	6594 12	5300 08

BY mtf

CASH CONTROL	
Beginning Cash On Hand	$ 100.00
Receipts Today (Col. B-1)	$ 44.97
Total	$ 55.03
Less Paid Outs	$
Less Bank Deposit	$ 44.97
Closing Cash On Hand	$ 100.00

TOTAL CASH	44 97
TOTAL CHECKS	151 15
TOTAL DEPOSIT	196 12

PROOF OF POSTING	
COL. D TOTAL	$ 1844.05
PLUS COL. A TOTAL	$ 930.18
SUB TOTAL	$ 2774.23
LESS COLS. B-1 & B-2	$ 202.12
MUST EQUAL COL. C	$ 2572.11

ACCOUNTS RECEIVABLE CONTROL	
PREVIOUS DAY'S TOTAL	$ 24822.00
PLUS COL. A	$ 930.18
SUB TOTAL	$ 25752.18
LESS COLS. B-1 & B-2	$ 202.12
TOTAL ACCTS. REC.	$ 25550.06

ACCOUNTS RECEIVABLE PROOF	
ACCTS. REC. 1ST OF MONTH	$ 25019.00
PLUS COL. A - MONTH TO DATE	$ 1898.18
SUB TOTAL	$ 26917.18
LESS B-1 & B-2 MO. TO DATE	$ 1367.12
TOTAL ACCTS. REC.	$ 25550.06

Figure 15-5. Completed daysheet, a record of charges and receipts

PROCEDURE 15-1

Prepare the Pegboard; Post Charges, Payments, and Adjustments, and Balance the Daysheet

Objective: To post charges, payments, and adjustments to a daysheet; verify that entries are correct and totals balance.

Equipment/Supplies: Pegboard, calculator, pencil, transaction slips, daysheet, receipts, ledger cards, and balances from the previous day.

Directions: Follow these step-by-step procedures, which include rationales, to learn this skill, which is presented in the *Workbook* (Job Skill 15-2, 15-3, 15-4, and 15-5) for practice.

Prepare the Pegboard

1. Prepare the pegboard by placing a daysheet on the pegs of the board.

2. Fill in the information at the top of the daysheet (current date and page number).

3. Carry all balances forward from the "Accounts Receivable Control" and "Accounts Receivable Proof" sections of the previous daysheet and enter the figures into the correct previous page Columns A–D. List "Previous Day's Total" and "Accounts Receivable 1st of Month" under the correct headings at the bottom of the daysheet.

4. Pull ledger cards for patients scheduled to be seen in the office, placing them in the order that each will arrive for his or her appointment.

5. Place transaction slips over the pegs. Be careful to align the posting line on the top slip with the first writing line on the daysheet.

Post Charges and Payments to the Daily Journal (Daysheet)

6. Place the first patient's ledger card under the first transaction slip; align it to the first writing line so correct posting entry occurs on the transaction slip and transfers to the ledger and daysheet.

7. Enter the patient's name (last name first), date, and transaction slip number.

8. Remove the transaction slip from the pegboard and clip it to the front of the patient's

medical record to be given to the medical assistant or physician when the patient is called into the back office. The physician will indicate the procedure and diagnostic codes for the service performed on the transaction slip and hand it to the patient to give to the medical assistant for final processing. Future appointments and other information may also be included.

9. Before the transaction slip is replaced on the pegboard, enter the appropriate fee from the fee schedule next to each procedure; calculate and write the total on the front of the transaction slip.

10. Replace and carefully realign the transaction slip on the pegboard, matching the transaction slip number, and insert the patient's ledger card under the last page of the transaction slip.

11. Post fees in the charge column, payment and adjustments in the credit column, old balance from the ledger card, and new balance from the transaction slip. All entries will automatically post to the patient's ledger and daysheet underneath. When posting a *payment only*, the following information is entered on the transaction slip: date, reference (date of service), description (who payment is from and check or voucher number), payment amount, and previous and new balance. The new balance is calculated by subtracting the payment amount from the previous balance.

12. Record all payments on the "Record of Deposits" slip in the correct column (cash or check). List the receipt number for cash payments and the ABA number for all checks.

13. Give the patient the completed transaction slip as a receipt.

14. Refile the patient's ledger card.

15. Repeat steps 6 through 14 as each patient concludes his or her appointment.

(continues)

PROCEDURE 15-1 *continued*

Balance the Daysheet

16. Total Columns A, B, C, and D of the daysheet at the end of the day in pencil. Use a calculator with paper strip and keep the printout.

17. Complete "Proof of Posting" for all totals by entering all figures from the "Totals This Page" column boxes to that section of the worksheet. Follow the directions of addition and subtraction to obtain subtotals and totals.

EXAMPLE 15-2

Proof of Posting

PROOF OF POSTING	
COL B TOTAL	$ 1844.05
PLUS COL A TOTAL	$ 930.18
SUB TOTAL	$ 2774.23
LESS COLS B 1 & B 2	$ 202.12
MUST EQUAL COL C	$ 2572.11

Balance the Month-to-Date Sections of the Daysheet

18. Note the previous day's total of the "Accounts Receivable Control." This amount does not change during a calendar month because it shows the A/R balance from the first day of the month.

EXAMPLE 15-3

Accounts Receivable Control

ACCOUNTS RECEIVABLE CONTROL	
PREVIOUS DAY'S TOTAL	$ 24822.00
PLUS COL A	$ 930.18
SUB TOTAL	$ 25752.18
LESS COLS B 1 & B 2	$ 202.12
TOTAL ACCTS REC	$ 25550.06

19. In the "Accounts Receivable Proof" section, enter other figures from the "Month-to-Date" column boxes. Then add, subtract, subtotal, and total as directed. If posted amounts, additions, and subtractions are correct, the "Total Accounts Receivable" figures in the "A/R Control" and "A/R Proof" boxes will match, indicating the daily journal (daysheet) is balanced.

EXAMPLE 15-4

Accounts Receivable Proof

ACCOUNTS RECEIVABLE PROOF	
ACCTS REC 1ST OF MONTH	$ 25019.00
PLUS COL A MONTH TO DATE	$ 1898.18
SUB TOTAL	$ 26917.18
LESS B 1 & B 2 MO TO DATE	$ 1367.12
TOTAL ACCTS REC	$ 25550.06

20. Verify the deposit section of the daysheet by totaling the cash column and the checks column. Enter the sum of both columns in the space marked "Total Deposit."

21. Verify that the "Total Deposit" amount and the total payments received in Column B-1 match.

Cash Control

22. Count and enter the amount of beginning cash on hand in the "Cash Control" section. List cash payments (receipts today) from Column B-1. Enter the subtotal and then subtract any amounts paid out and the amount of the bank deposit.

23. Total the "Closing Cash on Hand." Remember, the closing cash on hand should match the amount of beginning cash on hand.

EXAMPLE 15-5

Cash Control

CASH CONTROL	
Beginning Cash On Hand	$ 100.00
Receipts Today (Col B 1)	$ 44.97
Total	$ 144.97
Less Paid Outs	$
Less Bank Deposit	$ 44.97
Closing Cash On Hand	$ 100.00

After the Daily Journal (Daysheet) Is Balanced

24. Begin with Step 1 and transfer balances to a new daysheet for the following day.

of posting). Previous day totals are added to these figures to give month-to-date totals for each item. It is important for the assistant to check to see that the total of each day's cash and check receipts equals the day's total bank deposit.

ACCOUNTS RECEIVABLE CONTROL

Statements are sent every month to patients who have outstanding balances on their accounts. To ensure the balance of all outstanding accounts equals the total monies owed, it is important to have an accounts receivable control for verification of the records. To accomplish this, the medical assistant would:

1. Total the balances of all patient account records (ledgers) that indicate a balance due.

2. Compare that total with the ending total A/R figure on the daysheet (general ledger). If these two figures do not agree, there is an error in calculation or a ledger may be missing. The error must be found and corrected.

Computerized Reports

A variety of reports that provide a summary of the information stored in the database can be produced by a computerized system. A daysheet can be printed and used to balance the bank deposit, patient ledgers can be printed to verify activity on individual accounts, and other reports can be produced to track the money flow in and out of the office. At the end of the day, print the daysheet and crosscheck the day's transaction forms against the charges, payments, and adjustments to verify that all entries have been made correctly.

Locating Errors

To search for an error in posting, the assistant would look for a figure that was missed, a miskeyed number, or a transposition in figures; for example, a check for $830 may have been posted as $803. An amount divisible by nine may indicate a transposed number. Errors also occur when amounts are placed in wrong columns; for example, a credit in the debit column or vice versa. An amount divisible by two may indicate posting in the wrong column. Another type of error occurs from sliding a number; that is, writing 500 for 50 or writing 80 for 800. To minimize this possibility when posting, the assistant can eliminate writing zeros if there are no cents; for example, write $15— rather than $15.00.

CASH FUNDS

A medical practice has various needs for dispensing **cash** (currency and coins) on a daily basis. It is important to have two sources for access to cash and to keep them separate—a change drawer and a petty cash fund.

Change Drawer

Medical practices collecting copayments from patients may need to make change when patients pay by cash. This type of transaction should involve a *change drawer* and a receipt should be issued (Figure 15-6).

DATE	REFERENCE	DESCRIPTION	CHARGES	PYMNTS. CREDITS	ADJ.	BALANCE	PREVIOUS BALANCE	NAME
3-1-XX	142	99213 & 9078	44 97	44 97		35 00	35 00	Meadows, Terri

This is your RECEIPT for this amount
This is a STATEMENT of your account to date

Please present this slip to receptionist before leaving office.

Practon Medical Group, Inc.
4567 Broad Avenue
Woodland Hills, XY 12345-4700
Tel. 555/486-9002

Thank You!

ROA – Received on Account *Cash*

OT – Other

NEXT APPOINTMENT 4-15-XX   142

RB40BC-3-96

Figure 15-6. Completed receipt for a patient who paid cash on account

Cash/Change Drawer

Drawer contents: $100: five $10 bills, six $5 bills, and twenty $1 bills.

Patient's copayment: $15. The patient gives the receptionist a $20 bill, and the cashier places the $20 in the change drawer and gives the patient $5 in change.

End-of-day-change drawer: If no other cash transactions take place, at the end of the day, the change drawer would add up to $115 ($15 goes to the bank deposit and $100 remains in the drawer).

Cash proof: The day's cash received must match the cash control on the daysheet.

Bank deposit: The individual who does the banking should replenish the small bills from the larger ones in the drawer. It is best to separate the payments into an envelope and keep them apart from the money in the cash drawer. In this scenario, the receptionist would place $15 in an envelope.

The change drawer typically contains from $50 to $200 depending on the size of the practice in small bills at the beginning of each day. At the conclusion of each day after cash payments are received and change is made, the cash received should equal the cash amount on the deposit slip, and the remaining amount in the change drawer should be the same as the beginning amount (see Example 15-6).

When payment is made by the patient, write the word "check" or "cash" next to ROA on the receipt. If a payment is received by mail from the patient's insurer, list the name of the insurance carrier by OT (other).

For good bookkeeping practice, cash is usually handled by one individual. However, if the responsibility for the change drawer is shared by several individuals—more than one receptionist or bookkeeper—each person should reconcile the drawer and the monies received from patients during his or her shift.

Petty Cash

The term *petty* means small or little; hence, the purpose of a **petty cash fund** is to provide cash to make small, unanticipated purchases, such as coffee, small quantities of office supplies, postage-due fees, c.o.d.'s, office refreshments, or an employee's parking expense while on an errand for the physician. Use a petty cash fund only for minor expenses. Major expenses would always be paid by check.

The medical assistant may be responsible for the office petty cash and must account for each disbursement from the fund. Maintaining good cash procedures with firm control of funds is important to prevent cash being used in an unauthorized manner. Balancing, maintaining, and replenishing the cash drawer as well as petty cash fund is accomplished by keeping proper records for all transactions. Employees handling cash receipts should be bonded (see Chapter 3).

Setting Up Petty Cash Fund

Set up the petty cash fund initially with an amount of money large enough to cover small cash payments for two to four weeks—perhaps $100. A check is written payable to "Cash" or "Petty Cash," endorsed, and cashed. The currency is then placed in a drawer or cash box. When the fund is depleted to a predetermined amount, perhaps $25 or $50, another check is written to replenish it to the original amount of $100. Sometimes a fund is replenished weekly or monthly if there is continuous demand for the funds, regardless of the amount of expenditures. Judgment must be used so as not to allow the fund to become so low that it is entirely depleted before new funds can be obtained. A good rule is to replenish the fund when it goes below 25 percent of its full value. The medical assistant would reconcile the petty cash account and arrange for the fund to be replenished.

Petty Cash Record

A petty cash record of amounts received and expended may be permanently kept in a standard cash book or on a memo sheet with columns for dates, amounts received and expended, and an explanation of expenditures (Figure 15-7). An additional column could show a cumulative balance so that the amount in the fund is always known without having to total the list of expenditures. Additional columns would be of

PETTY CASH RECEIPT ENVELOPE

From _Sept 1_ **20XX To** _Sept 30_ **20XX** Paid by Check No. _100_

Entered	Audited	Approved	Paid

Date	No.	Paid to:	Item	Account	Amount	
9/1	45	ABC Drug Store	1 box rubber bands	ofc. supp	1	56
9/4	46	US Postal Service	stamps	postage	3	32
9/16	47	Bank Parking Downtown	parking 1 hour	misc	1	50
9/20	48	ABC Drug Store	3 boxes tissue	med supp	2	51
9/29	49	US Postal Service	50 stamps	postage	19	50
					28	39

Office Fund Amount $ _100.00_ **Receipts Paid** $ _28.39_
Total Receipts and Cash $ _100.00_ **Cash on Hand** $ _71.61_
(Over or Short) $ _0_ **TOTAL** $ _100.00_

DISTRIBUTION OF PETTY CASH

Ofc. Supp	Postage	Med. Supp	Misc.							Totals
1 56	3 32	2 51	1 50							
	19 50									
1 56	22 82	2 51	1 50							28.39

Figure 15-7. Completed monthly petty cash record printed on a small manila envelope

PROCEDURE 15-2

STEP 1 2 3

Establish, Record, Balance, and Replenish Petty Cash Fund

Objective: To establish, maintain a record of expenditures for, balance, and replenish a petty cash fund.

Equipment/Supplies: Calculator, petty cash record form, receipts (vouchers) for expenditures, check record (disbursement journal), checks, list of expenditures, and petty cash box.

Directions: Follow these step-by-step procedures, which include rationales, to learn this skill, which is presented in the *Workbook* (Job Skill 15-2, 15-3, and 15-4) for practice.

1. Determine the amount needed in the petty cash fund.

2. Write a check to "Petty Cash" in the amount determined to establish the fund.

3. Cash the check and put the money in the petty cash box.

4. Enter the beginning and ending dates on the petty cash record form.

5. Post the beginning balance (office fund amount) on the petty cash record form to indicate the original amount in the fund.

6. Post the amount of each petty cash receipt on the petty cash record form, listing the date, receipt number, to whom paid, item purchased, name of account, and amount.

7. Label the headings at the bottom of the petty cash record form and post the expenditure under the appropriate heading.

8. Add the "Amount" column and enter the total for "Receipts Paid."

9. Total all columns listed under the "Distribution of Petty Cash" on the petty cash record form.

10. Count the cash available and enter the amount in "Cash on Hand."

11. Add the "Receipts Paid" plus the "Cash on Hand" and list the "Total." This total should equal the amount established for the fund.

12. Enter the "Total of Receipts and Cash" (on hand) and subtract it from the original "Office Fund Amount" to determine if there is an overage or shortage.

13. Prepare a check made out to "Cash," "Petty Cash," or to the name of the bank cashing the check for the shortage amount. Write a check only for the amount that was used to bring it back to the original petty cash amount. Insert the check number on the petty cash record form.

14. Cash the check and add the money to the petty cash box.

value for categorizing expenditures for each petty cash account showing totals (see the bottom of Figure 15-7).

A large manila envelope containing the cash, vouchers, receipts, and receipted bills should be kept in a locked box, desk, or file, preferably fireproof. The envelope should contain petty cash transactions for a definite period. Borrowing from the petty cash fund should *not* be permitted. If the physician requests cash from the fund, a personal check or petty cash voucher should be written in exchange for the cash.

STOP AND THINK CASE SCENARIO

Determine a Bookkeeping System

Scenario: The physician is establishing a new medical practice and consults you regarding what type of bookkeeping system to use.

Critical Thinking: State what questions you would ask to obtain necessary information to make this decision. Name the advantages and disadvantages of each bookkeeping system:

Questions to ask:

_____

_____

_____

_____

_____

1. Single Entry System:

_____

_____

_____

_____

2. Double-Entry System:

_____

_____

_____

_____

3. Pegboard System:

_____

_____

_____

_____

4. Computerized System:

_____

_____

_____

_____

STOP AND THINK CASE SCENARIO

Obtain Change for a Patient

Scenario: You are the receptionist working at the front desk and have had to make change several times today. Your change drawer is depleted to one $10 bill and some coins. The deposit envelope has $200 cash. The petty cash drawer has been replenished and has three $20 bills, three $10 bills, and two $5 bills. A patient comes to the front desk to pay for the services he has received. The charge is $75 and he hands you a $100 bill; you cannot make change from the change drawer.

Critical Thinking: What would you do? Consider the suggestions listed and comment on each choice stating which action you would take and why.

1. Make change from the deposit if possible.

_____

_____

_____

_____

_____

2. Make change from the petty cash drawer and write an invoice indicating what you have done.

_____

_____

_____

_____

_____

3. Ask coworkers in the office if anyone has $25 or change for $100.

_____

_____

_____

_____

_____

4. Ask the patient to make a quick trip to the bank or go next door to the pharmacy to obtain change and then return.

_____

_____

_____

_____

_____

FOCUS ON CERTIFICATION*

CMA Content Summary

- Medical abbreviations
- Calculator
- Bookkeeping systems
- Demographic data
- Daysheets, charge slips, receipts, ledgers
- Financial transactions—charges, payments, and adjustments
- Identify and correct errors
- Petty cash
- Accounts receivable
- Write checks

RMA Content Summary

- Medical terminology and abbreviations
- Bookkeeping terminology
- Accounting procedures
- Balancing procedures

- Accounts receivable and payable
- Post charges, payments, adjustments
- Petty cash
- Bank deposits
- Patient account calculations

CMAS Content Summary

- Spell medical terms
- Basic accounting principles
- Bookkeeping procedures
- Financial computations
- Accounts receivable/payable
- Monthly trial balance
- Audit controls
- Patient accounts/ledgers
- Petty cash
- Software applications

REVIEW EXAM-STYLE QUESTIONS

1. Manual bookkeeping skills are:
   a. not needed since all physician's offices are computerized
   b. outdated and no longer apply
   c. helpful because they increase understanding of the basic computations a computerized system automatically does
   d. not related in any way to how debits and credits are recorded in a computerized system
   e. never used in the new millennium

2. Which bookkeeping system requires the transfer of information onto journals and ledgers?
   a. single-entry accounting
   b. double-entry accounting
   c. triple-entry accounting
   d. pegboard accounting
   e. computerized accounting

*This textbook and the accompanying Workbook meet the entry-level administrative and general competencies for the CMA outlined by the AAMA Examination Content Outline and Role Delineation Study and for the RMA and CMAS outlined by the AMT Competencies and Examination Specifications (see Competency Grid in Appendix B).

3. Monies that are owed to a medical practice are called:

   a. assets

   b. capital

   c. liabilities

   d. proprietorship

   e. equity

4. In a physician's practice, patient accounts are known as:

   a. restricted accounts

   b. open accounts

   c. closed accounts

   d. inactive accounts

   e. public accounts

5. A record that contains a cumulative listing of each patient seen in the office, services rendered, fees charged, payments made, and adjustments calculated on one day is called a/an:

   a. ledger or account

   b. accounts payable log

   c. accounts receivable log

   d. daysheet or daily journal

   e. check register

6. Select the correct statement regarding debits, credits, posting, and calculations on a ledger card.

   a. Credits are added and debits are subtracted from the account balance.

   b. Fees are posted in the credit column; payments and adjustments are posted in the charge column.

   c. Fees are posted in the charge column; payments and adjustments are posted in the credit column.

   d. Credits are fees charged by the physician.

   e. Debits are payments made by patients for services rendered.

7. To locate a transposition error, you would:

   a. divide the amount by 2

   b. divide the amount by 3

   c. divide the amount by 9

   d. look for an extra or missing zero

   e. round all numbers to the highest dollar amount

8. Totaling the balances of all patient accounts that indicate a balance due and comparing that total with the ending total A/R figure on the daysheet is referred to as:

   a. double-entry bookkeeping

   b. aging accounts

   c. ledger card balancing

   d. accounts receivable control

   e. end-of-month carry-over procedures

9. Monies kept in a physician's office for the purpose of making small cash purchases is called:

   a. a petty cash fund

   b. a change drawer

   c. a bank deposit

   d. patient payments

   e. payables

10. A petty cash fund would typically have:

   a. $50

   b. $75

   c. $100 to $200

   d. $50 to $200

   e. $500

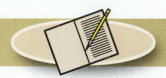

WORKBOOK ASSIGNMENT

To develop competency-based job skills, refer to the *Workbook* and complete the:

- Abbreviation and Spelling Review
- Review Questions

- Critical Thinking Exercises
- Job Skill activities, which are outlined at the beginning of this chapter under "Performance Objectives in the *Workbook*."

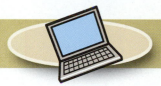

COMPUTER ASSIGNMENT

To review the concepts you have learned in this chapter, insert the *Student Practice* CD-ROM into a computer and work through the *StudyWARE* activities and games. Answer review questions in the practice mode and read the feedback, studying the questions you have missed. Take the chapter quiz until you achieve a minimum score of 90 percent. Successfully completing the *Critical Thinking Challenge* at the end of this course will help you think through scenarios and develop problem solving skills.

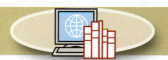

RESOURCES

Organizations

The American Institute of Professional Bookkeepers (AIPB)
Offers preparatory courses and certification for professional bookkeepers
6001 Montrose Road, Suite 207
Rockville, MD 20852
(800) 622-0121
Web site: http://www.aipb.com

CHAPTER 16

Health Insurance Systems

OBJECTIVES

After reading this chapter and learning step-by-step procedures to gain job skills,* you should be able to:

Learning Objectives

- Define frequently used insurance terms and abbreviations.
- Identify third-party payers and types of insurance.
- Explain methods of payment.
- Understand insurance plans and list various programs.
- Define precertification, predetermination, and preauthorization.
- Contrast and compare types of managed care organizations.
- Describe Medicare Parts A, B, C, and D.
- Indicate the three types of TRICARE coverage.
- Discuss different types of workers' compensation disability coverage.
- Code professional services and procedures using *CPT* and *HCPCS II.*
- Code diagnoses using *ICD-9-CM.*
- Complete health insurance claim forms.
- Trace unpaid insurance claims.

Performance Objectives (Procedures) in This Textbook

- Select correct procedure codes (Procedure 16-1).
- Select correct diagnostic codes (Procedure 16-2).
- Complete the Health Insurance Claim Form CMS-1500 using OCR guidelines (Procedure 16-3).

This textbook and the accompanying Workbook meet the educational components for entry-level administrative and general competencies outlined by CAAHEP and ABHES.

Performance Objectives (Job Skills) in the *Workbook*

▪ Review *Current Procedural Terminology* codebook sections (Job Skill 16-1).

▪ Code evaluation and management services (Job Skill 16-2).

▪ Code surgical services and procedures (Job Skill 16-3).

▪ Code radiology and laboratory services and procedures (Job Skill 16-4).

▪ Code procedures and services in the Medicine section (Job Skill 16-5).

▪ Code clinical examples (Job Skill 16-6).

▪ Code diagnoses from Chapters 1, 2, 3, 4, and 5 in *ICD-9-CM* (Job Skill 16-7).

▪ Code diagnoses from Chapters 6, 7, 8, 9, and 10 in *ICD-9-CM* (Job Skill 16-8).

▪ Code diagnoses from Chapters 11, 12, 13, 14, and 15 in *ICD-9-CM* (Job Skill 16-9).

▪ Code diagnoses from Chapters 16 and 17 and Supplemental Classification V and E codes in *ICD-9-CM* (Job Skill 16-10).

▪ Complete a managed care authorization form (Job Skill 16-11).

▪ Complete a health insurance claim form for a commercial case (Job Skill 16-12).

▪ Complete a health insurance claim form for a Medicare case (Job Skill 16-13).

▪ Complete a health insurance claim form for a TRICARE case (Job Skill 16-14).

OUTLINE WITH LECTURE NOTES

Introduction to Insurance

_____

_____

_____

_____

Third-Party Payers
Types of Insurance

_____

_____

_____

Insurance Benefits

_____

_____

_____

_____

The Insurance Policy

_____

_____

_____

_____

Methods of Payment

_____

_____

_____

Physician's Fee Profile

_____

_____

_____

Insurance Plans and Programs

Managed Care Plans

_____
_____
_____
_____

Medicaid

_____
_____
_____
_____

Medicare

_____
_____
_____
_____

TRICARE

_____
_____
_____
_____

CHAMPVA

_____
_____
_____
_____

State Disability Insurance

_____
_____
_____
_____

Workers' Compensation

_____
_____
_____
_____

General Guidelines for Handling Insurance Claims

Insurance Identification Card

_____
_____
_____
_____

Patient Registration Form

_____
_____
_____
_____

Assignments and Consent/Authorization

_____
_____
_____
_____

Completing the Claim

_____
_____
_____
_____

Posting to the Account

_____
_____
_____
_____

Provider Identification Numbers

_____
_____
_____
_____

Claims Submission

_____
_____
_____
_____

Coding for Professional Services

CPT Codebook

_____
_____
_____
_____

HCPCS Level II Codebook

_____
_____
_____
_____

RVS Codebook

_____
_____
_____

Terminology

_____
_____
_____

Codebook Sections

_____
_____
_____

Code Modifiers

_____
_____

Codebook Appendices

_____
_____
_____
_____

Unlisted Procedures

_____
_____
_____

Diagnostic Coding
Terminology

_____
_____
_____

Volumes I and II

_____
_____
_____

V Codes

_____
_____
_____

E Codes

_____
_____
_____

ICD-10-CM

_____
_____
_____

**Health Insurance
Claim Form CMS-1500**

_____
_____
_____

Tracing Insurance Claims
Appeals

_____
_____
_____

KEY TERMS

adjudicate
adjuster
assignment

capitation
claim
clearinghouse

(continues)

coinsurance
consent form
conversion privilege
coordination of benefits (COB)
copayment (copay)
deductible (deduc)
dependents
elimination period
exclusions
explanation of benefits (EOB)
fee-for-service
fiscal intermediary
grace period
health maintenance organization (HMO)
independent practice association (IPA)
insurance agent
insurance application
insured
limitations
major medical
Medicare Summary Notice (MSN)
National Provider Identifier (NPI)

nonparticipating physician (nonpar)
partial disability
participating physician (par)
permanent disability (PD)
physician's profile
point-of-service (POS) plan
preauthorization
precertification
predetermination
preexisting condition
preferred provider organization (PPO)
premium
provider
Remittance Advice (RA)
temporary disability (TD)
third-party payer
time limit
total disability
usual, customary, and reasonable (UCR)
waiting period (w/p)
waiver

HEART OF THE HEALTH CARE PROFESSIONAL

Service

Follow managed care guidelines to quickly obtain preauthorization so patients' health care is not delayed. Accurately complete and promptly submit insurance claim forms so timely reimbursement is received. By taking care of insurance requests or problems in an efficient and expedient manner, you will serve both the physician and the patient.

INTRODUCTION TO INSURANCE

With nearly 46 million Americans uninsured, medical costs continuing to escalate, and some of the largest employers in the United States cutting back on insurance benefits, it is important for the medical assistant to understand insurance plans and programs, accurately code procedures and diagnoses, and process insurance claim forms to gain maximum reimbursement for the physician and patient. The insurance **claim** is the tool used to request insurance payment under an insurance contract, and this process has developed into one of the most sophisticated and complex tasks an administrative medical assistant performs. In response to this health insurance crisis, two states, Massachusetts and Vermont, have enacted laws intended to create near-universal health coverage for their residents starting in 2007. No doubt we will continue to see drastic changes in the insurance world. Search "Center for Studying Health Insurance Change" via the Internet for updated information.

A thorough knowledge of all types of insurance and the ability to handle patients' insurance claims competently will not only increase the income and cash flow for the physician's practice but also enhance the medical assistant's position in a medical office.

As previously mentioned, some medical assistants specialize and become insurance claims and coding specialists. For further information about the organizations that have certification programs for this fast growing field, refer to the Resources at the end of Chapter 19.

In general, private health insurance and managed care claims follow similar patterns, with variations; therefore, this chapter will cover what the assistant needs to know: (1) the basic format and input requirements for claims processed manually and electronically, (2) the **time limits** involved when submitting claims to various programs, (3) the **deductibles (deduc)**, **coinsurance**, or **copayment (copay)** requirements for each program, and (4) insurance terminology.

In many practices, computer systems assist in insurance claims processing. The medical assistant usually is not expected to interpret fine points in health insurance policies and managed care plans. If questions arise, patients may be instructed to contact their insurance representative.

THIRD-PARTY PAYERS

The phrase **third-party payers** comes from the fact that three entities are involved in health care reimbursement:

1. patient—one who receives medical care

2. **provider**—physician or supplier who provides medical care and supplies

3. public or private payer—who bears the costs of medical services, such as the insurance company, government program, self-insured employer, or managed care plan

In other words, third-party payers are private insurance companies and insurance programs that pay personal liability claims, workers' compensation claims, and claims for patients seen under the government programs known as Medicaid, Medicare, TRICARE, and CHAMPVA.

America's Health Insurance Plans (AHIP) is a national association that represents health insurers on federal and state regulatory issues. Members offer insurance coverage for medical expenses, disability income, long-term care, and dental plans, as well as supplemental, stop-loss, and reinsurance to employers and other consumers. They provide informational services such as publications and online services and inform the public and policy makers about health care financing and delivery.

Types of Insurance

Health insurance may be purchased by a person under a group plan called a *group contract*, or a person may be insured under a private contract and pay the premium on an individual basis. A person can be included in a prepaid managed care health plan, such as a health maintenance organization (HMO), or may be a beneficiary under state or federal government programs.

Commercial Insurance

Commercial insurance plans are owned and run by private companies. Private plans consist of traditional indemnity benefit plans, self-insured plans, and managed care plans. Some examples are Aetna Casualty, Allstate, BlueCross/Blue Shield, Farmers Insurance, Medico, Prudential Insurance Company, United American, and so on.

Indemnity Insurance

Traditional *indemnity insurance* is protection against injury or loss of health and pays only when an individual is ill or injured. These individual or group plans may offer preventive care or share risk with providers or employers as optional benefits. Traditional indemnity and self-insured plans are moving toward structuring more managed care in their policies.

Group Insurance

Most group insurance is obtained through an employer. However, a patient may be eligible to obtain group insurance through an association or club to which he or she belongs (e.g., Lions Club, American Association for Retired Persons). If an individual under group coverage leaves the employer or organization or the group contract is terminated, the insured may continue the same or lesser coverage under an individual policy if the group contract has a **conversion privilege**.

Self-Insurance

Self-insurance is an arrangement in which an employer or other group, such as a labor union, assumes risk and pays for health care expenses usually covered by insurance. This is also known as *self-funding*. Some examples are the Procter and Gamble Company and the Teamsters Union. Self-insured employer groups are regulated by the federal government under the Employee Retirement Income Security Act of 1974 (ERISA). This act protects the interests of workers and their beneficiaries who participate in private pension and welfare plans and also allows an employee not covered by a pension plan other than Social Security to put money aside on a tax-deferred basis. Self-insured employers usually contract with an administrator who processes the claims.

Insurance Benefits

Basic health insurance coverage includes benefits for hospital, surgical, and other medical expenses. **Major medical** or *extended benefits* policies are created to help with compensation when an individual encounters large medical expenses caused by long illness or serious injury.

The Insurance Policy

The **insured** is the individual who contracts for a policy of insurance coverage; the insured is also known as a *member, policyholder, subscriber,* or *recipient* and may or may not be the patient seen for the medical service.

To obtain an insurance policy, the individual contacts an **insurance agent** who represents the insurance company and helps the candidate complete an **insurance application**. The *insurance carrier* is an organization that offers protection against losses in exchange for a premium. The application is a signed statement of facts used to determine whether to insure the individual. It becomes part of the health insurance contract if a policy is issued. Before a policy is written, the insurance company may ask the applicant to undergo a physical examination. Information is obtained about the applicant so the company can decide whether to accept the risk.

An insurance policy is a legally enforceable agreement, or contract. If a policy is issued, the applicant becomes part of the insurance contract or plan. Some policies may have a **waiting period (w/p)** (*excepted period* or **elimination period**), which is a time frame after the beginning date of a policy before benefits for illness or injury become payable. A policy might include **dependents** of the insured, which typically are children, spouses, and domestic partners. The policy becomes effective after the company offers it and the person accepts it and then pays the initial **premium**, which is the payment made periodically to keep the policy in force.

In some states policies do not provide benefits for conditions that existed and were treated before the policy was issued, called **preexisting conditions**. Health insurance policies also contain **exclusions** or **limitations**, which prohibit benefits for certain conditions such as pregnancy and self-inflicted injury.

Some policies have a **waiver**, which is an attachment to a policy that excludes certain illnesses or disabilities that would otherwise be covered. Waivers are used to eliminate benefits for specific preexisting conditions.

Coordination of Benefits

A **coordination of benefits (COB)** statement is included in most policies. If a patient has more than one insurance policy, this prevents duplication of benefits for the same medical expense and is called *nonduplication of benefits*.

Methods of Payment

Insurance companies and federal and state programs use various methods to determine payment, such as fee schedules in traditional plans (e.g., private, Medicare) and capitation in managed care plans. For inpatient services, payment may be under the diagnosis related group (DRG) system. See pages 516–519 for a discussion of DRGs.

Fee Schedule

A *fee schedule* is a list of services or procedures and the specific dollar amount that will be charged by the physician or paid by the insurance company for each service. A method of payment called **fee-for-service** is that in which the patient pays the physician for each professional service performed from an established schedule of fees. To see an example of mock fees and Medicare fees listed in a fee schedule, refer to Part IV: Appendix of the *Workbook to Accompany Administrative Medical Assisting*.

Usual, Customary, and Reasonable (UCR)—Reimbursement under the **usual, customary, and reasonable (UCR)** method is based on individual physician charge profiles and customary charge screens for similar groupings of physicians within a geographic area and with similar expertise. UCR definitions include:

- *Usual fee*—the fee normally charged for a given professional service by an individual physician to his or her patients (i.e., the physician's usual fee)

- *Customary fee*—the fee that is in the range of usual fees charged by physicians of similar training and experience for the same services within the same specific and limited socioeconomic area

- *Reasonable fee*—the fee that meets the two preceding criteria or is considered justifiable by responsible medical opinion, considering special circumstances of the particular case in question

Relative Value Studies (RVS)—Relative value studies consist of a list of five-digit procedure codes for professional services with unit values that indicate the relative value for each procedure. Workers' compensation and Medicare use their own RVS listings to establish fee schedules.

Capitation

Under managed care plans, the physician is paid by **capitation**, a method of payment for health services by which a health group is prepaid a fixed, per capita amount for each patient enrolled without considering the actual amount of service provided to each patient. This per capita amount is usually paid on a monthly basis.

Physician's Fee Profile

As each insurance claim form is received by the insurance company, the payment data is entered into permanent computerized records. This is called a **physician profile** or *fee profile* and becomes a statistical summary of the fee pattern (cost for services) of each physician for a defined population of patients. It is collected over time and compared with other practice patterns. The physician's profile effects periodic fee adjustments made by insurance carriers.

INSURANCE PLANS AND PROGRAMS

In order to process insurance claims, a thorough understanding of the various types of insurance plans and programs is necessary. Following is a discussion of managed care plans and types of managed care organizations, government programs such as Medicaid, Medicare, TRICARE, and CHAMPVA, as well as state disability and workers' compensation.

Managed Care Plans

As discussed in Chapter 2, numerous managed care plans operate under many different contracts with physicians and health facilities. These plans are called prepaid health plans. Patients pay monthly medical insurance premiums through their employer or individually. The physician renders service to the patient, and the patient pays copayments as required by the plan. The physician is reimbursed via capitation.

At every visit, verify insurance coverage with the patient because patients change plans frequently. Collect the copayment when the patient arrives for his or her appointment, because it is easy to forget to ask for payment when the patient is leaving the office and billing is not cost-effective.

Many plans require patients to have laboratory and x-ray tests performed at plan-specified (network) facilities. Always allow enough time to receive test results before scheduling a patient's return appointment.

Precertification, Predetermination, and Preauthorization

Precertification refers to finding out if a service or procedure is covered under a patient's insurance policy. **Predetermination** means finding out the maximum dollar amount that the insurance company will pay for the professional service to be rendered to the patient.

Most managed care programs and some private insurance plans require **preauthorization** for certain services, hospital admissions, inpatient or outpatient surgeries, elective procedures, or when the patient must be seen by someone other than the *primary care physician* also known as the *gatekeeper*. Preauthorization relates to whether a service or procedure is covered and whether the insurance plan approves it as medically necessary. If the preauthorization is not obtained when required, the insurance company may refuse to pay part or all of the fee (Figure 16-1).

Patients may not be aware of this stipulation, so be sure to check on preauthorization requirements. If the patient has received authorization for a service, obtain the authorization number, and remind him or her to bring in the form at the time of the scheduled visit. If the authorization is delayed and the patient comes in for the appointment, telephone the plan and obtain oral authorization documenting the date, time, and name of the authorizing person; otherwise, the patient's appointment may have to be rescheduled. If the specialist physician wishes to refer the patient to another provider, this must be documented in the patient's record and sent to the primary care physician. An organized office keeps a referral tracking log and does a weekly or biweekly follow-up.

MANAGED CARE PLAN
TREATMENT AUTHORIZATION REQUEST

**TO BE COMPLETED BY PRIMARY CARE PHYSICIAN
OR OUTSIDE PROVIDER**

Health Net	☐	Met Life	☐
Pacificare	☒	Travelers	☐
Secure Horizons	☐	Pru Care	☐

Patient Name: _Terisita Blanco_   Date: _6/13/xx_

M____ F _X_ Birthdate _10/23/47_   Home telephone number _(555) 487-7870_

Address _29 Seaview Lane, Woodland Hills, XY 12345-0439_

Primary Care Physician _Fran Practon, MD_   Member ID# _C 15038_

Referring Physician _Fran Practon, MD_   Member ID# _C15038_

Referred to _George Hansevoda MD_   Address _2000 Broad Avenue_

Woodland Hills, XY 12345-0001   Office telephone no. _(555) 486-7000_

Diagnosis Code _614.9_   Diagnosis _Pelvic inflammatory disease_

Diagnosis Code _789.34_   Diagnosis _LLQ Pelvicmass_

Treatment Plan: _Gynecology consultation for chronic pelvic inflammatory disease, left lower quadrant_
                     pain and palpable mass

Authorization requested for procedures/tests/visits:

Procedure Code _99244_   Description _New patient consultation_

Procedure Code _76856_   Description _Pelvic ultrasound_

Facility to be used: _College Hospital_   Estimated length of stay _0_

Office ☒   Outpatient ☒   Inpatient ☐   Other ☐

List of potential consultants (i.e., anesthetists, assistants, or medical/surgical):

George Hansevoda, MD - Gynecologist

Physician's signature _Fran Practon, MD_

TO BE COMPLETED BY PRIMARY CARE PHYSICIAN

PCP Recommendations: _See above_   PCP Initials _FP MD_

Eligibility checked _6/13/XX_   Effective date _1/1/XX_

TO BE COMPLETED BY UTILIZATION MANAGEMENT

Authorized_____ Not authorized_____

Deferred_____ Modified_____

Authorization Request #_____

Comments:_____

Figure 16-1. Example of a managed care plan treatment authorization request form completed by a primary care physician for preauthorization of consultation services and pelvic ultrasound

Following are several types of referrals that a plan may use for different levels of prior approval:

- Formal referral—An authorization request is required by the managed care plan contract to determine medical necessity. This preauthorization may sometimes be obtained via telephone, but usually a completed authorization form is mailed or transmitted via fax.

- Direct referral—Simplified authorization request form is completed and signed by the physician and handed to the patient at the time of referral. Certain services may not require a formal referral (e.g., obstetrical care, dermatology).

- Verbal referral—Primary care physician informs the patient that he or she would like to refer him or her to a specialist. The physician telephones the specialist and indicates the patient is being referred for an appointment.

- Self-referral—Patient refers himself or herself to a specialist. The patient may be required to inform the primary care physician.

If a patient refuses to be referred, this must be documented. If a referral (authorization) form is required, a letter may be written but only to supplement the mandatory form. When authorization is approved, make a copy of the form for each approved service. The form may be attached to the claim when billing for the services or sent electronically to accompany electronic claims. Some referral forms authorize several office visits or multiple procedures to be done by one provider. If so, when all copies are used, this indicates that all procedures that the patient's plan has approved have been done. If additional services are needed, a new authorization request must be made.

Medical Review

Managed care organizations (MCOs) must follow general federal guidelines when they are established, and the government requires that the quality of care be assessed. Regional *professional review organizations* (*PROs*) have been set up and are composed of physicians who evaluate the quality of professional care. They also settle disputes on fees and examine evidence for admission and discharge of hospital patients. PROs play an important role in Medicare inpatient cases.

Types of Managed Care Organizations

There are many types of managed care organizations (MCOs). They vary from plans that restrict patients from going outside the MCO group to plans that offer great flexibility. The definitions of such plans have changed throughout the years as plan guidelines have adjusted to patient demands and medical costs. Following are some basic types of MCO plans.

Health Maintenance Organizations—The oldest of all the prepaid health plans are **health maintenance organizations (HMOs)**. Under an HMO plan, certain medical services are rendered by **participating physicians (par)** (*member physicians*) to a group of enrolled people who make fixed periodic payments to the plan (Figure 16-2). The physician is typically paid by capitation and most HMOs require copayment, depending on the type of service rendered. A participating physician is one who agrees to accept an insurance plan's preestablished fee or reasonable charge as the maximum amount collected for services rendered. Patients pay a copayment and sometimes a cost share, deductible, or both. HMOs stress preventive care. Enrollees under government programs, such as TRICARE, Medicaid, and Medicare may also join HMOs if desired, and may assign their benefits to these prepaid health plans. The Blue Plans also have enrollees from large companies serviced by managed care plans. The following are three types of HMO plans:

1. *Group practice model.* Physicians form an independent group and contract with an HMO plan to provide medical treatment to members. The physicians are paid a salary by their own independent group, not by the administrators of the health plan. Health services are available at one or more locations from a group of physicians contracting with the HMO or from physicians who are employees of the HMO.

2. *Staff model.* This HMO plan hires physicians and pays them a salary instead of contracting with a medical group.

3. *Network model.* This plan contracts with two or more group practices to provide health services.

If the physician belongs to an Independent (or individual) practice association (IPA), preferred provider organization (PPO), or staff model HMO, he or she is usually required to submit a billing statement for auditing purposes.

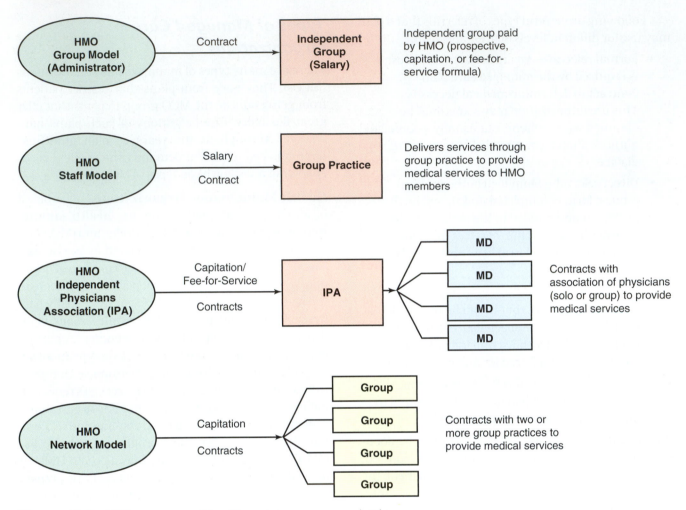

Figure 16-2. Different types of health maintenance organizations

Preferred Provider Organizations—A variation on the HMO theme is a **preferred provider organization (PPO)**. A formal agreement is drawn up among health care providers to treat a certain patient population, such as employees of a major corporation or members of a large union. Patients receive the highest level of benefits when seeking services from a preferred provider (participating provider). A PPO allows the subscriber more freedom of choice than does an HMO. Patients may go to nonparticipating physicians, but the fee will be covered at a lesser rate.

Independent Practice Association—An **independent** (or individual) **practice association (IPA)** is a type of MCO in which a program administrator contracts with several physicians who agree to provide treatment to subscribers in their own offices for a fixed capitation payment per month. Besides rendering services to subscribers of the IPA, the physician

also sees private-pay patients. The physicians are not employees and are not paid salaries. They are paid for their services on a capitation or fee-for-service basis from a fund drawn from the premiums collected from the subscriber, union, or corporation by the organization that markets the plan. A discount of up to 30 percent is withheld to cover operating costs. At the end of the year, the physicians share in any surplus or they must contribute if there is any deficit.

Physician Provider Groups—Physician provider groups (PPGs) are physician-owned businesses, which have flexibility built into them. One division may function as an IPA under contract to an HMO. A second division may act as the provider in a preferred provider organization (PPO) that contracts with hospitals as well as with other physicians to market services or medical supplies to employers and other third parties. A third division might be involved in joint ventures with hospitals, such as purchasing diagnostic equipment. The difference between an IPA and a PPG is that a PPG is physician-owned while an IPA is not owned by its member physicians. PPGs contain costs by combining services and by purchasing in bulk; appointments are made and billing is done at a central location. The member physicians give a small percentage of their income to the PPG for expenses.

Point-of-Service Plan—A managed care organization that combines elements of an HMO and a PPO and in addition offers some unique features is a **point-of-service (POS) plan**. It is basically an HMO consisting of a network of physicians and hospitals that provides an insurance company or an employer with discounts on its services. Members choose a primary care physician who manages specialty care and referrals. POS members have the flexibility, however, to go out of network but receive benefits at a greater level if they use member physicians.

Medicaid

Medicaid is a plan sponsored by federal, state, and local governments. It is an assistance program rather than an insurance program. Coverage and benefits vary widely among states. In California, this program is known as Medi-Cal.

In 1967, some states began bringing managed care to their Medicaid programs. Many states have adopted managed care systems as an effort to control escalating health care costs by curbing unnecessary emergency department visits and emphasizing preventive care. When the last state, Arizona, joined Medicaid, it started with prepaid care rather than following the way most states had structured their programs.

Eligibility

Eligibility requirements vary from state to state, but generally the Medicaid program is designed for certain needy and low-income people, the blind and disabled, and members of families receiving aid to dependent children.

A plastic or paper Medicaid identification card (or, in some states, coupons) are issued either monthly or at other intervals depending on the state laws. Some states allow the provider of service to verify eligibility and coverage in seconds via an electronic telecommunications system. A telephone system or special computer software program may also be used.

Photocopy the front and back sides of the card, and carefully check the expiration date and eligibility for the month of service each time the patient visits. The provider's name may also appear on the card, and if so, it would need to be verified monthly. Look to see if the patient has other insurance, copayment requirements, or restrictions (eligible for only certain types of service). Obtain any copayment when the patient comes in for the appointment.

In some instances, prior authorization is required before the service is rendered, unless it is a bona fide emergency. This may be done either via telephone, if urgent, or by completing a special request form (e.g., treatment authorization form) and sending it by mail.

Claims Submission

As of October 1, 1996, federal law mandates that Health Insurance Claim Form CMS-1500, formerly known as the HCFA-1500, be adopted for the processing of Medicaid claims in all states that optically scan their claims for payment. Always refer to the local Medicaid intermediary for guidelines on how the form should be completed. Claims must be signed by the physician and then be submitted either to a **fiscal intermediary** an *insurance carrier* who contracts to pay claims or to the local department of social services, depending on the rules of the state.

Time Limit

Every state has a time limit for the submission of claims; it can vary from two months from the date of service to one year. If submitted after the time limit, payment can be reduced, or the claim can be rejected unless there is valid justification recognized by state laws. Drugs and dental services may be billed to a different intermediary than services performed by a physician. The medical assistant can contact the local state department of public health or department of social services for further information.

Medicare

Medicare is funded by the federal government and administered by the Centers for Medicare and Medicaid Services (CMS). Depending on eligibility, a person may quality for only Part A, only Part B, or both. At the time of enrollment, a choice is made about how the health care coverage is delivered. The original Medicare plan is a fee-for-service plan, or coverage can be obtained by signing up for a Senior Advantage plan.

Eligibility

A person is eligible for Medicare health insurance coverage at age 65 and application is made through local Social Security Administration (SSA) offices. Medicare is also available to dependent widowers between ages 50 and 65; blind and disabled people; disabled workers of any age including widows, children, and adults who have chronic kidney disease requiring dialysis or end-stage renal disease (ESRD) requiring transplant; and kidney donors.

Part A—Part A of Medicare is hospital insurance benefits for people who are aged, disabled, or blind. The funds to furnish this health service come from the special contributions of employees and the self-employed and from employers who pay an amount equal to employees. The contributions are collected as Federal Insurance Contributions Act (FICA) contributions from wages and self-employed income earned during a person's working years.

A *benefit period* begins the day a patient enters a hospital and ends when the patient has not been a bed patient in any hospital for 60 consecutive days. Each time a patient begins a new benefit period, hospital insurance protection is renewed.

Part B—Part B of Medicare is referred to as supplementary medical insurance benefits covering outpatient medical services for people who are aged, disabled, or blind, because it supplements Part A, hospital coverage. The funds for this program come from premiums paid by those who sign up for it and from the federal government. The insurance premiums are deducted monthly from Social Security checks, from railroad retirement benefits, and from payments made to those receiving civil service annuities. Others not receiving Social Security benefits pay premiums directly to the Social Security Administration.

Due to the escalating costs of health care, the government has enforced many cost-containment features in the Medicare program. See Tables 16-1 and 16-2 for information on inpatient or outpatient Medicare cost-sharing benefits.

In a physician's office, medical assistants submit insurance claims to Medicare Part B fiscal intermediaries for participating or nonparticipating physicians. Under Medicare regulations, patients are not allowed to send in claims for reimbursement. Physicians may bill Medicare patients for noncovered services, that is, benefits that are not listed as covered in the Medicare program.

Part C—The Balanced Budget Act of 1997 created Medicare + Choice, which offers more health care options by allowing Medicare beneficiaries to join managed care plans instead of having Parts A or B. These plans are referred to as Senior Advantage plans, formerly known as HMOs. Some plans may require members to pay a premium similar to the Medicare Part B premium. Medicare + Choice plans receive a fixed amount of money from Medicare to spend on their Medicare members.

If a Medicare patient elects to join a Medicare + Choice managed care plan, there is no need for secondary coverage (e.g., Medigap). The patient agrees to go to doctors, hospitals, and other facilities on the plan's approved list. Small copayments are required for services rendered.

Another Medicare + Choice plan is a Medicare Medical Savings Account (MSA). The patient pays a high annual deductible for a catastrophic insurance policy approved by Medicare. Premiums for the policy are paid by the patient and deposits are made into the patient's MSA equaling the dollar amount difference between what is paid for the average beneficiary in the patient's area and the cost of the premium. The patient uses the money from the MSA to pay medical expenses until the high deductible is reached. Out-of-pocket payments may be necessary if the MSA money runs out before the deductible is met. Unused funds roll over to the next calendar year.

Part D—Medicare Part D is voluntary prescription drug coverage that became effective January 1, 2006. Private insurance companies offer a variety of plans; however, basic standardized benefits are set by the federal government and must be adhered to. Companies can offer benefits that exceed the basic standard, so premiums depend on the particular plan selected. The average premium was $32 per month in 2006. The patient also pays an annual deductible, not to exceed $250 in 2006 and will pay part of the cost of their prescriptions. Each plan has a list of covered generic and brand-name drugs and network pharmacies that must be used. Drugs are paid for by Medicare as follows:

- Part A—pays for medications related to hospital stays, skilled nursing facility stays (unless place of residence), and hospice care (see Table 16-1)

Table 16-1. Five Major Classifications of **Medicare Part A** Benefits: Hospital Insurance-Covered Services for 2007. (Modified from *Medicare & You 2007*, Washington, D.C., U.S. Government Printing Office, 2007.)

Services	Benefit	Medicare Pays	Patient Pays
HOSPITALIZATION Semiprivate room and board, general nursing and miscellaneous hospital services and supplies (Medicare payments based on benefit periods.)	First 60 days 61st to 90th day 91st to 150th day (60-reserve-days benefit paid at 100%)[1] Beyond 150 days	All but $992 All but $248 a day All but $496 a day Nothing	$992 deductible $248 a day $496 a day All costs
SKILLED NURSING FACILITY CARE Patient must have been in a hospital for at least 3 days and enter a Medicare-approved facility generally within 30 days after hospital discharge.[2] (Medicare payments based on benefit periods.)	First 20 days 21st to 100th day Beyond 100 days	100% of approved amount All but $124 a day Nothing	Nothing Up to $124 a day All costs
HOME HEALTH CARE Part-time or intermittent skilled care, home health aide services, durable medical equipment and supplies, and other services	Unlimited as long as Medicare conditions are met and services are declared "medically necessary"	100% of approved amount; 80% of approved amount for durable medical equipment	Nothing for services; 20% of approved amount for durable medical equipment
HOSPICE CARE Pain relief, symptom management, and support services for the terminally ill	If patient elects the hospice option and as long as doctor certifies need	All but limited costs for outpatient drugs and inpatient respite care	Limited cost sharing for outpatient drugs and inpatient respite care
BLOOD	Unlimited if medically necessary	All but first 3 pints per calendar year	For first 3 pints[3]

[1]*This 60-reserve-days benefit may be used only once in a lifetime.*
[2]*Neither Medicare nor private Medigap insurance will pay for most nursing home care.*
[3]*To the extent the blood deductible is met under Part B of Medicare during the calendar year, it does not have to be met under Part A.*

- Part B—covers medications that are administered by (or under the supervision of) the physician in the physician's office that cannot be self-administered; oral anti-cancer drugs, hemophilia clotting factors, drugs furnished by dialysis facilities, medication given as part of an outpatient procedure, intravenous immune globulin provided in home; flu, pneumonia, and Hepatitis B vaccines (see Table 16-2)

- Part D—is designed to cover drugs available only by prescription (exceptions apply)

An individual is eligible for Part D prescription drug coverage provided that he or she is entitled to Part A and/or enrolled in Part B and lives in the area of a Part D plan. Enrollment is not automatic unless the patient is dual-eligible, that is enrolled in Medicare and Medicaid. If the patient is eligible and does not enroll, a late enrollment penalty will be applied that equals 1 percent per month added to the premium. Those in original fee-for-service Medicare plans can enroll in a Part D Prescription Drug plan (PDP) that contracts with Medicare. This is considered a stand-alone drug plan. Those who are in Medicare Advantage managed care plans (HMO, PPO, etc.) can enroll in that plan's Part D Medicare Advantage Prescription Drug (MAPD) plan for combined medical and drug coverage. An annual election period is set aside for patients to change plans if desired.

Table 16-2. Six Major Classifications of **Medicare Part B** Benefits: Medical Insurance-Covered Services for 2007. (Modified from *Medicare & You 2007*, Washington, D.C., U.S. Government Printing Office, 2007.)

Services	Benefit	Medicare Pays	Patient Pays
MEDICAL EXPENSES Doctor's services (not routine physical exams), outpatient medical and surgical services and supplies, diagnostic tests, ambulatory surgery center facility fees for approved procedures, and durable medical equipment (such as wheelchairs, hospital beds, oxygen, and walkers). Also covers second surgical opinions, outpatient mental health care, and outpatient physical and occupational therapy, including speech-language therapy.	Unlimited if medically necessary	80% of approved amount (after $131 deductible); reduced to 50% for most outpatient mental health services	$131 deductible,[1] plus 20% of approved amount or limited charges
CLINICAL LABORATORY SERVICES Blood tests, urinalyses, and more	Unlimited if medically necessary	100% of approved amount	Nothing for services
HOME HEALTH CARE Part-time skilled nursing care, physical therapy, speech-language therapy, home health aide services, medical social services, durable medical equipment (such as wheelchairs, hospital beds, oxygen, and walkers), medical supplies, and other services.	Unlimited as long as patient meets conditions and benefits are considered medically necessary	100% of approved amount; 80% of approved amount for durable medical equipment	Nothing for services; 20% of amount for durable medical equipment
OUTPATIENT HOSPITAL TREATMENT Services for the diagnosis or treatment of illness or injury	Unlimited if medically necessary	Medicare payment to hospital based on hospital cost	$131 deductible, plus 20% of the hospital charges
BLOOD	Unlimited if medically necessary	80% of approved amount (after $131 deductible and starting with 4th pint)	First 3 pints plus 20% of approved amounts for additional pints (after $131 deductible)[2]
AMBULATORY SURGICAL SERVICES	Unlimited if medically necessary	80% of predetermined amount (after $131 deductible)	$131 deductible, plus 20% of predetermined amount

[1]*Once the patient has had $131 of expenses for covered services in the year, the Part B deductible does not apply to any further covered services received for the rest of the year.*

[2]*To the extent the blood deductible is met under Part A of Medicare during the calendar year, it does not have to be met under Part B.*

Plans are designed in three levels (see Example 16-1). The first level lists what the patient pays per prescription (copayment amount) up to a dollar amount (e.g., $2,000) for total drug costs. The second level is called the "donut hole" because the patient pays 100 percent of the cost of all prescriptions until the established yearly out-of-pocket drug cost is met (e.g., $3,600). The third level is what the patient pays per prescription (copay or percentage) *after* the yearly out-of-pocket drug costs have been met, until the year's end.

EXAMPLE 16-1

Part D Coverage Example

PLAN XXX $27/mo	Tier 1 Generic Drugs	Tier 2 Preferred Brand Drugs	Tier 3 Non Preferred Brand Drugs	Tier 4 Specialty Brand Drugs
LEVEL I Payment per prescription. *Total yearly drug cost up to $2,000.	$5 copay	$25 copay	$45 copay	25% coinsurance
LEVEL II Payment per prescription after reaching $2,000 total yearly drug costs until annual out-of-pocket expenses reach $3,600	100%	100%	100%	100%
LEVEL III Payment per prescription after yearly out-of-pocket drug costs reach $3,600	$2 or 5%	The Greater of . . . $5 or 5%	$5 or 5%	$5 or 5%

* This amount is when all drug costs reach $2,000; not the total of all copayments

Medicare Fee Schedule

Payment for all physicians' services are based on the Medicare fee schedule, which is determined by a Resource Based Relative Value System (RBRVS). Beginning in 1996, each Medicare local carrier annually sends each physician a Medicare fee schedule for his or her area or region listing three columns of figures for each procedure code number: participating amount, nonparticipating amount, and limiting charge. For an example, refer to the Mock Fee Schedule shown in Part IV: Appendix of the *Workbook to Accompany Administrative Medical Assisting*. Payment amounts are calculated by taking into account the following:

1. Work done by the physician (work RVU)
2. Practice expense (overhead RVU)
3. Malpractice insurance (malpractice RVU)

The RVU is adjusted by each Medicare local carrier, which determines a geographic adjustment factor (GAF) according to the cost of living in its region by using geographic practice cost indices (GPCIs—pronounced "gypsies"). To determine a payment amount, a conversion factor (CF) is used which is updated each year and published in Medicare Newsletters and the *Federal Register* in November. The formula looks like this: RVU × GAF × CF = $ amount of Medicare service.

RVUs are also helpful when negotiating the best contract available with managed care plans, so it is important for office managers or individuals assisting physicians to know and understand RBRVS data. See Example 16-2.

Participating Physicians

If a physician *participates* in the Medicare program, the physician agrees to accept payment from Medicare (*80 percent* of the *approved charges*) plus payment from the patient (*20% of the approved charges*) after the deductible has been met. When a physician participates, this is referred to as accepting **assignment** and the Medicare payment is sent directly to the physician. It is permissible but less confusing not to collect the Medicare copayment up front. The deductible should be collected after the claim has been paid.

Nonparticipating Physicians

Generally a **nonparticipating physician (nonpar)** is a physician who does not accept assignment, payment goes directly to the patient, and the patient is responsible to pay the bill in full. A nonparticipating physician has two options, however, of either not accepting

---

EXAMPLE 16-2

Medicare Formula Calculation for Payment of Each Service

Code		Work	Overhead	Malpractice
91000	RVUs	1.04	0.70	0.06
	GAF*	× 0.975	× 9.26	× 0.378
		1.014 +	0.6482 +	0.02268 = Total adjusted RVUs 1.68488

The 2007 conversion factor for nonsurgical care is $37.8975 × 1.68 = $63.67 allowed amount.

*The medical practice location is Winston-Salem, North Carolina.

---

assignment for all services or accepting assignment for some services and not accepting assignment for others. An exception to this policy is mandatory assignment for clinical laboratory tests and services.

Limiting charge is a percentage limit on fees that nonpar physicians may bill Medicare beneficiaries above the fee schedule allowed amount; therefore no charges are to be submitted to Medicare that are greater than this. Medicare pays 80 percent of the nonpar allowable fee. The physician can collect 20 percent of the allowable fee from the patient and the difference between the allowable fee amount and the limiting charge amount. For assignment claims, nonpar physicians may submit usual and customary fees; thus, two fee schedules are often maintained, one with usual fees and the other with limiting charges.

Claims Submission

Physicians use the new revised CMS-1500 claim form to submit their claims to Medicare. Charging for completing and submitting the claim form on an assigned claim violates the terms of the assignment. A template (Figure 16-3) may be used for reference when completing claims for patients on Medicare. Additional templates are shown in this chapter for other programs. A template makes it easier to learn which fields to complete and which to ignore (screened fields).

The patient's signature is required on this form. If the patient is unable to sign the CMS-1500 claim form—that is, if he or she is in a nursing home or hospital or is otherwise confined—his or her signature that is on file on a Lifetime Beneficiary Claim Authorization and Information Release will suffice. (See Figure 16-4 and its legend for particulars.) If the physician accepts assignment, an authorized person may sign the form or use a rubber stamp with the physician's signature.

Time Limit—The time limit for submitting Medicare claims is the end of the year following the fiscal year in which services were rendered. The fiscal year for claims begins October 1 and ends September 30.

Remittance Advice and Medicare Summary Notice

After a claim is submitted, the physician who submitted the claim receives a **Remittance Advice (RA)** (Figures 16-5A and B on pages 519 and 520), formerly known as Explanation of Medicare Benefits (EOMB) or Provider Claims Summary. This accompanies the Medicare payment check and breaks down the amount billed, amount approved (allowed), deductible, coinsurance requirement (patient responsibility), and amount of payment (see Figure 16-5A). The patient receives a separate simplified version of this called a **Medicare Summary Notice (MSN)**.

Medicare Cost Containment

The need to hold down rising health care costs was recognized by the government in the late 1970s, so a number of laws were passed to address cost containment and are discussed here.

Tax Equity and Fiscal Responsibility Act—In 1982, the Tax Equity and Fiscal Responsibility Act (TEFRA) was passed. It implemented a prospective payment system (PPS) for all hospitalization under the Medicare program. Reimbursement to hospitals is based on diagnosis related groups (DRGs). This system classifies patients who are medically related in regard to diagnosis and treatment and statistically similar in length of hospital stay. Instead of a fee-for-service system, the hospital receives a lump-sum, fixed-fee payment that is based on the diagnosis rather than on time or services rendered.

Figure 16-3. Example of a completed Health Insurance Claim Form CMS-1500 (revised 08/05) for a basic Medicare case with no other insurance coverage. Screened blocks do not need to be completed. The physician has accepted assignment. See Appendix A for step-by-step instructions on how to complete this form.

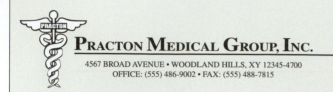

PRACTON MEDICAL GROUP, INC.

4567 BROAD AVENUE • WOODLAND HILLS, XY 12345-4700
OFFICE: (555) 486-9002 • FAX: (555) 488-7815

Fran Practon, M.D.
Gerald Practon, M.D.

LIFETIME BENEFICIARY CLAIM AUTHORIZATION AND INFORMATION RELEASE

Patient's
Name__**Busaba McDermott**__Medicare I.D. Number__**329-XX-6745**__

I request that payment of authorized Medicare benefits be made either to me or on my behalf to (name of physician/supplier) for any services furnished me by that physician/supplier. I authorize any holder of medical information about me to release to the Health Care Financing Administration and its agents any information needed to determine these benefits or the benefits payable to related services.

I understand my signature requests that payment be made and authorizes release of medical information necessary to pay the claim. If other health insurance is indicated in Item 9 of the CMS-1500 claim form or elsewhere on other approved claim forms or electronically submitted claims, my signature authorizes releasing of the information to the insurer or agency shown. In Medicare assigned cases, the physician or supplier agrees to accept Medicare's allowed amount. The carrier pays 80% of the allowed amount and the patient is responsible for the deductible, 2090 coinsurance, and noncovered services. Coinsurance is based upon the allowed amount of the Medicare carrier.

Busaba McDermott   _May 15, 20XX_
_____   _____
Patient's Signature   Date

Figure 16-4. Medicare Lifetime Beneficiary Claim Authorization and Information Release form. Patient's signature field on the CMS-1500 claim form should be submitted with this notation: "Signature on File" (SOF).

For the DRG system over 10,000 codes from the *International Classification of Diseases,* 9th Edition, *Clinical Modification (ICD-9-CM)* were divided into 25 basic major diagnostic categories (MDCs). These categories were each given a specific DRG number from 001 to 495 and a specific dollar amount that is the average of medical costs for treatment of patients with that

diagnosis in all geographic areas of the United States. There are six variables used for DRG classifications:

1. Patient's principal diagnosis

2. Patient's secondary diagnosis

3. Surgical procedures

4. Comorbidity* and complication

*Comorbidity means a preexisting condition that will cause an increase in length of stay in the hospital by at least one day.

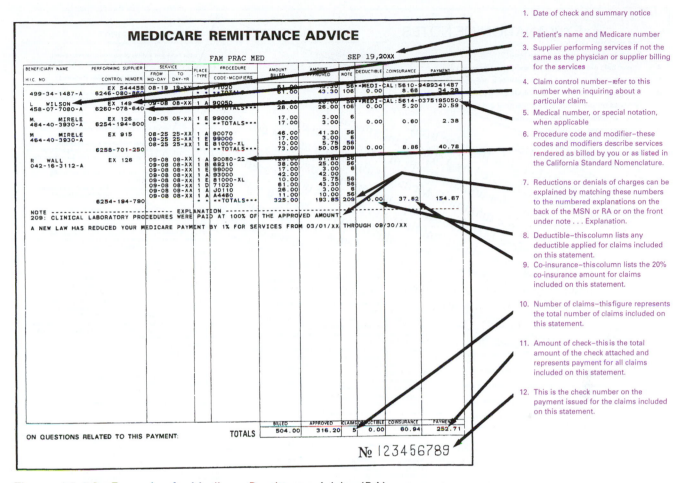

Figure 16-5A. Example of a Medicare Remittance Advice (RA)

5. Age and sex

6. Discharge status

Certain cases or cost outliers (extraordinarily high costs) that cannot be assigned to a DRG because they are considered atypical, such as leaving the hospital against medical advice, rare condition, death, and so forth, are paid the full DRG rate plus an additional amount.

Although DRGs affect Medicare hospital inpatients, the medical assistant plays an important role in DRG assignment when relaying the admitting diagnosis to the hospital. All of the diagnoses must be given if there are more than one; the hospital can sequence them as primary and secondary. If a hospital representative calls with questions about tests, length of hospital stay, or treatment ordered by the attending physician, the medical assistant should be prepared to furnish answers; this information will help determine the amount of the bill presented to Medicare by the hospital. The physician should be asked to review the treatment or procedure if there are questions.

Often, the physician will send a patient for preadmission testing (PAT). If the tests are done 48 to 72 hours before admission, they are included in the DRG amount on the inpatient bill.

Peer Review Organization—Under the prospective payment system, responsibility for maintaining quality of care is given to peer review organizations (PROs). PROs are composed of licensed doctors of medicine or osteopathy actively engaged in the practice of medicine or surgery. PROs review cases and focus on patient admission, readmission, transfer review, and review of procedures. They also study cases for additional Medicare reimbursement, day outlier (short and long lengths of hospital stay) review, the medical necessity of all services rendered, and cost outlier (extraordinarily high costs) review. In other words, they check to see if the DRG assignment is substantiated by the patient's clinical data.

Civil Monetary Penalties Law—To further contain costs, the government passed the Civil Monetary Penalties Law (CMPL) in 1983 to prosecute cases of

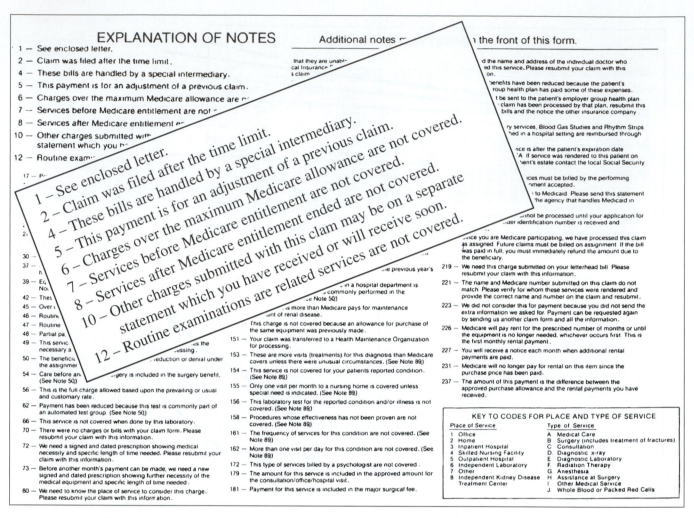

Figure 16-5B. Portion of Explanation of Notes on reverse side of Medicare Remittance Advice

Medicare and Medicaid fraud. A physician may be penalized for every requested payment that violates a Medicare assignment or a nonparticipating physician agreement. If an assistant submits false billings that the physician knows nothing about, the physician may be held liable. Incorrectly coded procedures can cause penalties to be imposed on a physician. It is the medical assistant's responsibility to keep up-to-date on all Medicare policies and perform related responsibilities capably and honestly.

Deficit Reduction Act—Another cost-containment plan was enacted in 1984: the Deficit Reduction Act. This act established a participating physician program giving incentives to physicians to accept assigned fees for Medicare patients. At that time, under this act, nonparticipating physicians were subject to a fee freeze and could not increase their fees.

Stark I and II Regulations*—In 1992 Stark I was enacted, prohibiting a physician or any member of a physician's family who has a financial relationship with a laboratory from referring patients to that facility. Then in 1995, an amendment was put into effect to expand prohibiting payments for other services where ownership interest is established, such as physical or occupational therapy, durable medical equipment, radiation therapy, and many other ancillary facilities and health-related services.

Medicare/Medicaid

In certain instances, some people qualify for both Medicare and Medicaid, simultaneously. In some states, this coverage is referred to as Medi-Medi. Usually these people are disabled, blind, or are over 65 and are entitled to Medicaid benefits, such as Old Age Security (OAS) assistance benefits. When patients are covered by both programs, Medicare is considered primary and Medicaid covers the residual not paid by Medicare. On such claims, the physician *must always accept assign-*

*There are numerous exceptions in the Stark statute and regulations. Be alert for CMS to issue the last phase of the final regulations.

ment or the payment goes directly to the patient and the Medicaid program does not pick up the residual.

Physicians use CMS-1500 forms to submit Medicare/Medicaid claims. It is not necessary to submit two claim forms, because a correctly completed claim form or an electronic claim will be automatically sent and processed by Medicaid after payment is completed by Medicare. The fiscal intermediary may refer to this as a *crossover claim*. It is not necessary for the patient to sign the claim form, but a physician or authorized person must sign the claim in ink; a stamped signature is not acceptable.

Time Limit—Claims should be submitted according to the time limit designated by the state Medicaid program. In some states, the fiscal intermediary for a Medicare/Medicaid claim may have a different address from that used for the processing of a Medicare-only claim. The assistant can contact the nearest Medicare fiscal intermediary for guidelines pertinent to the state or region.

Medicare/Medigap

Some Medicare beneficiaries purchase insurance policies regulated by the federal government to assist in paying left over medical services, such as deductibles and copayment amounts (i.e., $131 deductible and 20 percent of the Medicare allowed amount). Such policies are referred to as Medigap coverage for which the federal government has set regulations on what benefits may be offered. When the claim is completed correctly, it is automatically sent to the secondary Medigap plan. This is called "claims transfer" or "crossover." Figure 16-6 shows an example for submitting a claim when Medicare is primary and the patient has a Medigap (supplemental) policy. The assignment of benefits field on the claim form (Field 13) needs to be signed by the patient so the Medigap payment will go directly to participating physicians. Most Medicare carriers transmit Medigap claims electronically for participating physicians. In such cases, a signature on file (SOF) is necessary for the release of information and assignment of benefits. When an employee retires, Medicare becomes the primary coverage and the company's group health plan coordinates benefits with Medicare. These are conversion policies and are not considered "Medigap" as defined by federal law.

Medicare Secondary Payer (MSP)

Individuals age 65 years or over who are still employed may have insurance through an employer's health plan, which may be a private or managed care plan. In such cases, the employer's sponsored plan is billed as primary (first) and Medicare is billed second. These situations are referred to as a *Medicare Secondary Payer (MSP)*. Payments for these types of policies may not necessarily go to the physician but may go to the insured.

Another instance of an MSP claim is when liability insurance is primary to Medicare because the contractual agreement exists between the injured party and the liability insurance company, not Medicare.

Completing the CMS-1500 claim form for a patient who has Medicare and another insurance plan can be confusing. First find out whether Medicare is the primary or secondary payer, and then follow the directions on what information to enter in each field of the form depending on the primary payer.

TRICARE

TRICARE is a comprehensive health benefits program offering three (TRI) types of plans for dependents of men and women in the uniformed services (military). To control escalating medical costs and to standardize benefits for regions across the United States and Hawaii, TRICARE has also phased in managed care programs for eligible persons. The types of plans are:

- TRICARE Standard—fee-for-service cost-sharing plan
- TRICARE Extra—preferred provider organization plan
- TRICARE Prime—health maintenance organization plan with a point-of-service (POS) option

TRICARE Standard

The TRICARE program is designed to provide families of uniformed services personnel and service retirees a supplement to medical care in military and Public Health Service facilities. This program was previously entitled CHAMPUS (acronym for Civilian Health and Medical Program of the Uniformed Services), which still appears on the CMS-1500 claim form.

All those who qualify are automatically enrolled in the TRICARE Standard program with no enrollment fee.

Eligibility—All who qualify for TRICARE are known as *beneficiaries*. The active duty service member is referred to as the *sponsor*. Beneficiaries entitled to medical benefits under this government program are:

- Spouse and unmarried children up to age 21 (or 23 if full-time student) of uniformed

1500

HEALTH INSURANCE CLAIM FORM

APPROVED BY NATIONAL UNIFORM CLAIM COMMITTEE 08/05

Medicare/Medigap Claim

CARRIER

| | | PICA | | | PICA | | |

1. MEDICARE [X] (Medicare #) MEDICAID [ ] (Medicaid #) TRICARE CHAMPUS [ ] (Sponsor's SSN) CHAMPVA [ ] (Member ID#) GROUP HEALTH PLAN [X] (SSN or ID) FECA BLK LUNG [ ] (SSN) OTHER [ ] (ID)

1a. INSURED'S I.D. NUMBER (For Program in Item 1)
419XX7272A

2. PATIENT'S NAME (Last Name, First Name, Middle Initial)
BARNES AGUSTA E

3. PATIENT'S BIRTH DATE MM 08 DD 29 YY 1927 SEX M [X] F

4. INSURED'S NAME (Last Name, First Name, Middle Initial)

5. PATIENT'S ADDRESS (No., Street)
356 ENCINA AVENUE

6. PATIENT RELATIONSHIP TO INSURED
Self [ ] Spouse [ ] Child [ ] Other [ ]

7. INSURED'S ADDRESS (No., Street)

CITY
WOODLAND HILLS STATE XY

8. PATIENT STATUS
Single [X] Married [ ] Other [ ]

CITY STATE

ZIP CODE 12345 4700 TELEPHONE (Include Area Code) (555) 467 2646

Employed [ ] Full-Time Student [ ] Part-Time Student [ ]

ZIP CODE TELEPHONE (Include Area Code) ( )

9. OTHER INSURED'S NAME (Last Name, First Name, Middle Initial)
SAME

10. IS PATIENT'S CONDITION RELATED TO:

11. INSURED'S POLICY GROUP OR FECA NUMBER
NONE

a. OTHER INSURED'S POLICY OR GROUP NUMBER
MEDIGAP 419XX7272

a. EMPLOYMENT? (Current or Previous) YES [ ] NO [X]

a. INSURED'S DATE OF BIRTH MM DD YY SEX M [ ] F [ ]

b. OTHER INSURED'S DATE OF BIRTH MM DD YY SEX M [ ] F [ ]

b. AUTO ACCIDENT? YES [ ] NO [X] PLACE (State)

b. EMPLOYER'S NAME OR SCHOOL NAME

c. EMPLOYER'S NAME OR SCHOOL NAME

c. OTHER ACCIDENT? YES [ ] NO [X]

c. INSURANCE PLAN NAME OR PROGRAM NAME

d. INSURANCE PLAN NAME OR PROGRAM NAME
CALFCA 002

10d. RESERVED FOR LOCAL USE

d. IS THERE ANOTHER HEALTH BENEFIT PLAN?
YES [ ] NO [ ] If yes, return to and complete item 9 a-d.

READ BACK OF FORM BEFORE COMPLETING & SIGNING THIS FORM.

12. PATIENT'S OR AUTHORIZED PERSON'S SIGNATURE I authorize the release of any medical or other information necessary to process this claim. I also request payment of government benefits either to myself or to the party who accepts assignment below.
SIGNED _Agusta E Barnes_ DATE 11 / 21 / XX

13. INSURED'S OR AUTHORIZED PERSON'S SIGNATURE I authorize payment of medical benefits to the undersigned physician or supplier for services described below.
SIGNED _Agusta E Barnes_

14. DATE OF CURRENT: MM DD YY ILLNESS (First symptom) OR INJURY (Accident) OR PREGNANCY(LMP)

15. IF PATIENT HAS HAD SAME OR SIMILAR ILLNESS. GIVE FIRST DATE MM DD YY

16. DATES PATIENT UNABLE TO WORK IN CURRENT OCCUPATION FROM MM DD YY TO MM DD YY

17. NAME OF REFERRING PROVIDER OR OTHER SOURCE
GASTON INPUT MD

17a.
17b. NPI 3278 3127 XX

18. HOSPITALIZATION DATES RELATED TO CURRENT SERVICES FROM MM DD YY TO MM DD YY

19. RESERVED FOR LOCAL USE

20. OUTSIDE LAB? YES [ ] NO [X] $ CHARGES

21. DIAGNOSIS OR NATURE OF ILLNESS OR INJURY (Relate Items 1, 2, 3 or 4 to Item 24E by Line)
1. 786 59
2.
3.
4.

22. MEDICAID RESUBMISSION CODE ORIGINAL REF. NO.

23. PRIOR AUTHORIZATION NUMBER

24. A. DATE(S) OF SERVICE From MM DD YY To MM DD YY	B. PLACE OF SERVICE	C. EMG	D. PROCEDURES, SERVICES, OR SUPPLIES (Explain Unusual Circumstances) CPT/HCPCS MODIFIER	E. DIAGNOSIS POINTER	F. $ CHARGES	G. DAYS OR UNITS	H. EPSDT Family Plan	I. ID. QUAL.	J. RENDERING PROVIDER ID. #
1 11 21 20XX	11		93350	1	146 83	1		NPI	65499947XX
2								NPI	
3								NPI	
4								NPI	
5								NPI	
6								NPI	

25. FEDERAL TAX I.D. NUMBER SSN [ ] EIN [X]
7340313XX

26. PATIENT'S ACCOUNT NO.
060

27. ACCEPT ASSIGNMENT? (For govt. claims, see back) YES [X] NO [ ]

28. TOTAL CHARGE $ 146 83

29. AMOUNT PAID $

30. BALANCE DUE $

31. SIGNATURE OF PHYSICIAN OR SUPPLIER INCLUDING DEGREES OR CREDENTIALS (I certify that the statements on the reverse apply to this bill and are made a part thereof.)
FRAN PRACTON MD
SIGNED _Fran Practon MD_ DATE 11 22 20XX

32. SERVICE FACILITY LOCATION INFORMATION
a. NPI b.

33. BILLING PROVIDER INFO & PH # (555) 486 9002
PRACTON MEDICAL GROUP
4567 BROAD AVENUE
WOODLAND HILLS XY 12345 4700
a. 36640210XX b.

NUCC Instruction Manual available at: www.nucc.org

APPROVED OMB-0938-0999 FORM CMS-1500 (08-05)

Figure 16-6. Template of revised Health Insurance Claim Form CMS-1500 (08/05) indicating Medicare as primary payer and Medigap as the supplemental insurance policy. Shaded fields do not need to be completed.

service members who are in (1) active duty*, (2) the United States Coast Guard, (3) Public Health Service, or (4) the National Oceanic and Atmospheric Administration

- Eligible children over age 21 with disabilities
- Uniformed service retirees and their eligible family members
- Unremarried spouses and unmarried children of deceased, active, or retired service members
- Former spouses of Uniformed Service personnel who meet certain length-of-marriage criteria and other requirements
- Physically or emotionally abused spouses, former spouses, or dependent children of uniformed service personnel who were found guilty and discharged for the offense
- Spouses and children of North Atlantic Treaty Organization (NATO) nation representatives (outpatient services only)
- Disabled beneficiaries younger than 65 years of age who have Medicare Parts A and B

Those *not* eligible for TRICARE are:

- Medicare-eligible beneficiaries age 65 and over not enrolled in Medicare Part B
- Veterans eligible for CHAMPVA
- Uniformed service member parents or parents-in-law (unless eligible under Supplemental Health Care Program)
- Secretarial designees who are entitled to care at a military treatment facility (MTF) or from a civilian provider.

Defense Enrollment Eligibility Reporting System—The sponsor's responsibility is to make sure all TRICARE-eligible persons in his or her family are enrolled in the *Defense Enrollment Eligibility Reporting System (DEERS)* computerized database. The sponsor's Social Security number (SSN) is used to access DEERS and file claims. Before processing claims, TRICARE claims processors check DEERS to verify beneficiary eligibility.*

Providers do not access DEERS, instead they verify a TRICARE beneficiary's eligibility by using the *Voice Response Unit (VRU)* system, which is manned 24 hours a day. To use this system, call the toll-free number and follow the commands, which will connect to DEERS and provide eligibility information.

Benefits—Those on the TRICARE Standard program may receive a wide range of civilian health care services with a portion of the cost paid by the federal government. Patients usually seek care from a military hospital near their home. In certain areas or in certain situations, they can seek care through a private physician's office. The patient pays a deductible for outpatient care and cost-sharing percentages. If the provider participates and accepts assignment, he or she accepts the TRICARE allowable fee as the full amount for the services rendered.

Effective as of October 1, 1996, the nonparticipating physician is required to file the claim and may charge no more than 15 percent above the TRICARE maximum allowable charge for his or her services. The check goes directly to the patient, and the patient pays the bill in full. Benefits under this program are shown in Figures 16-7 and 16-8. Study these figures carefully. They give an overall picture of cost-sharing (deductibles and copayments) for the TRICARE Standard, TRICARE Extra, and TRICARE Prime programs.

TRICARE Extra

TRICARE Extra is a preferred provider organization. In this option, the TRICARE beneficiary does not have to enroll or pay an annual fee. On a visit-by-visit basis, the individual may seek care from a provider who is part of the TRICARE Extra network and receive a discount on services and reduced cost-shares. Therefore, a beneficiary may bounce back and forth between network and non-network providers on a visit-by-visit basis and receive benefits from both TRICARE Standard and TRICARE Extra options. No identification card is issued, because the individual presents a military identification card as proof of eligibility when receiving care.

TRICARE Prime

TRICARE Prime is a managed care (HMO-type) option. Retirees, family members, and survivors pay an annual fee per person or per family but active duty service members and their families do not. As shown in Figures 16-7 and 16-8, benefits and covered services include preventive and primary care. Medical care is rendered from within a Prime network of civilian and military providers. The beneficiary has the option of

---

Active duty service members are entitled to medical benefits in a program called TRICARE Prime Remote.

ADFM = active duty family members RFMS = retires, family members and survivors	**Benefit and Coverage Chart**					
OUTPATIENT SERVICES	**Programs and Beneficiary Costs**					
Program and Classification	**TRICARE Prime**		**TRICARE Extra**		**TRICARE Standard**	
	ADFM	**RFMS**	**ADFM**	**RFMS**	**ADFM**	**RFMS**
Annual Enrollment Fee* (per fiscal year)	None	$230/person $460/family	None ⟶		None ⟶	
Annual Deductible (per fiscal year 10/1 to 9/30) (applied to outpatient services before cost-share is determined)	None (except when using point-of-service option)		E-4 and below $50/person $100/family E-5 and above $150/person $300/family	$150/person $300/family	E-4 and below $50/person $100/family E-5 and above $150/person $300/family	$150/person $300/family
Physician Services	None	$12	15% of contracted fee	20% of contracted fee	20% of maximum allowable charge	25% of maximum allowable charge
Ancillary Service (certain radiology, laboratory, & cardiac services)	None (RFMS may have 412 copay if test provided independent of office visit)					
Ambulance Services	None	$20				
Home Health Services	None	$12				
Family Health Services	None	$12				
Durable Medical Equipment (greater than $100)	None	20% cost-share				
Emergency Services (network and non-network)	None	$30 copayment				
Outpatient Behavioral Health (limitations apply)	None	$25 copayment $17 group visits				
Immunizations (for required overseas travel)	None	Not covered		Not covered		Not covered
Ambulatory Surgery (same day)	None	$25 copayment (applied to facility charges only)	$25 copayment for hospital charges	20% of contracted fee	$25 copayment for hospital charges	*Professional:* 25% of maximum allowable charge *Facility:* 25% of maximum allowable charge OR billed charges, whichever is less
Eye Examinations (limitations apply)	None	Clinical Preventive Service	15% of contracted fee	Not covered	20% of maximum allowable charge	Not covered
Prescription Drugs– Network Pharmacy	$3 copayment for each 30–day supply of **generic** medication $9 copayment for each 30–day supply of **brand name** medication					
Prescription Drugs– National mail Order Pharmacy	$3 copayment for each 90–day supply of **generic** medication $9 copayment for each 90–day supply of **brand name** medication (Note: If the beneficiary has primary insurance that covers prescription medication, the beneficiary is not eligible for the mail–order pharmacy benefit)					
Prescription Drugs– Non-network Pharmacy	$9 or 20% of total cost (whichever is greater) plus deductible					

*No enrollment fee for those who are eligible for Medicare (enrolled in Part B) on the basis of disability or end–stage renal disease

NOTE: TRICARE Prime Remote–benefits are similar to TRICARE Prime program; however, ADSMs have no copayment, costshare, or deductible

Program for Persons with Disabilities–no deductible; monthly cost–share varies from $25 to $250, depending on sponsor's rank

Figure 16-7. TRICARE Prime, Extra, and Standard Outpatient Service Benefits and Coverage Chart

ADFM = active duty family members RFMS = retires, family members and survivors	**Benefit and Coverage Chart**					
INPATIENT SERVICES	**Programs and Beneficiary Costs**					
Program and Classification	**TRICARE Prime**		**TRICARE Extra**		**TRICARE Standard**	
	ADFM	**RFMS**	**ADFM**	**RFMS**	**ADFM**	**RFMS**
Hospitalization* including **Maternity Benefits***	No copayment	$11.45/day; civilian care $11/day or $25 min charge per/admission, whichever is greater	$11.45/day; civilian care $11/day or $25 min charge per/admission, whichever is greater	$11.45/day; civilian care $250/day or 25% cost-share (contracted fee), whichever is less, plus 20% cost-share for separately billed professional charges	$11.45/day; civilian care $11/day or $25 min charge per/admission, whichever is greater	$11.45/day; civilian care $512/day or 25% cost-share (contracted fee), whichever is less, plus 25% cost-share (maximum allowable charge) for separately billed professional charges
Skilled Nursing Care					$25/admission, or $11.45/day whichever is greater	25% cost-share (billed charges), plus 25% cost-share (maximum allowable charge) for separately billed professional charges
Mental Illness Hospitalization* and **Substance Use treatment*** (inpatient, partial hospital program)	None	$40/day (no copayment or cost-share for separately billed professional charges)	$20/day	20% cost-share (contracted fee), plus 20% cost-share (contracted fee) separately billed professional charges)	$20/day	25% cost-share (max allowable charge), for separately billed professional charges plus: 25% of (1) per diem, (2) fixed daily amount or billed charges, or (3) 25% of allowed amount (RTC & partial hospitalization)
Partial Hospitalization* (mental illness)	None	$40/day or $25/admission, whichever is greater	$20/day	20% cost-share (contracted fee) plus 20% cost-share for separately billed professional charges	$20/day	25% of allowed amount, plus 25% maximum allowable charge for separately billed professional charges
Hospice care	**Available in lieu of other TRICARE benefits (provided by Medicare–approved program).**					
*Preauthorization required						

Figure 16-8. TRICARE Prime, Extra, and Standard Inpatient Service Benefits and Coverage Chart

choosing or being assigned a primary care manager (PCM) for each family member. This provider furnishes and manages all aspects of the patient's health care, including referrals to specialists. For active duty service members (ADSMs) and their families who work and live more than 50 miles or 1 hour from an MTF, the TRICARE Prime Remote program is available, which enables these individuals to receive care from any TRICARE-certified civilian provider.

Active-duty service members are enrolled automatically in TRICARE Prime and use local military providers and, when directed, the civilian portion of the TRICARE network. There are no annual deductibles and copayments vary (see Figure 16-7). A dental plan is available for an additional monthly premium. Outpatient or ambulatory surgery must be on the approved procedure list in the TRICARE Policy Manual before it is performed.

Enrollees are issued a TRICARE Prime identification card, but this does not guarantee eligibility. Providers must call the local health care finder (HCF) or check the military identification card for effective and expiration dates, and call the automated Voice Response Unit system to verify eligibility. Photocopy both the military identification card and the TRICARE Prime card, and retain them in the patient's file. Check both cards at every visit. Beneficiaries who are not enrolled as members in TRICARE Prime may continue to receive services through TRICARE Extra from network providers or through TRICARE Standard using non-network providers.

Nonavailability Statement—A Nonavailability Statement is a certification by a Uniformed Services Medical Treatment Facility (USMTF), usually a hospital, when a specific type of non-emergency care is not available at that facility, at a specific time, to a patient who needs care and who lives within the hospital's ZIP code service area; also called a *catchment* area. For all *outpatient* services from civilian sources provided on or after September 23, 1996, TRICARE patients no longer need *Nonavailability Statements* (NASs).

NASs are still required for nonemergency *inpatient* care from civilian sources for those people who live within the service areas of one or more uniformed services hospitals and who get their civilian care under TRICARE or TRICARE Extra. An inpatient NAS is not required for persons enrolled in TRICARE Prime or who use the POS option and live within the service area of a uniformed services hospital.

The only exception is that in areas where TRICARE contracts are in operation, providers who see TRICARE-eligible persons must obtain preauthorization for three procedures: (1) cardiac catheterization, (2) laparoscopic cholecystectomy (gallbladder removal), and (3) magnetic resonance imaging (MRI), or the amount of payment will be reduced by 10 percent.

Call the health benefits advisor (HBA) at the nearest military medical facility to verify the procedures, the approved facility, and the need for an NAS before scheduling surgery. If no preauthorization is obtained, a POS option is available featuring an annual outpatient deductible and 50 percent cost-share. Patients may need prior authorization for nonemergency care received while away from the area in which they are enrolled.

TRICARE for Life

TRICARE for Life (TFL) is a health care program funded by the Department of Defense (DOD) offering additional TRICARE benefits as a supplementary payer to Medicare.

Eligibility—Those eligible are uniformed service retirees, their spouses, and survivors age 65 and over. Most beneficiaries must be eligible for Medicare Part A and enrolled in Medicare Part B to qualify for TFL. An exception is Uniformed Services Family Health Plan (USFHP) members. TFL beneficiaries do not have to enroll, but they do need to be enrolled in DEERS. Beneficiaries who qualify for TFL do not need a TRICARE enrollment card. There are no preauthorization requirements for the TFL program. For coverage, all services and supplies must be a benefit of the Medicare program, TRICARE program, or both.

Payment Guidelines—Payment guidelines are as follows:

1. Generally Medicare is the primary payer and TRICARE is the secondary payer.

2. Services covered under Medicare and TRICARE: Medicare pays the Medicare rate and TRICARE covers the beneficiary's deductible and cost-share. No copayment, cost-share, or deductible is paid by the TFL beneficiary.

3. Services covered under Medicare, but not TRICARE: Medicare pays the Medicare rate and the beneficiary pays the Medicare cost-share and deductible amounts.

4. Services covered under TRICARE, but not Medicare: TRICARE pays the TRICARE allowed amount and Medicare pays nothing. The beneficiary is responsible for the TRICARE cost-share and the deductible amounts.

TRICARE Plus

TRICARE Plus is for persons eligible for care in MTFs and not enrolled in TRICARE Prime or a commercial HMO. TRICARE Plus allows some Military Health System (MHS) beneficiaries to enroll with a military primary care provider. There is no enrollment fee.

Enrollees of TRICARE Plus receive an identification card and are identified in the DEERS. TRICARE

Plus offers the same benefits as TRICARE Prime when using an MTF.

TRICARE Claims Submission

The TRICARE fiscal year is from October 1 to September 30, so medical assistants collecting deductibles and copayments need to post reminder notices to TRICARE patients in the waiting room prior to October 1. The beneficiary does not file claims under TRICARE Standard, TRICARE Extra, or TRICARE Prime. The TRICARE program is administered by the Department of Defense, TRICARE Management Activity (TMA) in Aurora, Colorado; however, the provider submits the claim either electronically or manually using the CMS-1500 claim form (Figure 16-9). The physician or an authorized person must sign it; however, a stamped signature is acceptable. The service member or a responsible family member must sign the form.

The physician must agree to accept assignment, thereby consenting to accept what TRICARE states are "reasonable charges," plus 20 percent or 25 percent of these charges after the deductible has been met. The payment goes to the physician. If the physician does not accept assignment, the payment goes directly to the patient and the patient pays the total bill.

When patients have other insurance in addition to TRICARE, by law TRICARE is last to pay except when the other insurance is:

1. A plan administered under Title XIX of the Social Security Act (Medicaid)

2. Coverage specifically designed to supplement TRICARE benefits

If the patient is in an automobile accident or receives an injury that may have third-party involvement, TRICARE Form 691 (Statement of Personal Injury— Possible Third-Party Liability) must be sent in with the regular claim form for cost-sharing of the civilian medical care.

Time Limit—TRICARE claims must be filed on time. The time limit for submitting a TRICARE claim is within 60 days from the date of service or, for inpatient care, within 60 days from the patient's date of discharge from the inpatient facility.

CHAMPVA

The Civilian Health and Medical Program of the Veterans Administration (CHAMPVA), now known as the Department of Veterans Affairs is a service benefit program, therefore no premiums are paid. A *veteran* is anyone who has served in the United States armed forces and has received an honorable discharge.

Eligibility

The Veterans Health Care Expansion Act of 1973 (PL93082) authorized a TRICARE-like program for the spouses and children of veterans with total, permanent, service-connected disabilities, and for the surviving spouses and children of veterans who die as a result of service-connected disabilities. These beneficiaries have comparable benefits and cost-sharing, as do dependents of retired and deceased uniform service personnel under TRICARE.

Claims Submission and Time Limit

For CHAMPVA claims, VA Form 10-7959A is completed and submitted when billing for professional services. The time limit for submission of CHAMPVA claims is the same as that for the TRICARE program.

State Disability Insurance

State Disability Insurance (SDI) is insurance that gives coverage for off-the-job injury or sickness and is paid for by deductions from a working individual's paycheck. This program is administered by a state agency and is sometimes known as *Unemployment Compensation Disability (UCD)*. SDI programs are available in five states (California, Hawaii, New Jersey, New York, and Rhode Island) and Puerto Rico. SDI deductions are discussed briefly in Chapter 18.

Benefits begin after the seventh consecutive day of disability. An employee is also entitled to disability benefits from a previous disability or illness if he or she has returned to work for 15 days and then becomes ill with the same ailment. Most states mentioned have maternity benefits that may be applied for when maternity leave is taken. There are some limitations, so it is important for the medical assistant to contact the state agency regarding current regulations. With the exception of Hawaii and Puerto Rico, most states' programs do not allow hospital benefits.

The definition of **total disability** varies in each of the five states, but a general definition might be that the insured must be unable to perform the major duties of his or her specific occupation. This may be temporary or permanent. The term **partial disability** may be defined as when an illness or injury prevents an insured person from performing one or more of the

---

1500

HEALTH INSURANCE CLAIM FORM
APPROVED BY NATIONAL UNIFORM CLAIM COMMITTEE 08/05

TRICARE Claim

| | | PICA | | | | | | | PICA | | |

1. MEDICARE ☐ (Medicare #) MEDICAID ☐ (Medicaid #) TRICARE CHAMPUS ☒ (Sponsor's SSN) CHAMPVA ☐ (Member ID#) GROUP HEALTH PLAN ☐ (SSN or ID) FECA BLK LUNG ☐ (SSN) OTHER ☐ (ID)

1a. INSURED'S I.D. NUMBER (For Program in Item 1)
581XX7211

2. PATIENT'S NAME (Last Name, First Name, Middle Initial)
FORBES SUSAN M

3. PATIENT'S BIRTH DATE MM 03 DD 16 YY 1976 SEX M ☐ F ☒

4. INSURED'S NAME (Last Name, First Name, Middle Initial)
FORBES WILLIAM O

5. PATIENT'S ADDRESS (No., Street)
882 SHARP STREET

6. PATIENT RELATIONSHIP TO INSURED
Self ☐ Spouse ☒ Child ☐ Other ☐

7. INSURED'S ADDRESS (No., Street)
SAME

CITY WOODLAND HILLS **STATE** XY

8. PATIENT STATUS
Single ☐ Married ☒ Other ☐
Employed ☐ Full-Time Student ☐ Part-Time Student ☐

CITY **STATE**

ZIP CODE 12345 4700 **TELEPHONE** (Include Area Code) (555) 789 9698

ZIP CODE **TELEPHONE** (Include Area Code) ( )

9. OTHER INSURED'S NAME (Last Name, First Name, Middle Initial)

10. IS PATIENT'S CONDITION RELATED TO:

11. INSURED'S POLICY GROUP OR FECA NUMBER

a. OTHER INSURED'S POLICY OR GROUP NUMBER

a. EMPLOYMENT? (Current or Previous)
YES ☐ NO ☒

a. INSURED'S DATE OF BIRTH MM 06 DD 12 YY 1974 SEX M ☒ F ☐

b. OTHER INSURED'S DATE OF BIRTH MM DD YY SEX M ☐ F ☐

b. AUTO ACCIDENT? PLACE (State)
YES ☐ NO ☒

b. EMPLOYER'S NAME OR SCHOOL NAME
USN

c. EMPLOYER'S NAME OR SCHOOL NAME

c. OTHER ACCIDENT?
YES ☐ NO ☒

c. INSURANCE PLAN NAME OR PROGRAM NAME
TRICARE

d. INSURANCE PLAN NAME OR PROGRAM NAME

10d. RESERVED FOR LOCAL USE

d. IS THERE ANOTHER HEALTH BENEFIT PLAN?
YES ☐ NO ☒ *If yes,* return to and complete item 9 a-d.

READ BACK OF FORM BEFORE COMPLETING & SIGNING THIS FORM.
12. PATIENT'S OR AUTHORIZED PERSON'S SIGNATURE I authorize the release of any medical or other information necessary to process this claim. I also request payment of government benefits either to myself or to the party who accepts assignment below.
SIGNED _SOF_ DATE _____

13. INSURED'S OR AUTHORIZED PERSON'S SIGNATURE I authorize payment of medical benefits to the undersigned physician or supplier for services described below.
SIGNED _____

14. DATE OF CURRENT: MM 09 DD 19 YY 20XX ILLNESS (First symptom) OR INJURY (Accident) OR PREGNANCY(LMP)

15. IF PATIENT HAS HAD SAME OR SIMILAR ILLNESS. GIVE FIRST DATE MM DD YY

16. DATES PATIENT UNABLE TO WORK IN CURRENT OCCUPATION
FROM MM 06 DD 28 YY 20XX TO MM 08 DD 09 YY 20XX

17. NAME OF REFERRING PROVIDER OR OTHER SOURCE
ADAM LANGERHANS MD
17a.
17b. NPI 665783 2XX

18. HOSPITALIZATION DATES RELATED TO CURRENT SERVICES
FROM MM 06 DD 28 YY 20XX TO MM 07 DD 01 YY 20XX

19. RESERVED FOR LOCAL USE

20. OUTSIDE LAB? YES ☐ NO ☒ $ CHARGES

21. DIAGNOSIS OR NATURE OF ILLNESS OR INJURY (Relate Items 1, 2, 3 or 4 to Item 24E by Line)
1. 650
2.
3.
4.

22. MEDICAID RESUBMISSION CODE ORIGINAL REF. NO.

23. PRIOR AUTHORIZATION NUMBER

24. A. DATE(S) OF SERVICE From MM DD YY — To MM DD YY	B. PLACE OF SERVICE	C. EMG	D. PROCEDURES, SERVICES, OR SUPPLIES (Explain Unusual Circumstances) CPT/HCPCS MODIFIER	E. DIAGNOSIS POINTER	F. $ CHARGES	G. DAYS OR UNITS	H. EPSDT Family Plan	I. ID. QUAL.	J. RENDERING PROVIDER ID. #
1	06 28 20XX	21		59400	1	1864 30	1		NPI	65499947XX
2									NPI	
3									NPI	
4									NPI	
5									NPI	
6									NPI	

25. FEDERAL TAX I.D. NUMBER SSN ☐ EIN ☒
7340313XX

26. PATIENT'S ACCOUNT NO.
080

27. ACCEPT ASSIGNMENT? (For govt. claims, see back)
YES ☒ NO ☐

28. TOTAL CHARGE $ 1864 30

29. AMOUNT PAID $

30. BALANCE DUE $ 1864 30

31. SIGNATURE OF PHYSICIAN OR SUPPLIER INCLUDING DEGREES OR CREDENTIALS (I certify that the statements on the reverse apply to this bill and are made a part thereof.)
FRAN PRACTON MD
Fran Practon MD
SIGNED DATE 06 29 20XX

32. SERVICE FACILITY LOCATION INFORMATION
COLLEGE HOSPITAL
4500 BROAD AVENUE
WOODLAND HILLS XY 12345 4700
a. 54378601XX b.

33. BILLING PROVIDER INFO & PH # (555) 486 9002
PRACTON MEDICAL GROUP
4567 BROAD AVENUE
WOODLAND HILLS XY 12345 4700
a. 36640210XX b.

NUCC Instruction Manual available at: www.nucc.org APPROVED OMB-0938-0999 FORM CMS-1500 (08-05)

Figure 16-9. Template of a revised Health Insurance Claim Form CMS-1500 for a TRICARE Standard case when billing for professional services

functions of his or her regular job either temporarily or permanently.

Claims Submission

A claim form is supplied by the state and may appear in two or three parts to be completed by the claimant, employer, and physician. The claim must be documented with the signatures of both the patient and the physician before the claimant can begin receiving benefits. It is important that the Social Security number of the patient be accurate on the claim, because without it the claim cannot be properly researched to establish wages earned in the last quarter. Claims are submitted to:

California	Branch office of Employment Development Department
Hawaii	Department of Labor and Industrial Relations, Disability Compensation Division
New Jersey	Department of Labor and Industry, Division of Unemployment and Disability Insurance
New York	Workmen's Compensation Board, Disability Benefits Bureau
Puerto Rico	Department of Labor and Human Resources, Bureau of Employment Security, Disability Insurance Division
Rhode Island	Department of Labor and Training, Temporary Disability Insurance Division

Addresses of these offices can be found in the telephone directory. Those working in states that do not have disability programs may contact a local private insurance carrier about such coverage. Some state laws provide that a voluntary plan may be adopted instead of the state plan if a majority of company employees consent to private coverage.

Time Limit—A claim for disability insurance should be filed within the time limit for your state—there is a **grace period** of seven to eight days after the deadline. Maximum payments in a benefit year, time limits for filing claims, deductions from salaries, and a listing of what the benefits are based on appear in Table 16-3.

Workers' Compensation

An industrial accident or disease is an unforeseen, unintended event arising out of one's employment. Workers' compensation is a form of insurance paid by the employer and provides cash benefits to a worker injured or disabled in the course of his or her employment. The worker is also entitled to benefits for some or all of the medical services necessary for treatment and restoration to resume a useful life, and in some instances, the worker is rehabilitated and trained for a new job.

Workers' Compensation Laws

Workers' compensation programs are mandatory under state laws in all states. Some of their goals are to provide the best medical care to achieve maximum recovery, to get the ill or injured individual back to work, and to provide income to prevent the injured from having to go on welfare. The following are a number of federal workers' compensation laws that have been enacted:

1. Workmen's Compensation Law of the District of Columbia provides benefits for workers in Washington, D.C.

2. Federal Coal Mine Health and Safety Act provides benefits to coal miners

3. United States Longshoremen's and Harbor Workers' Compensation Act provides benefits for private or public employees engaged in maritime work

4. Federal Employees' Compensation Act (FECA) provides benefits for on-the-job injuries to all federal workers

In industrial injuries (workers' compensation) cases, the contract exists between the physician and the insurance carrier. When an insurance company **adjuster** telephones for information on a case, the medical assistant should verify who the adjuster is before providing medical information. Such cases do not require a signed consent from the patient to release information.

Types of Disability

There are three types of workers' compensation claims: *nondisability*, **temporary disability (TD)**, and **permanent disability (PD)**. A nondisability claim is

Table 16-3. Disability Information Summary for Five States and Puerto Rico

State	Name of State Law	Maximum Weekly Payments in Benefit Year	Time Limit for Filing Claims	2006 Deductions from Salary (%)	Benefits
California	California Unemployment Insurance Code	52	49 days from disability	0.8	Based on earnings in a 12-month base period, which begins approximately 18 months prior to disability
Hawaii	Temporary Disability Insurance Law	26	90 days from disability	0.5	Based on 58% of average weekly wage
New Jersey	Temporary Disability Benefits Law	26	30 days from disability	0.5	Based on average weekly wage
New York	Disability Benefits Law	26	30 days from disability	0.5 (max. 60 cents/wk)	Based on 50% of average weekly wage, maximum $170 per week
Puerto Rico	Disability Benefits Act	26	3 months from disability	Employee, 0.3; employer, 0.3	Based on wages earned during base year
Rhode Island	Temporary Disability Insurance Act	30	1 year from disability	1.4	4.62% of wages in the base period quarter in which wages were the highest

one in which the patient is seen by the physician but may continue to work. TD claims are those in which the injured cannot perform all the functions of his or her job for a limited period of time. Weekly TD benefits are based on the employee's earnings at the time of the injury. PD claims are those in which the injured worker is left with residual disability. Sometimes, such a person can be rehabilitated in another occupation, however, recent reforms in workers' compensation in some states replaced vocational rehabilitation with a voucher system that is not issued until after the case is settled. When the employee's condition becomes *permanent and stationary (P and S)* and no further improvement is expected, the industrial case is rated as to the percentage of permanent residual disability and **adjudicated** so a monetary settlement can be made, called a *compromise and release (C and R)*. This settlement can be awarded as a lump sum or in the form of monthly payments.

Reports

In most states, an initial report of an industrial injury is submitted by both the employer and the physician; it is a requirement of the law. The form and time limit to submit the report varies with each state. Copies of the first report (Figure 16-10) go to the insurance carrier, the state, and the employer, and one copy is retained by the physician. The initial report contains the history of the accident, present complaints (subjective information), past history, findings on physical examination (objective observations), laboratory and x-ray results, diagnosis, recommended treatment, disability (type and length), and prognosis.

STATE
COMPENSATION
INSURANCE
FUND

**DOCTOR'S FIRST REPORT OF
OCCUPATIONAL INJURY
OR ILLNESS
STATE OF CALIFORNIA**

Within 5 days of your initial examination, for every occupational injury or illness, send original and one copy of this report to the employer's workers' compensation insurance carrier or the self-insured employer. Failure to file a timely doctor's report may result in assessment of a civil penalty. **In the case of diagnosed or suspected pesticide poisoning,** send a copy of this report to Division of Labor Statistics and Research, P.O. Box 420603, San Francisco, CA 94142-0603, and notify your local health officer by telephone within 24 hours.

	PLEASE DO NOT USE THIS COLUMN
1. INSURER NAME AND ADDRESS STATE COMPENSATION INSURANCE FUND P.O. BOX 9045, OXNARD, CA 93031-9045	Case No.
2. EMPLOYER NAME Tri color Paint Company Policy # 189-2467-344	
3. Address: No. and Street City Zip 4200 Main Street, Woodland Hills, XY 12345-0000	Industry
4. Nature of business (e.g., food manufacturing, building construction, retailer of women's clothes) commercial painting company	County
5. PATIENT NAME (First name, middle initial, last name) Jack P. Hiner 6. Sex [X] Male [ ] Female 7. Date of Mo. Day Yr. Birth 11 - 02 - 45	Age
8. Address: No. and Street City Zip 789 Stanton Avenue, Woodland Hills, XY 12345-0000 9. Telephone number (555) 509-8760	Hazard
10. Occupation (Specific job title) house painter 11. Social Security Number 540 - XX - 1298	Disease
12. Injured at: No. and Street City County 5409 West First Street, Woodland Hills, Los Angeles	Hospitalization
13. Date and hour of injury or onset of illness Mo. Day Yr. 10 - 20 - 20XX Hour _____ a.m. 4:00 p.m. 14. Date last worked Mo. Day Yr. 10 - 20 - 20XX	Occupation
15. Date and hour of first examination or treatment Mo. Day Yr. 10 - 20 - 20XX Hour _____ a.m. 5:30 p.m. 16. Have you (or your office) previously treated patient? [ ] Yes [X] No	Return Date/Code

Patient please complete this portion, if able to do so. Otherwise, doctor please complete immediately. Inability or failure of a patient to complete this portion shall not affect his/her rights to workers' compensation under the California Labor Code.

17. DESCRIBE HOW THE ACCIDENT OR EXPOSURE HAPPENED (Give specific object, machinery or chemical. Use reverse side if more space is required.)

While painting a room ceiling, I slipped and fell from a ladder and hit the left side of my body and my head.

18. SUBJECTIVE COMPLAINTS (Describe fully. Use reverse side if more space is required.)

Left shoulder pain, head pain, dizziness, blurred vision

19. OBJECTIVE FINDINGS (Use reverse side if more space is required.)

A. Physical Examination

Abrasions, multiple contusions and sprain of the left shoulder, 2.5 cm head laceration; 2 views each AP & lat of lt hip, lt femur, and cervical spine, all negative.

B. X-ray and laboratory results (State if none or pending.)

20. DIAGNOSIS (If occupational illness, specify etiologic agent and duration of exposure.) Chemical or toxic compounds involved? [ ] Yes [X] No

Abrasions, multiple contusions, and sprain of the left shoulder. Head laceration. ICD-9 Code __ ____ . __

21. Are your findings and diagnosis consistent with patient's account of injury or onset of illness? [X] Yes [ ] No If "no", please explain.

21A. Based on your evaluation, is the injury/illness work related? [X] Yes [ ] No [ ] Further investigation needed

22. Is there any other current condition that will impede or delay patient's recovery? [ ] Yes [X] No If "yes", please explain.

23. TREATMENT RENDERED (Use reverse side if more space is required.)
Examination, x-rays, treated for abrasions and contusions, 2.5 cm head laceration sutured, to be kept under observation in hospital to rule out head trauma.

24. If further treatment required, specify treatment plan/estimated duration.

Hospital observation

25. If hospitalized as inpatient, give hospital name and location. Date admitted Mo. Day Yr. 10-20-20XX Estimated stay 1 day
College Hospital, 4500 Broad Ave., Woodland Hills

26. WORK STATUS – Is patient able to perform usual work? [ ] Yes [X] No
If no, date when patient can return to: Regular work 11/ 1 / 20XX
Modified work 10/ 29 / 20XX Specify restrictions No lifting

Doctor's Signature *Gerald Practon, MD* Date 10-22-20XX CA License Number C 4821X
Doctor Name and Degree (please type) Gerald Practon, MD IRS Number 95-366402XX
Address 4567 Broad Avenue, Woodland Hills, XY 12345-0000 Telephone Number (555) 486 9002

wtf
SCIF 3110 (REV. 2-93) FORM 5021 (Rev. 4) 1992

Figure 16-10. Example of a completed Doctor's First Report of Occupational Injury or Illness form for a workers' compensation case

Subsequent progress reports informing the carrier of the progress of the injured or ill worker are submitted each time the patient is seen or monthly. These reports are submitted either by completing forms, writing a letter, or copying the patient's chart.

Fee Schedule

Some states have adopted an RVS, which is used for coding and a fee schedule. In these states, a different conversion factor of dollars and cents is used for each of the six sections of the RVS codebook as seen in Example 16-3.

EXAMPLE 16-3

Workers' Compensation RVS Fee Schedule

$7.15/unit	Evaluation and Management section
$6.15/unit	Medicine section
$34.50/unit	Anesthesia section
$153.00/unit	Surgery section
$1.50/unit	Pathology section
$12.50/unit	Radiology section (total unit value column)
$1.95/unit	Radiology section (professional component unit value column)

The unit value is multiplied with the relative value amount for each procedure to determine the actual payment (see Example 16-4 on page 537).

Claims Submission

An itemized billing statement is usually submitted at the time the report is sent to the insurance company. All forms and letters must be signed in ink by the physician. A stamped signature is not acceptable. If payment is not received, the assistant should contact the employer to find out if the employer's report has been submitted. The physician does not bill the patient directly unless the insurance carrier will not accept the claim as an industrial case. Physicians accept payment from insurance carriers as payment in full.

If the patient is a private patient of the physician, a separate medical record and financial account (ledger) should be maintained for the industrial accident or illness. If the injured or ill person has several different industrial accidents on different dates, separate financial accounts and medical records are required for each situation.

Time Limit—Each state has a different time limit and form for reporting an accident or illness.

Timely filing of claim forms will keep the carrier informed about the ongoing cost of medical care. Contact the Workers' Compensation Board to inquire about your state's time limit for sending supplemental reports and filing claims.

GENERAL GUIDELINES FOR HANDLING INSURANCE CLAIMS

The medical assistant should verbally communicate information and provide a brochure to each patient outlining specific office policies regarding insurance procedures. This avoids misunderstandings and helps increase cooperation for claims processing.

Insurance Identification Card

Ask the patient to show his or her health insurance card, and note the effective date and pertinent information (Figure 16-11). Sometimes the reverse side of the card provides information on deductible, copayment, preapproval provisions, and insurance company name, address, and telephone number. Always copy front and back sides of the card and date the photocopy, as this provides error-free insurance data.

Patient Registration Form

The complete, accurate, and up-to-date information obtained on the patient registration form discussed in Chapter 5 and illustrated in Figure 5-5 is the same

---

PATIENT EDUCATION

On each visit, remind the patient to bring in his or her insurance identification card. Ask to see the card and verify the name and address of the insurance company and the policy number. If different, photocopy and date it, relaying the new information to the individual processing insurance claims.

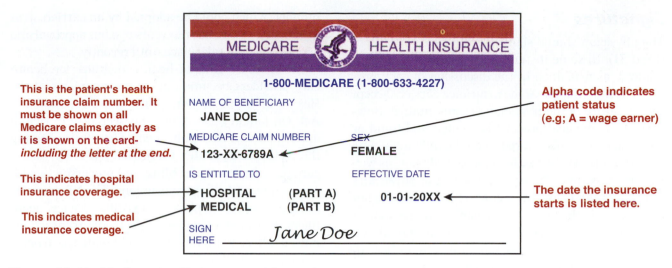

This is the patient's health insurance claim number. It must be shown on all Medicare claims exactly as it is shown on the card—*including the letter at the end.*

This indicates hospital insurance coverage.

This indicates medical insurance coverage.

Alpha code indicates patient status (e.g; A = wage earner)

The date the insurance starts is listed here.

MEDICARE HEALTH INSURANCE

1-800-MEDICARE (1-800-633-4227)

NAME OF BENEFICIARY
JANE DOE

MEDICARE CLAIM NUMBER   SEX
123-XX-6789A   **FEMALE**

IS ENTITLED TO   EFFECTIVE DATE
HOSPITAL   **(PART A)**   **01-01-20XX**
MEDICAL   **(PART B)**

SIGN
HERE _____ *Jane Doe* _____

Figure 16-11. Medicare health insurance claim card

data abstracted and included on an insurance claim form. This information needs to be re-verified frequently for claims to be processed efficiently.

Assignments and Consent/Authorization

The CMS-1500 claim form includes an assignment of benefits (Field 12 for government programs and Field 13 for private insurance) and a consent to release medical information statement (Field 12). All patients should sign a consent to release medical information either on the claim form or on a separate **consent form** kept in their file. If the physician has a contract with the insurance company or wishes to have the insurance check sent to the office, the patient is asked to sign the assignment of benefits statement either on the form or on a separate form kept in his or her file.

Completing the Claim

If it is office policy to complete and submit the insurance claim form for the patient, the assistant should do so even in situations when coverage of specific services are in question. An official rejection from the carrier may be the best explanation to present to the patient. Electronic submission is preferred; however, if paper claims are being processed, the assistant should use the revised CMS-1500 (08/05) Health Insurance Claim Form (Figure 16-4). This form is accepted by nearly all private insurance, managed care plans, and government programs (i.e., TRICARE, Medicaid, and Medicare). Instructions for individual

COMPLIANCE

Inform the patient of his or her right to know how health information is used, when asking for a signature on a consent/authorization form. Refer to Chapter 3 for a complete discussion on this HIPAA requirement.

fields on the CMS-1500 claim form for the major programs are included in Appendix A of this textbook. By learning field requirements on paper claims, these learned-components can be used while inputting information into a computerized system for electronic submission.

Proofreading

Proofread every paper claim, especially longer and more complex claims, as they involve larger sums of money and are more difficult to complete. Try to be as accurate as possible when inputting data. Review the data, and check for transposition of numbers (group, policy, claim, physician's identification, diagnostic and procedural codes), misspelled name(s), incorrect gender, missing date of birth, and blanks appearing in mandatory fields.

When submitting electronically, software code edit checks (in the physician's or insurance company's computer) can identify invalid codes, age conflicts, gender conflicts, procedure and diagnostic code linkage conflicts, and other problematic data before claims are processed or paid.

Signatures

The physician should sign the insurance claim form (Field 31). In some instances a stamped signature is allowed, as explained in the discussion of each program in this chapter. Some insurance carriers accept the signature of the physician's representative. However, if the medical practice is audited and fraud or embezzlement is discovered, then the individual who had signature authorization can be held liable as well as the physician. The assistant keys the physician's name above or below the signature if the name is not preprinted on the form. A removable adhesive indicator tab may be placed where the physician should sign the claim. The medical assistant inserts his or her initials in the bottom lower left corner of the claim to eliminate confusion as to who completed the form, in case a claim is returned because of errors.

Posting to the Account

All charges are posted individually on the patient's account or ledger with the date and a brief description of the service. An entry is made with the current date indicating the insurance has been billed and stating the name of the carrier (see Chapter 15, Figure 15-3A). Inclusive dates of service should also be shown so money received can be applied accurately. The assistant then files the office copy of the completed insurance form in a separate insurance file (preferred method) or in the back of the patient's medical record.

When the insurance payment is received, the assistant posts the payment to the account or ledger as well as the daysheet or journal, indicating the date received, received on account (ROA), name of the insurance company, check voucher number, amount of payment, and name of the patient if the account contains family members.

Provider Identification Numbers

The physician's or medical group's Internal Revenue Service employer identification number (EIN) or Social Security number (SSN) must appear on the insurance claim (Field 25) for tax purposes.

In years past, medical practices who submitted claims to a number of different health plans had to keep track of multiple provider numbers. Provider Identification Numbers (PINs), Unique Physician Identification Numbers (UPINs), state license numbers, and other insurance-assigned numbers were all used on claim forms to identify physicians, specialties, medical groups, and office locations. A standardized

number, which could be adopted by all carriers, was introduced more than ten years ago but approval and adoption did not take place until recently.

A standard unique health identifier for health care providers became one of the mandates of the Health Information Portability and Accountability Act. On January 23, 2004, the Secretary of Health and Human Services published a Final Rule adopting the **National Provider Identifier (NPI)** for health care providers to use in filing and processing health care claims and other transactions. The NPI is a new number that will replace all existing "legacy" identifiers. Providers completing electronic transactions must use the NPI by May 23, 2007. Small health plans must use the NPI by May 23, 2008.

The NPI requirement applies by law to covered entities such as health care providers, clearinghouses, and health plans in the United States when exchanging electronic transactions for which a national standard has been adopted under HIPAA. Other health care plans may elect to require use of the NPI in submission of paper claims and for non-HIPAA transaction purposes. At present, the Centers for Medicare and Medicaid Services (CMS) have adopted the NPI for the Medicare program and it should also be used when reporting Medicaid, TRICARE, and CHAMPVA claims.

The NPI is an all-numeric intelligence-free identifier consisting of 10 digits (9 plus a check digit in the last position). The numbers do not carry other information about the health care providers, such as the state in which they live or their medical specialty. The NPI is a lifetime number that will not change if the provider changes location or specialty. The implementation of this number is a step forward in standardizing electronic health care transactions; providers will be able to submit transactions to any health plan in the United States. Transactions, such as the remittance advice and referral authorizations will also be transmitted using this number.

COMPLIANCE

All HIPAA covered health care providers, whether individuals (e.g., physicians, nurse practitioners, chiropractors), or organizations (e.g., hospitals, home health agencies, clinics, group practices) must obtain an NPI for use to identify themselves in HIPAA standard transactions.

Claims Submission

Insurance claims can be sent on paper using the new revised CMS-1500 claim form (08/05) or electronically using a modem.

Paper Submission

The paper claim form (CMS-1500) is only accepted from physicians and suppliers who are excluded from mandatory electronic claim submission as required by law. It has been revised as of August 2005 to include room for the new NPI 10-digit number as well as "legacy" identifiers.

A transition period, from October 1, 2006, to March 31, 2007, has been set to start receiving the new form with the new identifier (NPI). During this time there will be a dual acceptability period of the current and revised forms. The old form (12/90) will be discontinued April 1, 2007, and only the revised form (08/05) will be accepted. There is a strong possibility that the Center for Medicare and Medicaid Services will revise the CMS-1500 insurance claim form again after the NPI is in place, so that all fields used for the legacy numbers during the transition can be renamed or replaced and more fields allowed for diagnostic codes.

There are a number of methods for submitting paper insurance claims after they have been either manually completed (typed) or printed (generated) via computer. The medical practice may send them by mail, transmit them via fax machine, or employ a billing service for submitting insurance claims.

It must be noted that there will be increased delays in paper claims—some will be held for 28 days and only paid if the payment reserves have not been exhausted once the claim is eligible for determination.

Electronic Submission

Another method for submission of claims is using an *electronic claims transmission (ECT)* computer software system. This method requires the physician's computer to communicate directly to the insurance carrier's computer using a modem via the telephone or a DSL line. This paperless method allows for fewer errors and omissions when compared with manual processing, and provides a quicker turnaround time (7 to 14 days) from submission to payment. The insurance carrier automatically issues a check unless an error or omission occurs causing the claim to be set aside for manual review.

Electronic transmission can also occur in several ways. An insurance biller on site can transmit; the

COMPLIANCE

On July 1, 2005, electronic Medicare claim submission became mandatory for all physicians, practitioners, and suppliers unless they have fewer than ten full-time employees; some other exceptions apply.

physician can employ a billing service to input information, transmit, and follow up; or the practice can employ a **clearinghouse**. This service receives claims in a central location, usually electronically from the medical practice. Claims are sorted, processed through a computer claims error check, and electronically transmitted to the appropriate insurance carriers. The clearinghouse may charge for its services by claim, month, or amount billed. This service is also used by offices that are not computerized or do not have a modem for electronic billing. An *Attachment Control Form* (*ACF*) has been developed and is available on government Web sites to assist the process of linking paper attachments to electronic claims.

Regardless of the system used, the computer-generated or electronic insurance claim must comply with national electronic standards. Prior to billing electronically, the medical practice must transmit a sample claim or send samples of proposed forms to insurance carriers and ask them to examine the format and coding for compatibility with their system.

Provider's Signature—Each medical practice must have a signed agreement with individual carriers so claims can be submitted electronically. The physi-

COMPLIANCE

The Health Insurance Portability and Accountability Act (HIPAA), passed by Congress in 1996, legislated that the federal government adopt national electronic standards for automated transfer of certain health care data between health care payers, plans, and providers, thus eliminating all nonstandard formats. The standard code set is ANSI ASC X12N v4010 837 and was implemented in 2001 with compliance by October 2002. This electronic claim may be referred to as the Health Care Claim: Professional. The field data is almost identical to data required on the CMS-1500 claim form.

cian's signature on the agreement is a substitute for his or her signature on the claim form.

Patients' Signatures—Each patient must have a signature on file (SOF) in his or her medical record if the patient's claims are to be processed by ECT. This consent authorizes information to be sent to the insurance carrier.

CODING FOR PROFESSIONAL SERVICES

When coding insurance claims the diagnosis code will determine whether the physician gets paid and the procedure code will determine how much the practice receives. Codes from a Standard Code Set should be used, which has been developed by the Centers for Medicare and Medicaid Services (CMS), formerly known as the Health Care Financing Administration (HCFA) and mandated by HIPAA (Figure 16-12). Codes within this standard that apply to billing outpatient medical claims include:

- *International Classification of Diseases*, 9th Edition, *Clinical Modification (ICD-9-CM)* (diagnostic codes)
- *Current Procedural Terminology (CPT)* (also referred to as *HCPCS Level I* codes for procedures and services)
- *Healthcare Common Procedure Coding System (HCPCS) Level II* codes

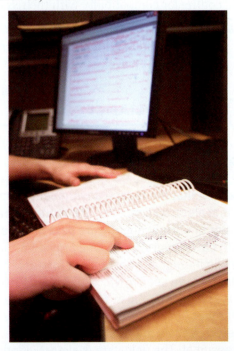

Figure 16-12. Medical assistant at the computer completing and coding an insurance claim

The approved code set was implemented by all providers October 2003 and October 2004 for small health care plans. *HCPCS Level III* codes, which were codes developed by local and regional health plans, have been phased out.

CPT Codebook

The most common reference used to code procedures is the annual publication entitled *Current Procedural Terminology (CPT)** published by the American Medical Association. This code system uses five-digit numbers with two-digit modifiers. New codes are added, deleted, and descriptions revised each October, so it is important to obtain the current edition to code accurately. Mini *CPT* codebooks are available for specialty practices, and coding software may be purchased to assist in the assignment of codes.

Computerized assisted coding (CAC) automatically assigns codes to clinical procedures and services. CAC can integrate with other systems like document imaging and transcription, making remote coding a possibility; however, as this becomes integrated in medical offices, the coder's responsibilities may change to include such things as editing and analyzing data, outcomes, and coding trends. Personal digital assistants (PDAs) are also being used in the coding and billing process. They can easily capture, store, and manipulate a variety of information, helping to secure charges and track, record, and access patient data while reducing paperwork. Use of the *CPT* codebook will be emphasized in this chapter.

HCPCS Level II Codebook

HCPCS Level II codes are used to code those services, products, supplies, drugs, and procedures generally not fully listed in the *CPT* codebook. There are both temporary and permanent codes. This second level is composed of alphanumeric codes from A through V (e.g., AD021 = ambulance service) and is used by all regional Medicare fiscal agents or carriers along with many other insurance programs. Special alpha modifiers (e.g., AA = anesthesia services performed personally by anesthesiologist), and alpha-numeric modifiers (e.g., A1 = dressing for one wound) have been developed by CMS to clarify unusual services or procedures not fully described by *HCPCS* codes. An example list of *HCPCS* codes with alpha modifiers may be found in the Mock Fee Schedule shown in Part IV: Appendix of the *Workbook*.

---

*2007 Current Procedural Terminology © 2006 American Medical Association. All rights reserved.

RVS Codebook

Another code system commonly used in workers' compensation billing is the relative value scale [schedule] (RVS). This code system falls outside of the standard code set mandated via the HIPAA. Five-digit codes and two-digit modifiers are also used with this coding system, but it includes unit values for each service and procedure. The unit value indicates the relative value for each service performed, taking into account the time, skill, and overhead cost required (see Example 16-4). The units in this scale are based on median charges of all physicians during the period in which the *RVS* was published. Conversion factors are used to translate the abstract units in the scale to dollar fees for each service. A commonly used annual publication is entitled *Relative Values for Physicians* by Ingenix. For information on where to obtain all codebooks mentioned, refer to Resources at the end of this chapter.

EXAMPLE 16-4

Relative Value Scale Fee Formula

Procedure Code	Description	Units
10000	Incision and drainage of cyst	0.8

Using a hypothetical figure of $153/unit, this procedure would be valued at $122.40.

Math: $153.00 \times 0.8 = 122.40

Terminology

The medical assistant needs to be familiar with terminology used in codebooks as well as reimbursement and medical terminology to process and follow up on insurance claims. Acronyms, symbols, and abbreviations must be interpreted for efficient coding and claim form completion. Coding is an art, not an exact science.

Codebook Terms

The *Current Procedural Terminology** codebook uses medical and surgical terminology to accurately describe professional services so correct codes can be assigned and maximum payment from insurance carriers can be obtained.

Codebook terms also relate to the type of care the patient receives. As mentioned in Chapter 7, a *new patient* is one who has not received any professional services from the physician, or another physician of the same specialty who belongs to the same group practice, within the past three years. An *established patient* is one who has received professional services from the physician, or another physician of the same specialty who belongs to the same group practice, within the past three years.

Concurrent care is the provision of similar services (e.g., hospital visits) to the same patient by more than one physician on the same day. The physicians are typically from different specialties, taking care of different medical problems. When concurrent care is provided, each physician is cross-referenced on the claim form.

Critical care is the care of an unstable, acutely ill or injured patient requiring constant bedside attention by a physician (e.g., cardiac arrest, shock, bleeding, respiratory failure, postoperative complications, a seriously ill neonate, and so forth). Critical care may sometimes but not always be rendered in a critical care area, such as the coronary care unit, intensive care unit, respiratory care unit, or emergency care facility.

Emergency care differs from critical care in that it is provided to prevent serious impairment of bodily functions or a serious dysfunction to a body part or organ. It is typically provided in an emergency department and codes 99281 through 99285 are used. Code 99288 is used when advanced life support is required during emergency care. If office services are provided on an emergency basis, code 99058 from the medicine section may be used in addition to a code from the evaluation and management section.

Counseling is a discussion with a patient and family concerning one or more of the following:

1. Diagnostic results, impressions, and recommended diagnostic studies
2. Prognosis
3. Risks and benefits of treatment options
4. Instructions for treatment and/or follow-up
5. Importance of compliance with chosen treatment options
6. Risk factor reduction
7. Patient and family education

It may be billed separately if a complete history and physical examination does not take place.

Consultations can occur in a home, office, hospital, extended care facility, and so forth. A physician consultant gives a second opinion regarding a con-

---

*2007 Current Procedural Terminology © 2006 American Medical Association. All rights reserved.

dition or need for surgery and may initiate diagnostic or therapeutic services. Remember the three "Rs" when *coding consultations:* services must be *requested* by another physician, findings and recommendations must be *recorded,* and a *report* must be sent to the referring physician. Codes* for consultations are as follows:

- Office or other outpatient consultations (new or established patient) 99241 through 99245
- Initial inpatient consultations (new or established patient) 99251 through 99255

If an insurance company (except Medicare) states that a second opinion is necessary prior to approval for a surgery, modifier -32 (mandated services) should be applied to the consultation code. If a physician performs a follow-up consultation in a hospital setting, the appropriate subsequent hospital care code should be selected. For each admission, only one initial consultation should be reported. If a physician performs a follow-up consultation in an office setting, the office consultation codes may be used again. If follow-up visits in the consultant's office take place, the appropriate new patient or established patient evaluation and management code should be used.

A *referral* is the *transfer* of the total or specific care of a patient from one physician to another. It is not a consultation. However, a patient may be referred from one physician to another for a consultation.

Codebook Symbols

With each annual edition of *CPT,** there are new codes and description changes indicated by the use of symbols, as seen in Figure 16-13. Other symbols are used to alert the coder when codes can or cannot be used in certain situations. It is important to be mindful of these symbols and become familiar with the new codes and any description changes. Appendix B in the *CPT* codebook gives a summary of the additions, deletions, and revisions.

Key Terms in Documentation

As discussed previously, all services and procedures must be documented in the medical record. To code, obtain a copy of the patient's operative report and review it carefully. Look for key terms that may change the code or determine the need for the assignment of a modifier, such as "very difficult," "extensive," "complicated," "hemorrhage," "blood loss of over 600 cc," "unusual findings or circumstances," "multiple,"

"ordinary," "simple," "uncomplicated," "unilateral," or "bilateral." If unsure about a code assignment, ask the physician to clarify the case. Medical terminology is very technical and can puzzle even the most knowledgeable medical assistant. A good medical dictionary can help. If the case is complex, send copies of the operative report, discharge summary, or any test reports to the insurance carrier.

If the physician verbally says "extensive complications," make sure this appears in the report to validate the codes chosen.

Reimbursement Terminology

When processing claims, certain terms are used to communicate situations when services and procedures may be suspended, paid less than charged, or denied because of the codes selected or other medically necessary criteria. Following are common situations and terminology used when they occur.

Down Coding—When *down coding* occurs, the computer system changes the submitted code to a lower level code. This can occur in the following instances.

1. When the coding system used on the insurance claim does not match the coding system used by the insurance company receiving the claim. The computer converts the code submitted to the closest code in use. Payment generated is typically less.

2. When the claims examiner in a workers' compensation case must convert the *CPT* code submitted to an RVS code. The claims examiner will pick the lowest-paying code. Before billing, find which RVS system is used by the carrier and find the best match for the *CPT* code.

3. When a claims examiner reviews an attached document and compares the code used with the written description of the procedure. If the two do not match, the insurance carrier will reimburse according to the lowest-paying code that fits the description stated.

To detect down coding and prevent further occurrences, always monitor reimbursement and become knowledgeable about which codes are affected. Call the insurance carrier and verify that the standard code set is being used.

Upcoding—The term *upcoding* is the practice of billing a health plan for a procedure that reimburses the

---

*2007 Current Procedural Terminology © 2006 American Medical Association. All rights reserved.

Current Procedural Terminology Codebook Symbols

New code

● 64650   Chemodenervation of eccrine glands; both axillae

Revised code (altered procedure descriptor)

▲ 44310   Ileostomy or jejunostomy, non-tube

New or revised text (other than the procedure descriptors)

▶◀ 90760   Intravenous infusion, hydration; initial, up to 1 hr
            ▶(Do not report 90760 if performed as a concurrent
              infusion service)◀

Add–on code

+11732   Avulsion of nail plate, each additional nail plate (list separately in addition
          to code for primary procedure)

Modifier –51 exempt

⊘ 17004   Destruction (e.g., laser surgery) of 15 or more lesions

Conscious Sedation

⊙ 33233   Removal of permanent pacemaker pulse generator

Product Pending FDA Approval

⫽ 90736   Zoster (Shingles) vaccine, live, for subcutaneous injection

Reference to *CPT Assistant*, Clinical Examples in Radiology and *CPT* Changes book

47000   Biopsy of liver, needle: percutaneous
      ➥ *CPT Assistant* Fall 93:12

2007 Current Procedural Terminology © 2006 American Medical Association. All rights reserved.

Figure 16-13. *Current Procedural Terminology** codebook symbols

physician at a higher rate than a procedure actually done; also know as *code creep, overcoding,* or *overbilling.* Because computer software has built-in edits referred to as post-payment screens in the Medicare program, this may be easily spotted and can lead to an audit and penalties.

Bundled Codes—A bundled code contains a grouping of several services that are related to a procedure. Sometimes a payment notice will state "Benefits have been combined." The Medicare program has many procedures considered bundled. For example, a sterile tray (99070) is typically bundled with the service unless a second tray is needed due to complications so it is not billed separately. Services such as telephone calls, surgical dressings, and reading of test results are typically bundled into evaluation and management codes.

Unbundling—*Unbundling* is breaking down a procedure into separate billable codes with charges to increase reimbursement; also know as *fragmentation, exploding,* or *à la carte* medicine. To code a bilateral procedure using two codes when one code includes it in the description is a good example of unbundling (see *CPT Code* 77056). Insurers use special software to detect unbundling. This practice is considered fraud and can lead to audit and costly penalties. The use of out-of-date codes often result in unbundling so it is important to use current codebooks.

Codebook Sections

There are six sections in *CPT*.* Within each main section, there may be subsections, categories, and subcategories divided according to anatomic body systems, procedure, condition, description, and specialty.

At the beginning of each section are guidelines relating to that section. Read these thoroughly prior to coding as they contain helpful definitions and directions. *CPT* codes are considered Category I codes. At the end of all Category I codes are Category II and III codes, which have been developed to improve the coding system. Category II codes (performance measurements) are optional and are used to help decrease the need for record abstraction and chart review. Category III codes are temporary codes used for emerging technologies and new services or procedures.

Table 16-4 lists the main sections for the 2007 edition of *CPT*.

Evaluation and Management Section

The evaluation and management (E/M) section has subsections, categories, and subcategories that have codes with three to five levels for reporting purposes. These levels are represented by the last digit (9920**1**) and are based on key components and contributory factors. To code, first determine the following:

- place of service (POS)
- type of service (TOS)
- patient status (new versus established)

Then familiarize yourself with the section divisions by looking at Table 1 (Categories and Subcategories of Service) found in the Evaluation and Management

Table 16-4. Sections of the *Current Procedural Terminology* Codebook with Code Ranges

Section	Code Range
Evaluation and Management (E/M)	99201 to 99499
Anesthesia	00100 to 01999
	99100 to 99150
Surgery	10021 to 69990
Radiology	70010 to 79999
Pathology and Laboratory	80048 to 89356
Medicine	90281 to 99602
Category II	0001F to 6005F
Category III	0016T to 0170T

(E/M) Guidelines at the beginning of the E/M section. Once you have located the right POS, TOS, and patient status, read the description thoroughly to match the *key components*:

- history
- physical examination
- medical decision making

Note the *contributory factors*, counseling, coordination of care, nature of presenting problem, and face-to-face time for the service. For detailed information about the key components and contributory factors refer to Chapter 9, "Patient Medical History," Physical Examination," and "Complexity of Medical Decision Making."

For a new patient, all three of the key components must be present to assign a code; otherwise code to the lowest key component mentioned by the physician. For an established patient, two out of three key components must be present to assign a code.

An additional subsection on preventive medicine is categorized according to new or established patients and patient ages to be used for such services as routine physical examinations and well body checkups.

In the majority of E/M services where counseling or coordination of care dominates (more than 50 percent) the face-to-face physician/patient encounter, *time* is considered the key component to qualify for a particular level of service. As learned in Chapter 9, documentation is required in the patient's record to substantiate the chosen level. Tables 16-5 and 16-6 give a concise view of the components for the most common E/M code numbers. In the *CPT* codebook, medical case scenarios are presented in Appendix C, as clinical examples to assist in the correct selection of codes.

Anesthesia Section

The anesthesia section is divided into subsections according to the anatomic site where the surgery is performed. After locating the correct site, you must determine what type of anesthetic was administered and by whom, (e.g., anesthesiologist, nurse anesthesist).

After the code selection is made, anesthesia modifiers are assigned to indicate patient status (e.g., P3 = patient with severe systemic disease). Special add-on codes are used in addition for qualifying circumstances if they exist, such as 99100, "Anesthesia for patient of extreme age, under 1 year and older than 70."

Surgery Section

The surgery section is the largest section in *CPT*.* It is divided into subsections according to body systems, (e.g., integumentary, musculoskeletal). In the integumentary system, lacerations (wounds) are treated as *simple, intermediate,* or *complex* repairs. Simple lacerations are superficial, whereas intermediate lacerations involve subcutaneous tissue and require layered closure. Complex repairs require more than layered closure (e.g., reconstructive surgery). Repairs are coded according to the type of repair, location, and the length in centimeters (cm) rather than inches. When multiple wounds of the same type (e.g., simple) occur in the same area (e.g., scalp, neck, axillae) add together the lengths of all and report them with a single code. If the wound repairs are not of the same type and area, list the most complex first or that with the highest dollar value. The first code will be given the highest payment and the payments for the subsequent codes will be substantially decreased.

Surgical code descriptions may define a correct coding relationship when one code is part of another (see Example 16-5).

EXAMPLE 16-5

Descriptive Surgical Code Language

Partial or *complete,* which means the partial procedure is included in the complete procedure.

56620	Vulvectomy simple; *partial*
56625	*complete*

Partial or *total,* which means the partial procedure is included in the total procedure.

58940	Oophorectomy, *partial* or *total*

Unilateral and *bilateral,* which means the unilateral procedure is included in the bilateral procedure.

58900	Biopsy of ovary, *unilateral* or *bilateral* (separate procedure)

Single and *multiple,* which means the single procedure is included in the multiple procedure.

49321	Laparoscopy, surgical; with biopsy (*single* or *multiple*)

How to Code from the Surgery Section—To code from the surgery section, look in the index under the service or procedure, organ or anatomic site, condition, synonym, eponym, or abbreviation. Then look for subterms until you identify the procedure or service. You will find either a single code (e.g., Abdomen, Abdominal Wall, Removal, *Mesh . . . 11008*), several code listings (e.g., Abdomen, Abscess, *Incision and Drainage . . . 49020, 49040*), or a code range (e.g., Abdomen, Drainage, *Fluid . . . 49080—49081*). Be sure to look up all codes listed after index subterms by turning to the correct codebook section and then reading the code descriptions (e.g., 26011). To read the description, start with the stand-alone code that is nonindented (see 26010); it appears above the indented code. Read the first part of the code description up to the semicolon (i.e., Drainage of finger abscess), then continue reading the indented description of the chosen code (i.e., complicated). The indented language is used to save space in the codebook.

Surgical Supplies—Typically the surgical tray is included in the procedure code for the surgery being performed. However, if a sterile surgical tray is used for office surgery and the materials are over and above those usually included for such a surgery, *CPT* code 99070 from the medicine section may be used and supplies may be itemized on an attachment and given a separate fee.

Surgical Package Rules—Surgical package rules apply to major and minor surgical procedures and include bundled services with the surgery code. This concept means the surgical code includes the operation, local infiltration, digital block or topical anesthesia, and normal, uncomplicated postoperative care (follow-up hospital visits, discharge, and follow-up office visits) for a number of designated follow-up days. This is referred to as a "package" for surgical procedures, and one fee covers the entire package. Preoperative services (consultations, office visits, and initial hospital care) are usually billed and paid for separately if they occur more than 24 hours prior to surgery. The Centers for Medicare and Medicaid Services (CMS) and the American Medical Association (AMA) provide different definitions of what is included in the package fee, so it is wise to determine whether the carrier is following CMS or AMA guidelines.

Follow-Up Days—A variable number (10, 30, or 90) of follow-up days after surgery is included in the surgical code depending on whether it is minor or major surgery. Postoperative (*text continues on page 545*)

Table 16-5. Selection of E/M Codes for Office/Other Outpatient and Inpatient Services

E/M Code	History	Exam	Medical Decision Making	Problem Severity	Coordination of Care; Counseling	Time Spent (avg.)
Office or Other Outpatient Services						
New Patient*						
99201	Problem-focused	Problem-focused	Straightforward	Minor or self-limited	Consistent with problem(s) and patient's needs	10 min. face to face
99202	Expanded Problem-focused	Expanded Problem-focused	Straightforward	Low to moderate	Consistent with problem(s) and patient's needs	20 min. face to face
99203	Detailed	Detailed	Low complexity	Moderate	Consistent with problem(s) and patient's needs	30 min. face to face
99204	Comprehensive	Comprehensive	Moderate complexity	Moderate to high	Consistent with problem(s) and patient's needs	45 min. face to face
99205	Comprehensive	Comprehensive	High complexity	Moderate to high	Consistent with problem(s) and patient's needs	60 min. face to face
Established Patient*						
99211	—	—	Physician supervision but presence not required	Minimal	Consistent with problem(s) and patient's needs	5 min. face to face
99212	Problem-focused	Problem-focused	Straightforward	Minor or self-limited	Consistent with problem(s) and patient's needs	10 min. face to face
99213	Expanded Problem-focused	Expanded Problem-focused	Low complexity	Low to moderate	Consistent with problem(s) and patient's needs	15 min. face to face
99214	Detailed	Detailed	Moderate complexity	Moderate to high	Consistent with problem(s) and patient's needs	25 min. face to face
99215	Comprehensive	Comprehensive	High complexity	Moderate to high	Consistent with problem(s) and patient's needs	40 min. face to face
Hospital Observation Services						
99217	Observation care discharge services—use with codes 99218–99220					
99218	Detailed or Comprehensive	Detailed or Comprehensive	Straightforward or low complexity	Low	Consistent with problem(s) and patient's needs	—
99219	Comprehensive	Comprehensive	Moderate complexity	Moderate	Consistent with problem(s) and patient's needs	—

*Key component: For new patients with initial office and other outpatient services, all three components (history, exam, and medical decision making) are essential in selecting the correct code. For established patients, at least two of these three components are required.

Table 16-5 (*continued*). Selection of E/M Codes for Office/Other Outpatient and Inpatient Services

E/M Code	History	Exam	Medical Decision Making	Problem Severity	Coordination of Care; Counseling	Time Spent (avg.)
Hospital Observation Services (*continued*)						
99220	Comprehensive	Comprehensive	High complexity	High	Consistent with problem(s) and patient's needs	—
99234	Detailed or Comprehensive	Detailed or Comprehensive	Straightforward or low complexity	Low	Consistent with problem(s) and patient's needs	Admit and discharge on same day
99235	Comprehensive	Comprehensive	Moderate	Moderate	Consistent with problem(s) and patient's needs	Admit and discharge on same day
99236	Comprehensive	Comprehensive	High	High	Consistent with problem(s) and patient's needs	Admit and discharge on same day
Hospital Inpatient Services: Initial Care*						
99221	Detailed or Comprehensive	Detailed or Comprehensive	Straightforward or low complexity	Low	Consistent with problem(s) and patient's needs	30 min unit/floor
99222	Comprehensive	Comprehensive	Moderate complexity	Moderate	Consistent with problem(s) and patient's needs	50 min. unit/floor
92223	Comprehensive	Comprehensive	High complexity	High	Consistent with problem(s) and patient's needs	70 min. unit/floor
Hospital Inpatient Services: Subsequent Care*						
99231	Problem-focused interval	Problem-focused	Straightforward or low complexity	Stable, recovering, or improving	Consistent with problem(s) and patient's needs	15 min. unit/floor
99232	Expanded problem-focused interval	Expanded problem-focused complication	Moderate complexity	Inadequate response to treatment; minor	Consistent with problem(s) and patient's needs	25 min. unit/floor
99233	Detailed interval	Detailed	High complexity	Unstable; significant new problem or complication	Consistent with problem(s) and patient's needs	35 min. unit/floor
99238	Hospital discharge day management	—	—	—	—	30 min. or/ less
99239	Hospital discharge day management	—	—	—	—	more than 30 min.

Key component: For new patients with initial office and other outpatient services, all three components (history, exam, and medical decision making) are essential in selecting the correct code. For established patients, at least two of these three components are required.

Table 16-6. Code Selection Criteria for Consultations

E/M Code	History	Medical Decision Exam	Problem Making	Severity	Coordination of Care; Counseling	Time Spent (avg.)
			Consultations			
Office and Other Outpatient						
99241	Problem-focused	Problem-focused	Straightforward	Minor or self-limited	Consistent with problem(s) and patient's needs	15 min. face to face
99242	Expanded	Expanded problem-focused	Straightforward	Low problem-focused	Consistent with problem(s) and patient's needs	30 min. face to face
99243	Detailed	Detailed	Low complexity	Moderate	Consistent with problem(s) and patient's needs	40 min. face to face
99244	Comprehensive	Comprehensive	Moderate Complexity	Moderate to high	Consistent with problem(s) and patient's needs	60 min. face to face
99245	Comprehensive	Comprehensive	High Complexity	Moderate to high	Consistent with problem(s) and patient's needs	80 min. face to face
Initial Inpatient*						
99251	Problem-focused	Problem-focused	Straightforward	Minor or self-limited	Consistent with problem(s) and patient's needs	20 min. unit/floor
99252	Expanded problem-focused	Expanded problem-focused	Straightforward	Low	Consistent with problem(s) and patient's needs	40 min. unit/floor
99253	Detailed	Detailed	Low complexity	Moderate	Consistent with problem(s) and patient's needs	55 min. unit/floor
99254	Comprehensive	Comprehensive	Moderate complexity	Moderate to high	Consistent with problem(s) and patient's needs	80 min. unit/floor
99255	Comprehensive	Comprehensive	High complexity	Moderate to high	Consistent with problem(s) and patient's needs	110 min. unit/floor

*Key component: For initial care, all three components (history, exam, and medical decision making) are essential in selecting the correct code. For subsequent care, at least two of these three components are required.

2007 Current Procedural Terminology © 2006 American Medical Association. All rights reserved.

services pertaining to the surgery may not be billed separately during this period. Since the codebook does not specify how many follow-up days should be given to a specific surgical procedure, a separate reference is needed. A source that lists the follow-up days (global fee period) for each surgical procedure is the Medicare fee schedule published annually in the *Federal Register*. See Resources at the end of this chapter for the Web site address.

Medicare Global Package—The surgical package concept is used by Medicare (CMS) with varying rules. It is referred to as the Medicare global surgery policy for surgeries and includes the following:

1. Preoperative: E/M office visit or hospital visit one day (24 hours) prior to hospital admit

2. Intraoperative: Services that are a usual and necessary part of a surgical procedure, such as local infiltration, digital block, or topical anesthesia

3. Postoperative: Routine postoperative care and any complications not requiring return to the operating room 10, 30, or 90 days after surgery

Services provided for a Medicare patient not included in the global surgery package are:

1. Initial consultation or evaluation regardless of when it occurs (apply modifier -57 if within 24 hours prior to surgery)

2. Postoperative visits unrelated to diagnosis for which surgical procedure was performed (modifier -24 would apply)

3. Treatment required to stabilize a seriously ill patient before surgery

4. Diagnostic tests and procedures

5. Related procedure for postoperative complications that requires a return trip to operating room (modifier -78 would apply)

6. Immunosuppressive therapy following transplant surgery

Radiology Section

Diagnostic radiology, ultrasound, radiation oncology, and nuclear medicine are listed in the radiology section but are coded separately. When coding x-rays, take into consideration the part of the body viewed, number of views, and type of view, such as AP (anteroposterior), Lat (lateral), Obl (oblique), and so on. If the radiology procedure was complicated and not sufficiently described by a code, attach a copy of the x-ray report.

Pathology and Laboratory Section

A pathologist working in a hospital or freestanding laboratory will use codes from this section for tests performed. When the physician performs laboratory work in a physician office laboratory (POL), it is coded separately from office visits. Locate codes in subsections that describe the type of test (e.g., urinalysis, chemistry, hematology). If the physician collects a specimen, such as a pap smear, biopsy, or throat culture, and sends it to an outside laboratory, assign code 99000 from the medicine section for collection and handling of a specimen. If the medical assistant performs a phlebotomy and obtains a blood sample, assign code 36415 (venipuncture).

Medicine Section

The medicine section includes codes representing diagnostic and therapeutic services that are generally not surgically invasive. These codes may be used in conjunction with codes from all different sections of *CPT.** The *CPT* table of contents may be reviewed to determine various subsections (e.g., vaccines, toxoids, psychiatry, ophthalmology, and so forth).

Injections are found in the medicine section and the type of injection (therapeutic, prophylactic, diagnostic), as well as the route—IA (intra-arterial), IM (intramuscular), IV (intravenous), SC or SQ (subcutaneous), ID (intradermal), or parent (parenteral)—needs to be determined prior to code assignment. When documenting injections, the physician records the name of the medication, the amount of injection in cubic centimeters or grams, and the route of administration. When coding injections, use one code for the product and one for the administration.

Code Modifiers

A modifier is used in addition to the procedure code to indicate circumstances in which a procedure as performed differs in some way from that described by the *CPT* five-digit code. In some billing scenarios, it is necessary to use two-digit modifiers to give a more accurate description of the services rendered. Use of modifiers prevents a physician's fee profile from being affected. Refer to Table 16-7 for a complete list of

---

*2007 Current Procedural Terminology © 2006 American Medical Association. All rights reserved.

Table 16-7. *Current Procedural Terminology* Modifier Codes. (CPT codes, descriptions, and material are taken from 2007 Current Procedural Terminology © 2006 American Medical Association. All rights reserved.)*

Modifier Code	Explanation
-21	**Prolonged Evaluation and Management Services:** *When the face-to-face or floor/unit service(s) provided is prolonged or otherwise greater than that usually required for the highest level of evaluation and management service within a given category, it may be identified by adding modifier -21 to the evaluation and management code number. A report may also be appropriate.**
	Example: A physician spends an hour with a spouse and new patient, then an additional hour reviewing laboratory studies and x-ray films and reports, setting up a treatment plan and coordinating care by two other specialists. The history and exam were comprehensive with high medical decision making. Code 99205-21
-22	**Unusual Procedural Services:** *When the services provided are greater than that usually required for the listed procedure, they may be identified by adding modifier -22 to the usual procedure number. A report should be included.*[†]
	Example: Removal of foreign body from stomach, which usually takes about 45 minutes, takes 2 hours on a particular patient; use modifier -22. A discharge summary or specially dictated statement should be attached to the claim form. This modifier increases the payment.
-23	**Unusual Anesthesia:** *Occasionally, a procedure that usually requires either no anesthesia or local anesthesia must be done under general anesthesia because of unusual circumstances. This circumstance may be reported by adding the modifier -23 to the procedure code of the basic service.*[†]
	Example: A proctoscopy might require no anesthesia. A skin biopsy or excision of a subcutaneous tumor might require local anesthesia. If general anesthesia is needed, append the procedure code with modifier -23.
-24	**Unrelated Evaluation and Management Service by the Same Physician during a Postoperative Period:** *The physician may need to indicate that an evaluation and management service was performed during a postoperative period for a reason(s) unrelated to the original procedure. This circumstance may be reported by adding the modifier -24 to the appropriate level of E/M service.*[†]
	Example: A patient seen for a postoperative visit after an appendectomy complains of a lump on the leg. The physician takes a history and examines the site, and a biopsy is scheduled. The E/M code 99024 is used for the postsurgery examination and the modifier -24 is added for unrelated service rendered during a postoperative period.
-25	**Significant, Separately Identifiable Evaluation and Management Service by the Same Physician on the Day of a Procedure or Other Service:** *The physician may need to indicate that on the day a procedure or service identified by a CPT code was performed, the patient's condition required a significant, separately identifiable E/M service above and beyond the other service provided. The E/M service may be prompted by the symptom or condition for which the procedure and/or service was provided. As such, different diagnoses are not required for reporting the E/M service on the same date.*
	Example: A patient is seen for a diabetic follow-up and the physician discovers a suspicious mole on the patient's neck (0.4 cm), which is removed. The physician makes a minor adjustment of the oral diabetes medication. This case illustrates a significant E/M service provided on the same day as a procedure, so -25 is added to the E/M code. Code 11420 is used for removal of the benign lesion.
	Note: *This modifier is not used to report an E/M service that resulted in a decision to perform surgery. See modifier -57.*[†]

*2007 Current Procedural Terminology © 2006 American Medical Association. All rights reserved.

Table 16-7 (continued). *Current Procedural Terminology* Modifier Codes. (CPT codes, descriptions, and material are taken from 2007 Current Procedural Terminology © 2006 American Medical Association. All rights reserved.)*

Modifier Code	Explanation
-26	**Professional Component:** *Certain procedures are a combination of a professional physician component and a technical component. When the professional (physician) component is reported separately, the service may be identified by adding the modifier -26 to the usual procedure number.**
	Note: The professional component comprises only the professional services performed by the physician during radiologic, laboratory, and other diagnostic procedures. These services include a portion of a test or procedure that the physician does, such as interpretation of the results. The technical component includes personnel, materials, and equipment (excludes the cost of radioisotopes). When billing for the technical component, use the usual five-digit procedure number with modifier -TC.
	Example:
	70450-26 Computerized axial tomography, head or brain; without contrast material. The modifier -26 indicates the physician interpreted this test only.
	70450-TC Computerized axial tomography, head or brain; without contrast material. The modifier indicates the facility is billing only for the use of the equipment, and technician.
-27	**Multiple Outpatient Hospital E/M Encounters on the Same Date:** *For hospital outpatient reporting purposes, utilization of hospital resources related to separate and E/M encounters performed in multiple outpatient hospital settings on the same date may be reported by adding the modifier -27 to each appropriate level outpatient and/or emergency department E/M code(s). This modifier provides a means of reporting circumstances involving E/M services provided by physician(s) in more than one (multiple) outpatient hospital setting(s) (e.g., hospital emergency department, clinic). Do not use this modifier for physician reporting of multiple E/M services performed by the same physician on the same date. See E/M, emergency department, or preventive medicine services codes.*
	Example: Patient is seen in a hospital outpatient clinic. The patient falls in the treatment room and receives a cut on the right arm. The patient is taken to the emergency department for two stitches and a dressing.
-32	**Mandated Services:** *Services related to mandated consultation and/or related services (e.g., PRO, third-party payer, governmental, legislative or regulatory requirement), may be identified by adding the modifier -32 to the basic procedure.†*
	Example: A patient is referred to the physician by an insurance company for an unbiased opinion regarding permanent disability after a year of treatment following an accident. Add modifier -32 to the E/M code because the second opinion is mandated by the insurance company.
-47	**Anesthesia by Surgeon:** *Regional or general anesthesia provided by the surgeon may be reported by adding the modifier -47 to the basic service (this does not include local anesthesia).†*
	Note: Modifier -47 would not be used for anesthesia procedures 00100 through 01999.
	Example: A gastroenterologist performs an endoscopy for removal of esophageal polyps using the snare technique. The physician sedates the patient with Versed to perform the procedure.
	43217-47 Esophagoscopy with removal of polyps by snare technique; administered versed.

(continues)

Table 16-7 (continued). *Current Procedural Terminology* Modifier Codes. (CPT codes, descriptions, and material are taken from 2007 Current Procedural Terminology © 2006 American Medical Association. All rights reserved.)*

Modifier Code	Explanation
-50	**Bilateral Procedure:** *Unless otherwise identified in the code descriptions, bilateral procedures requiring a separate incision performed during the same operative session should be identified by the appropriate five-digit code describing the first procedure and either appended with modifier -50 or listed as a second procedure with modifier -50.* **Note:** It is important to read each surgical description carefully to look for the word "bilateral." **Example A:** 71060　　Bronchography, bilateral (would be listed with no modifier) **Example B:** 19200　　mastectomy, radical 19200-50　mastectomy, radical; bilateral
-51	**Multiple Procedures:** *When multiple procedures, other than E/M services, are performed at the same session by the same provider, the primary procedure or service may be reported as listed. The additional procedure(s) or service(s) may be identified by adding the modifier -51 to the additional procedure or service code(s).* **Note:** This modifier should not be appended to designated "add-on" codes (see Appendix D and E of CPT). Always list the procedure of highest dollar value first. **Example:** Patient had herniated disk in lower back with stabilization of the area where the disk was removed. 63030　　Lumbar laminectomy with disk removal 22612-51　Arthrodesis 　　(modifier used after the lesser of the two procedures)
-52	**Reduced Services:** *Under certain circumstances a service or procedure is partially reduced or eliminated at the physician's election. Under these circumstances the service provided can be identified by its usual procedure number and the addition of the modifier -52 signifying that the service is reduced. This provides a means of reporting reduced services without disturbing the identification of the basic service.§* **Note:** This means there will be no effect on the physician's fee profile in the computer data. It is not necessary to attach a report to the claim when using this modifier, because it indicates a reduced fee. When a physician performs a procedure but does not charge for the service, such as a post-operative follow-up visit that is included in a global service, remember to use code 99024 (postoperative follow up visit included in surgical package). Some physicians prefer to bill the Insurance carrier the full amount and accept what the carrier pays as payment in full. In such cases, a modifier would not be used. If only part of a procedure is performed and the physician feels a reduction in the service is warranted, to develop a reduced fee try calculating the reduced service by time. Calculate the amount (cost) per minute of the complete procedure by dividing the amount (cost) by the usual time it takes to complete the procedure. To determine how long the reduced procedure took, multiply the amount (cost) per minute by the time it took to do the reduced procedure. **Example:** A patient is not able to participate or cooperate in a minimal psychiatric interview (90801) and the physician decides to attempt this at a later date. Modify the code with -52.

Table 16-7 (continued). *Current Procedural Terminology** Modifier Codes. (*CPT* codes, descriptions, and material are taken from *2007 Current Procedural Terminology* © 2006 American Medical Association. All rights reserved.)

Modifier Code	Explanation
-53	***Discontinued Procedure:*** *Under certain circumstances, the physician may elect to terminate a surgical or diagnostic procedure. Due to extenuating circumstances or those that threaten the well-being of the patient, it may be necessary to indicate that a surgical or diagnostic procedure was started but discontinued. This circumstance may be reported by adding the modifier "-53" to the code for the discontinued procedure.* **Note:** This modifier is not used to report the elective cancellation of a procedure before the patient's anesthesia induction and/or surgical preparation in the operating suite. For outpatient hospital or ambulatory surgery center (ACS), see modifiers -73 and -74. **Example:** The physician is beginning a laparascopic cholecystectomy on a patient. An earthquake of great magnitude occurs and the electricity is shut off. The backup generator comes on and electricity is restored; however, because of the disarray in the operative suite, the physician decides to discontinue the surgery. Code 47562 is used with -53 appended to it.
-54	***Surgical Care Only:*** *When one physician performs the surgical procedure portion of a surgical package, and another provides preoperative and/or postoperative management, surgical services may be identified by adding the modifier -54 to the usual procedure number.** **Note:** Because many surgical procedures encompass a "package" concept that includes normal uncomplicated follow-up care, the surgeon will be paid a reduced fee when using this modifier. **Example:** A patient presents in the emergency department with severe abdominal pain. Dr. A, the on-call surgeon, examines the patient and performs an emergency appendectomy. Dr. A is leaving on vacation the next morning so he calls his friend and colleague Dr. B. He asks him to visit the patient in the hospital the following day and take over the postoperative care. Dr. A bills using the appendectomy procedure code 44950 and modifies it with -54.
-55	***Postoperative Management Only:*** *When using a surgical package code and one physician performs the postoperative management and another physician performs the surgical procedure, the postoperative component may be identified by adding the modifier -55 to the usual procedure number.* **Note:** The fee to list would be approximately 30% of the surgeon's fee. **Example:** The Dunmires are relocating to Memphis, Tennessee, when she discovers a lump on her arm. She visits her family physician, Dr. A, who tells her it needs to be excised. She wants her physician (Dr. A) to do the surgery and Dr. A agrees if she promises to arrange for a physician in Memphis to follow her postoperatively. She makes arrangements with Dr. B in Memphis. Dr. B bills using the correct excision code that he obtained from Dr. A and modifies it with -55.
-56	***Preoperative Management Only:*** *When using a surgical package code, and one physician performs the preoperative care and evaluation and another physician performs the surgical procedure, the preoperative component may be identified by adding the modifier -56 to the usual procedure number.*† **Example:** Dr. A sees Mrs. Jones and determines she needs to have a lung biopsy. He admits her to the hospital and Dr. A becomes ill. Dr. B is called in and performs the surgery. Dr. A bills for the preoperative care using the surgical code he obtained from Dr. B and modifies it with -56.

(continues)

Table 16-7 (continued). *Current Procedural Terminology** Modifier Codes. (*CPT* codes, descriptions, and material are taken from *2007 Current Procedural Terminology* © 2006 American Medical Association. All rights reserved.)

Modifier Code	Explanation
-57	***Decision for Surgery:*** *An evaluation and management service that resulted in the initial decision to perform the surgery may be identified by adding the modifier -57 to the appropriate level of E/M service.*[†] **Note:** Use this modifier only if the E/M service occurs with in 24 hours of surgery. **Example:** A patient is referred to a surgeon for a consultation to determine whether surgery is necessary. The patient consents to surgery for the following day. The surgeon bills the E/M consultation code and adds the -57 modifier. By adding this modifier, the third party payer is informed that the consultation is not part of the global surgical procedure. Medicare will pay if it is for major surgery that requires a 90-day postoperative follow-up but not for a minor surgical procedure (0- to 10-day postoperative follow-up).
-58	***Staged or Related Procedure or Service by the Same Physician during the Postoperative Period:*** *The physician may need to indicate that the performance of a procedure or service during the postoperative period was (a) planned prospectively at the time or the original procedure (staged), (b) more extensive than the original procedure, or © for therapy after a diagnostic surgical procedure. This circumstance may be reported by adding the modifier -58 to the staged or related procedure.*[‡] **Example:** A patient has breast cancer, and a surgeon performs a mastectomy. During the postoperative global period, the surgeon inserts a permanent prosthesis. The -58 modifier is added to the code for inserting the prosthesis, indicating that this service was planned at the time of the initial operation. If the modifier is not used, the insurance carrier may reject the claim because surgery occurred during the surgery's global period.
-59	***Distinct Procedural Service:*** *Under certain circumstances, the physician may need to indicate that a procedure or service was distinct or independent from other services performed on the same day. Modifier -59 is used to identify procedures/services that are not normally reported together but are appropriate under the circumstances. This may represent a different session or patient encounter; different procedure or surgery, different site or organ system, separate incision or excision, separate lesion, or separate injury (or area of injury in extensive injuries) not ordinarily encountered or performed on the same day by the same physician. However, when another already established modifier is appropriate it should be used rather than modifier -59. Only if no more descriptive modifier is available, and the use or modifier -59 best explains the circumstances, should modifier -59 be used.* **Example:** The patient is scheduled for a hysterectomy. She asks the physician if he will remove a lipoma (2.2 cm) from the right upper thigh area while she is under anesthesia. The surgeon bills for the hysterectomy, and bills for the lipoma removal (11403) modifying it with -59.
-62	***Two Surgeons:*** *When two surgeons work together as primary surgeons performing distinct parts or a single reportable procedure, each surgeon should report his/her distinct operative work using the same procedure code and adding the modifier -62. If additional procedures (including add-on procedures) are performed during the same surgical session, separate codes may be reported without the modifier -62.* **Note:** If the co-surgeon acts as an assist in the performance of additional procedure(s) during the same surgical session, those services may be reported using separate procedure code(s) with modifier -80 or -81. **Example:** A procedure for scoliosis is performed by a thoracic surgeon who does the anterior approach and an orthopedic surgeon who does the posterior approach and repair.

Table 16-7 (continued). *Current Procedural Terminology* Modifier Codes. (CPT codes, descriptions, and material are taken from 2007 Current Procedural Terminology © 2006 American Medical Association. All rights reserved.)*

Modifier Code	Explanation
-63	***Procedure Performed on Infants Less Than 4 kg:*** *Procedures performed on neonates and infants up to a present body weight of 4 kg may involve significantly increased complexity and physician work commonly associated with these patients. This circumstance may be reported by adding the modifier -63 to the procedure number.* **Note:** Unless otherwise designated, this modifier may only be appended to procedures/services listed in the 20000-69999 code series. Modifier -63 should not be appended to any *CPT* codes listed in the evaluation and management services, anesthesia, radiology, pathology and laboratory, or medicine sections. **Example:** A premature neonate has heart surgery for tetrology of Fallot
-66	***Surgical Team:*** *Under some circumstances, highly complex procedures (requiring the services of several physicians, often of different specialties, plus other highly skilled, specially trained personnel and various types of complex equipment) are carried out under the "surgical team" concept. Such circumstances may be identified by each participating physician with the addition or the modifier -66 to the basic procedure number used for reporting services.** **Example:** A kidney transplant, requiring use of a vascular surgeon, urologist, and nephrologist, with the assistance of anesthesiologist and pathologist, or a complex open heart surgery using perfusion personnel, three cardiologists, and an anesthesiologist.
-76	***Repeat Procedure by Same Physician:*** *The physician may need to indicate that a procedure or service was repeated subsequent to the origin a service. This circumstance may be reported by adding modifier -76 to the repeated service.†* **Example:** A femoral-popliteal bypass graft (35556) is performed, the graft clots later that day, and the entire procedure is repeated. The original procedure is reported and the repeat procedure is reported using modifier -76. A report should be attached to the insurance claim when using this modifier.
-77	***Repeat Procedure by Another Physician:*** *The physician may need to indicate that a basic procedure performed by another physician had to be repeated. The situation may be reported by adding modifier -77 to the repeated service.* **Example:** A femoral-popliteal graft (35556) is performed in the morning and in the afternoon it becomes clotted. The original surgeon is not available and a different surgeon performs the repeat operation later in the day. The original surgeon reports 35556. The second surgeon reports 35556-77.
-78	***Return to the Operating Room for a Related Procedure during the Postoperative Period:*** *The physician may need to indicate that another procedure was performed during the postoperative period of the initial procedure. When this subsequent procedure is related to the first, and requires the use or the operating room, it may be reported by adding the modifier -78 to the related procedure. (For repeat procedures on the same day see -76.)†* **Example:** A patient has an open reduction with fixation of a fracture of the elbow. While still hospitalized, the patient develops an infection and is returned to surgery for removal of the pin because it appears to be the cause of an allergic reaction. The original procedure would be billed for the open treatment of the fracture. The pin removal would be billed with modifier -78 because it is a related procedure.

(continues)

Table 16-7 (continued). *Current Procedural Terminology** Modifier Codes. (*CPT* codes, descriptions, and material are taken from *2007 Current Procedural Terminology* © 2006 American Medical Association. All rights reserved.)

Modifier Code	Explanation
-79	**Unrelated Procedure or Service by the Same Physician During the Postoperative Period:** *The physician may need to indicate that the performance of a procedure or service during the postoperative period was unrelated to the original procedure. This circumstance may be reported by using the modifier -79. (For repeat procedures on the same day, see -76.)*[†] **Example:** A patient in the hospital has colon resection surgery and is discharged home. After 7 days, the patient develops acute renal failure, is hospitalized, does not recover renal function, and hemodialysis is ordered. A nephrologist inserts a cannula for the dialysis. When billing for the nephrologist, the code for hemodialysis is shown with a -79 modifier indicating that this is unrelated to the initial surgery. If modifier -79 is not used, the insurance carrier may not realize the service is not related to the initial surgery and may reject the claim.
-80	**Assistant Surgeon:** *Surgical assistant services may be identified by adding the modifier -80 to the procedure number(s).** **Note:** Some insurance policies do not include payment for assistant surgeons, such as for 1-day surgery, but do pay for major or complex surgical assistance. Medicare will not pay assistant surgeons for operations that are not life threatening. Therefore, Medigap insurance will not pay on this service because the service is nonallowable. Assisting surgeons usually charge 16% to 30% of the primary surgeon's fee. **Example:** The primary surgeon performs a right ureterectomy submitting code 50650-RT. The assistant surgeon would bill using the primary surgeon's code with modifier -80 (50650 -80).
-81	**Minimum Assistant Surgeon:** *Minimum surgical assistant services are identified by adding the modifier -81 to the usual procedure number; the assistant does not have to be in the operating room the entire time.* **Note:** Payment is made to physicians but not registered nurses or technicians who assist during surgery.* **Example:** A primary surgeon plans to perform a surgical procedure but during the operation circumstances arise that require the services of an assistant surgeon for a relatively short period of time. In this scenario, the second surgeon provides minimal assistance and may report using the procedure code with the -81 modifier appended.
-82	**Assistant Surgeon:** *(When qualified resident surgeon is not available.) The unavailability of a qualified resident surgeon is a prerequisite for use of modifier -82 appended to the usual procedure code number(s).** **Note:** This modifier is used for services rendered at a teaching hospital. **Example:** A resident surgeon is scheduled to assist with an anorectal myomectomy (45108). Surgery is delayed due to the previous surgery, the shift rotation changes, and the resident (nor any other resident) is not available. A non-resident assists with the surgery and reports the procedure appending it with modifier -82 (45108-82).
-90	**Reference (Outside) Laboratory:** *When laboratory procedures are performed by a party other than the treating or reporting physician, the procedure may be identified by adding the modifier -90 to the usual procedure number.*[†] **Note:** Use this modifier when the physician bills the patient for the outside laboratory work and the laboratory is not doing its own billing.

*2007 Current Procedural Terminology © 2006 American Medical Association. All rights reserved.

Table 16-7 (continued). *Current Procedural Terminology* Modifier Codes. (CPT codes, descriptions, and material are taken from 2007 Current Procedural Terminology © 2006 American Medical Association. All rights reserved.)*

Modifier Code	Explanation
	Example: Dr. Input examines the patient, performs venipuncture, and sends the specimen to an outside laboratory for a lipid panel. The physician has an arrangement with the laboratory to bill for the test, and, in turn, he bills the patient. Dr. Input bills for the examination (E/M code), venipuncture (36415), and lipid panel (80061), using modifier -90 (80061-90) to append to the lipid panel code.
-91	**Repeat Clinical Diagnostic Laboratory Test:** *In the course of treatment or the patient, it may be necessary to repeat the same laboratory test on the same day to obtain subsequent (multiple) test results. Under these circumstances, the laboratory test performed can be identified by its usual procedure number and the addition of modifier -91.*
	Note: This modifier may not be used when tests are rerun to confirm initial results; due to testing problems with specimens or equipment; or for any other reason when a normal, one-time, reportable result is all that is required. This modifier may not be used when other code(s) describe a series of test results (e.g., glucose tolerance tests, evocative/suppression testing). This modifier may only be used for laboratory test(s) performed more than once on the same day on the same patient.
	Example: A patient is scheduled for a nonobstetrical dilation and curettage for dysfunctional uterine bleeding. When the patient arrives at the office, a routine hematocrit is obtained. During the procedure, the patient bleeds excessively. After the procedure, the physician orders a second hematocrit to check the patient for anemia due to blood loss. The first hematocrit is billed using *CPT* code 85014. The second hematocrit is billed using the same code appended with modifier -91 (85014-91).
-99	**Multiple Modifiers:** *Under certain circumstances, two or more modifiers may be necessary to delineate a service completely. In such situations modifier -99 should be added to the basic procedure, and other applicable modifiers may be listed as part of the description of the service.*[‡]
	Note: Multiple modifiers can be listed on the new CMS-1500 claim form.

*This modifier may have an effect on reimbursement.

[†]This modifier may affect reimbursement, depending on the payer.

[‡]Modifier is informational in nature. Do not ask for an adjustment in reimbursement.

[§]This modifier affects reimbursement but not the physician's fee profile.

Modified with permission from the American Medical Association, Chicago, Illinois

CPT modifiers, descriptions of when to use them and examples.

Codebook Appendices

The *CPT* codebook has appendices located after Category III codes and before the index. Following is a brief list of each appendix and what it includes for the 2007 edition of *CPT*:

- Appendix A—Complete list of modifiers with descriptions

- Appendix B—Summary of new codes, coding language changes, and deletions

- Appendix C—Clinical examples for Evaluation and Management codes

- Appendix D—Summary of add-on codes

EXAMPLE 16-6

Multiple Modifiers

The patient is grossly obese, and the operative report states that a bilateral sliding-type inguinal herniorrhaphy was performed. The procedure took two hours, fifteen minutes to perform.

A.

24. A. DATE(S) OF SERVICE From MM DD YY To MM DD YY	B. PLACE OF SERVICE	C. EMG	D. PROCEDURES, SERVICES, OR SUPPLIES (Explain Unusual Circumstances) CPT/HCPCS MODIFIER	E. DIAGNOSIS POINTER	F. $ CHARGES	G. DAYS OR UNITS	H. EPSDT Family Plan	I. ID. QUAL.	J. RENDERING PROVIDER ID. #
1			49525 50 22					NPI	

B.

19. RESERVED FOR LOCAL USE
1 = 50 22

20. OUTSIDE LAB? ☐ YES ☐ NO   **$ CHARGES**

21. DIAGNOSIS OR NATURE OF ILLNESS OR INJURY (Relate Items 1, 2, 3 or 4 to Item 24E by Line)

1. ____ . ____   3. ____ . ____

2. ____ . ____   4. ____ . ____

22. MEDICAID RESUBMISSION CODE   **ORIGINAL REF. NO.**

23. PRIOR AUTHORIZATION NUMBER

24. A. DATE(S) OF SERVICE From MM DD YY To MM DD YY	B. PLACE OF SERVICE	C. EMG	D. PROCEDURES, SERVICES, OR SUPPLIES (Explain Unusual Circumstances) CPT/HCPCS MODIFIER	E. DIAGNOSIS POINTER	F. $ CHARGES	G. DAYS OR UNITS	H. EPSDT Family Plan	I. ID. QUAL.	J. RENDERING PROVIDER ID. #
1			49525 99					NPI	

- Appendix E—Summary of codes exempt from modifier -51

- Appendix F—Summary of codes exempt from modifier -63

- Appendix G—Codes that include moderate (conscious) sedation

- Appendix H—Alphabetic index of performance measures by clinical condition or topic

- Appendix I—Genetic testing code modifiers

- Appendix J—Electrodiagnostic medicine listing of sensory, motor, and mixed nerves

- Appendix K—Code for products pending FDA approval

- Appendix L—Vascular family branches

- Appendix M—Crosswalk to deleted codes

Unlisted Procedures

When a service is rendered and a code number cannot be found for the procedure, check Category III codes found after the medicine section. These are temporary codes and may be assigned, if available. If no Category III code is found, proceed to the end of the appropriate category, subsection, or section and locate a five-digit code for "unlisted procedures." Use this code with the description stating "unlisted" (see Example 16-7). Send in a report that details the nature and extent of the procedure and the supporting diagnosis.

EXAMPLE 16-7

Unlisted Services and Procedures

99429	Unlisted preventive medicine service (E/M section)
19499	Unlisted procedure, breast (integumentary subsection)

DIAGNOSTIC CODING

After the medical assistant has learned some basics of procedural coding, the next step is to learn how to code diagnoses. All diagnoses that affect the current status of the patient must be assigned a code. Sometimes two or more codes are necessary to completely describe a given diagnosis, be sure to list all of the code numbers (see Example 16-10 on page 556). The insurance carrier's computer software cross-checks claims to match procedure codes with diagnostic codes. This is referred to as *code linkage*, and if there are discrepancies, the insurance claim is held up and becomes questionable for payment.

The *International Classification of Diseases, Ninth Revision, Clinical Modification (ICD-9-CM)* Volumes 1 and 2 are used to code diagnoses in physicians' practices. See Resources at the end of this chapter for information on where to obtain this codebook. Volume 3 is used to code procedures in the hospital setting. Psychiatric disorders are coded using the *Diagnostic and*

STEP 1 2 3

Select Correct Procedural Codes

Objective: Accurately locate and select codes for procedures and services.

Equipment/Supplies: *Current Procedural Terminology* codebook, medical dictionary, and pen or pencil.

Directions: Follow these step-by-step procedures to learn this skill, which is presented in the *Workbook* (Job Skills 16-2 through 16-6) for practice.

1. Read the Introduction section at the beginning of the codebook. This information may change with each annual edition.

2. Select the term to look up and use the Index at the back of the codebook. Listings may be looked up according to names of procedures or services, organs, anatomic site, conditions, synonyms, eponyms, and abbreviations.

3. First look under the procedure performed. If it is not listed, check for the organ involved. If the procedure or organ is difficult to find, look up the condition. Keywords, such as synonyms or eponyms, and abbreviations may also help you find the appropriate code.

4. Mark down all codes listed. Codes may be listed as single codes, multiple codes, or code ranges (see Example 16-8). Page numbers are not listed.

5. Turn to the beginning of the section for the code(s) given in the index and read the guidelines. They give general information and instructions on coding certain procedures within each section.

6. Look at the size of the title to find out the area you are in. Some codebooks have color-coded titles, making this determination easier. In the surgery section, each subsection is further

---

EXAMPLE 16-8

Procedure Codes Listed in the Index

Biopsy (procedure)

Abdomen (anatomic site)	49000	→	Single Code
Colon (anatomic site)	44025, 44100	→	Multiple Codes
Hip (anatomic site)	27040–27041	→	Code Range

---

divided into categories based on anatomic site. Within each category are subcategories listed by type of procedure (e.g., excision, repair, destruction, graft) or condition (burn, fracture).

7. Turn to the correct section, subsection, category, or subcategory, and thoroughly read through all notes pertaining to that area.

8. Read all descriptions carefully.

9. Notice punctuation and indentions. Descriptions for stand-alone codes begin at the left margin and have a full description. Read the description of an indented code by reading the portion of the description of the stand-alone code that appears above it and comes before the semicolon (;); then continue reading the description after the semicolon. No matter how many indented codes are listed, always go back to the stand-alone code to begin reading the description (see Example 16-9).

10. Select the code. Remember, the service or procedure description should match the code's narrative description before an assignment is made.

EXAMPLE 16-9

Reading CPT Code Descriptions

11055	**Paring or cutting of benign hyperkeratotic lesion; single lesion**	→	stand-alone code
11056	two to four lesions	→	indented code
11057	more than four lesions	→	indented code

(continues)

PROCEDURE 16-1 *continued*

11. Determine if one or more modifiers are needed to give a more accurate description of the services rendered or the circumstances in which they were performed.

12. Enter a five-digit code(s) and modifier (if applicable) in the proper field(s) (24D) on the insurance claim form for each procedure or service rendered. Take care not to transpose numbers.

EXAMPLE 16-10

Two Diagnoses

The patient's diagnosis is *dyspepsia* with heartburn.

536.8	dyspepsia
787.1	heartburn

Statistical Manual of Mental Disorders, Fourth Edition (DSM IV),* which is not discussed in this text.

To complete a CMS-1500 claim form, abstract the correct diagnosis from the patient's medical record or transaction slip, code it, and insert the code in Field 21 on the claim form. There is room for four diagnoses; however, Medicare will process up to eight diagnostic codes on paper and electronic claims effective July 1, 2007. Write "IMP" (impression), or "DX" (diagnosis) when recording the diagnoses. The diagnosis must agree with the treatment rendered.

If the final diagnosis is qualified by any of the following terms (*suspected, suspicion of, questionable, likely, probably, or possible*), do not code these conditions as if they existed or were established. Instead, code signs, symptoms, abnormal test results, or other reasons for the encounter. If the statement "rule out" is used, *do not code*. This refers to a condition that is suspected and is being ruled out after tests are performed (see Example 16-11).

Table 16-8 contains a chapter outline of Volumes 1 and 2 of *ICD-9-CM*.

Terminology

It is imperative to have a working knowledge of medical terminology to become an efficient diagnostic coder. When learning, study the codebook terminology, then read all of the information at the beginning of Volumes 1 and 2 before coding. The following are some of the abbreviations, punctuation, and symbols encountered in Volume 1.

Abbreviations

NEC   Not Elsewhere Classifiable (in the codebook); category number for the diagnosis including NEC is used only when the coder cannot find the description necessary to code the diagnosis in a more specific category.

NOS   Not Otherwise Specified means "unspecified" by the physician. The coder may need to ask the physician for more specific information.

Punctuation

[ ]   Brackets are used to enclose synonyms, alternative wordings, or explanatory phrases (see Example 16-12).

( )   Parentheses are used to enclose supplementary words that may be present in the statement of a disease or procedure without affecting the code number to which it is assigned.

EXAMPLE 16-11

Qualified Diagnosis

A patient presents in the office complaining of excessive thirst. A urinalysis indicates excessive sugar in the urine. The physician documents, "Rule out diabetes mellitus."

Code: polydipsia (783.5) and glycosuria (791.5)

EXAMPLE 16-12

Additional Diagnostic Code

Volume 2

Arthropathy (see also Arthritis) 716.9
    Behçet's 136.1 [711.2]

---

*2007 Current Procedural Terminology © 2006 American Medical Association. All rights reserved.

Table 16-8. Chapter Outline of Volumes 1 and 2 of the *International Classification of Diseases—9th Revision—Clinical Modification (ICD-9-CM)*, 2008

Volume 1 Contains the Numeric Index

Chapter	Codes
1. Infectious and Parasitic Diseases	001–139
2. Neoplasms	140–239
3. Endocrinologic, Nutritional, and Metabolic Diseases and Immunologic Disorders	240–279
4. Diseases of the Blood and Blood-Forming Organs	280–289
5. Mental Disorders	290–319
6. Disease of the Nervous System and Sense Organs	320–389
7. Diseases of the Circulatory System	390–459
8. Diseases of the Respiratory System	460–519
9. Diseases of the Digestive System	520–579
10. Diseases of the Genitourinary System	580–629
11. Complications of Pregnancy, Childbirth, and the Puerperium	630–677
12. Diseases of the Skin and Subcutaneous Tissue	680–709
13. Diseases of the Musculoskeletal System and Connective Tissue	710–739
14. Congenital Anomalies	740–759
15. Certain Conditions Originating in the Perinatal Period	760–779
16. Symptoms, Signs, and Ill-Defined Conditions	780–799
17. Injury and Poisoning	800–999

Supplementary Classification

Classification of Factors Influencing Health Status and Contact with Health Service	V01-V86
Classification of External Causes of Injury and Poisoning	E800-E999

Appendices

A. Morphology of Neoplasms

B. Glossary of Mental Disorders

C. Classification of Drugs by American Hospital Formulary Service List Number and Their *ICD-9-CM* Equivalents

D. Classification of Industrial Accidents According to Agency

E. List of Three-Digit Categories

Volume 2 Contains the Alphabetic Index

Section 1. Table of Hypertension
Table of Neoplasms

Index to Diseases and Injuries

Section 2. Table of Drugs and Chemicals

Section 3. Alphabetic Index to External Causes of Injury and Poisoning (E Codes)

: Colons are used in the tabular list after an incomplete term that needs one or more of the modifiers that follow to make it assignable to a given category.

{ } Braces are used to enclose a series of terms, each of which is modified by the statement appearing at the right of the brace.

Symbols

☐ Lozenge symbol printed in the left margin preceding the disease indicates the content of a four-digit category has been moved or modified.

§ Section mark symbol preceding a code denotes the placement of a footnote at the bottom of the page that is applicable to all subdivisions in that code.

[ ] Volume 2: The alphabetic index for disease classification uses slanted brackets to indicate the need for another code. A code is listed after a diagnosis, which is followed by slanted brackets that enclose an additional code. Always list both codes in the same sequence as indicated in the index.

Volumes I and II

To code using *ICD-9-CM* always start in Volume II, and locate the main term (condition) in the alphabetic index. In some codebooks the index may be located in the front, others have it in the back. After locating the code(s) in Volume II, turn to Volume I, the tabular list. Refer to Procedure 16-2 for step-by-step instructions.

V Codes

V codes are a supplementary classification of coding located at the end of Volume 1 (tabular list). V codes are used when a person who is not currently ill uses health services for some specific purpose, when a patient receives treatment for a known condition or disease, or when a patient's health status is influenced by a circumstance that is not in itself a current injury or illness. Examples might be a vaccination, chemotherapy, cast change, dialysis, circumcision, sterilization (contraception), consultation for family planning, organ donation, and so on. V codes are also used when a problem is present that influences the person's health status but is not in itself a current illness or injury, such as allergy to a specific drug or a history of cancer. In such cases, the V code would be secondary to a primary diagnostic code.

When selecting V codes, locate main terms in Volume 2 (alphabetic index); V codes are included in the major section entitled Index of Diseases.

E Codes

E codes are also a supplementary classification listed after the V codes in a separate section at the end of Volume 1 (tabular list). However, when selecting E codes, go to the end of Volume 2 to locate the main term in a separate E code index, "Index to External Causes of Injury and Poisoning," located after the alphabetic index. E codes are used to code external causes of injury and poisoning rather than disease. In addition, E codes are used in coding adverse reactions to medications. The *cause, intent,* and *place* where the injury or poisoning occurred are provided in code descriptions. Typically, E codes are not used to code outpatient claims submitted by physicians' offices. An E code is used after a primary or other acute secondary diagnosis to inform the insurance carrier of the source of the injury in a hospital setting. Some insurance companies do not accept E codes; however, some physicians for comprehensiveness may elect to use them when documenting, such as in workers' compensation and personal injury cases.

ICD-10-CM

ICD-9-CM diagnostic coding has been in use for 30 years. Because of advances in technology, discovery of new diseases, development of new procedures, and the need to report more details for statistical purposes, adoption of a new system is inevitable. The updated system (*ICD-10-CM*) is actually two systems.

- *International Classification of Diseases,* 10th Revision, *Clinical Modification (ICD-10-CM—diagnostic codes)* used for inpatient and outpatient diagnostic coding, replaces *ICD-9-CM,* Volumes 1 and 2

- *ICD-10 Procedure Coding System (ICD-10-PCS)* used to code procedures in an inpatient setting replaces *ICD-9-CM* Volume III (will not replace *CPT*)

ICD-10-CM differs from *ICD-9-CM* in the following ways:

1. Major changes in codebook organization

2. Additional categories and chapters have been added

3. Six-digit alphanumeric codes rather than all numeric

PROCEDURE 16-2

Select Correct Diagnostic Codes

Objectives: To accurately select and insert diagnostic codes on insurance claim forms.

Equipment/Supplies: Diagnostic codebook (Volumes 1 and 2), medical dictionary, and pen or pencil.

Directions: Follow these step-by-step procedures to learn this skill, which is presented in the *Workbook* (Job Skills 16-7 through 16-10) for practice.

1. Locate the main term or condition (not the anatomic site) in the alphabetic index (Volume II). It is important to identify the main term in the diagnostic statement that relates to what is wrong with the patient (condition) (see Example 6-13).

2. Look for subterms and sub-subterms indented under the main term (see Example 16-14).

3. If the condition or disease is not listed, rearrange the root portions of the medical terms (see Example 16-15).

4. Refer to any notes under the main term, and read terms closed in parentheses.

5. Follow any cross-reference instructions.

EXAMPLE 16-14

Identifying Terms

Lumbar fracture of the vertebra due to senile osteoporosis

Main Term	Subterm	Sub-subterm	Code Assignment
↓	↓	↓	↓
Fracture,	vertebra,	pathologic (any site)	733.10

EXAMPLE 16-15

Medical Terminology Components

gastro / esophag / itis

↑	↑	↑
root	root	suffix

or

esophago / gastr / itis

| root | root | suffix |

EXAMPLE 16-13

Main Terms

Diagnostic Statement	Main Term	Code Selection	Additional Term
muscle atrophy	atrophy	728.2	muscle—where?
chronic bronchitis	bronchitis	491.9	chronic—time frame
allergic conjunctivitis	conjunctivitis	372.14	allergic—type
recurrent depression	depression	296.30	recurrent—time frame
nasal (bone) fracture	fracture	802.0	nasal—where?

Note: To identify the main term, ask what is wrong with the patient. The additional term may state where the problem is, how long the patient has experienced the problem (e.g., acute, subacute, chronic), or further define the problem.

(*continues*)

PROCEDURE 16-2 *continued*

6. Write the code number.

7. Locate the code number in Volume 1 (tabular list), and read any instructional terms. Always use both Volume 2 (alphabetic index) and Volume 1 (tabular/numeric list) of *ICD-9-CM* before assigning a code. Never use only one volume.

8. Always code to the highest level of specificity; that is, code to the highest number of digits (three, four, or five) in the classification. When a fourth or fifth digit is listed, *its use is NOT optional.* A three-digit code is considered a category unless no fourth or fifth digit appears

after it. Five-digit codes appear either at the beginning of a chapter, section, three-digit category, or within the four-digit subcategory. A symbol (e.g., ⑤) may be included in your codebook to signify the need for a fourth or fifth digit (see Example 16-16).

9. Do not arbitrarily use a zero as a filler character when listing a diagnostic code number. This may nullify the code or indicate a different disease. The codebook includes decimal points, but these are not required on optically scanned insurance claims.

10. Assign the code.

EXAMPLE 16-16

Fifth Digits

Post-term pregnancy delivered – 645.11

⑤ 645   Late pregnancy
     645.1   Post-term pregnancy [0, 1, 3]
     645.2   Prolonged pregnancy [0, 1, 3]

COMPLICATIONS MAINLY RELATED TO PREGNANCY (640-649)
INCLUDES the listed conditions even if they arose or were present during labor, delivery, or the puerperium
The following fifth-digit subclassification is for use with categories 640-649 to denote the current episode of care. Valid fifth-digits are in [brackets] under each code.

0 **unspecified as to episode of care or not applicable**
1 **delivered, with or without mention of antepartum condition**
     Antepartum condition with delivery
     Delivery NOS (with mention of antepartum complication during current episode of care)
     Intrapartum obstetric condition (with mention of antepartum complication during current
        episode of care)
     Pregnancy, delivered (with mention of antepartum complication during current episode of care)
2 **delivered, with mention of postpartum complication**
     Delivery with mention of puerperal complication during current episode of care
3 **antepartum condition or complication**
     Antepartum obstetric condition, not delivered during the current episode of care
4 **postpartum condition or complication**
     Postpartum or puerperal obstetric condition or complication following delivery that occurred:
        during previous episode of care outside hospital, with subsequent admission for
        observation or care

The symbol indicates a need for a fifth digit. Go to the beginning of the category "Complications Mainly Related to Pregnancy (640-649)," and select a code from the eligible choices (i.e., 0, 1, 3). The correct way of listing the code on the claim form in Field 21 would be without a decimal. The decimal is included on the form. (64510, 64511, 64513 or 64520, 64521, 64523)

4. Old injury (800-999) codes have been changed to S and T codes

5. Explanatory notes and instructions have been greatly expanded

6. Dagger and asterisk symbols of dual classification in *ICD-10* have been expanded

7. E and V codes are now Chapters XX and XXI

8. Room for expansion as new codes are assigned

Because a coder must have a higher level of clinical knowledge to work with *ICD-10-CM,* it is imperative to attend an anatomy and physiology course to be able to select codes proficiently. Implementation of *ICD-10-CM* is expected by October 1, 2010.

HEALTH INSURANCE CLAIM FORM CMS-1500

The new revised Health Insurance Claim Form CMS-1500 (08/05) is accepted by most health insurers for outpatient services. It is the basic form prescribed by the Center for Medicare and Medicaid Services (CMS) for the Medicare and Medicaid programs. It has also been adopted by the TRICARE programs and has received the approval of the American Medical Association (AMA) Council on Medical Services. The Health Insurance Association of America (HIAA) endorses the CMS-1500 and recommends that their members (private insurance companies) accept the form.

Using the CMS-1500 claim form eliminates completing insurance forms brought into the office by patients. It is typically used in lieu of other forms; however, the medical assistant may complete the CMS-1500 and attach it to the patient's form, ensuring the patient's portion and employer's portion of the private insurance form are complete and accurate and that the patient has signed the release-of-information box and the assignment if applicable. Both forms go to the insurance carrier.

COMPLIANCE

Be alert for an upgrade to the new revised CMS-1500 (08/05) claim form. Once the shaded areas are no longer needed for the legacy provider numbers, the Centers for Medicare and Medicaid Services plan another revision.

If the patient is insured with two companies, the medical assistant obtains assignments for both insurance carriers and bills the primary carrier first. When the primary carrier pays, the secondary carrier is submitted a claim with an attached photocopy of the **explanation of benefits (EOB)** from the primary carrier. The EOB is a document that accompanies the payment check from the carrier, showing the breakdown of the amounts charged, allowed, paid, and denied. In some states, the CMS-1500 claim form can be used for industrial claims.

The red printed version of this form was developed so insurance carriers could process claims by optical character recognition (OCR) for speed and efficiency. The scanner transfers the typed or printed insurance claim information directly to a computer's memory thus eliminating the need to key it separately. Keying a form for OCR scanning requires different techniques than preparing one for standard claims submission. Quantities of the CMS-1500 can be purchased from many medical office supply companies or from the American Medical Association (see Resources at the end of this chapter). The forms may be personalized to the medical practice.

The medical assistant should follow the guidelines presented in the next procedure to complete OCR claims.

Instructions for each field of the CMS-1500 claim form for private insurance carriers, Medicare, Medicare/Medicaid, Medicare/Medigap, and Medicare Secondary Payer (MSP) are included in Appendix A. Information is color-coded so you can quickly locate data related to a specific program or plan. Only general guidelines are stated since claim requirements may differ between private carriers and from state to state.

Templates are provided in this chapter to illustrate data entered properly in each field. Shaded areas indicate when not to complete the field for the insurance program.

TRACING INSURANCE CLAIMS

To assure timely reimbursement, the assistant should establish a well-organized follow-up procedure for insurance claims. When an insurance form is completed and sent to the carrier, it is chronologically filed in an insurance-claims follow-up accordion file indexed with dates of service or names of insurance companies. Place a copy of the insurance claim in a pending file so that the unpaid claims can be retrieved

PROCEDURE 16-3

Complete the Health Insurance Claim Form CMS-1500 Using OCR Guidelines

Objective: To manually complete the CMS-1500 claim form.

Equipment/Supplies: CMS-1500 claim form (08/05), electronic typewriter, procedural and diagnostic codebooks, medical dictionary, and pen or pencil.

Directions: Follow these step-by-step procedures, which include a rationale, to learn this skill, which is presented in the *Workbook* (Job Skill 16-12, 16-13, and 16-14) for practice.

1. Use original claim forms printed in red ink; photocopies cannot be scanned.

2. Use clean equipment (typewriter or computer) and laser or inkjet printers. Clean line printers frequently. Adjust hammer density to prevent shadows. Pica (10 pitch) is preferred for OCR claims. *Do not* handwrite information on the document.

3. Leave the field blank when information is not applicable. *Do not* use N/A or DNA. *Do not* insert data in the shaded areas, as shown in claim templates.

4. Align the typewriter or printer correctly so characters appear in the proper fields. Keep the characters within the borders of each field, and do not touch the box lines.

5. Enter all information in uppercase (CAPITAL) letters. *Do not* use a script typing element; use an OCR or manifold typing element so shifting for capitals is unnecessary.

6. *Do not* strike over any errors when correcting; OCR equipment does not read corrected characters on top of correction tape or correction fluid.

7. *Do not* use highlighter pens or colored ink on claims, because OCR equipment will not pick these up. *Do not* use stickers or rubber stamps such as those that print "tracer," "resubmitted," "corrected billing," or the provider's name and address.

8. Use alpha or numeric symbols. *Do not* use symbols such as $, #, -, /, periods, commas, ditto marks, or parentheses, nor use decimals in the money columns.

9. List diagnostic codes in Field 21 and procedure codes in Field 24D. *Do not* use narrative descriptions of diagnoses, procedures, or modifiers.

10. Indicate in Field 19 "See attachment" or "See attached operative report" when documents are attached. Accompanying documents must include the patient's name, claim number, and insurance identification number typed near the top. *Do not* use paper clips, cellophane tape, or staples to affix attachments to the left upper corner of the form.

11. Enter date using 8-digit format: (050120XX).

12. If using continuous forms use care in separating. *Do not* overtrim or undertrim forms when bursting.

13. Have patients sign Field 12, the consent to release information, so data may be given to a third party.

14. Have patients sign Field 13 for assignment of benefits to the physician when applicable.

15. Have the physician sign the claim and keep the signature within Field 32. Rubber stamps may be used if they are accepted by the insurance company and produce complete, clean images without smudges or missing letters.

16. Mail forms in large manila envelopes. *Do not* fold forms because they will not properly feed into OCR equipment if creased.

for easy follow-up. This method permits placing one telephone call or addressing multiple outstanding claims in one letter to an insurance carrier each month rather than placing multiple calls or submitting many letters covering individual claims.

Following are recommendations for unprocessed or unpaid claims:

Unprocessed:

- Telephone the insurance carrier to inquire about the claim
- Send inquiry letter
- Fax or send electronic claim noting "second submission"
- If additional document requests (ADRs) are made by the insurance carrier, they should be responded to immediately; within 30 days for Medicare claims

Unpaid:

- Gather documentation, which might include history of similar claims that have been paid
- Present logic for time spent and skill of physician
- Obtain "position papers" from a specialty society (e.g., OB-GYN) or FDA regarding procedure or service

- Send letter from physician giving summary of circumstances that relate directly to the patient
- Send the operative report; make sure it presents an accurate story of the procedure

When payment has been received, claims can be pulled and the explanation of benefits attached. After posting payment in the patient account/ledger, daily journal, and deposit slip, file the claim and EOB in a file drawer or box labeled "paid claims" with the month and year of payment noted.

Appeals

If payment is not received after inquires have been made, an appeal may need to be filed. Refer to guidelines for each carrier's appeal process. Medicare has five levels of appeals:

1. Redetermination
2. Reconsideration
3. Administrative Law Judge
4. Department Appeals Board Review
5. Federal Court Review

STOP AND THINK CASE SCENARIO

Determination of Benefits

Scenario: A patient is seen in the office and the physician determines that a bronchoscopy is needed. You are asked to make sure the procedure is a covered benefit, determine what the payment will be, and find out whether prior approval is necessary.

Critical Thinking: Consider which process is necessary to determine the following:

1. What process will you go through to determine whether a bronchoscopy is a covered benefit?

_____

_____

2. What process will you go through to determine the maximum dollar amount that the insurance company will pay for this procedure?

_____

_____

3. What process will you go through to determine if prior approval is necessary?

_____

_____

STOP AND THINK CASE SCENARIO

Submission of a Late Medicare Claim

Scenario: You have recently begun to work for Dr. Practon's office and discover an old claim that has not been submitted. The date of service on this Medicare claim is May 16, 2006.

Critical Thinking: Using the date November 22, 2007, is it too late to submit this claim?

_____

What is the billing limitation of this claim; in other words, what is the deadline date by which the claim must be submitted?

_____

_____

_____

STOP AND THINK CASE SCENARIO

Determine TRICARE Coverage and Benefits

Scenario: A patient calls the doctor's office and states that she is covered under the TRICARE program; her husband is serving in the United States Air Force, his rank is E4. Doctors Fran and Gerald Practon are contracted physicians with the TRICARE Extra network but do not participate in the TRICARE managed care plan.

Critical Thinking: The patient asks the following questions about how the claim will be processed and what her payment responsibilities will be.

1. Will the physician's office be submitting the claims?

_____

2. What is her responsibility for the deductible?

_____

3. How will the patient's eligibility be checked?

_____

_____

STOP AND THINK CASE SCENARIO

Determine the Responsible Party in an Injury Case

Scenario: An established patient has arrived at Dr. Practon's office with an injury to his head.

Critical Thinking: What questions should you ask the patient (or person accompanying the patient) to determine who will be paying the medical bill?

_____

_____

_____

FOCUS ON CERTIFICATION*

CMA Content Summary

- Medical abbreviations
- Medicare/Medicaid regulations
- HIPAA
- Personal injury
- Workers' compensation
- Coding systems (*CPT, ICD-9-CM,* and *HCPCS II*)
- Code linkage
- Capitation
- Medicare, Medicaid, TRICARE, CHAMPVA
- Prepaid health plans (HMO, PPO, POS)
- Manual and electronic claim processing
- Tracing claims, inquiry, and appeals
- Primary/Secondary claims
- Reconciling payments
- Referrals and precertification
- Fee schedules (RVS, RBRVS, DRG)

RMA Content Summary

- Insurance terminology and abbreviations
- Medical, disability, accident insurance plans
- HMO, PPO, EPO, indemnity plans
- Workers' compensation

- Medicare, Medicaid, TRICARE
- Paper and electronic insurance claims
- HIPAA
- Explanation of benefits
- Claim rejection and follow-up procedures
- Code *ICD-9-CM, CPT, HCPCS II*
- Contractural requirements of insurance plans (time-limits)
- Track unpaid claims
- Referral and authorization process

CMAS Content Summary

- Medical and insurance terminology
- Private and managed care plans
- Medicare, Medicaid, Veteran's Administration, TRICARE
- Insurance claims (time-limits)
- Workers' compensation and state disability
- Paper and electronic claim submission
- Procedure and diagnostic coding
- Use *CPT, ICD-9-CM,* and *HCPCS II* codebooks
- Process insurance payments
- Track unpaid claims

REVIEW EXAM-STYLE QUESTIONS

1. The insured is also known as a:

   a. member

   b. policyholder

   c. subscriber

   d. recipient

   e. all of the above

2. In an insurance contract, the waiting period is:

   a. also called the elimination period

   b. a time frame after the beginning date of a policy before benefits for illness or injury become payable

   c. the time frame the applicant is waiting to be approved

   d. in force only if there are preexisting conditions

   e. both a and b

This textbook and the accompanying Workbook meet the entry-level administrative and general competencies for the CMA outlined by the AAMA Examination Content Outline and Role Delineation Study and for the RMA and CMAS outlined by the AMT Competencies and Examination Specifications (see Competency Grid in Appendix B).

3. Unit values for each procedure code are used in the following payment method:

   a. capitation

   b. UCR

   c. RVS

   d. fee-for-service

   e. DRG

4. Medical necessity is insured when the insurance carrier mandates:

   a. precertification

   b. preauthorization

   c. predetermination

   d. a formal referral

   e. a direct referral

5. The oldest of all prepaid health plans are:

   a. HMOs

   b. PPOs

   c. IPAs

   d. PPGs

   e. POS

6. Medicaid is sponsored by:

   a. the federal government

   b. the state government

   c. local governments

   d. federal and local governments

   e. federal, state, and local governments

7. When working in a physician's office, you will be billing:

   a. Medicare Part A

   b. Medicare Part B

   c. Medicare Part C

   d. Medicare Part D

   e. all of the above

8. Which system does Medicare use to calculate fees?

   a. Usual, Customary, and Reasonable charges

   b. Relative Value Scale

   c. Capitation

   d. Resource-Based Relative Value System

   e. Physician's Fee Profile

9. In the TRICARE program, an enrollment fee is sometimes charged for:

   a. TRICARE Standard

   b. TRICARE Extra

   c. TRICARE Prime

   d. all TRICARE programs

   e. none of the TRICARE programs

10. State disability is available in Puerto Rico and in the states of:

   a. California, Hawaii, New Jersey, New York, and Rhode Island

   b. California, Nevada, Hawaii, New Jersey, and New York

   c. Arizona, Florida, New Hampshire, New York, and Texas

   d. Alaska, California, Florida, New York, and Texas

   e. Hawaii, Nebraska, Oregon, New York, and Washington

11. In a workers' compensation case, who does the medical assistant communicate with?

   a. claims representative

   b. insurance representative

   c. adjuster

   d. authorization desk

   e. social worker

12. The CMS-1500 claim form has an assignment of benefits for government programs in:

   a. field 12

   b. field 13

   c. field 14

   d. field 31

   e. field 33

13. The new standarized number used to identify the physician, which replaces all old "legacy" numbers on the claim form, is the:

    a. PIN

    b. UPIN

    c. state license number

    d. ECT

    e. NPI

14. How many sections are there in *Current Procedural Terminology?*

    a. 3

    b. 5

    c. 6

    d. 8

    e. 10

15. When coding from the surgery section of *CPT*, the first thing you should do is:

    a. start at the beginning

    b. go to the index

    c. go to the table of contents

    d. go to the appendices

    e. determine the section the procedure or service is in

16. Checking a diagnostic code against a procedure code is referred to as:

    a. cross-checking

    b. proofreading

    c. code linkage

    d. code correlation

    e. spot-checking

17. When coding diagnoses, start by looking:

    a. in Volume I

    b. in the Tabular List

    c. up the anatomic body part

    d. in Volume II

    e. in the table of contents

18. The reason that the CMS-1500 claim form is printed in red ink is:

    a. to make the inserted information stand out

    b. to make it easier to read

    c. to comply with OCR machines

    d. to comply with copyright laws

    e. to make sure no one copies the form

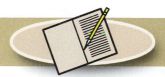

WORKBOOK ASSIGNMENT

To develop competency-based job skills, refer to the *Workbook* and complete the:

- Abbreviation and Spelling Review
- Review Questions

- Critical Thinking Exercises
- Job Skill activities, which are outlined at the beginning of this chapter under "Performance Objectives in the *Workbook.*"

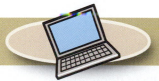

COMPUTER ASSIGNMENT

To review the concepts you have learned in this chapter, insert the *Student Practice* CD-ROM into a computer and work through the *StudyWARE* activities and games. Answer review questions in the practice mode and read the feedback, studying the questions you have missed. Take the chapter quiz until you achieve a minimum score of 90 percent. Successfully completing the *Critical Thinking Challenge* at the end of this course will help you think through scenarios and develop problem solving skills.

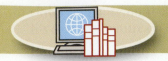

RESOURCES

Claim Forms

American Medical Association
Order Department
PO Box 930876
Atlanta, GA 31193-0876
(800) 621-8335
Web site: http://www.amabookstore.com
Key Term: Resources; References and Forms
Bibbero Systems, Inc.
(800) 242-2376
Web site: http://www.bibbero.com
Medical Arts Press
(800) 328-2179
Web site: http://www.medicalartspress.com
Veterans Affairs (VA) Government forms
Web site: http://www.va.gov/search

Codebooks

Current Procedural Terminology (CPT) (published annually)
American Medical Association
(800) 621-8335
Web site: http://www.amabookstore.com
Health Care Financing Administration Common Procedure Coding System (HCPCS) National Level II Codes, published by:
American Medical Association (800) 621-8335
Ingenix Publishing Group (800) 464-3649
Practice Management Information Corporation (PMIC) (800) MED-SHOP
Wasserman Medical Publishers, Limited (800) 669-3337
International Classification of Diseases, Ninth Revision, Clinical Modification (ICD-9-CM), published by:
American Medical Association (800) 621-8335
Channel Publishing Ltd. (800) 248-2882
Ingenix Publishing Group (800) 464-3649
Practice Management Information Corporation (PMIC) (800) MED-SHOP

Coding and Billing Questions

Part B News
Subscribe to listserv, ask questions and communicate with insurance billers via e-mail
Web site: http://www.partbnews.com

Coding Guidelines

Central Office on *ICD-9-CM* of the American Hospital Association (312) 422-3000
National Center for Health Statistics
Web site: http://www.cdc.gov/nchs/icd9.htm

Internet

Health Insurance Portability and Accountability Act
Health Savings Account (HAS)
Allows consumers to pay for qualified medical expenses with pre-tax dollars
Web site: http://www.ehealthinsurance.com
Search: HSA
HIPPA regulations
Key Term: Regulations and Guidelines
Web site: http://www.cms.hhs.gov
Standard Code Set (rules and information for electronic claim submission)
Search: Electronic billing
Web site: http://www.aspe.hhs.gov
CHAMPVA
Key Term: Benefits
Web site: http://www.va.gov/hac
Medicaid
Web site: http://www.cms.hhs.gov/Medicaid
Medi-Cal
Web site: http://www.medi-cal.ca.gov
Medicare
Web site: http://www.medicare.gov
Medicare Education and Training
Web site: http://www.cms.hhs.gov/medlearn
Medicare Prescription Help
Web site: http://www.ssa.gov/prescriptionhelp
State Disability Insurance Programs
Web site: http://www.vpainc.com
TRICARE
Web site: http://www.tricare.osd.mil
Workers' Compensation
Web site: http://www.workerscompensation.com

Surgical/Global Package Books

Federal Register
Web site: http://www.archives.gov
Medicare Correct Coding and Payment Manual for Procedures and Services, (includes unbundling information)
Ingenix Publishing Group
(800) 464-3649

UNIT 6

Managing the Office

CHAPTER 17

Office Managerial Responsibilities

OBJECTIVES

After reading this chapter and learning step-by-step procedures to gain job skills,* you should be able to:

Learning Objectives

- Discuss ways to promote patient satisfaction and communication.
- Describe ways of increasing office productivity.
- List reasons for office staff meetings.
- State components of an employee handbook.
- Recite employment laws.
- Understand safety and health standards in the medical office.
- Assemble items for an office policy and procedures manual.
- Identify techniques used for recruitment, screening, interviewing, hiring, and training new employees.
- Write a plan for building and equipment maintenance.
- Select a system for ordering and controlling inventory.
- Design a basic travel itinerary and locate travel help sites on the Internet.

Performance Objectives (Procedures) in This Textbook

- Set up a staff meeting (Procedure 17-1).
- Prepare a staff meeting agenda (Procedure 17-2).
- Develop and maintain an employee handbook (Procedure 17-3).
- Compile and maintain an office policies and procedures manual (Procedure 17-4).
- Recruit an employee (Procedure 17-5).

*This textbook and the accompanying Workbook meet the educational components for entry-level administrative and general competencies outlined by CAAHEP and ABHES.

- Orient a new employee (Procedure 17-6).
- Prepare an order form (Procedure 17-7).
- Pay an invoice (Procedure 17-8).
- Establish and maintain inventory (Procedure 17-9).
- Prepare a travel expense report (Procedure 17-10).

Performance Objectives (Job Skills) in the *Workbook*

- Write an agenda for an office meeting (Job Skill 17-1).
- Prepare material for an office procedures manual (Job Skill 17-2).
- Abstract data from a catalog and key an order form (Job Skill 17-3).
- Complete an order form for office supplies (Job Skill 17-4).
- Perform mathematic calculations of an office manager (Job Skill 17-5).
- Prepare two order forms (Job Skill 17-6).
- Prepare a travel expense report (Job Skill 17-7).

OUTLINE WITH LECTURE NOTES

Office Manager
The Work Environment

_____
_____
_____
_____

Promoting Patient Satisfaction and Communication

_____
_____
_____
_____

Increasing Office Productivity

_____
_____
_____
_____

Staff Meetings

_____
_____
_____
_____

Office Guidebooks
Employee Handbook

_____
_____
_____
_____

Employment Laws and Management Plans

_____
_____
_____
_____

Office Policies and Procedures Manual

_____
_____
_____
_____

Employer Responsibilities
Recruitment and Hiring

_____
_____
_____
_____

Employee File

_____

_____

_____

Orientation and Training

_____

_____

_____

Staff Development

_____

_____

_____

_____

Working with Various Personality Types

_____

_____

_____

_____

Evaluation of Performance and Salary Review

_____

_____

_____

_____

Termination of Employees

_____

_____

_____

_____

Facility Oversight

Building Maintenance

_____

_____

_____

Equipment

_____

_____

_____

Office Supplies

_____

_____

_____

Business Travel

Travel Arrangements

_____

_____

_____

Foreign Travel

_____

_____

_____

Travel Help on the Internet

_____

_____

_____

Medical Meeting Expenses

_____

_____

_____

KEY TERMS

agenda

back ordered (B/O)

employee handbook

inventory cards

invoice

itinerary

job descriptions
office manager (OM)
office policies and procedures manual
practice information brochure

sharps containers
staff meetings
visa

HEART OF THE HEALTH CARE PROFESSIONAL

Service

The office manager (OM) can set the scene of service within the medical office by exemplifying a responsible and caring attitude. Opportunities to model a professional image and positive work ethic characteristics are numerous and should be observed and adopted by employees. Demonstrate initiative to render prompt service and quality care.

OFFICE MANAGER

One of the most prestigious yet demanding positions associated with the medical office is that of an **office manager (OM)**. When the medical practice grows to a point where there are several employees or more than one physician sharing a facility, it may be prudent to assign one person to oversee employees and all activities, both administrative and clinical. Proven competence in the role of administrative medical assistant can be rewarded with promotion to office manager. If you are ambitious and enjoy a fast-paced atmosphere, ongoing challenges, and unpredictable shifting responsibilities you may want to consider pursuing management. Managing people and projects takes a creative approach as well as leadership, organizational abilities, and interpersonal skills. A good manager needs to manage time wisely, prioritize responsibilities, and be able to accept that a task may not be completed at the close of the day.

The line of authority would be established as: first, the physician; next, the OM; and finally, the staff members. The OM acts as a liaison between employees and physician(s). This is graphically shown in Chapter 2, Figure 2-4. The administrative assistant who has gained sufficient experience and has been promoted to this responsible position needs to prepare and implement an effective management plan that will foster a team spirit of cooperation among all employees with an equitable division of the workload. He or she must be able to take the initiative and exer-

cise independent judgment, which reflects accurately the attitude of the physician.

Once the chain of command has been established, the OM should be firm, yet flexible and fair, in his or her decisions to ensure respect, promote teamwork, and avoid friction and tension within the office. Responsibilities may include hiring and training, performance and salary review, supervision, and disciplining or dismissal of employees when necessary.

The OM usually delegates the maintenance of equipment and ordering of supplies to promote the efficient running of the office. Another responsibility might include making travel arrangements for the physician to attend medical conventions. Tracking continuing education units for the physician, sending in documentation to assure that the physician's state license is current, and maintaining liability coverage for malpractice insurance are also responsibilities of the OM. The duties of managing the office are challenging, but there are rewards and immense personal satisfaction knowing that the office operates efficiently for the physician. Updating skills, attending seminars, and reading medical periodicals will enable the manager to keep current, excel in his or her position, and possibly attain a higher career goal as the manager of an outpatient facility or multiphysician clinic. Other managerial responsibilities may include generating and analyzing financial reports and preparing payroll; these topics are discussed in the next chapter.

The Work Environment

It is important for the OM to create a work atmosphere that is free of barriers and bias. A multicultural staff can help strengthen an office, attract new patients, and connect with a rapidly growing immigrant population that may be wary of seeking medical care. Laws concerning equal pay, age discrimination, and Americans with disabilities should all be enforced.

The OM should be a model to all employees and should hold staff members to a high standard. Set performance goals, seek input from employees, utilize individual talents, and update standards yearly. Align desired behaviors with the goals of the practice and maintain an upbeat spirit, always thanking employees for the work they have done while displaying a cooperative attitude.

Be a mentor and coach to those who are learning how to be good employees. Plan strategies together, foster problem-solving skills, delegate responsibility, and ask employees how things are going. Be authentically committed to each person's achievement and support the staff so they know that help is available if and when they need it.

Promoting Patient Satisfaction and Communication

Promote patient satisfaction by utilizing good communication skills. Be observant, listen carefully, and develop a complaint protocol that includes procedures to document the complaint and a mechanism to resolve it. A patient complaint form may be adapted to prompt staff to pay close attention to patient relations and to learn where policies and procedures need

improvement (Figure 17-1). A patient survey form may be another tool used to gain insight regarding problematic areas.

When there is a problem, staff members should feel free to openly discuss their concerns, thus avoiding

PATIENT EDUCATION

Patients need to be kept informed about office policies that management has changed or developed to enhance patient services. For example, if a physician wants to reduce incoming telephone calls and conclude all business at the time of the office visit, signs need to be placed in reception and examination rooms to inform patients that prescriptions will not be handled by telephone.

PRACTON MEDICAL GROUP, INC.

4567 BROAD AVENUE • WOODLAND HILLS, XY 12345-4700
OFFICE: (555) 486-9002 • FAX: (555) 488-7815

Fran Practon, M.D.
Gerald Practon, M.D.

PATIENT COMPLAINT DOCUMENT

Date of complaint ___5/13/XX___   Account number ___006935___

Patient name ___Kevin Skuza___   Account balance ___$750.00___

Complaint ___Pt states authorization was obtained for services, but insurance pd as if he went "out of plan" and applied $500 to the deductible. Pt called ofc and "someone" told him to work it out c̄ his insurance.___

Action taken to resolve complaint ___Track autho and rebill insurance c̄ hard copy and explanation.___

___Norma Vasquez___   ___5/13/XX___
Employee signature   Date

Figure 17-1. Patient complaint document

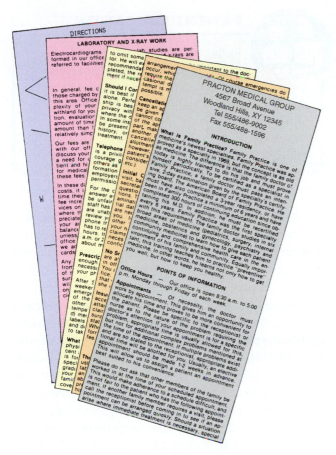

Figure 17-2. Sample pages from a medical practice information brochure

unexpected confrontations. This is often referred to as having an open-door policy. Problematic situations can be discussed at the staff meeting or privately.

Practice Information Brochure

Management consultants have determined that the easiest way to close the communication gap and reduce the number of patient questions is to present each new patient with a printed **practice information brochure** describing the basic office policies and procedures of the physician's practice (Figure 17-2). It is best designed by the physician's OM and office staff, should avoid technical language, and should emphasize points relevant to the practice. To personalize, the brochure could be written as if it were addressed to a friend. Patients could be referred to as "you" and the staff as "we." The brochure is intended to act as an effective instrument for communication with patients, to provide the answers to patients' most commonly asked questions, and to prevent relationships from deteriorating to the point of termination. It reduces questions by introducing the physician and the specialty and the office's policies and proce-

dures as well as presenting an image of a practice that is professional in every aspect. Physicians who have used information brochures report marked improvement in rapport, and they know that the brochure serves as an effective marketing tool because patients often share them with friends and relatives.

Brochure Format—Paragraphs can be typed on 8½ by 11-inch letterhead stationery or can be printed in a multipage pamphlet or brochure to fit into a standard office size envelope. If the office has a logo, it can appear on the cover. General information can include office hours, appointment scheduling, telephone procedures, and so forth. In a multiphysician office, a short biography of each doctor might be included. In a family practice, a line on the front of the brochure with a space for the patient's name might read, "This booklet prepared especially for the _____ family." If booklets are printed, it is advisable to order a six-month supply at a time, allowing sufficient time for both printing and delivery. The information presented in the brochure helps inform patients of their responsibilities and helps train them to work with the office staff and physician to provide the best medical care possible.

Brochure Headings—Paragraph headings in the patient brochure may include some or all of the following:

- Emergencies
- Office Hours
- Privacy Policy
- Appointments
  - Cancellations
  - Holiday Schedules
  - House Calls
- Telephone
- Physician Information
- Specialty Information
- Staff Information
- Services and Procedures
- Prescriptions
- Medical Records
  - Consent for Medical Treatment
  - Authorization for Release of Records
- Managed Care and Insurance Participation
- Billing and Collection Procedures
  - Payments
  - Past-Due Accounts
- Maps
  - Transportation
- Smoking
- Miscellaneous

Distribution of the Brochure—Much of the information detailed in the brochure for new patients is related to that in the office procedures manual. Therefore, any change in the manual will probably necessitate an updating of the patient information brochure.

The brochure can be mailed with a detachable medical questionnaire before the first appointment. Or, after a patient has completed the patient information form, the physician or medical assistant may personally hand the brochure to the patient, taking that opportunity to review pertinent items. An adequate supply of information brochures should also be available in all examination rooms, in the physician's office, and at the front desk.

Medical Practice Web Site

A Web site for the medical practice can be a marketing and communication tool. It should be simply designed so that navigation is easy. Items mentioned in the medical practice brochure can be included. It should attract new patients, educate existing patients, answer general questions, and include office hours, location, and driving directions. Following is a list of basic headings that may be included:

- *About Us*—State who you are. For example: Practon Medical Group is a family practice established in 1987 (list physician biographies and a brief statement about each staff member)

- *Our Mission*—The medical practice's vision and philosophy

- *Our Services*—Primary care, hospital care, surgery, nursing home visits, home visits

- *FAQ*—Frequently asked questions may be included with straightforward answers

- *Our Locations*—Include all office locations and directions from north, south, east, or west and a map

- *Contact Us*—Address, telephone, and fax numbers with a mechanism for patients to send e-mails

A Web site can streamline or eliminate tasks if registration and history forms can be filled out and printed or e-mailed to the office. Privacy notices can be read and signed, and information sites can be linked (e.g., American Heart Association, American Diabetes Association, American Cancer Association).

Designing a Web Site—After the decision is made to launch a Web site, a domain name must be selected,

---

PATIENT EDUCATION

Patient education articles may be included on the medical practice Web site and changed weekly or monthly. Subjects such as "Healthy Living," "Diabetes," "Obesity," "Women's Health Concerns," Men's Health Concerns, "Parents and Kids," and "Seniors" could be included.

---

registered, and paid for with a nominal fee. This process involves logging onto a domain name registration service and entering the name to be sure it is not already in use. Next, all Web pages must be created and the information written. Special software programs are designed to help with this task. Services such as Webmonkey, which provide step-by-step authoring procedures and developing tips, can also be used. If the OM does not have the time or technical skill to design the Web site, a professional designer may be contacted who has experience creating a clean, attractive-looking site, linking other sites, and offering technical enhancements. Whether a medical office designs a Web site in-house or outsources the job, all staff members should be asked to contribute some time and effort to the cause.

After the Web site is created, it needs to be published. A *hosting service* can be purchased; however, it is best to avoid sites that host for free. Finally, maintenance of the site must be considered. Maintenance is an ongoing process in which someone browses the site frequently to make sure all links are working and updates content as needed. See Resource section at the end of this chapter for specific Web site information.

Increasing Office Productivity

The administrative medical assistant should strive to boost office productivity so as to improve efficiency and increase income for the physician. To accomplish this goal, suggestions to the physician might include:

1. Promote specialization; for example, assign one person to handle all insurance claims, who, as a result, will acquire expertise, become known personally to claims processors, to file claims more efficiently, follow up on unpaid claims, and, thus increase reimbursement.

2. Employ part-time personnel to help during peak hours, file documents, transcribe reports,

or assist the insurance biller when there is not enough work to warrant hiring a full-time person.

3. Hire two part-time employees to share one job, known as "job sharing," to decrease overhead.

4. Initiate flextime. Adopt flexible work hours by having some personnel arrive before normal office hours to prepare for the day's patients, while others start later and stay after office hours to handle additional tasks or prepare for the next day. Offer the option of one-hour lunch breaks to be reduced to one-half hour, thus allowing the employee to arrive late or leave early. Flextime reduces tardiness and sick time substantially and is an effective recruiting tool and morale booster.

5. Encourage continuing education for the staff by paying tuition wholly or in part.

6. Ensure employees have the most current knowledge by subscribing to the latest reference material, paying registration fees for attendance at workshops and seminars, and covering dues for membership in medical societies.

7. Cross-train all staff to allow substitution for each other to reduce boredom, increase efficiency, encourage professional growth, and make the staff more versatile when personnel are absent.

8. Promote in-house expertise in financial matters; for example, develop a follow-up collection routine to handle difficult collection cases or find ways to earn top interest on cash reserves.

9. Suggest that each employee keep a notebook of hints on how to perform office tasks more efficiently and effectively.

10. Make clear to all employees that attendance is extremely important and is one of the criteria used in evaluating performance; also reduce absenteeism by paying back unused sick time or giving bonuses to those who have the best attendance records.

11. Minimize distractions in open-space offices by facing desks away from high-traffic areas.

12. Measure the physician's productivity level by determining the patient-per-hour rate. Select eight to ten recent half-day office sessions, total the number of patients seen during those sessions, and divide by the total number of office

hours in all sessions. This will help determine patient scheduling, staffing needs, and space design.

Staff Meetings

The importance of establishing a pattern of good communication among all members of the staff cannot be overstated. Regularly scheduled **staff meetings** with organized topics for discussion are a necessity; usually a 15- to 30-minute session once a week will provide a pattern of positive staff interaction (Figure 17-3). Start and stop all meetings on time; this is a courtesy to those who are punctual. Proceed at a fast pace so that inattention will not be a problem and discourage repetitious dialogue by using phrases such as, "I am sure everyone agrees that . . ." or "We have concluded that . . ." Involve employees in solving staff problems and generating outcomes or assignments from decisions that have been made. Once a decision is final, it is important for those who may disagree to refrain from carrying their dissatisfaction out of the meeting room. Allow dissatisfied employees to vent their frustration and then move on to other business. Remind everyone that all decisions are made for the good of the whole and they are sometimes restricted by financial limitations or other barriers.

Small or established offices may schedule meetings less often than large or new offices that have multiple staff members or start-up concerns. Monthly meetings around the noon hour, either in a private meeting room of a restaurant or in the office with catered food—with the physician occasionally paying for lunch—can create an atmosphere of informal-

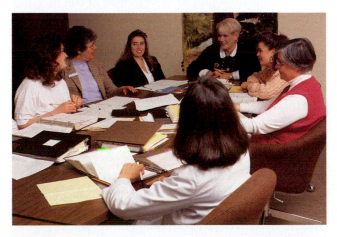

Figure 17-3. Routine staff meetings between the office manager and coworkers helps improve patient care and maintain good rapport

PROCEDURE 17-1

Set Up a Staff Meeting

Objective: To arrange a staff meeting for the physician's employees.

Equipment/Supplies: Physician, employees, meeting place, purpose, agenda, and computer.

Directions: Follow these step-by-step procedures, which include rationales, to learn this skill.

1. Verify the proposed date and time for the meeting to ensure the room will be available.

2. Gather details for the meeting, such as:

   a. Purpose of the meeting

   b. Attendees

   c. Program agenda

   d. Expected duration of the meeting

3. Arrange for the meeting room.

4. Prepare the agenda.

5. Obtain necessary equipment; for example, microphone, projector, screen, VHS player, and hand outs.

6. Compose a memo to the employees and physician to notify them of the following:

   a. Date

   b. Time

   c. Place of the meeting

   d. Program agenda

ity and camaraderie. Emphasize a team attitude, offer praise for jobs well done, and say thank you to boost performance.

Agenda

Even though staff meetings are usually informal, a prepared **agenda** will speed discussion and diffuse office conflicts. When a time has been set for a staff meeting, the OM is usually assigned to compose an agenda with input from the staff and physician. The agenda outlines topics to be reviewed at the meeting to create a plan of action. The agenda should focus on specific points but be open-ended to allow for changes. After it has been written, copies are distributed to everyone in the office for review two or three days before the meeting. A well-organized agenda will improve the quality of a staff meeting because it will provide sufficient time for a new proposal to be studied, keep topics well-focused, enable participants to prepare for discussion of office concerns, and provide time to research various aspects of office functions. Brainstorming sessions or informal meetings should have agendas for direction and to make sure time is used wisely in accomplishing goals. Figure 17-4 shows a sample agenda.

Meetings can also be used to educate or to share information acquired at workshops and seminars with a free interchange of ideas as they relate to office matters. Effective training can take place with a captured audience, and outside experts can be invited to speak or demonstrate use of new equipment or software.

Minutes

Often the administrative assistant will be asked to take minutes at staff or professional meetings. Notes have to be taken even if everyone at the meeting is in agreement that the discussion can be taped. Generally, the minutes will follow the outline of the agenda with the assistant noting the most important information. As soon as possible after the meeting, the minutes should be typed concisely and accurately while fresh in mind to avoid any omissions. Appropriate terminology, content, and format for taking minutes can be found in *Robert's Rules of Order Newly Revised.* If no action was taken on an item discussed, reference to the discussion should be omitted. Copies of the minutes should be distributed to those who attended the meeting and a copy placed with the agenda and any handouts in a file folder. Acceptable content and sequence of topics for writing minutes would be:

1. Name of parties holding meeting

2. Type of meeting (staff) and interval (weekly, monthly) with time, date, and place indicated

---

AGENDA FOR STAFF MEETING
February 2, 20XX
1:00 p.m.
Conference Room
Bag Lunch—Drinks and Dessert Provided

Call to order—Jane Paulsen, office manager

Minutes of January 21 meeting

Committee Reports:
   a. Jane Paulsen—cleaning service estimates from Todd's Cleaning and Dave's Dusters
   b. Mike O'Shea—bookkeeper, year-end financial summary

Unfinished business:
   a. Fran Practon, MD—Flex-time discussion and vote to implement April 1

New business:
   a. Carla Haskins—file clerk, advantages of alphabetic filing system vs. numeric system
   b. Amy Fluor—transcriptionist, costs of transcription machines vs. overhaul of 8-year-old model
   c. Jane Paulsen—February holiday schedule, 4-day weekend versus two 3-day weekends

Adjournment until February 25 meeting

Figure 17-4. Example of a typed agenda for a staff meeting

PROCEDURE 17-2

Prepare a Staff Meeting Agenda

Objective: To prepare a staff meeting agenda to be discussed and acted on for the smooth and efficient operation of the medical practice.

Equipment/Supplies: Minutes from previous meeting, order of business, names of individuals giving reports, notes for rough draft of agenda, new business items, and computer.

Directions: Follow these step-by-step procedures, which include rationales, to learn this skill, which is presented in the *Workbook* (Job skill 17-1) for practice.

1. Review the previous meeting's minutes to determine which old business topics need to be included.

2. Check with employees for reports on various job duties.

3. Identify new business subjects.

4. Compose a rough draft of the agenda with the gathered information.

5. Ask the physician to view the agenda for content and to make sure the agenda is correct and complete.

6. Key the final draft of the agenda and print copies for all meeting attendees.

7. Distribute the agenda to the staff meeting participants so each one can prepare for the meeting by completing any required tasks and preparing necessary documentation for reports.

3. Name of chairperson

4. Number of people present or names of absentees (sign-in sheet can be used)

5. Reading of minutes of previous meetings

6. Reports of committees, departments, or individuals

7. Old, unfinished business

8. New business

9. Adjournment, with date and place of next meeting indicated

10. Signature of chairperson or person recording minutes

If the office staff has part-time employees who seldom come together at one time, keep everyone informed on office matters by distributing minutes from the meeting, outlining decisions or action taken. A "communications book" with "need-to-know" information can be set up where each entry would be dated and addressed to specific staff members, who initial it after it has been read.

OFFICE GUIDEBOOKS

Office guidebooks are used in a medical practice as reference books for employer policies and procedures, to outline job descriptions, describe office routines, and detail job tasks. Everything an employee should know about the place of employment should be included in an employee handbook.

Employee Handbook

An **employee handbook**, also known as a personnel manual, is a compilation of data that provides standards and guidelines for work conditions (e.g., time cards, vacation, and sick leave policies). It also

PATIENT EDUCATION

Promote the medical practice through positive public relations by offering quality medical care and an efficient business environment with staff members that express the 4 Cs (care, concern, compassion, and competence). This will have a domino effect and patients will tell others.

outlines **job descriptions** and lists the responsibilities of each position and the qualifications needed to fulfill them. This can be used as a guide for each staff member's work assignments and is an excellent hiring and evaluation tool for practice management. Figure 17-5 shows the importance of a job description in various areas of office management. It assists in training, enhances morale, and fosters a cooperative spirit by making clear to employees exactly what their jobs entail. A generic job description for an entry level administrative medical assistant may be found in Chapter 1, Figure 1-3. A job description can also be useful when candidates are interviewed for a position because it effectively ensures that the applicant will understand the individual tasks and responsibilities of the position.

All employees should sign a statement indicating the handbook has been read. See Table 17-1 for suggested contents of an employee handbook.

Employment Laws and Management Plans

Employers must adhere to many statutes and regulations that are administered by the Department of Labor (DOL) and other federal agencies. The Employer Law Guide published by the DOL is a resource that can be used to determine which statutes apply to a particular business. Following some content areas of an employee's handbook are described in more detail, including the laws that relate to them. An attorney should review the handbook for wording and content to avoid future legal problems. See Resources at then end of this chapter for Web site information on agencies mentioned. Laws pertaining to wages, hours worked, and payroll are covered in Chapter 18.

American with Disabilities Act

The Americans with Disabilities Act of 1990 (ADA) is legislation that addresses the needs of employees or patients with physical or mental problems. A disabled person is a person who has a physical or mental condition that limits at least one major life activity such as walking, seeing, learning, and breathing, or a person who has a history of disability resulting from such things as a stroke or severe burns. This law affects medical offices, hospitals, and nursing homes that employ 15 or more persons. To accommodate disabled employees, for example, job descriptions and work schedules might need to be modified to

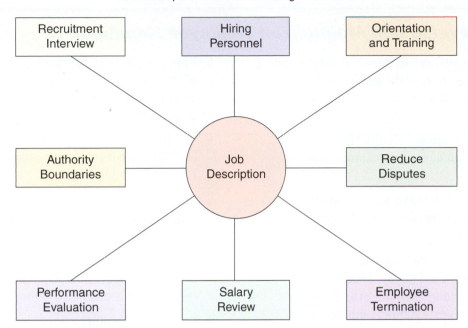

Job Description Used As a Management Tool

Figure 17-5. Job descriptions can be used in a variety of ways as a tool for good business management

Table 17-1. Recommended Contents of an Employee Handbook (Not All-Inclusive)

Introduction: Welcome to Practon Medical Group, Inc.

Absenteeism and Tardiness (excessive, excused, unexcused)

Americans with Disabilities Act

Attendance

Benefit Plans

Bereavement

Cash Shortage

Code of Ethics

Confidentiality (employer information, electronic mail, computer data, fax machine, medical records, telephone)

Continuing Education and Tuition Reimbursement

Disability: Short-Term, Long-Term, and Disability Insurance Benefits

Discrimination Issues

Disciplinary Policies

Dress Code and Regulations

Drug Abuse, Alcoholism, and Smoking Policies

E-mail, Internet, and Intranet Policies

Employment Application

Equal Opportunity Employment

Equipment and Facility Use Policy (computer software or hardware, vehicles)

Family and Medical Leave Act Policy

Forms

Full-Time Schedule and Part-Time Schedule

Grievance Procedure and Discipline

Health Insurance (COBRA rights)

Holidays

Hours of Work, Lunch, Rest Breaks

Job Descriptions

Leaves of Absence: Condolence, Sick Leave, Emergency, Maternity, Family, Jury Duty

Orientation Period and Training

OSHA Compliance

Overtime Policy

Paychecks and Paydays

Payroll Deductions

Performance Reviews

Personal Telephone Calls

Personnel Records

Privacy Policy

Probationary Period

Promotions

Resignations, Terminations, Grounds for Dismissal

Retirement Plan

Safety Policy

Salary/Wage Increases and Adjustments

Security Guidelines for Personnel

Sexual Harassment Guidelines

Smoking Policy

State Disability Insurance

Time Cards, Time Sheets, Time Clocks

Vacations: Eligibility, Accrual, Capping

Work-Related Injury (Workers' Compensation) (procedures and forms)

Right to Revise Policy

STEP 1 2 3 PROCEDURE 17-3

Develop and Maintain an Employee Handbook

Objective: To develop and maintain a comprehensive, up-to-date employee handbook to establish employment guidelines to be followed.

Equipment/Supplies: Computer, three-ring binder, paper, job descriptions, and employee handbook.

Directions: Follow these step-by-step procedures, which include rationales, to learn this skill.

1. Compile information and compose detailed step-by-step guidelines with rationales for each employment policy. These policies help staff understand the office rules and procedures pertaining to employees.

2. Write detailed and comprehensive job descriptions for each position in the medical practice.

3. Distribute appropriate job descriptions to employees within the office.

4. Title each item and key the data into a computer file, which can be easily modified when updates are needed.

5. Print the file, then alphabetize, collate, and place the pages into a three-ring reference binder. The binder lends itself to periodic updates as changes are made.

6. Identify sections by placing colored indexing tabs, and use transparent sheet covers to protect all pages.

7. Add examples where appropriate to facilitate understanding and act as a reference guide.

8. Put the employee handbook in an easily accessible location to all employees; it is only relevant if it is used as a reference.

9. Review the employee handbook annually. Keep it current by adding any new policies and deleting or modifying as necessary. This should be the task of one person.

10. Indicate a revision date at the top or bottom of each new policy when added; for example, Rev. 11/14/07. This shows that the handbook is being maintained and is up to date.

---

fit the person's limitations. Structural changes might include making drinking fountains and bathrooms easily accessible, widening aisles, raising the desk height to accommodate a wheelchair, and equipping telephones for use by the deaf. Steps to take to comply with the act would include documenting actions taken or not taken, training current employees to erase biases, revising job applications, and creating detailed job descriptions.

Benefit Plans

Title I of the Employee Retirement Income Security Act (ERISA) covers most employee benefit plans in the private sector. Such plans are voluntary and ERISA sets uniform minimum standards to ensure the plans are maintained in a fair and financially sound manner. Benefits are ensured via the statutes and authority of the Employee Benefits Security Administration (EBSA) and the Internal Revenue Service (IRS).

Disaster Response Plan

A disaster response plan is a blueprint for evacuating the premises and recovery of valuable documents and property should a catastrophe strike. To prepare an evacuation plan, draw a diagram of the medical office and mark all exits, determine a chain of command, and list each staff member's responsibilities. Familiarize staff with location of flashlights, fire extinguishers, and other emergency equipment and offer training on how to use them.

When constructing a plan for loss of use of the facility, assume that patient records and other valuable documents will not be available and describe how they can be retrieved from a remote location. Define the nature of all possible disasters (e.g., earthquake, electrical outage, explosion, fire, and so forth), then establish a priority list of what must be done. Determine an alternate site or means of operating if the present site is compromised or destroyed. Indicate the means of informing patients and staff of how the practice is recovering or of a new location. List important contacts such as employee information, government and emergency agencies, creditors, insurance carriers, suppliers, utility companies, and so forth. Prepare a script for a telephone answering machine to inform patients of why the practice has temporarily shut down, who they should call for medical emergencies, and other pertinent contact information. Duplicate and store in a fire proof safe or off site these items and other important contracts or agreements that are vital to the operation of the practice.

Involve all physicians and staff members in the planning stage and revise the plan yearly. Coordinate your plan with your neighbors if you are in an office building with other businesses. Calculate how long your practice can survive financially and determine your insurance needs; research coverage for all possible disasters.

Equal Opportunity Employment

The federal Equal Employment Opportunity (EEO) laws prohibit job discrimination based on race, color, religion, sex, or national origin. The Equal Pay Act of 1973 protects men and women who perform the same type of work in the same establishment from sex-based wage discrimination. Protection for age discrimination for individuals 40 years or older is provided by the Age Discrimination in Employment Act of 1967.

Family and Medical Leave Act

The Family and Medical Leave Act was adopted in 1993 and applies when there are more than 50 employees on staff. A few policies that would affect hospital or medical facilities are:

- Employers must offer as much as 12 weeks of unpaid leave after childbirth, adoption, or serious illness or when it is necessary to care for a seriously ill child, spouse, or parent.

- A doctor must verify a serious illness and indicate the planned duration of medical treatment.

- Health care insurance covering the employee at the time of an illness must be continued during the leave.

- Employees will be able to return to the same or comparable position.

- Employees may be exempt from leave if they have not worked at least a year or 1,250 hours or 25 hours a week in the previous 12 months.

- Employees are required to give 30 days' notice for a future planned leave.

Office Security

Medical offices may be the target of theft because of the presence of expensive equipment and drugs. The medical assistant can encourage the entire staff to be aware and take steps to prevent thievery. Insurance carriers recommend the following security steps:

1. Encourage all staff members to keep valuables such as beepers, cellular telephones, purses, and cash locked in desk drawers or cabinets to alleviate temptation.

2. Minimize the number of prescription pads to one per doctor and lock the remaining pads in a desk drawer.

3. Never leave the reception room unattended; leave one or two lights on in the reception room and hallways and close all blinds and curtains tightly at the end of the day.

4. Lock filing cabinets, cash boxes, and cupboards containing medical records, financial records, and controlled substances.

5. Install burglar alarms with digital coding that can be changed periodically and activate them each evening.

6. Keep careful records of keys that have been distributed, and be sure employees leaving the practice return all keys. Locks may need to be changed if theft is a problem.

7. Ensure inside and outside doors lock with separate keys; do not facilitate access by using a single master key.

8. Make certain all unattended doors cannot be opened from the outside during the day.

9. Lock office doors and secure all windows, if you are the last staff person leaving the office, even if the physician remains on the premises.

10. Install cylinder guards on locks and dead bolts with at least a one-inch throw, and hang doors on inside hinges.

11. Use mercury and metallic vapor lamps, which are unbreakable, for outside lighting, keeping entrances and parking areas well lit.

12. Install burglar-resistant glass.

13. Advertise office security measures by applying stickers with the name of the security alarm service to doors and windows.

14. Notify the answering service when the office is closed.

15. Keep shrubbery outside the building trimmed to no higher than 3 feet, this keeps the building well lit at night and reduces places for burglars to hide.

16. Install a system that can be activated if there are problems with unauthorized persons wandering into the back office; for example, a wireless paging system.

17. Suggest staff members leave the office together after dark.

18. Be alert for loiterers when leaving the office to make a bank deposit; vary times and patterns to avoid predictability.

19. Install a firewall and router or disconnect computer modems at the end of each day to prevent electronic theft to patient and personal records.

20. Mark all equipment with identifying marks, especially computers and computer-related items; record serial numbers and take pictures of items to store in a safe.

21. Contact the local police department for additional office security recommendations.

Safety and Health Standards (OSHA Compliance)

Safety and health conditions in the medical office are regulated by the Occupational Safety and Health Act administered by the Department of Labor's Occupational Safety and Health Administration (OSHA). Employers must be knowledgeable about all job safety issues and health standards that apply to their work situation. They must be responsible for complying with the OSH Acts 'general duty' clause (Section 5(a)(1), which states that each employer "shall furnish . . . a place of employment which is free from recognized hazards that are causing or are likely to cause death or serious physical harm to his employees." Training to protect the medical staff from on-the-job health and safety hazards and to learn proper disposal of medically related hazardous materials is usually managed by the safety officer, who is often the OM. This person is also responsible for developing a safety manual and compliance plan, performing inspections, keeping records, and correcting hazards. Employees must comply with all rules and regulations and employers who fail to meet the government standards established by OSHA are subject to fines of thousands of dollars. Offices may be checked for violations by an inspector who arrives unannounced or by advance appointment.

Medical Waste Management—The employer shall ensure the office is maintained in a clean and sanitary condition with a written schedule outlining cleaning and decontamination procedures that will include the following guidelines:

1. All equipment such as pails, bins, receptacles, and work surfaces must be cleaned and decontaminated with an appropriate disinfectant.

2. Any protective covering must be removed and replaced when contaminated.

3. Broken glassware shall not be picked up directly with the hands.

4. Any regulated waste such as liquid or semiliquid blood or infectious material must be contained and disposed of in a manner ensuring the protection of the employee.

5. Contaminated needles, blades, and glass must be placed in **sharps containers** that are labeled and are closable, puncture-resistant, sturdy, and leakproof. They must be located in designated areas, easily accessible to employees, maintained upright during use, and closed immediately prior to moving, storage, or transport.

6. Contaminated laundry must be handled as little as possible with a minimum of agitation and a color-coded label attached. It must be bagged or containerized at the location it was used and not sorted or rinsed. Employees handling contaminated laundry must wear gloves or other protective equipment.

7. Waste containers in treatment rooms should be out of reach of children.

8. Waste must be hauled by a registered hauler or an approved person and it must be properly identified.

Federal and state laws affect physicians who generate, store, haul, or treat biohazardous waste. Examples of medical waste include cultures; specimens; blood products; sharps such as needles, blades, and glass; and items with rigid corners or edges. These waste items might be generated as a result of diagnosis, testing, treatment, and immunization. In some states physicians are required to register as either a small or a large quantity generator. Usually, an accumulation of over 200 pounds of waste per month is considered to be a large generator. (Refer to Chapter 10 about disposal of controlled or uncontrolled substances.)

Waste may be treated on-site or at an approved medical waste treatment facility by incineration, discharge into a public sewage system if it meets specific requirements, or by steam sterilization.

Some of the specific regulations regarding the medical office staff and outlined by OSHA will be summarized briefly; for more detailed fact sheets, booklets, and guidelines on bloodborne pathogens, contact the nearest state OSHA office or write to OSHA Publications Office, 200 Constitution Avenue, N.W., Room N3101, Washington, DC 20210.

Exposure Control Plan—An employer must have a written plan accessible to employees and updated and reviewed annually to eliminate or minimize employees' exposure to contaminated items.

When a new employee is hired and will be exposed to bloodborne pathogens, he or she must receive formal training at the medical practice's expense during regular working hours; current employees assigned tasks that risk exposure must also receive training once a year in May. A control plan would include occupational exposure such as:

- When skin, eye, or mucous membrane comes in contact with blood or infectious materials
- When pathogenic microorganisms are present in human blood that can cause disease in humans, such as hepatitis B virus (HBV) and human immunodeficiency virus (HIV)
- When there can be contact with body fluids such as saliva, semen, vaginal secretions or contact with unfixed tissue or organs from a living or dead human

Personal Protective Equipment (PPE)—Appropriate personal protective clothing such as gloves,

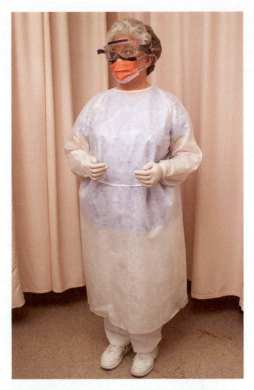

Figure 17-6. This medical assistant is wearing PPE (face shield, gown, and gloves) in preparation for assisting with a procedure that may involve contact with blood or body fluids

gowns, lab coats, face shields, mouth guards, masks, and latex gloves shall be provided by the employer at no cost to the employee with assurance that the protective item is accessible to the employee (Figure 17-6). Protective clothing shall be cleaned, replaced, repaired, or disposed of at no cost to the employee. Gloves must comply with indicated standards, and surgical caps and shoe coverings shall be worn when

COMPLIANCE

To comply with the Occupational Safety and Health Administration regulations, employers must display the Department of Labor poster informing employees of the protections of OSHA. In a medical practice, the employer must also post standard precautions for bloodborne pathogens, exposure to hazardous chemicals, and job safety and health protection guidelines in areas accessible to all employees.

contamination is anticipated and should be removed before the employee leaves the work area. Masks or eye protection equipment should be worn when droplets or splashes of blood or body fluids might be anticipated.

Immunizations—Employers must offer (free of charge) the Hepatitis B virus (HBV) vaccine to all employees who are exposed to blood or other potentially infectious materials as part of their job duties. Hepatitis B is a potentially life-threatening pathogen that is transmitted through exposure to blood or other infectious body fluids and tissues. Inoculations occur in a series of three injections; the first should be offered within ten days of hire, the second approximately thirty days later, and the third six months after the initial dose. Booster shots may be required depending on the level of immunity provided. If an employee declines the vaccination, this must be documented on the OSHA form.

Exposure Employee Records—The employer must establish and maintain accurate records for each employee indicating those who are at risk to exposure by bloodborne pathogens or other infectious agents. Each record must include:

1. Employee name and Social Security number

2. Copy of vaccination record

3. Copies of all information provided to health care professionals

4. Copies of all examinations, testing, and follow-up procedures

5. Employer's copy of the health care professionals' written opinions

Employers must ensure confidentiality of all records, and records must be maintained for the duration of employment plus 30 years. Training records are retained for five years and are not confidential; they must include training session dates, summary of session, and the trainer's name with qualifications. Training records must be provided by the employer upon request from employees, employees' representatives, Assistant Secretary of Labor for OSHA, Director of NIOSH, U.S. Department of Health and Human Services, and designated representatives. Any work-related injuries or illnesses must be documented on OSHA Form No. 200 and kept on file for five years for employee and compliance officer requests.

Sexual Harassment

Any conduct in the workplace that occurs because of a person's gender is sex discrimination, and is prohibited by Title VII of the Civil Rights Act of 1964. If an employee regards the conduct as undesirable or offensive and does not solicit or initiate the conduct then it is considered unwelcome. If employment conditions are altered so an abusive work environment is created by sexual harassment then the work environment is considered hostile. The legal definition of sexual harassment includes several types of sexual conduct in the workplace:

- *Quid pro quo harassment* (something for something)—Someone in authority offers a benefit in return for something else (e.g., a boss says, "Come to dinner with me if you want to get that raise").

- *Hostile environment*—Continual, relentless, and unwelcome sexual conduct in the workplace that interferes with an employee's work performance or creates an abusive, intimidating, and hostile work environment (e.g., sexual flirtation, vulgar language).

- *Sexual favoritism*—Sexual favors are granted by an employee to a boss in exchange for a promotion. A second employee can claim harassment because of the favoritism.

- *Harassment by nonemployees*—Customers, suppliers, or other third-parties perform some form of sexual harassment and the employer has some degree of control to stop the improper behavior but does not.

The OM should take every complaint seriously. All complaints should be documented and investigated. Never assume or make judgments based on reputation or looks. Everyone is at risk for sexual harassment, not just young and attractive women. If a case should go to court the following questions may be asked:

- Did the practice know or should it have known that harassment was taking place?

- Did the practice take any action to stop the harassment?

To reduce liability, the medical practice should establish a written policy prohibiting harassment. The language of the policy should:

- State that sexual harassment will not be tolerated

<table>
<tr><td>

EXAMPLE 17-1

Sexual Harassment

Sexual Advances by a Manager
The physician said repeatedly, "You look good in those tight white pants" to Jeanne each time she walked passed him in the office. Jeanne ignored the statement hoping he would stop.

Sex as a Condition for Promotion
An administrator of a large group medical practice called female subordinates while they were at work and bragged about sexual encounters he supposedly had with several other female workers. One time he stated, "Maggie will get the promotion because she really knows how to make me feel good."

</td></tr>
</table>

- Define various types of harassment
- Outline complaint procedures and list the person of authority with whom to file the complaint
- Guarantee that all complaints will be treated confidentially
- Guarantee that employees who file a complaint will not suffer adverse job consequences
- State that any employee who engages in sexual harassment is subject to discipline and possible discharge

Plan a staff meeting to present and explain the policy and have employees sign a form indicating they have read and understand it. The OM should seek training on how to enforce the policy and establish an effective complaint procedure.

Office Policies and Procedures Manual

An **office policies and procedures manual** is a written guide describing office routines and practices. It may contain a compilation of sample forms to be used for reference when executing office tasks. It can be used for orientation of new employees and as a handbook for people substituting for absent personnel. Figure 17-7 shows a sample page from an office policies and procedures manual.

For some offices, a more limited manual may be desirable-one that contains task sheets only, covering the work assignments of each assistant, and arranged in the sequence in which the duties are performed during a typical office day. Or, if using a computer, a "Job-File-Disk," easily updated and modified, can be prepared and filed under each subject and then printed in hard copy.

EMPLOYER RESPONSIBILITIES

This section includes recruiting new employees, conducting personal interviews, hiring, maintaining employee records, orientation, training, and staff development. Strategies for working with various personality types are discussed as well as disciplining employees, handling employee evaluations, and employee termination.

Recruitment and Hiring

A key responsibility of the OM is locating a qualified individual to fill a job that has become vacant or finding the right person for a new position. Frequently advertisements are placed in the local newspaper; however, ads may not attract the most qualified candidates. Job openings may be posted at nearby medical facilities and vocational training schools, employment agencies may be contacted, and online job notices may be placed. Sometimes a staff member may wish to apply for the open position. When resumés are received and application forms are completed, then the job of screening the applicants is performed. This is followed by doing initial interviews of the individuals chosen.

To avoid legal problems when hiring aliens, the office must be certain all job applicants are U.S. citizens with identity and eligibility to work in the United States verified within three days of hiring. Applicants born outside the United States must show a naturalization certificate or an alien registration receipt card, temporary resident receipt card, or an employment authorization card. A completed verification Form I-9, kept for three years or for one year after the person leaves employment, is required (see Procedure 17-5).

Applicant Screening

Applicants may send in a resumé or complete an application form. Review resumés and applications carefully by looking at handwriting, spelling, and sentence structure in addition to education, work experience, and skills. Read through those received to see if they are correctly typed, include essential information, and contain the qualifications needed to fill the

APPOINTMENTS

Appointment Office Hours _____
_____
_____

Time Allotment For Services and Procedures

Initial Office Visit, Complete History
and Physical Examination _____

Office Visit, Established Patient _____

Consultation _____

Office Surgery _____

_____

_____

_____

Preoperative Visit _____
Postoperative Visit _____

Questions Asked When Appointment Is Made Over the Telephone

1. Has patient been seen by any doctor in this practice within the past 3 years? _____
2. What is the primary complaint? _____
3. Is the patient covered by insurance? _____
4. Is the doctor contracted with the insurance plan? _____

Additional Information Regarding Appointments In This Office

1. If patient is new, patient should arrive at least _____ minutes prior to appointment
to complete patient information form.
2. If patient cannot keep appointment, he or she should notify the office at least _____
hours in advance to ensure no charge.
3. Uncancelled appointments scheduled for more than __ minutes will be billed at
_____ .
4. Elective appointments should be made at least _____ weeks in advance.
5. Preprinted notices are mailed as reminders for the following types of appointments:
_____

A sample of this notification is shown in this manual.

Figure 17-7. Appointment page for an office procedure manual

Table 17-2. Front-Office Procedures Manual Assignment Headings

Areas that might be discussed in a front-office procedures manual are:			
Accounts payable	Daysheet	Inventory	Photocopy
Agenda samples	Dismissal of patient letter	Laboratory procedures	Physician's bibliography
Appointment scheduling, cancellations, and recalls	Emergency and referral telephone list	Ledger	Prescriptions
Authorization forms	Equipment and maintenance	Letter samples	Professional courtesy
Banking	Fee schedule and financial policy	Mail incoming/outgoing	Recycling paper products
Billing	Filing guidelines	Manuscripts, abstracts, publications	Security measures (fire and theft)
Bonding		Medicolegal forms	Staff meetings
Bookkeeping instructions	Hospital admission sheet	Memo samples	Supply orderbook
Cash and check policy	Housekeeping duties	Narcotic records	Telephone protocol
Collection follow-up	Insurance claim forms	Patient information form	Travel information
		Petty cash	Waste management

STEP 1 2 3 PROCEDURE 17-4

Compile and Maintain an Office Policies and Procedures Manual

Objective: To develop and maintain a comprehensive, up-to-date policies and procedures manual for each administrative procedure performed in the medical office, with step-by-step instructions and rationales for performing each task to establish consistent guidelines to be followed.

Equipment/Supplies: Computer, three-ring binder, paper, and procedure manual.

Directions: Follow these step-by-step procedures, which include rationales, to learn this skill.

1. Ask each staff member to outline detailed instructions for work assignments. The job instructions can be reviewed by the OM and all office personnel for modification before being written as office policy. Clinical assistant's tasks can provide guidelines on patient care, contents of an emergency or crash cart, sterilizing procedures, laboratory and x-ray techniques, ECG procedures, and so forth. See Table 17-2 for contents of a front-office policies and procedures manual.

2. Compose and compile complete, detailed step-by-step instructions with rationales for each administrative function. These policies help maintain organized, efficient, and effective operation of the office, and employees understand why a task is performed in a specific manner.

3. Title each job assignment.

4. Key data onto standard loose-leaf sheets.

5. Alphabetize under assignment headings.

6. Collate, and place into a reference three-ring binder. This lends itself to periodic update as changes are made.

COMPLIANCE

To adhere to the Health Insurance Portability and Accountability Act of 1996 (HIPAA), a medical practice must have an appointed privacy official who drafts privacy policies and procedures, and implement a program to educate and train physicians and all employees to the mandates of HIPAA. This person could be the OM. These policies and procedures become part of the office procedure manual.

7. Identify sections by placing colored indexing tabs.

8. Use transparent sheet covers to protect all pages.

9. Add samples or examples where appropriate to facilitate learning and act as a reference guide.

10. Put one office policies and procedures manual in an easily accessible location to all employees because it is only relevant if it is used.

11. Distribute appropriate sections to various departments within the office.

12. Review the office policies and procedures manual annually. Keep it current by adding any new procedures and deleting or modifying as necessary. This should be the task of one person.

13. Indicate a revision date at the top or bottom of each new assignment when added, for example, Rev. 11/14/07, because this shows that the manual is being maintained and is up to date.

open position. Can you read the handwriting on the application? Is the form thoroughly or partially completed? Did the applicant follow the form's instructions? Screen all the applicants according to those most suited to the open position and then arrange personal interviews. If you telephone the applicant to schedule an appointment, you will have the opportunity to critique his or her telephone voice, which may be helpful if the position requires that skill. If a prospective candidate stops by the office to personally

PROCEDURE 17-5

STEP 1 2 3

Recruit an Employee

Objective: To fill a new position or replace a vacant position.

Equipment/Supplies: Job description, computer, telephone, paper, and pen.

Directions: Follow these step-by-step procedures, which include rationales, to learn this skill.

1. Discuss with the physician and staff members the required skills of the new position, or, if filling a vacancy, review the existing job description to make sure it meets the needs and is current.

2. Discuss the hourly rate for the open position with the physician even though it may be listed in the job description.

3. Compose an advertisement describing the job and submit it to the classified section of the local newspaper; indicate what response is to be made (e.g., mail resumé, fill out application, and so forth).

4. Telephone the local college or technical school and inquire from the career placement service or instructor of the medical assisting courses if he or she has any suitable candidates.

5. Attend local job fairs to let attendees know about the available position.

6. Call a local employment agency to obtain help in getting applicants interested in the open position.

7. Network with colleagues to inquire if he or she knows of someone who might be qualified for the open position.

---

hand in an application or resumé, take the opportunity to see how they are dressed and determine whether they project a professional image.

Personal Interview

Prepare for interviewing an applicant by composing a standard list of questions you wish to ask. Be careful not to make inquiries that would be prohibited by the Equal Employment Opportunity Act of 1972, such as an applicant's race, color, country of origin, sex, religion, medical history, debts, arrest records, former drug use, sexual preference, whether married, or has children. Use open-ended questions that cannot be answered with a simple "yes" or "no" answer, such as:

1. "What were the duties at your last job?"

2. What challenges have you encountered when trying to get to work on time, and how have you dealt with the situation?

3. What kind of experience have you had handling multiple tasks at once without getting frustrated or loosing your temper with patients and coworkers?

4. How are you qualified to perform this job?

5. What are two of your strengths and two weaknesses?

Refer to Chapter 19 for a list of interview questions for the job seeker, which could be used as a reference aid in developing the office manager's interview dialogue.

Another list to be developed would pertain to the observation of the applicant's grooming, eye contact, interest in and motivation for the position, mannerisms, and so on. Explain the office policies regarding working hours, pay scale, future raises, and mention sick leave, time off, vacations, fringe benefits, and dress code; detail expected duties.

Ask the applicants for the names and telephone numbers of references you may have permission to call. Research at least two references and compose a list of questions prior to telephoning.

Let the applicants ask you questions also. This may give you some idea of their communication style. Conclude the interview on a positive note if you are seriously considering an applicant for the position.

Testing

After selecting several prospective employees, test their knowledge and skills to determine whether they are capable. For grammar, spelling, composition, and tact, have them compose a letter discharging a patient from the practice. For typing, 10-key, and computer skills, give a timed test. For telephone etiquette, prepare several brief role-playing situations; you can be the patient and the applicant the receptionist, and for an insurance and coding position, devise a quiz asking specific questions about *CPT, ICD-9-CM,* and insurance carrier information.

Employee File

When hiring an employee, he or she must have a Social Security number and specific employment forms must be completed. File the original application and resumé, noting the hire date. Hand out all job descriptions that pertain to the position and obtain a signed policies and procedures agreement form. Collect all certificates of training, document dates of tuberculosis and hepatitis tests and note any exposure to blood-borne pathogens. Obtain the employee's emergency contact information and give the insurance enrollment form to the new employee for completion. Obtain signatures on other forms such as sign-off sheets for office keys and the confidentiality agreement. Financial forms related to payroll are discussed in Chapter 18.

Orientation and Training

The new employee should be introduced to everyone in the office and given a tour of the facility. To acquaint the employee with office policy, he or she is given a copy of the office policies and procedures manual to read. An explanation of the types of patients seen gives the employee some insight into who to expect to interact with as well as how to handle some of the problems that might occur. The employee's immediate supervisor usually walks the employee through the daily routine to make the employee feel more comfortable.

Specific training to use the office's medical software program should be conducted by the OM or a knowledgeable and patient coworker. The employee should be allowed to take on responsibilities one at a time and not be expected to perform all tasks immediately.

Staff Development

Offer staff development opportunities to employees and encourage staff members to attend workshops, seminars, and medical conventions. Provide read-

---

STEP 1 2 3

PROCEDURE 17-6

Orient a New Employee

Objective: To direct a new employee through job orientation and initial training of procedures required in a medical office.

Equipment/Supplies: Office policies and procedure manual, timesheet, paper, and pen.

Directions: Follow these step-by-step procedures, which include rationales, to learn this skill.

1. Meet with the new employee; be friendly, courteous, and introduce him or her to all employees.

2. Familiarize the new employee with the entire facility, showing location of coat closets, supply cabinets, staff meeting room, laboratory, physician offices, restrooms, lunchroom, and so on.

3. Inform the new employee of the duties he or she is expected to perform.

4. Give the new employee a copy of the office policies and procedures manual and advise him or her to read it. Ask the employee to note any questions down on paper for discussion at a later time.

5. Periodically check with the new employee during the first two weeks to find out if the work is going smoothly or if there are additional questions.

6. Meet weekly during the probationary period (typically the first three months) to address any problems or concerns and to give positive feedback on duties performed.

7. Check with the physician and other staff members to find out how the new employee is doing the required job duties and working as a team member.

8. Note items discussed at any meetings with the new employee and comments from other staff members. This may be of some help when the employee comes up for job performance evaluation.

ing material from newsletters, bulletins, government carriers, and professional publications. Encourage employees to attend continuing education classes at local community colleges and to join professional organizations. The more knowledgeable your staff is, the more pride they will take in their work and the better job they will do.

Working with Various Personality Types

The OM has the opportunity to work with a number of different types of people. Similar methods can be used when dealing with patients, coworkers, vendors and others as long as expectations are communicated. Always project a positive attitude and learn to work with different personalities, not against them. Empower employees by giving them encouragement, compliments, recognition and respect. Although work styles may vary, remember they were hired because they were qualified and have the right attitude to fit into the work team. Allow their differences to become assets.

Employee Disagreements and Discipline Approaches

Outline expectations and enforce them with a verbal warning, note in the employee's file or more extreme action when necessary. Your response to employees who come to you with a disagreement will be directed by the circumstances at hand. Take the time to learn wise responses. Although there is no guarantee for success, a positive change in employee's attitudes might result. Following are various approaches that can be used:

- *Advisory Approach*—When an employee complains about a coworker's problematic behavior try to help the employee solve the problem without intervening. Recall times when the employee acted appropriately and discuss how to reinforce this behavior.

- *Direct Approach*—When an employee leaves the reception desk unattended and another employee has to cover, speak directly to the employee stating, "Please let your coworker know at least 5 minutes in advance if you have to leave your job post so that coverage can be arranged."

- *Dismissive Approach*—When an employee complains about all the foot traffic passing by the door, you may want to let him or her vent and not take any action. A response could be, "It sound like this is disturbing you; however, I see you are trying to work through it and doing a good job of it."

- *Investigative Approach*—If an employee comes to you stating he or she overheard the receptionist talking back to a patient, this may involve improper behavior. Your response may be to formally investigate the situation by asking, "Can you describe how the conversation started and recite what each party said?"

- *Mediation Approach*—When two employees do not see "eye to eye" on how their shared job duties are being carried out, it may be the result of an interpersonal conflict, poor communication, or a lack of clear responsibilities. Your response may be to bring in an objective third person (another experienced employee) to help successfully resolve the disagreement.

- *Performance Approach*—When an employee does not like a coworker's personality and is disgruntled with the way he or she performs the job, try to provide work habit coaching with a performance objective: "Let's discuss three things that can be done to build a more effective working relationship, then we will assess your performance in carrying out these actions during your upcoming evaluation."

- *Planning Approach*—When one employee blames another for contributing to a problem at hand, it may be an interpersonal problem, a problem processing the information, or just sloppy work. Try outlining a work plan that requires both employees to work together to accomplish the task. Let each know that they are responsible for making the plan work and getting the task done.

- *Team Approach*—When two employees disagree on how a new task is to be done, your response might be to put together a team made up of the two employees and two others who will discuss all the possible ramifications of doing the task in several different ways then the team will decide on which way will be best.

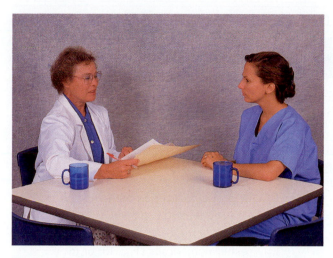

Figure 17-8. The office manager and medical assistant have established good rapport by maintaining open communication during the performance evaluation

Evaluation of Performance and Salary Review

Most employers give a 60- to 90-day probationary period to determine whether a new employee is able to work well with patients and as a team member and perform all job duties in a satisfactory manner. A date and time should be set at the end of the probationary period to review positive observations as well as areas of deficiency (Figure 17-8). The employee may ask questions and be given the opportunity to respond to a negative performance evaluation by giving his or her version of the facts. The evaluation should be candid but constructive. It should include quality and quantity of work, personal grooming, attitude, team spirit, dependability, self-discipline, motivation, and attendance. It is at this time that any problems should be mentioned and a discussion on how to resolve them conducted using problem-solving techniques and helpful criticism. Specific goals should be developed to improve any deficient areas.

Refer to Table 17-3 for various types of performance appraisals with definitions and examples.

Formal performance evaluations should be continued at regular intervals (quarterly or semiannually) because this is helpful in determining increased responsibilities as well as salary review and future promotion. The evaluation should be signed by one or two appraisers (office manager) and the employee so there is proof that the employee received the evaluation. The written evaluation should be kept con-fidential with one copy given to the employee and the original locked in the personnel file. Chapter 19 gives additional information on performance evaluation from an employee's perspective, and Figure 19-11 shows an example of a performance evaluation form.

Termination of Employees

Sometimes it becomes necessary to dismiss an employee.

Causes for dismissal include:

1. Willful disobedience

2. Violation of company policies

3. Business downturn

Prior evaluations should be reviewed to make sure the employee was informed of the performance deficiencies and the evaluations match the reasons for the employee's dismissal. A well-documented file citing specific incidents and attempts to improve the situation will provide the facts required if it should be necessary to discharge an employee; then the physician cannot be sued for defamation or libel.

The office policies and procedures manual should have a section listing the ground rules for terminating an employee. However, the final decision is left to the physician-employer based on recommendations by the OM. The OM is the one who should do the firing if he or she did the hiring. An employee who does poorly during the probationary period should be terminated using tact and giving him or her a complete explanation of the reasons for the dismissal during an exit interview. Documented episodes of underperformance and conversations regarding the need to improve will ensure no retaliatory action or potential for future legal claims.

An employee who has worked in the medical office for some time but is not performing satisfactorily should be fairly evaluated and counseled regarding the problem. A long-term attempt to cure the problem should be well documented. If he or she does not improve, then dismissal would follow.

It is recommended by practice consultants that a discussion about termination with the employee be scheduled at the end of the day after all employees have left. When asked by a prospective employer for details, the OM or physician can simply state, "I would not hire the ex-employee again."

According to the Fair Labor Standards Act, severance pay is a matter of agreement between an

Table 17-3. Types of Performance Evaluations With Definitions and Examples

Type of Evaluation	Definition	Example
Behavioral Evaluation	Assess specific actions and conduct (on-the-job behavior) to weigh job success	The supervisor sits at the side of the employee while doing computer functions and accesses his or her attitude toward technology
Critical Incident Evaluation	Specific events and actions are used to access employee's performance	The employee calmed down a patient at the front desk who was out of control. The appraisal focuses on the elements used in the successful encounter
Duties Evaluation	The job description is used as a basis for assessment	Each duty of the job description is rated, either numerically (1 to 10) or in narrative form
Forced Choice Evaluation	Both employee and OM rate skills and performance as opposites	Assessment of the employee's ability to solve problems: Are solutions individually analyzed or are others involved in discussion of the problem?
Management-By-Objective Evaluation (MBO)	Compares actual performance and results against predetermined benchmarks	A certain number of insurance claims should be processed daily; daily results are accessed
Metric Evaluation	Various areas of performance are reduced to quantitative scales or standards and accessed by coworkers	Assessing how well an employee can multitask: Coworkers are asked to rate the employee on a numerical scale (1 to 10)
Performance Review Form	List of statements are included on a form with an area to check off "Excellent," "Satisfactory," "Needs Improvement," "Unacceptable"	List might include: (1) Conducts self in professional manner with patients, (2) Performs well under pressure, (3) Workis neat and legible
Periodic Evaluation	Supervisor appraises the employee's work at regular intervals throughout the year (weekly, monthly) in conference style	Annually, the evaluation is a compilation and summary of previous appraisals
Process Evaluation	Attempts to access how well the employee follows procedures	Uses standards for such duties as posting to ledgers, totaling daysheets, or submitting authorization requests
Rating Evaluation	Classifies performance on a number of job attributes using a numerical scale with room for comments	(1) Continuing education, (2) Efficient use of time, (3) Motivation, (4) Neatness, (5) Punctuality
Self-Appraisal	Employee initially evaluates his or her work by preparing a narrative summary of accomplishments; used as a basis for discussion	Accounts receivable was decreased by 3 percent during the last quarter
360-Degree Evaluation	Attempts to obtain feedback from everyone who works with the employee	How well does the employee communicate with patients? . . . Handle stress? . . . Interact with coworkers?

employer and an employee. It is usually based on how long an employee has been employed when he or she is terminated.

FACILITY OVERSIGHT

The OM is in charge of all aspects of the facility and the medical practice, including building maintenance, service contracts, utilities, insurance, equipment, and supplies. Keeping the office in good running order involves overseeing housekeeping duties and making purchasing decisions, although some tasks can be delegated to staff members.

Building Maintenance

Whether the building is owned by the medical practice or rented, it should be well maintained. If owned, the OM will deal directly with outside contractors and should arrange for periodic inspections to check the condition of the water heater, roof, carpet, parking lot, and so forth. Termite and fire inspections will need to be arranged. If the office space is rented, the OM will contact the landlord when problems occur.

Housekeeping

The OM will determine which housekeeping duties will be performed by the staff and which ones will be done by a professional cleaning service. The staff may be asked to pick up loose objects and make sure everything is in its place, dust furniture, wipe glass tables, clean mirrors, spot-clean furniture and carpets, and disinfect portions of the reception area (see Chapter 5). Before selecting a service, minimum cleaning requirements must be established and standards set. Janitorial duties usually include vacuuming rugs, mopping floors, washing woodwork, scrubbing sinks and toilets, and emptying wastepaper baskets. Cleaning services are often reluctant to wipe treatment room counters and perform cleaning near unfamiliar equipment; these tasks are best left to staff members. The clinical medical assistant is usually assigned to disinfect treatment rooms and the office laboratory. This person should pay particular attention to counter tops and doorknobs. Leave a note for the cleaning staff when special tasks need to be done. Arrange a schedule for additional services such as window washing, laundering drapes, cleaning carpet, and other types of deep cleaning. Before a contract can be negotiated, several price bids should be solicited for comparison. If during the contract period, the service proves to be

inadequate and discussion fails to solve the problem, seek new bids and hire a new cleaning service.

Cleaning Equipment and Supplies—Cleaning equipment and supplies must be readily available for staff members so that they can keep the facility clean throughout the day. Protective gloves should be worn when cleaning and try to perform tasks out of the sight of patients when possible. A vacuum cleaner (upright with handheld attachments), dust mop, and broom are essential equipment along with cleaning solutions, window cleaner, furniture polish, trash bags, cleaning washclothes, and a bucket. A carpet sweeper may be kept on hand to quickly pick up items that have been dropped or dirt that has been tracked into the office.

Equipment

Office and medical equipment must be serviced and maintained and may periodically need to be replaced. The OM can order new instruments, furniture, or expensive pieces of equipment only with the physician's express approval. Communication equipment such as the telephone system, fax machine, pagers, and beepers are offered by many vendors, so it is wise to do comparison shopping. Solicit staff input when purchasing such things as typewriters, dictating/transcribing equipment, adding machines, and calculators. The performance of staff members often depends on the type of equipment used, so it is good to involve them in purchasing decisions. Photocopy machines receive a lot of use in a medical office, and their selection should be based on the size of the machine needed, as well as volume, speed, ease of use, and cost. A postage meter and scale proves to be a good investment, saving both time and money. A paper shredder should be available; however, all final decisions to shred documents should be directed by the OM or physician. Computer hardware is considered a major expense and a thorough investigation should take place prior to deciding to purchase this type of equipment. Medical software can be expensive, and it is wise to spend a day at another facility where the software under consideration is being used. This will allow you to see it in action and ask questions prior to making the decision to buy.

When evaluating a piece of equipment, examine all of the special features and consider the benefits they will provide. Determine which ones are necessary and how easy the equipment is to use. Note the size, weight, appearance, warranty, and price. When replacing equipment, evaluate how the old piece of equipment served the office needs. If the equipment performed well and lasted a long time, consider replacing it with a newer model of the same name brand.

Purchasing

When large pieces of equipment are needed, decide first whether to purchase it outright or to lease it. Look in the yellow pages, visit local retail stores, and search online for the best prices and sales information. Have sales representatives demonstrate the product and operate it yourself prior to the final purchase. Take your time to analyze the product and compare it to others before selecting what you think best meets the needs of the office. You may want to get a recommendation from the physician and or discuss the purchase with him or her. Each piece of equipment comes with a limited warranty, usually for one year. Find out what is included and what is not, along with the length of time covered. Consider an extended warranty to increase the length of time if it is an item that demands frequent service (e.g., copy machine). Consult an accountant about depreciation and tax consequences of all major purchases.

Leasing

Consider leasing equipment if keeping costs low is a priority or if the physician replaces equipment frequently. Before leasing, examine the terms of the lease agreement, find out the initial cost, and determine what the monthly payment will be. Consider how much you will pay over the time-frame listed in the agreement and compare it with the outright purchase price. Find out if the lease includes service and if the lease payments are deductible on the physician's income tax return. Weigh the advantages and disadvantages of leasing and buying prior to making a decision.

Equipment Maintenance

Keep office equipment in working order so that it will provide high-quality service. Vacuum dust particles from computer components and the copy machine, change ink cartridges and toner when needed, and treat all equipment as if you owned it personally. Become familiar with each piece of equipment so simple problems can be resolved without service calls. Solicit the help of a staff member who enjoys technology and put him or her in charge of equipment maintenance.

For all electronic equipment plugged into outlets, surge suppressors should be used to prevent damage by power spikes. A special type of surge suppressor should be obtained for facsimile equipment.

Repairs may be facilitated by keeping a service file folder containing maintenance records and operation instructions on all office and medical equipment. Major equipment repairs should be handled by qualified repair people. Guarantees, instruction manuals, information pamphlets, and service contracts are placed in the service file folder; and guarantee cards should be mailed as soon as the equipment has been delivered. To manage equipment maintenance, the assistant should:

1. Assign one person to request repairs on all equipment, thus eliminating the possibility of everyone, or no one, calling for service.

2. Arrange for equipment to be serviced immediately when failures occur.

3. Deal only with respected service companies that respond quickly to requests for service.

4. Keep an up-to-date list of all equipment and repair costs; this information will help determine when the cost of maintaining a piece of equipment might justify its replacement. These figures will be necessary and readily available for making up the operating budget.

5. Understand the service agreement before the equipment is purchased. A service agreement is a form of insurance against future repair costs and as such contains certain specifications that should be thoroughly understood by the staff person in charge of managing the maintenance of the equipment.

6. Stockpile frequently replaced parts.

If the medical assistant performs a well-organized approach to equipment repairs, delays due to downtime will be minimized, and many of the problems that can destroy operating efficiency will be avoided.

Office Supplies

Ordering supplies and maintaining an adequate inventory is usually the responsibility of the OM, but the task may be delegated to those who use the supplies daily. The clinical assistant is primarily concerned with keeping on hand medical supplies and equipment related to patient care, whereas the administrative assistant orders clerical supplies, forms, and items used in running the business side of the practice. A sign-out procedure that establishes who checked out supplies listing dates will help the buyer track actual usage and will discourage waste and theft.

Reducing Supply Expenses

Some suggestions for maintaining inventory and reducing expenses are:

- Establish a baseline amount spent previously on a specific item and then track price trends.

- Set a budget for supplies based upon the average amounts spent during the past year or two.

- Comparison shop about twice a year, researching prices on major items.

- Buy selected items in bulk if storage is available, and consider pooling purchases if there are other physicians in the building.

- Take advantage of special discounts and free shipping incentives.

- Maintain a friendly attitude with the local stationer who can get items immediately even if most items are ordered from catalogs.

- Track inventory in the storage room at regular intervals.

Ordering Supplies

The frequency of ordering supplies will depend on storage space and cash flow. Availability of products and approximate delivery time also need to be considered when ordering.

Clinical supplies must be evaluated depending on the office policy and procedures; for example, every two weeks or every month. Supplies should be ordered to last for several months, and the ordering should be done on a preset schedule.

Important points to consider when selecting a supplier are: quality, price, and service; that is, how the sales representative will work with you to get the item when needed. When it is decided which stationery or business supply houses to patronize, it is wise for the assistant to establish and maintain good credit and business relations with the designated firms. If a problem develops, work with the merchant to solve it. There is generally no reason to change to another supplier unless the service has deteriorated, items are inferior in quality, or a better price can be consistently obtained by another retailer. Most firms try to please their established customers by expediting

orders and by allowing a new product to be sampled before purchase.

Orders for supplies from out-of-town dealers may be placed directly with a sales representative or by fax, telephone, or completing and mailing a purchase order form (Figure 17-9). If necessary, delivery in one or two days can be arranged with United Parcel Service (UPS) or other delivery services. Typical office supplies ordered are paper goods (e.g., Kleenex, paper towels), computer disks, paper, and printer cartridges; copy toner and paper for typewriters, printers, fax, and copy machines; appointment sheets, daysheets, ledger cards, file folders, and labels; letterhead stationery, envelopes, pens, pencils, rubber stamps, paper clips, and so forth.

Consider ordering online if you are in a remote area or if your storage space is small. Supplies ordered over the Internet can be shipped within 24 hours, less cash is tied up in inventory, and less space is devoted to storing supplies.

Consider a group purchase organization (GPO) if you manage a small office and are paying high prices for goods. A GPO is an organization that joins businesses to increase negotiating and purchasing power. Experts provide information to its members and handle the purchasing. The limitations of using a GPO might include limited choices of products (usually only one line of each product type is carried) and decreased information on new products.

Purchase Orders—A *purchase order* is a written authorization to a merchant to deliver merchandise, materials, or services at an agreed-upon price. Once accepted by the supplier, the purchase order becomes a legally binding purchase contract. Purchase orders are used by large businesses, such as hospitals and clinics. When supplies are delivered, the purchase order number is included on the invoice as verification of the order.

Payment of Invoices

Businesslike purchasing habits are fundamental to the efficient management of the medical office. Purchasing supplies in bulk and paying invoices, itemizing merchandise ordered, within the 10- to 30-day discount period will save the physician money. However, overstocking of items to obtain a discount can mean extra costs if the items become obsolete, deteriorate with age, get dirty on the shelf, or monopolize shelf space; for example, rubber bands stiffen if kept too long, and some liquids evaporate.

ORDER FORM 67000_B

medical arts press

SOURCE CODE	CUSTOMER NUMBER
B2PX	6796030

1-A BILL TO: Party responsible for payment. If name and address are not correct, please make changes below. We cannot ship to a P.O. Box. If P.O. Box is shown, please fill in street address in "Ship To" area at right.

PRACTON MEDICAL GROUP, INC
4567 BROAD AVENUE
WOODLAND HILLS, XY 12345-4700

Office Phone (555) 486-9002   FAX Phone (555) 488-7815
E-Mail Address: PMG@AOL.COM

For questions...
Call BECKY
Phone (555) 486-9002

To serve you better
Practice Specialty Family/General practice
No. of Doctors 2

1-B SHIP TO: (Fill in only if different from "BILL TO".) For delivery, we must have a street address. We cannot ship to a P.O. Box.
Name(s) _____
Address _____
_____
City _____
State/Zip _____

3 PLEASE SEND ME: Fill in only those areas that apply to your order.

Please Fill In As Applicable

QUANTITY	CATALOG NUMBER	DESCRIPTION	MESSAGE	INK COLOR(S)	TYPE STYLE	LAYOUT NO.	LOGO NO.	PRODUCT COLOR	SIZE	YEAR	START NO.	TOTAL AMOUNT
3 ea	36B	Correction pens										9.75
4 boxes	98IT	Plastic clip ball point pens										15.92
1 pk	337P	Post-it pop-up dispenser pack										12.73
5 reams	811P	16 # White bond paper						white				51.25
3 reams	989J	Yellow second sheet paper						yellow				6.75

COUPON CODE(S) If you have any coupon or discount codes, please enter them here:

*For Rush Delivery specify: ☐ UPS Next Day   ☐ UPS 2nd Day
Check the box at left if desired. You will be billed for rush shipping and handling charges.

☐ **RX BLANKS** (Complete the following information as it pertains to your state requirements.)
DEA No. _____
License No. _____

☐ **MEDICAL INSURANCE CLAIM FORMS** (Only complete the following if you want it printed on your forms.)
Box 25:   Box 33:
SSN No. _____   PIN No. _____
or   or
Group No. _____   EIN No. _____

MERCHANDISE TOTAL	96.40
Handling Fee	FREE
Sales Tax: Medical Arts Press collects tax in all states that have a sales/use tax. Please add tax at applicable rate.	4.82
*Rush Delivery	
TOTAL	101.22

Figure 17-9. Purchase order form for office supplies. (Courtesy of Medical Arts Press, PO Box 43200, Minneapolis, MN 55443-0200; Telephone: (800) 328-2179; Web site: http://www.medicalartspress.com.)

If an item is temporarily out of stock, the supplier indicates on the invoice **"back ordered (B/O)"** and returns a copy to the office; then, when shipment is received from the manufacturer, the supplier sends it on to the office. A date may be included to indicate when the back-ordered item is available. When an order needs to be followed up on, an item is defective, or a mistake has been made, notify the supplier and indicate the invoice number, the date of the order or shipment, and the complaint. When an order is received, each item should be checked off on the packing list (slip), which is a statement of the contents of a container. Then the *packing list (slip)* is filed, awaiting arrival of the **invoice**, a statement of amounts owed that is prepared by the seller of the supplies or

(*text continues on page 602*)

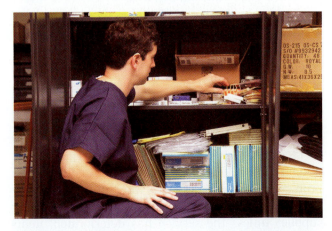

Figure 17-10. Medical assistant organizing supplies on a shelf in the medical office

STEP 1 2 3

PROCEDURE 17-7

Prepare an Order Form

Objective: To prepare an order form for ordering office or medical supplies.

Equipment/Supplies: Order form, inventory reorder notice, catalog, and computer or typewriter.

Directions: Follow these step-by-step procedures, which include rationales, to learn this skill, which is presented in the *Workbook* (Job Skill 17-3 and 17-4) for practice.

1. Obtain all inventory reorder notices and make a list of all supplies and items low in inventory.

2. Use an order form and insert the "ship to" address where the items ordered should be sent by the supplier.

3. Insert the address where the supplier needs to send the billing statement (invoice) for payment, if the "bill to" address is different from the office location.

4. Note the customer (order) number, which may be preprinted on the order form. This number may be used for tracking a lost order and appear on the invoice when billing.

5. For some medical supplies, you may need a physician's signature, a copy of his or her medical license, or a copy of the doctor's DEA certificate.

6. Insert the vendor or supplier name and the address (if not provided) where the order needs to be faxed or sent.

7. Insert the date on the order, which is the date when placing the order.

8. Insert the method of payment (cash, check, credit card) agreed upon under "terms."

9. Key in the method of shipping (United Parcel Service, Federal Express, Airborne Express, U.S. Postal Service) agreed upon, and indicate whether express delivery is required.

10. List the quantity of each item ordered and type of unit (e.g., box, ream, package).

11. List the stock, catalog, or item number.

12. Give a brief description of the ordered item to ensure accuracy; the supplier may need to refer to the description if an item number is obsolete or entered incorrectly.

13. Insert special order information (e.g., color, style, size) if applicable, and the unit price in the designated areas on the form, stating whether it is sold individually (each), box, case, dozen, or gross.

14. Calculate and enter the total cost of all units for each item (multiply the number of units ordered by the unit price).

15. Insert a subtotal of all of the items ordered.

16. Calculate and list the sales tax required by the state.

EXAMPLE 17-2

Calculate Sales Tax

Using a sales tax percentage multiply the total cost by the sales tax rate:

5%	7.25%
$125	$125
× .05	× .0725
$6.25	$9.06

17. Enter the shipping and handling fee.

18. Enter the "total amount due" for all items, including tax, shipping, and handling.

19. Either insert the name of the person requesting the item or sign the order.

20. Double-check figures and proofread the order before submitting it to the supplier.

(continues)

PROCEDURE 17-7 *continued*

21. Submit the order by fax, telephone, mail, or transmit electronically over the Internet. If ordering by fax, telephone to verify that the order was received and understood, and confirm the delivery date and payment requirements. If ordering by telephone, obtain the order or confirmation number.

22. Indicate on the inventory cards the date the order was placed so as not to duplicate the order when using an inventory system.

23. File a copy of the order in the appropriate file for easy access when the merchandise is received.

PROCEDURE 17-8

Pay an Invoice

Objective: To verify receipt of an order and pay the invoice using appropriate accounting procedures.

Equipment/Supplies: Invoice, packing list (slip), check, envelope, and pen.

Directions: Follow these step-by-step procedures, which include rationales, to learn this skill.

EXAMPLE 17-3

Invoice Terms

Terms	Meaning
• Terms	Refers to timing of payment
• Net 30	Buyer has 30 days in which to pay the total amount
• 1 Percent 10 Days Net 30	A savings of 1 percent of the total sales amount by paying the balance within 10 days (or 2 to 5 percent 30 Days Net)
• F.O.B	"Free on Board" relates to responsibility for paying the carrier
• F.O.B. Point	Customer will have responsibility for the charge and claim if the material is lost in transit
• F.O.B. Destination	Vendor will bear the responsibility

1. Acknowledge receipt of merchandise ordered by signing the shipping receipt and listing the date received.

2. Check the original order against the packing list (slip) to determine that all items ordered have been received in good condition at the quoted price.

3. Verify that dated drugs or supplies are current.

4. Confirm that quantity discounts and discount dates have been observed.

5. Compare the invoice with the packing list (slip).

6. Authenticate that invoice calculations and figures are correct.

7. Verify that the invoice has not already been paid.

8. Write a check for the balance due amount of the invoice. "For Deposit Only" may be written on the back of any check to be mailed. Then if the check is stolen, the thief cannot cash it.

9. Write the invoice number in the memo section on the front of the check to provide identification on the canceled check should any question arise at a later date.

10. Present the check to the physician for his or her signature.

11. Post an entry in the check register.

PROCEDURE 17-8 *continued*

12. Rubber-stamp or write a notation on the invoice that indicates the invoice has been paid (Pd or PIF-paid in full) and include the date, amount of payment, check number, and the assistant's or physician's initials (Figure 17-11).

13. Staple the packing list (slip) to the invoice and file with other accounts payable receipts (in an accordion A to Z file folder) to be kept a minimum of three years.

INVOICE   No. 1972

Sold to:	Ship to:
Practon Medical Group, Inc.	Practon Medical Group, Inc.
4567 Broad Avenue	4567 Broad Avenue
Woodland Hills, XY 12345-4700	Woodland Hills, XY 12345-4700

Date	Order No.	Terms	Weight	Store No.	Dept No.	Shipped Via
05/01/20XX	97231	C.O.D.		15	23	United Parcel Service

BEST-BUY MEDICAL SUPPLY COMPANY

Quantity	Unit	Size/Color	Description	Unit Price	Amount	Total
12	boxes	medium	Non-latex exam gloves	9.49	113.88	113.88
2	cartons	white	Table paper	34.99	69.98	183.86
					Sales tax	9.19
					TOTAL DUE	**$193.05**

DATE PD   6/2/20XX
CK.#   4289
AMT.   193.05
APPROVED BY: MS

CUSTOMER COPY

Figure 17-11. Completed invoice with a paid notation

services listing quantity, item, shipping date, and price.

Types of Systems for Controlling Inventory

A continuing ample stock of supplies depends on an effective inventory control system. A good system should include current office supply catalogs, an up-to-date list of all supplies, the number of items on the shelf, the reorder point, and time required to fill an order.

Many supply companies include a reorder form with shipments so it is important to check the amount of remaining stock each time items are removed from the shelf or storage area in case an order needs to be placed.

Manual System—One method for maintaining adequate office supplies is to label each inventory item with a strip of plastic adhesive tape on which is written the name of the item and the minimum number of units constituting a safe reserve. Each time stock is withdrawn, the units remaining are checked against the reorder point; when the reserve supply matches the number on the label, an order is placed.

A similar system is to put colored markers or index cards on shelves between boxes or supplies at the reorder point and to attach a rubber band to the last stock item. A red marker or card might signal that an item needs to be reordered; a yellow marker is substituted to indicate the order has been placed. When staff members remove the item just in front of the marker, they notify the OM so the supplier can be contacted or the card placed in a "to be ordered" envelope. When the order arrives, the yellow marker is removed and a red marker is reinserted at the point where reordering is necessary. Orders can be made by placing a call to the supplier's toll-free 800 number, by fax, via e-mail, or at their Web site. Preplanning will avoid costly rush orders.

Another way to use a manual system is to list each inventory item on individual sheets of notebook paper or on **inventory cards** arranged in alphabetic order. Entries, written in pencil because some data will change, record the following information:

1. Name of the item
2. Identification or catalog number
3. Supplier's or manufacturer's name, address, and telephone number
4. Quantity ordered
5. Reorder point
6. Price
7. Dates when each order was placed, received, and paid for

The amount of an item to purchase can be determined by evaluating and comparing information dealing with the consumption rate, cost, and the amount of storage space available. If an item proves unsatisfactory, it can be identified by a notation on the card. Inventory cards are usually kept in a file near the cabinet (storage area) or at the assistant's desk.

A running-inventory card provides preprinted columnar headings for listing quantity, reorder point, and the location of supplies (Figure 17-12). Each time items are removed from the shelf or storage area, the amount taken is crossed off leaving the correct amount remaining, this provides sufficient warning to reorder. Running-inventory cards should be kept near the supply cabinets.

ITEM	QUANTITY	REORDER POINT	LOCATION	
Black felt-tip pens	6 bx. ~~6 5 4 3~~ 2 1	2	Drawer	#2
9 x 12 manila file folders (center cut)	6 bx. ~~5~~ 4 3 2 1	2	Cupboard	#4
Blue adhesive file folder labels	8 bx. ~~7 6 5~~ 4 3 2 1	5	Cupboard	#4
3" center metal fasteners	6 bx. ~~5~~ 4 3 2 1	3	Drawer	#3

Figure 17-12. Running-inventory card for office supplies

```
DATE: 09/30/XX   STOCK LIST      PAGE:1
TIME:   01:13 PM


STOCK
NUMBER    DESCRIPTION      AMOUNT
DEPT
-------------------------------------------

  3       ACE 1" WRAP         10
  2       ACE 3" WRAP         10
  1       BANDAGE             10
  5       SHEETS               3
  4       TONGUE DEPRESSORS    2


      5 ITEMS ON FILE
```

Figure 17-13. Computer printout of an inventory sheet for office supplies

Computerized Systems—Computer software is available for creating a database of inventory for equipment as well as clinical and office supplies. When an item is purchased, sold, traded, or replaced, the information is keyed into the inventory database. It is easy to add or delete items as necessary. For tax purposes, it is important to keep a list that shows all equipment and any items that have been replaced. A current inventory list can be printed at any time (Figure 17-13). The computer can be programmed to automatically alert when to order supplies. If the office uses a modem, the order can be placed directly with the supply house, which speeds delivery and reduces mistakes.

In a multiphysician practice, supplies are usually checked and stocked in a major supply room once a week, with the OM maintaining control and another staff member assigned as backup. Replenishing items on a regular basis prevents unanticipated shortages.

Regardless of the inventory system used, all supplies must be counted regularly and labeled with expiration dates when applicable. The scheduling of inventory will be governed by the rate at which items are used.

Storing Office Supplies

When shelves are being restocked, older supplies go in front and newer items at the rear. If a central supply area is not provided, similar items of inventory can be grouped and placed at various locations in the office.

The following are tips for storing office supplies:

1. Leave all bond paper sealed in original boxes; use older paper first and open new packages only as needed.

2. Avoid storing paper products in cold, damp rooms; do not expose to direct sunlight.

3. Stack boxes horizontally because standing paper packages on end will cause paper to curl.

4. Install wooden dividers to separate items stored on one shelf.

5. Attach identifying labels to shelves indicating the items that are stored there.

6. Store information pamphlets and maintenance brochures vertically to save space.

7. Position small items at eye level.

8. Place large, bulky supplies on lower rear shelves.

9. Never keep on hand more than a year's supply of inventory unless space is of no concern and the discount was terrific.

10. Check all incoming orders to make certain that items ordered have been received, and then place them beneath or behind other similar items.

Sterile, disposable paper products have virtually eliminated the need for an inventory of linen supplies. If, however, the physician owns linens or contracts to have sheets, gowns, or uniforms cleaned, each item should be labeled with permanent ink. When linen supplies are delivered to the office, the medical assistant is responsible for checking the invoice to be sure that everything sent out has been returned.

BUSINESS TRAVEL

The OM may be asked by the physician to formulate and expedite arrangements for business trips or travel to medical conventions held in this country or abroad. A worry-free trip depends on systematic and prudent planning to eliminate the frustrating problems

STEP 1 2 3

PROCEDURE 17-9

Establish and Maintain Inventory

Objective: To establish and maintain an inventory of all expendable supplies and follow an efficient well-organized plan of order control using a card system.

Equipment/Supplies: File box, inventory control cards, list of supplies on hand, metal tags, reorder tags, and pen or pencil.

Directions: Follow these step-by-step procedures, which include rationales, to learn this skill.

1. Compose a list of administrative and clinical supplies and insert a copy in the office policies and procedures manual.

2. Make a file for supply invoices, and completed order forms. These documents must be retained for three years.

3. Create an inventory system of 3-inch × 5-inch file cards and list the following data on each card.

   a. Name of the item and quantity on hand.

   b. Name, address, and telephone number for the supplier or sales representative.

   c. Number for the reorder point, place a reorder tag at the location where the supply should be replenished.

   d. Place the movable metal tag over the order section of the file card to act as a reminder when placing the next order.

   e. Place the order and note the date and quantity of each order in the appropriate location on the file card; move the metal tag to the "on order" section of the card.

   f. When the shipment is received, insert the date received, unit cost or price per piece in the appropriate location on the file card, remove the metal tag, and refile the card. For orders only partially filled, let the metal tag remain until the order is complete.

4. Take inventory every one to two weeks to check stock and reorder. Mark data when inventory is checked on your calendar, or make a tickler file in the computer.

---

that haphazard arrangements can bring. No matter what the distance or duration of the trip, the manager should be able to make arrangements when the physician announces his or her plans.

Travel Arrangements

As soon as a convention site is announced and a decision is made to attend, the OM must see that applications for attendance are returned. On receiving written confirmation, the OM may be asked to make travel and hotel arrangements. Any delay or procrastination in initiating reservations may mean the physician will be unable to stay at the hotel where the convention is being held, and it might affect the chance of securing the most direct transportation at an affordable cost.

Use an atlas if you are unfamiliar with geography and need to determine mileage. Accumulate the physician's preferences in a travel file folder noting favorite airlines, hotel/motel accommodations, and car rental agencies. Also included might be discount and credit card identification numbers, passport and visa numbers, frequent flyer numbers, class of travel preferred, airline aisle or window seating choice, and special meal or dietary preferences. The OM can discuss with the physician the purpose of the trip, the dates of departure and arrival, as well as a daily business schedule and the accommodation preferred for a specific trip. When the basic details are arranged to the physician's satisfaction, the OM can proceed to make the arrangements via the Internet or telephone, or by contacting a travel agent who will handle all the details for a small fee.

Travel Agent

If the physician plans to be out of town on numerous occasions during the year or is planning a convention trip with multiple stopovers, the OM should select a reputable veteran local travel agent. A travel agent uses a computerized system to obtain availability information and has the expertise to assist in all areas of travel (airline, hotel, car rental) and can handle changes or problems if they occur.

To work productively with a travel agent, the assistant should gather all information and determine a basic itinerary. In addition to making reliable arrangements for transportation and accommoda- tions, a travel agent will arrange for shuttles to and from the airport, procure visa application forms, obtain insurance information, make sight-seeing res- ervations, and handle special arrangements related to diets. The final **itinerary** is supplied by the travel agent. It must be accurate because it will be distrib- uted to other physicians and medical personnel who might need to contact the physician in an emergency (Figure 17-14).

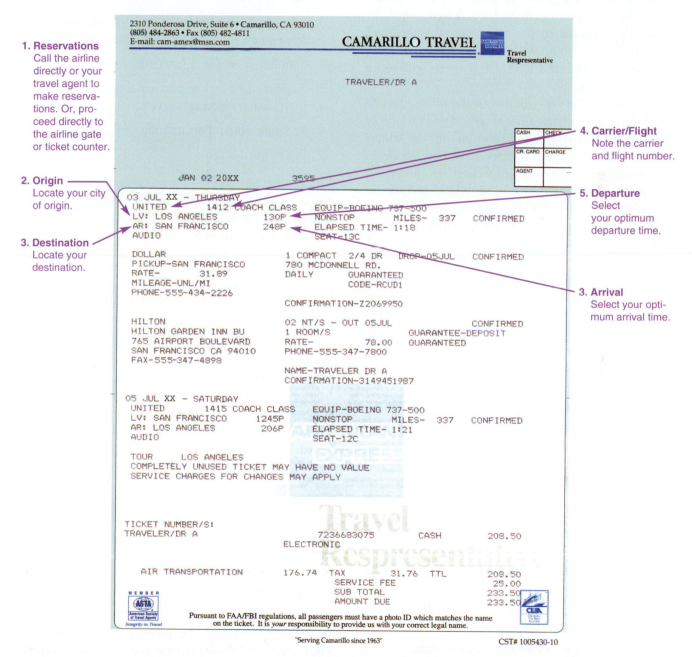

Figure 17-14. A travel itinerary and invoice. (Courtesy of Janet LaMacchia, Camarillo Travel, Camarillo, California.)

Airline Travel Reservations

When making airline reservations by telephone note the name of the reservation clerk and record the confirmation number. If another call is necessary, the reservation can be quickly retrieved. The assistant should know if the physician prefers first class or coach accommodations prior to making the telephone call. Connecting flight reservations can be made with the airline through which the trip is initiated. Plane arrival and departure times are printed as local times. Multi-legged trips usually require confirmation at every point of departure. A non-stop flight means the airplane makes *no* stops, while a direct flight means the plane will stop at least once before reaching the final destination but there will be no change of planes.

If airline tickets are mailed to the office, the OM should promptly check arrival and departure dates and times against the information on the itinerary work sheet to see that they have been made as requested. It is extremely important to clarify the charge for cancellation or change when making the reservations. Airline tickets are nontransferable and may be totally refundable, reusable within one year, or have penalties to reuse.

Many airlines offer serve-yourself check-in at the airport and e-mail check-in to eliminate misplaced tickets and expedite check in. When making the reservation, request an e-ticket with a confirmation number and itinerary.

Hotel and Motel Accommodations

Most hotel and motel chains have toll-free 800 numbers that can be used to make and verify reservations. A hotel room is typically "reserved" until 6 p.m. If arrival time is to be after 6 p.m., it is necessary to notify the reservation clerk ahead of time. If the physician is attending a convention, the assistant should convey this to the clerk to obtain special group rates. Before making the room reservation, the OM should have a knowledge of the physician's preferences, and be prepared to ask the hotel clerk the following questions:

1. Are there "business-class" rooms or floors with fax and computer hookup facilities?

2. Are there express check-in and checkout procedures?

3. Is there a deadline for cancellation? (If yes, it should be in writing.)

4. What is the checkout time and is there a charge or penalty for early checkout?

When making a room reservation, the assistant should be ready with the following information:

1. Type of room desired (single, double, queen, king, suite)

2. Specific features desired (studio, tub, shower, hairdryer, iron)

3. Special requests such as nonsmoking, away from an elevator, lower floor room, and so forth

4. Number of people registering

5. Approximate arrival and departure times based on transportation schedules.

6. Probable dates of occupancy

7. Price rate desired

Electronic Services—Many modern hotels, at an additional charge, have designed conference rooms that are available with special electronic equipment for the working traveler. Individual guest rooms may also be furnished with an adjustable-height desk, chair on wheels, a modem jack, two power outlets, and movable lighting. Workstations designed to look like armoires often provide a personal computer, telecommunication equipment for in-room conferencing, a printer, and fax machine.

Car Arrangements

The physician may request a reservation be made with a local door-to-door shuttle service to eliminate driving and parking a car at the airport. Telephone numbers for such services may be found in the telephone book under "Airport Transportation Services."

If the physician plans to rent a car in the city of his or her destination, car rental discounts are usually given if they show their American Medical Association (AMA) or other association card at the check-in counter. If advance car reservations are made, reserve the car based on arrival time.

Foreign Travel

Numerous steps must be taken to arrange for foreign travel. Passport applications may be obtained from travel agents, major post offices, or from a local county clerk. The applicant must appear in person. Renewal of a passport can be accomplished by mailing the current passport, the fee, new photos, and a completed application, Form DS-11 (available at a post office), to the nearest passport agency or to the U.S. State Department, Passport Services, Washington, DC 20524. Applications for U.S. passports can be downloaded from the Internet and printed (see Resources at the end of this chapter). Once filled in they must be submitted in person or by mail. Copies should be made of all documents and kept in the travel file. A notation of the passport number should be made in the travel file folder before it is stored in a safe place.

A **visa**, which is written permission to enter a country, is required to visit some areas of the world. It is an endorsement made on the passport indicating the traveler has been examined by the proper authorities—usually the local consulate—and is permitted to enter the country. The Congressional Directory gives the addresses of consular offices. Because visa applications are subject to the idiosyncrasies of individual embassy personnel, it may be advisable to secure the services of a visa agency. These agencies, which are located in Washington, DC, and in many major U.S. cities, charge a small fee to process visas and to secure passports. The travel agent may recommend a visa company that he or she works with.

Travel Help on the Internet

It is possible to use the Internet to find the lowest fares. Internet navigational services such as Infoseek, Lycos, Magellan, or Yahoo (See Resources) can help locate travel sites. First, enter a word or words describing a topic (e.g., air travel) and then a list of related Web sites will appear. Click on the address or the underlined or highlighted words to get to a site. Check out sites like American Express Travel, Internet Travel Network, or Travelocity, which cover major and some smaller airlines and employ the same booking software that travel agents use. To be safe, always call a credit card number to a merchant when dealing on the Internet because the number could be intercepted by someone who has no right to it.

Use of a hotel broker (e.g., Accommodations Express, Hot Rooms, Hotel Reservations Network, or Travel Concepts) can cut a lodging bill substantially. Hotels use brokers to fill empty rooms. Some brokers make the reservation and the client pays the hotel on checkout. Others require a prepayment fee. The broker either mails a voucher to the client or it may be waiting at the hotel on check-in. If the reservation is canceled, there may be a penalty issued by the prepaid broker to the client.

Medical Meeting Expenses

Attendance of the physician or medical assistant at medical conferences is considered a legitimate expense and can be tax deducted if properly documented. Some expenses can be used as itemized income tax deductions if courses are classified as professional and if credits are granted for attendance. Medical meetings are divided into two categories, those held in the United States and those held in foreign countries. Tax rules covering expenses for meetings held in this country are more lenient than for those held abroad. The Tax Reform Act of 1986 requires that detailed written records support all deductions and that receipts are kept for expenditures. Basic information to support deductions includes date and time of departure and return, place of the event, the purpose of the event, and the benefit expected from attendance at the event. Travel expenses include lodging and meals subject to the 50 percent rule, which limits deductions to 50 percent of the cost. A photocopy of the signed registration sheet and a record of the place, dates, and time spent at each meeting will verify attendance.

The best way to document expenses is to use major credit cards and to complete the reverse side of the voucher each time an expense is incurred, listing the date, name, and location of the establishment, and the reason for the expense.

The rules and requirements for deducting expenses connected with seminars and conventions are complex, and the recordkeeping requirements are demanding. Some type of daily record detailing the expenses of an entire trip should be maintained (Figure 17-15). The tax implications can be attended to by the OM and the accountant.

TRAVEL EXPENSE REPORT

for _Gerald Practon, MD_

TRIP BEGINNING _June 10, 20XX_   TRIP ENDING _June 17, 20XX_

NAME OF EVENT _American Medical Assn. national convention_

DATE	SAT 6/10	SUN 6/11	MON 6/12	TUES 6/13	WED 6/14	THURS 6/15	FRI 6/16	SAT 6/17	TYPE OF EXPENSE TOTALS
LODGING	175.00	175.00	175.00	175.00	175.00	175.00	200.00		$1,250.00
BREAKFAST		15.00	10.00	15.00	9.00	15.00	10.00		74.00
LUNCH		15.00	16.00	15.00	13.00	12.00	15.00		86.00
DINNER		38.00	35.00	39.00	41.00	36.00	35.00		224.00
AUTO FUEL		25.00					25.00		50.00
PARKING FEE		40.00	40.00	40.00	40.00	40.00	40.00		240.00
PHONE/FAX		10.00	10.00	15.00	15.00	10.00	10.00		70.00
ENTERTAINMENT									
TIPS		5.00			5.00		6.00		16.00
MISCELLANEOUS									
AIR TRANSPORTATION							500.00		500.00
DOOR TO DOOR SHUTTLE							200.00		200.00
DAILY SUBTOTAL	175.00	323.00	286.00	299.00	298.00	288.00	341.00	700.00	

GRAND TOTAL $ _2710.00_

Description of business purpose/locations

Attend annual AMA convention (lecture on June 12, 20XX) in Chicago, Illinois

Figure 17-15. A completed travel expense report

STEP 1 2 3   PROCEDURE 17-10

Prepare a Travel Expense Report

Objective: To complete a travel expense report by listing dates, details of the purpose of the trip, and related business trip expenditures.

Equipment/Supplies: Travel expense report form (see Figure 17-15) calculator, and pen or pencil.

Directions: Follow these step-by-step procedures, which include rationales, to learn this skill.

1. Insert the name of the individual taking the business trip.

2. Insert the dates of departure and return of the business trip.

3. List the name of the event.

4. State the purpose of the business trip.

5. Describe the benefit expected from attendance at the event to justify the business trip.

6. Insert all of the dates showing itemization of costs for transportation, lodging, meals, parking fees, telephone and fax fees, business entertainment, tips, tolls, and other miscellaneous business expenses.

7. Total each column showing the type of expense as subtotals.

8. Calculate all of the expenditures together for a grand total of business expenditures.

STOP AND THINK CASE SCENARIO

Determine the Agenda for a Staff Meeting

Scenario: You are preparing for an end-of-year staff meeting and need to establish an agenda.

Critical Thinking: What items might you select to place on the agenda for discussion? List at least three items to talk about.

1. _____
   _____
   _____

2. _____
   _____
   _____

3. _____
   _____
   _____

STOP AND THINK CASE SCENARIO

Calculate Prices for an Order Form

Scenario: You are preparing to order the following items from a supply company.

Critical Thinking: (1) Calculate the price of each item ordered, (2) add them all together to determine a total price, (3) subtract the discount of 2 percent if paid in 10 days, (4) calculate sales tax at 5.25 percent, (5) add the shipping charge of .25 percent of total sale, and (6) calculate a total.

1. Ten cases of paper @ $23.92/case _____
2. Three 6-inch desk rulers @ $.69/each _____
3. Five packages of transparent _____
   tape @ $5.85/package
4. Ten glue sticks @ $1.89/each _____
5. Twenty highlight pens @ $1.94/each _____
6. Twenty-five red roller pens, five _____
   to a box at $6.98/each
7. Twelve adhesive flags at $4.69/each _____
8. Two print cartridges for the Laser _____
   Jet copy machine @ $99.49/each
9. Eighteen single ink cartridges _____
   for the color copy machine
   @ $12.99 each
10. Fifteen reams of colored paper _____
    @ $6.64/ream
11. Total of all items ordered: _____
12. Discount: _____
12. Sales tax: _____
13. Shipping charge: _____
14. Total of all items ordered _____
    including sales tax and shipping

CMA Content Summary

- Medical abbreviations
- Professional organizations
- Group dynamics
- Office policies
- Professional communication and behavior
- Interviewing techniques
- Legal restrictions
- Personnel standards, hiring, and termination
- OSHA compliance
- Americans with Disabilities Act
- HIPAA
- Employment laws
- Maintenance agreements and repairs of equipment
- Management report generation
- Managing physician's professional schedule and travel
- Maintain physical plant
- Office environment
- Recruit, interview, hire, evaluate, discipline, and terminate employees
- Inventory control; purchasing and storage
- Liability coverage
- Time management
- Office policies and procedures manual
- Patient brochure
- Personnel manual
- Ordering goods, monitoring invoices, tracking merchandise, paying accounts
- Maintain employee immunization records
- Preplanned emergency actions

RMA Content Summary

- HIPAA
- Laws, regulations, and acts pertaining to the practice of medicine
- Professional development; continuing education

- Interpersonal relations
- Patient brochures
- Office policies and procedures
- Family medical leave act
- Maintain practice accounts
- Supplies and equipment management
- OSHA regulations
- Computer hardware and software
- Office sanitation, safety, and comfort
- Emergency protocols and procedures
- Training employees
- Biohazardous waste controls
- Procedures to prevent infectious pathogens by employees

CMAS Content Summary

- Medical and insurance terminology
- Basic laws pertaining to the medical practice
- Continuing education
- Prevention of disease transmission
- Medical office emergencies
- Patient information materials
- Business functions
- Vendors and supplies
- Manage and supervise staff
- Performance reviews and disciplinary action
- Office procedural manual
- Recruit, orient, and train new staff members
- Manage employee benefits
- Office safety and emergency instructions
- Biohazardous waste
- OSHA
- Supply, ordering, and inventory
- Office equipment, maintenance, and repair
- Medical office environment
- Oversee facility
- Staff meetings and in-service

(This textbook and the accompanying Workbook *meet the entry-level administrative and general competencies for the CMA outlined by the AAMA Examination Content Outline and Role Delineation Study and for the RMA and CMAS outlined by the AMT Competencies and Examination Specifications (see Competency Grid in Appendix B).*

REVIEW EXAM-STYLE QUESTIONS

1. One easy and practical way of closing the communication gap and reducing patient questions is to:

   a. design a Web site and put information on the Internet

   b. present each new patient with a practice information brochure

   c. schedule and conduct new patient interviews

   d. maintain a separate telephone line for frequently asked questions (FAQ)

   e. encourage patients to talk to others within the practice

2. Adoption of flextime is one way to:

   a. keep the physician happy

   b. assure employees come to work on time

   c. increase office productivity

   d. discourage overtime

   e. cross-train staff

3. An employee handbook is also knows as a/an:

   a. office policy manual

   b. office procedure manual

   c. office routine's manual

   d. personnel manual

   e. work assignment manual

4. A contract with a cleaning service would fall under:

   a. ordering office supplies and other miscellaneous expenditures

   b. facility oversight performed by the office manager

   c. the office manager's inventory responsibilities

   d. the administrative medical assistant's housekeeping duties

   e. purchasing and leasing

5. A purchase order is:

   a. used by all medical practices

   b. only used by small medical practices

   c. a way to reduce supply expenses

   d. a written authorization that assures an agreed-upon price

   e. used instead of an invoice

6. "Net 30" means:

   a. the vendor is offering a percentage reduction on the purchased goods

   b. the buyer has 30 days in which to pay the total amount of an order

   c. the physician has a 30 month price contract

   d. the vendor will be responsible to deliver the order within 30 days

   e. the price of an item is good for 30 days

7. OSHA stands for:

   a. Occupational Safety and Health Administration

   b. Occupational Safety and Health Authorities

   c. Oversight Safeguards and Health Acts

   d. Operations Safety and Health Administration

   e. Operations Security and Health Authorities

8. Employment applications should be:

   a. disregarded if a resumé is provided

   b. reviewed by the receptionist when the applicant brings it to the office prior to an interview

   c. reviewed with resumés for handwriting, spelling, and sentence structure

   d. typed

9. The OM should consider leasing equipment if:

    a. the medical practice cannot afford the equipment

    b. the physician has bad credit

    c. the office manager has bad credit

    d. the physician does not agree that a piece of equipment is needed

    e. money is tight and the physician likes to replace equipment frequently

10. An exposure control plan must be:

    a. kept in the office safe

    b. kept with the personal protective equipment (PPE)

    c. in writing, reviewed and updated yearly

    d. ordered through OSHA

    e. signed by all clinical and administrative medical assistants regardless of their duties

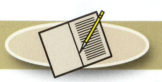

WORKBOOK ASSIGNMENT

To develop competency-based job skills, refer to the *Workbook* and complete the:

- Abbreviation and Spelling Review
- Review Questions
- Critical Thinking Exercises
- Job Skill activities, which are outlined at the beginning of this chapter under "Performance Objectives in the *Workbook*."

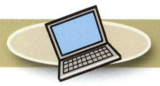

COMPUTER ASSIGNMENT

To review the concepts you have learned in this chapter, insert the *Student Practice* CD-ROM into a computer and work through the *StudyWARE* activities and games. Answer review questions in the practice mode and read the feedback, studying the questions you have missed. Take the chapter quiz until you achieve a minimum score of 90 percent. Successfully completing the *Critical Thinking Challenge* at the end of this course will help you think through scenarios and develop problem solving skills.

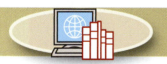

RESOURCES

Books

Healthcare Marketplace (Online bookstore)
  Website: http://www.hcmarketplace.com
Online Library Services
  Search: Topics (e.g., Sexual Harassment Manual)
  Web site: http://www.worldcat.org
Physician Office Safety Guide
  ECRI publisher
  Plymouth Meeting, PA
  Telephone: (610) 825-6000 Ext. 5888

Internet

AllBusiness
  Resources for businesses (management articles)
  Web site: http://www.allbusiness.com
Compliance (Employment Law Guide)
  Web site: http://www.dol.gov/compliance
Employer Advice
  Search: topics of choice (e.g., sexual harassment)
  Web site: http://www.employeradvice.com

Employment laws
Web site: http://www.dol.gov/elaws
Medical Economics
Topics: Career/Legal areas, personal development, malpractice, practice management
Web site: http://www.memag.com
National Labor Relations Board
Web site: http://www.nlrb.gov
Occupational Safety & Health Administration
Web site: http://www.osha.gov
Web site: http://www.cdc.gov/niosh/homepage.html
United States Department of Labor
Search: topics and agencies
Web site: http://www.dol.gov
United States Equal Employment Opportunity Commission
Web site: http://www.eeoc.gov

Medical Supplies—Online Vendors

Esurg
Telephone: (877) 443-7874
Web site: http://www.esurg.com
Everything4Mds (Kern Surgical Supplies)
Telephone: (800) 500-9145
Web site: http://www.everything4mds.com
Henry Schein Inc.
Telephone: (800) 772-4346
Web site: http://www.henryschein.com
Neoforma
Web site: http://www.neoforma.com
Medical Buyer.Com
Web site: http://www.medicalbuyer.com
MedicalSuppliesUSA.Com
Web site: http://www.medicalsupliesusa.com
Physician Sales and Service
Telephone: (904) 332-3000
Web site: http://www.pssd.com

Travel

Airline Travel
Web site: http://www.bestfares.com (Tom Parsons' Best Fares)
Complete Trip Information
Web site: http://www.aaa.com (American Automobile Association)

Web site: http://www.americanexpress.com (American Express)
Web site: http://www.expedia.com
Web site: http://www.travelocity.com
Web site: http://travelweb.com
Currency
Web site: http://www.xe.net/currency (XE Corporation's Universal Currency Converter)
Food
Web site: http://www.restaurantrow.com (The Diners' Grapevine)
Inoculations (Travel Health)
Web site: htt://www.cdc.com (Center for Disease Control and Prevention)
Passport and Visa Information
Web site: http://travel.state.gov (U.S. Department of State Bureau of Consular Affairs)
Transportation Security Administration (luggage regulations)
Web site: http://www.tsa.gov/public
Travel Accommodations
Web site: http://www.accommodationsexpress.com (Accommodations Express)
Web site: http://www.hotelaccommodations.com
Web site: http://www.travelnow.com (discounts)
Web site: http://www.hoteldiscount.com (discounts)
Travel Tips
Web site: http://www.foders.com (Fodors)
Weather
Web site: http://www.weather.com

Web Design

JKC Publishing
Web site: http://www.jkcpublishing.net
Web Site Design
Internet safety (intelligent infrastructure services)
Web site: http://www.VeriSign.com
Web Site Sample
Web site: http://www.intmedonline.com
Web Development
DEA Web Designs
Web site: http://www.deawebdesigns.com
Webmonkey
Web site: http://www.webmonkey.com

CHAPTER 18

Financial Management of the Medical Practice

OBJECTIVES

After reading this chapter and learning step-by-step procedures to gain job skills,* you should be able to:

Learning Objectives

▌ Distinguish between types of financial reports.

▌ Explain gross and net income.

▌ List accounts payable categories.

▌ Define payroll terminology and use the abbreviations.

▌ Obtain and record payroll information.

▌ Describe how to obtain a tax identification number.

▌ Name deductions withheld and state how they are determined when preparing payroll.

▌ Identify tax reports and forms used in payroll.

▌ State when quarterly and annual reports are due.

▌ List components of an employee's earnings record and payroll register.

Performance Objectives (Procedures) in This Textbook

▌ Create headings and post entries in an accounts payable system; write checks (Procedure 18-1).

▌ Create category headings, determine deductions, calculate payroll, and make entries to a payroll register (Procedure 18-2).

Performance Objectives (Job Skills) in the *Workbook*

▌ Write checks for disbursement (Job Skill 18-1).

▌ Record expenditures, pay bills, replenish and balance petty cash fund (Job Skill 18-2).

This textbook and the accompanying Workbook meet the educational components for entry-level administrative and general competencies outlined by CAAHEP and ABHES.

- Reconcile a bank statement (Job Skill 18-3).
- Prepare payroll (Job Skill 18-4).
- Complete a payroll register (Job Skill 18-5).
- Complete an employee earning record (Job Skill 18-6).
- Complete an employee's withholding allowance certificate (Job Skill 18-7).
- Complete an employee benefit form (Job Skill 18-8).

OUTLINE WITH LECTURE NOTES

Computerized Financial Management

Medical Office Budget

_____

_____

_____

_____

Financial Status Reports

_____

_____

_____

_____

Analyzing Practice Productivity

Collection Ratio

_____

_____

_____

_____

Overhead Expenses

_____

_____

_____

_____

Cost of Procedures and Services

_____

_____

_____

_____

Managed Care Analysis

_____

_____

_____

_____

Accounts Payable

Check Controls

_____

_____

_____

_____

Payroll

Wages and Hours of Work

_____

_____

_____

_____

Payroll Procedures

_____

_____

_____

_____

Employer Identification Number

_____

_____

_____

_____

Social Security Number

_____

_____

_____

_____

Employee Withholding Allowance Certificate

_____

_____

_____

_____

Payroll Deductions

_____

_____

_____

Federal Unemployment Tax

_____

_____

_____

_____

State Unemployment Tax

_____

_____

_____

Tax Reports

_____

_____

_____

_____

KEY TERMS

balance sheet
closed accounts
deductions
disbursement record
Employee Withholding Allowance Certificate (Form W-4)
employer identification number (EIN)
Employer's Quarterly Federal Tax Return
exemptions
Federal Insurance Contributions Act (FICA)
Federal Unemployment Tax Act (FUTA)
federal withholding tax (FWT)
gross income

net income
payroll
payroll tax
Social Security (FICA) Taxes
State Disability Insurance (SDI)
state income tax
Temporary Disability Insurance (TDI)
Transmittal of Wage and Tax Statement (Form W-3)
Unemployment Compensation Disability (UCD)
Wage and Tax Statement (Form W-2)
wage base

HEART OF THE HEALTH CARE PROFESSIONAL

Service

Analyzing practice productivity involves scrutinizing financial reports, assessing medical care, and evaluating patient satisfaction. It takes a well-rounded medical practice to be successful, one that patients will talk about with high regard.

COMPUTERIZED FINANCIAL MANAGEMENT

In previous chapters you learned about the financial administration of a medical practice, including setting fees, credit and collection of accounts receivable, processing insurance claims, banking procedures, posting and balancing patient accounts or ledgers and the daysheet, and petty cash procedures. In this chapter, you will learn how to generate financial management reports, analyze practice productivity, make disbursements for invoices and record them in an accounts payable system, calculate payroll, make entries to a payroll register, and prepare tax reports for the employer.

In a medical practice, financial management is the most widely used of all computer applications. It provides an accurate business analysis of a medical practice and improves cash flow by accelerating the collection process. This system relieves time-consuming activities such as preparing billing statements, completing insurance claims, preparing monthly reports, and so on.

Medical Office Budget

In a medical practice, financial problems may develop and not be realized until it is too late. The office manager (OM) needs to have a good idea of how much _avail-_

able cash is needed for the operations of the practice each month (e.g., rent, utilities, payroll, insurance). Actual cash available is different from income shown on the daily journal. To project the actual cash that will be needed, a written budget is essential. The OM needs to keep a close eye on the balance of the check book. His or her experience in the area of preparing a realistic budget will be valuable to the success of the medical practice. The budget is derived from analyzing the previous year's income and expenses and then projecting the needs of the practice for the upcoming year. Many tools are available that can track income and expenses and therefore indicate the financial health of a practice. Financial status reports help managers and physicians plan and make corrections to avoid expensive problems.

Financial Status Reports

In many areas of a medical office, it is essential to obtain computerized reports. A quality accounts receivable system is most important and the practice's analysis of systems should begin in this area. Figure 18-1 is a computer-generated daily transaction regis-

---

DAILY TRANSACTION REGISTER

Run Date: 01/13/20XX

Includes all transactions posted today

New patients are marked with *

Report only includes transactions posted 12/18/XX

PRACTION MEDICAL GROUP INC

Patient Name	Rec No	Ins-Type	Date/Ser	Code	Tx/Proc	Chg	Pd	Date/Ref	AA
BOND MARK	430	Medicaid	12/16/XX	99233	HV L-3	130.00		Y	
			12/17/XX	99232	HV L-2	100.00		Y	
			12/18/XX	99231	HV-L1	75.00		Y	
CHAN ERIC*	431	Medicare	12/16/XX	99204	OV-L4	106.11		Y	
ESTRADA JOSE*	146	Medi-Medi	12/16/XX	99202	OV-L2	51.91		Y	
NGUYEN KIN*	435	Medi-Medi	12/16/XX	99204	OV-L4	106.11		Y	
SCHMIDT CARL	311	PPO	12/16/XX	99233	HV-L-3	130.00		Y	
SOUZA JOE	13	Medicare	12/16/XX	99231	HV-L1	75.00		Y	
SMITH FRED*	43	HMO	12/16/XX	99203	OV-L3	70.92		Y	
TALMAN AL	432	Medicaid	12/16/XX	99291	CC 1st HR	250.00		Y	
URICH BUD	509	BC	12/16/XX	99215	OV-L5	96.97		Y	
WEST ALAN	213	BS	12/16/XX	99213	OV-L3	40.20		Y	
WONG CHI	234	Medicare	12/16/XX	99212	OV-L2	28.55		Y	
WYNN KEN	450	PPO	12/16/XX	99211	OV-L1	16.07		Y	

Totals	Transaction Type	Patients	Number	Debit Amt	Credit Amt
	Production	12	14	1276.83	
	Collections	0	0		0.00
	Debit Adjustments	0	0	0.00	
	Credit Adjustments	0	0		0.00
	Grand Totals	12	14	1276.83	0.00
	New Change to A/R			1276.83	
	Total New Patients	4			

Figure 18-1. Computer printout of a daily transaction register

ter that shows all the transactions posted for one day, including the name of each patient seen, the medical record number, type of insurance, date of service, procedure code number, type of service, fee charged, and whether assignment has been accepted (AA).

Each medical practice financial management software system generates a variety of reports but the names of these reports vary depending on the software used. Some vendors provide inferior accounts receivable packages, therefore, the system selected should include the following basic information.

Accounts Receivable

An accounts receivable (A/R) management system creates and maintains database files containing demographic and billing information used in the preparation of patient statements, insurance forms, and management reports including a breakdown of the A/R.

A detailed aged *accounts receivable report* is a list of all account balances and is usually printed at the end of the month. It is an important document that shows all money owed to the medical practice and is used in the collection process.

A *financial report generator* is the accounts receivable in a concise format. The report in Figure 18-2 is printed from a financial report generator and allows a physician to quickly view and analyze financial data. It shows beginning and ending A/R in columns, which represent the current month, previous month, and year-to-date charges, the breakdown of the charges, total payments, where payments originated, and types of credit adjustments made. If the total

12/31/20XX   **FINANCIAL REPORT GENERATOR**

	For Posting Dates From 12/01/20XX To 12/31/20XX		For Posting Dates From 11/01/20XX To 11/30/20XX		For Posting Dates From 01/01/20XX To 12/31/20XX	
Office E & M Codes	2	540.00	27	3,460.00	43	5,980.00
Procedures	0	0.00	2	125.00	2	125.00
Hospital	565	85,725.00	991	167,765.00	2284	410,875.00
Inj (oth)	1	10.00	2	20.00	5	280.00
Inj (mcl)	0	0.00	0	0.00	0	0.00
Transitional Care	0	0.00	0	0.00	0	0.00
Nursing Homes	0	0.00	0	0.00	0	0.00
Medical Procedures	0	0.00	0	0.00	0	0.00
Hospice	0	0.00	0	0.00	0	0.00
Unassigned Prod	0	0.00	0	0.00	0	0.00
Total Productions	**568**	**86,275.00**	**1022**	**171,370.00**	**2334**	**417,260.00**
Balance Forward	0	0.00	2	410.75	41	11,031.70
Credit Balance Fwd	0	0.00	0	0.00	0	0.00
Medicare Check	620	<47,640.96>	700	<55,928.83>	1391	<109,216.87>
Medicaid Checks	41	<4,924.80>	186	<22,663.40>	253	<30,749.80>
Ins Check #1	79	<10,973.84>	56	<6,018.21>	262	<31,792.37>
Ins Check #2	94	<1,758.82>	178	<3,237.97>	304	<5,649.34>
Patient Payments	2	<635.04>	3	<231.56>	5	<866.60>
Unassigned Coll	0	0.00	0	0.00	0	0.00
Total Collections	**836**	**<65,933.46>**	**1123**	**<88,079.97>**	**2215**	**<178,274.98>**
Debit Adj/Refund	3	0.78	3	0.03	7	0.82
Unassigned Deb Adj	0	0.00	0	0.00	0	0.00
Total Debit Adj	3	0.78	3	0.03	7	0.82
Credit Adjustments	749	<47,329.36>	984	<73,722.27>	1945	<135,728.77>
Unassigned Cred Aj	0	0.00	0	0.00	0	0.00
Total Credit Adj	749	<47,329.36>	984	<73,722.27>	1945	<135,728.77>
P P O Payments	0	0.00	0	0.00	0	0.00
P P O Credit Adj	0	0.00	0	0.00	0	0.00
Beginning A/R		141,275.81		131,297.27		0.00
Ending A/R		114,288.77		141,275.81		114,288.77
(ending A/R Chk)		114,288.77		141,275.81		114,288.77

Figure 18-2. Computer printout of a financial report entitled Financial Report Generator. The report is from the practice of an internal medicine physician with a subspecialty of infectious diseases.

<table>
<tr><td colspan="2">

EXAMPLE 18-1

Accounts Receivable Ratio

June 1, 20XX

Year-to-date revenue charged:	$300,000
Year-to-date revenue received: (includes write-offs)	$220,000
Year-to-date outstanding A/R:	$ 80,000
Monthly average revenue received:	$ 36,666

Formula: 2 (or 2.5) $\times$ average monthly revenue = dollar figure used for comparison $2 \times 36,666 = 73,332$ ($80,000 - 73,332 = \$6,668$) this is under the cut-off point for successful collections

</td></tr>
</table>

A/R figure exceeds between two and two and a half times the revenue received on an average per month, a check of the person who is responsible for following up on accounts should be made, and policies should be developed to improve collections and reduce this ratio (Example 18-1).

Aging Summary Analysis

An insurance aging analysis is a report showing the age of the physician's accounts receivable. The current balance may be divided by account type so the physician can analyze how patients and various insurance carriers are paying and take appropriate action on unpaid accounts (Figure 18-3).

Insurance Aging Report

Computer software can be utilized to separate accounts according to past due balances, zero balances (**closed accounts**), credit balance accounts, or by insurance carrier. And the accounts receivable report can be printed showing all overdue accounts and the amounts overdue with a breakdown of the length of time (or age) the account is overdue (0–30 days, 31–60 days, 61–90 days, 91–120 days, and 120 days or more) as shown in Figure 18-4. Also, it is possible to generate a delinquent account record or activity report that shows the percentage of accounts in each category, only the accounts that are delinquent over 90 days, or accounts that are delinquent by a certain dollar amount.

Financial Summary

A *financial summary* is a monthly report that shows in detail the diagnoses and the frequency of cases treated by the physician, the amount of income generated each month, and the percentage each doctor generated. The cost of treating each diagnosis is listed to help with office management, inventory of supplies, and fee profile studies (Figure 18-5).

Periodic Transaction Summary

A periodic transaction summary report presents the financial position of the medical practice at a particular point in time, usually the last day of the accounting period. It may be compiled into an annual report to discover the financial condition of the practice, for the completion of tax forms, for analysis of insurance needs, for loan applications, and for management planning. This report is referred to by other names depending on the medical software program used, such as *practice management report*, *annual summary sheet*, or **balance sheet**. Although they may be prepared by the medical practice's accountant, it is important the office manager (OM) understand the reason why summaries are kept and why figures must be accurate.

In a manual bookkeeping system, the balance sheet consists of the three elements of the double-entry equation:

Assets		**Capital**		**Liabilities**
$415,000	=	$325,000	+	$90,000

The two sides of the equation must total the same amount in order for all accounts to be in balance. If they do not, they are out of balance and this is a good indication that something is not recorded correctly.

To utilize a computerized periodic transaction summary, the physician should circle procedures and diagnoses on each patient's encounter form. At the end of each day, the OM should then compare the total charges and payments from the manual forms with those from the computer-generated management report. If they do not agree the OM should locate and correct any errors and then post the reconciled total to a control log. At the end of the month, charges are added from the control log and compared with the computer's monthly total. This is not to check arithmetic but to reveal other problems. Sometimes after the date a transaction was keyed into the computer, it may have been adjusted incorrectly or the computer itself may be mishandling something.

Run Date: 12/31/20XX

AGING SUMMARY ONLY
FOR PATIENTS INCLUDED IN THIS REPORT (ONLY)

TOTALS FOR FRAN PRACTON MD

INSURANCE TYPE	PATIENTS	DEBITS	CREDITS	BALANCE DUE	CURRENT	AS OF 11/01/20XX	AS OF 10/02/20XX	AS OF 9/02/20XX
NO INS	7	23,850.00	0.00	23,850.00	23,850.00	0.00	0.00	0.00
MEDICARE	43	72,650.00	3,811.97	68,838.03	65,632.86	3,015.17	190.00	0.00
MEDICAID	22	35,880.00	1,000.00	34,880.00	33,140.00	1,740.00	0.00	0
MEDI-MEDI	45	86,785.00	3,567.13	83,217.87	80,080.00	2,715.02	260.00	162.85
PRIVATE	16	20,985.00	5,643.18	15,341.82	11,749.13	3,592.50	0.00	0.00
WORK COMP	1	5,950.00	4,810.00	1,140.00	1,140.00	0.00	0.00	0.00
PPO/HMO	34	45,140.00	17,102.45	28,037.55	25,803.86	2,233.69	0.00	0.00
TOTALS	168	291,240.00	35,934.73	255,305.27	241,396.04	13,296.38	450.00	162.85

TOTALS FOR GERALD PRACTON, MD

INSURANCE TYPE	PATIENTS	DEBITS	CREDITS	BALANCE DUE	CURRENT	AS OF 11/01/20XX	AS OF 10/02/20XX	AS OF 9/02/20XX
NO INS	2	4,750.00	0.00	4,750.00	4,750.00	0.00	0.00	0.00
MEDICARE	83	100,698.69	82,295.74	18,402.95	6,029.14	66.54	0.00	12,307.27
MEDICAID	34	79,555.00	63,755.00	15,800.00	4,880.00	3,750.00	0.00	7,170.00
MEDI-MEDI	72	131,520.01	108,973.55	22,546.46	2,453.34	0.00	0.00	20,093.12
PRIVATE	40	65,843.75	24,111.87	41,731.88	5,843.86	27,310.00	0.00	8,578.02
WORK COMP	3	5,240.00	3,640.00	1,780.00	790.00	0.00	0.00	950.00
PPO/HMO	30	40,505.07	31,227.59	9,277.48	1,880.00	702.13	0.00	6,695.35
TOTALS	264	428,292.52	314,003.75	114,288.77	26,626.34	31,828.67	0.00	55,833.76

Includes transactions with posting dates through 12/31/20XX.
Report compiled using all of the patients.
Includes patients with all insurance types.
There were no condition codes selected or de-selected for this report.
Includes the patients of both treating physicians.
Includes patients with all balances.
Aged by date of first billing with an aging date of 12/31/20XX.

Figure 18-3. Computer printout of an aging summary report divided by physician and insurance type

Insurance Aging

Friday, January 02, 20XX

MEDICAID

Clyde E. Williams (WILLIA0010) Date of Birth: 03/17/1933 Insured: Self
Insurance: Secondary Policy: 5133031815 ID: 5133031815

Billing	Date	Code/CPT	Billed	Amount	Current	31 - 60	61 - 90	91 - 120	> 120	Total
Patient Total				95.00	95.00	0.00	0.00	0.00	0.00	95.00

				Amount	Current	31 - 60	61 - 90	91 - 120	> 120	Total
Insurance Total				111.40	111.40	0.00	0.00	0.00	0.00	111.40

MUTUAL—Mutual of Omaha Mutual of Omaha Plaza, Omaha, NB 68175 (555) 327-8870

James K. Froist (FROIST0000) Date of Birth: 07/11/1972 Insured: Self
Insurance: Primary ID:CMZX1C-193591-97

Billing	Date	Code/CPT	Billed	Amount	Current	31 - 60	61 - 90	91 - 120	> 120	Total
5170233	12/05/20XX	99204/99204	01/03/20XX	175.00	175.00					175.00
5170233	12/05/20XX	87070/87070	01/03/20XX	35.00	35.00					35.00
5170233	12/05/20XX	36415/36415	01/03/20XX	20.00	20.00					20.00
5170233	12/05/20XX	81002/81002	01/03/20XX	21.00	21.00					21.00
517305	12/11/20XX	99213/99213	01/03/20XX	95.00	95.00					95.00
Patient Total				346.00	346.00	0.00	0.00	0.00	0.00	346.00

				Amount	Current	31 - 60	61 - 90	91 - 120	> 120	Total
Insurance Total				346.00	346.00	0.00	0.00	0.00	0.00	346.00

PAC POS—Pacificare POS P. O. Box 6099, Cypress, CA 90630 (555) 316-9776

Dorothy J. Blan (BLAN0000) Date of Birth: 02/23/1950 Insured: Self
Insurance: Primary Policy: 90158778 ID: 463808651 01

Billing	Date	Code/CPT	Billed	Amount	Current	31 - 60	61 - 90	91 - 120	> 120	Total
5170434	12/20/20XX	99214/99214	01/03/20XX	150.00	150.00					150.00
5170434	12/20/20XX	93000/93000	01/03/20XX	85.00	85.00					85.00
5170434	12/20/20XX	36415/36415	01/03/20XX	20.00	20.00					20.00
5170434	12/20/20XX	81002/81002	01/03/20XX	21.00	21.00					21.00
5170434	12/20/20XX	Patient co-pay	01/03/20XX	-10.00	-10.00					-10.00
Patient Total				266.00	266.00	0.00	0.00	0.00	0.00	266.00

Alice Oganesyan (OGANES0000) Date of Birth: 06/17/1960 Insured: Self
Insurance: Primary Policy: 00010085 ID: 564972684

Billing	Date	Code/CPT	Billed	Amount	Current	31 - 60	61 - 90	91 - 120	> 120	Total
5166555	06/04/20XX	99213/99213	06/13/20XX 08/29/20XX	95.00					95.00	95.00
5166555	06/04/20XX	Patient co-pay		-10.00					-10.00	-10.00
5170283	12/09/20XX	99213/99213		95.00	95.00					95.00
5170283	12/09/20XX	Patient co-pay		-10.00	-10.00					-10.00
Patient Total				170.00	85.00	0.00	0.00	0.00	85.00	170.00

Mona Vargas (VARGAS0001) Date of Birth: 07/23/1973 Insured: Self
Insurance: Primary Policy: 00010659 ID: 584-69-5112 01

Billing	Date	Code/CPT	Billed	Amount	Current	31 - 60	61 - 90	91 - 120	> 120	Total
5167164	05/16/20XX	99213/99213	07/12/20XX	95.00					95.00	95.00
5167164	08/07/20XX	IA		-25.69					-25.69	-25.69
5167164	05/16/20XX	Patient co-pay		-15.00					-15.00	-15.00
Patient Total				54.31	0.00	0.00	0.00	0.00	54.31	54.31

				Amount	Current	31 - 60	61 - 90	91 - 120	> 120	Total
Insurance Total				490.31	351.00	0.00	0.00	0.00	139.31	490.31

PRU - Prudential HMO

Patty J. Smith (SMITH0002) Date of Birth: 09/12/1946 Insured: Robert Smith, Sr. (SMITH0000)
Insurance: Primary Policy: 23236 ID: 54650875702

Billing	Date	Code/CPT	Billed	Amount	Current	31 - 60	61 - 90	91 - 120	> 120	Total
5166497	04/30/20XX	99213/99213	06/13/20XX	95.00					95.00	95.00
5166497	04/30/20XX	Patient co-pay		-10.00					-10.00	-10.00
5167710	07/09/20XX	99214/99214	07/12/20XX	150.00					150.00	150.00
5167710	07/09/20XX	Patient co-pay		-10.00					-10.00	-10.00
Patient Total				225.00	0.00	0.00	0.00	0.00	225.00	225.00

				Amount	Current	31 - 60	61 - 90	91 - 120	> 120	Total
Insurance Total				225.00	0.00	0.00	0.00	0.00	225.00	225.00

Provider Totals

	Amount	Current	31 - 60	61 - 90	91 - 120	> 120	Total
Fran Practon, M.D.	45979.01	29743.84	2851.42	1114.13	600.94	11668.68	45979.01
Gerald Practon, M.D.	17885.34	7476.27	1413.79	414.85	805.00	7776.43	17855.34

	Amount	Current	31 - 60	61 - 90	91 - 120	> 120	Total
Report Totals	63864.35	37219.11	4265.21	1528.98	1405.94	19445.11	63864.35

		Current	31 - 60	61 - 90	91 - 120	> 120	Total
Percent of Total		58.28%	6.68%	2.39%	2.20%	30.45%	100.00%

Figure 18-4. Computer printout of an insurance aging analysis report

RUN DATE: 12/31/20XX			FINANCIAL SUMMARY					
ALL DOCTORS								
DESCRIPTION	PROC FREQ	% PRACTICE	12/01/20XX TO 12/31/20XX DOLLARS	% PRACTICE	PROC FREQ	% PRACTICE	DOLLARS	% PRACTICE
OPEN WOUND ABDOMINAL WALL	3	0.2	345.00	0.1	31	0.8	5,005.00	0.7
CANDIDIASIS OF MOUTH	14	1.0	1,940.00	0.8	27	0.7	3,795.00	0.5
ENDOCARDITIS VALVE UNSPFD	10	0.7	2,050.00	0.8	15	0.4	2,700.00	0.4
MYCOBACTERIA DISEASE UNSP	0		0 .00		1	0.0	100.00	0.0
EMBOLISM/THROMBOSIS OTHER	2	0.1	260.00	0.1	2	0.0	260.00	0.0
TOXIC EFFECT OF VENOM	1	0.1	130.00	0.1	1	0.0	130.00	0.0
ACUTE FACILITIES								
COLLEGE HOSPITAL	380	25.9	60,795.00	25.0	1,046	25.5	172,615.00	24.0
GRANADA HILLS COMMUNITY HOSP	566	38.6	91,750.00	37.8	1,433	34.9	245,865.00	34.2
CONVALESCENT FACILITIES								
VISTA GRANADA SKILLED NRSG	57	3.9	11,150.00	4.6	79	1.9	16,185.00	2.2
HOLY CROSS HOSPITAL SNF	22	1.5	5,550.00	2.3	23	0.6	5,750.00	0.8
PLACE OF SERVICE CATEGORIES								
INPATIENT HOSPITAL	1,382	94.3	225,520.00	92.8	3,907	95.1	679,030.00	94.4
OUTPATIENT HOSPITAL	0		0 .0		2	0.0	380.00	0.1
DOCTOR'S OFFICE	5	0.3	810.00	0.3	55	1.3	7,155.00	1.0
SKILLED NURSING FACILITY	79	5.4	16,650.00	6.9	102	2.5	21,935.00	3.0
INSURANCE TYPES								
NO INSURANCE	43	2.9	9,040.00	3.7	221	5.4	49,900.00	6.9
MEDICARE	439	29.9	69,195.00	28.5	1,135	27.6	176,679.46	24.6
MEDICAID	115	7.8	25,400.00	10.0	458	11.2	106,885.00	14.9
MEDI-MEDI	725	49.5	112,540.00	46.3	1,356	33.0	209,594.18	29.1
PRIVATE INSURANCE	40	2.7	7,775.00	3.2	327	8.0	63,562.99	8.8
WORKMAN'S COMP	6	0.4	1,020.00	0.4	85	2.1	11,500.00	1.6
PPO/HMO	8	6.7	19,010.00	7.8	525	12.8	101,410.07	14.1
REFERRING PHYSICIANS								
NO REFERRING SOURCE	96	6.5	17,490.00	7.2	394	9.6	67,755.44	9.4
66 SINGH DENT MD	84	5.7	14,580.00	6.0	174	4.2	31,825.00	4.4
82 NAHED BALBIR MD	82	5.6	13,715.00	5.6	207	5.5	41,465.00	5.8

Figure 18-5. Computer printout of a monthly and year-to-date financial summary of a medical practice. The first part of the summary connects outpatient services to diagnoses indicating the number of cases treated by the physician, amount of income generated, and the percent of each type of case relative to all diagnostic cases. Other parts of the summary show number of patients treated, income generated, and percentages for acute care hospitals, convalescent facilities, insurance types, and patients referred by other physicians.

Profit and Loss Statement

A *profit and loss statement* is a financial report for a specific period of time summarizing income received and expenses paid with an indication of the resulting profit or loss (Figure 18-6). It may also be called an income and expense statement or operating statement. Generally this report is required at the end of an accounting period (i.e., fiscal or calendar year) to determine if the business has made a profit or loss or to find out the net worth of the business when selling a practice. The total income is called *gross* income or *earnings*. Subtract the expenses from that figure to obtain the *net* income.

ANALYZING PRACTICE PRODUCTIVITY

There are many areas in a medical practice that can be analyzed and various ways to evaluate them. Following are several formulas to obtain information about such things as: how effectively outstanding accounts are being collected, how to calculate overhead expenses to determine what it costs to run a medical practice, how much specific procedures and services cost, and how to determine whether managed care contracts are profitable.

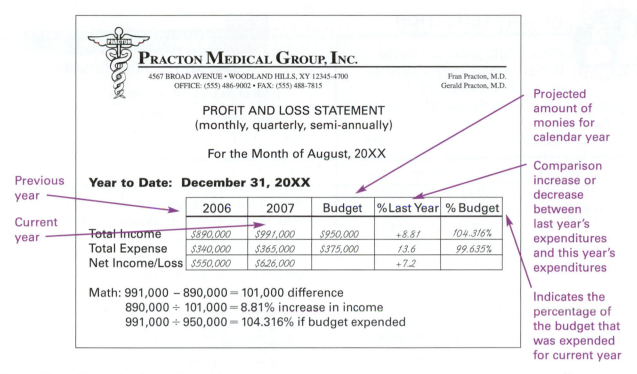

Figure 18-6. Example of a profit and loss statement

Collection Ratio

As explained in Chapter 15, an *accounts receivable (A/R)* control is done to verify that the balance of all outstanding accounts equals the total monies owed. A collection ratio is the formula for illustrating the percentage of monies collected for outstanding accounts and the performance or effectiveness of the billing department (See Example 18-2). This reveals the status of collections and possible potential losses in a medical practice. Many practices have busy and slow seasons so it is wise to obtain these data periodically rather than use average annual data. Determining other services to render to patients during those times may help raise revenue by increasing activity. As learned in Chapter 13, the longer an account remains delinquent, the harder it is to collect.

EXAMPLE 18-2

Collection Ratio Formula

This example illustrates the monthly collection ratio formula, which shows the total monthly payment figure that is divided by the total monthly charges minus the total monthly adjustment figure when payments are received and posted.

$$\frac{\text{Total monthly payments}}{\text{Total monthly charges minus adjustments}} = \text{Monthly collection ratio}$$

The following formula may be used to determine an annual collection ratio:

$$\frac{\text{Total payments for 20XX}}{\text{Total yearly charges minus adjustments}} = \text{Annual collection ratio}$$

PATIENT EDUCATION

When overpayment is received in the physician's office, patients need to be educated regarding refund practices. By explaining office protocol for management of the accounts receivable, patients will better understand why payments cannot be made immediately and accept waiting until a specific time of the month to get their refund checks. Otherwise, you will be left dealing with disgruntled patients calling repeatedly and insisting on their refunds before the day designated to write checks.

Overhead Expenses

The overhead ratio shows what the cost is to run a medical practice on a monthly basis (Example 18-3). It is figured by taking the total of all expenses for the month and subtracting the expenses of items that benefit the physician such as medical insurance, auto expense, meals and entertainment, salary, and travel and lodging, and then dividing this sum by the adjusted receivable (monthly write-offs) amount. This ratio should be monitored monthly as well as annually so that a trend will be recognized if the overhead increases.

EXAMPLE 18-3

Overhead Expense Formula

$$\frac{\text{Total expenses} - \text{Physician benefits}}{\text{Adjusted receivables}} = \begin{array}{l}\text{\% of income}\\\text{used for over-}\\\text{head expense}\end{array}$$

Cost of Procedures and Services

To find out the cost of performing a specific procedure or service in the office, divide the total expenses for the procedure for one month by the number of procedures performed that month (see Example 18-4).

Managed Care Analysis

While under contract to managed care plans, it is always important to track capitated monthly payments with systematic audits. This is done by com-

EXAMPLE 18-4

Cost per Procedure Formula

$$\frac{\text{Total expenses for procedure}}{\text{Total number of procedures}} = \begin{array}{l}\text{Cost per}\\\text{procedure}\end{array}$$

paring the actual amount per patient contracted for against the incoming capitation eligibility list of current members. As mentioned previously, monthly capitation revenue means what the medical practice receives as a dollar amount per patient whether the patient is seen or not. The contracted rates by benefit plan are matched against the monthly capitated payment received. There may be errors discovered because of retroactivity of membership and inaccurate payments.

It is also important to have certain data available when a medical practice is making a decision to sign a contract to participate in a managed care plan because contracts may operate in a variety of ways, for example, monthly capitation amounts, copayments, discounted fees, withholds, and so on. The following are helpful ratios for tracking information:

- *Encounters per member per year*—Divide annual total visits of managed care members by the average number of members seen per month:

$$\frac{\begin{array}{l}\text{Annual total number of}\\\text{visits by capitated members}\end{array}}{\begin{array}{l}\text{Average number of}\\\text{members seen per month}\end{array}} = \begin{array}{l}\text{Average}\\\text{encounters per}\\\text{member per year}\end{array}$$

- *Revenues per member per month*—Divide total capitation revenues by total number of members seen each month:

$$\frac{\text{Total capitation receipts}}{\begin{array}{l}\text{Total members seen}\\\text{per month}\end{array}} = \begin{array}{l}\text{Revenues per}\\\text{member per}\\\text{month}\end{array}$$

- *Revenues per visit*—Divide total capitation revenues by total capitation visits:

$$\frac{\text{Total capitation revenues}}{\text{Total capitation visits}} = \text{Revenues per visit}$$

- *Total managed care revenue*—Add total capitation payments received, total copayment receipts, and any fee-for-service revenues received from capitation members:

Total capitation + Total + Fee-for-
   payments   copayments   service
   received   receipts

= Total managed care revenue

- *Capitation to fee-for-service ratio*—Divide total capitation revenues by total fee-for-service (non-capitation) revenues:

$$\frac{\text{Total capitation revenues}}{\substack{\text{Total fee-for-service} \\ \text{(non-capitation) revenues}}} = \substack{\text{Capitation to} \\ \text{fee-for-service} \\ \text{ratio}}$$

- *Capitation stop loss*—*Stop loss* limits are set in the physician contract and limit the dollar amount of prepaid services that can be incurred by any one patient during the plan year. For example, the plan may have a stop loss limit of $7,000 per patient. In addition to the capitated amount paid for this patient, charges beyond this stop loss limit would be paid on a reduced fee-for-service basis. The physician must therefore keep track of all charges incurred for each patient. By maintaining good tracking, the physician knows when to bill on a fee-for-service basis for each patient.

- *Withhold*—When physicians participate in a capitated plan, a percentage of the monthly payment from the managed care plan is withheld until the end of the year or contract period. This is done to create additional incentives to provide efficient care and lower utilization. Physicians who exceed utilization norms will not receive the full amount. Withholds are also used to pay for administrative costs for the plan.

  To determine the percentage withheld, take the total amount of withhold and divide by the amount paid by each managed care plan in which the medical practice participates (see Example 18-5).

- *Risk pools*—In addition to withholds, some health plans have created risk pools.

  These risk pools are used to pay for nonprimary care services and are a further incentive to control utilization. If utilization is controlled, part of the risk pool will be distributed among the referring physicians.

EXAMPLE 18-5
Withhold

Charges	$100.00
Patient's copayment	$10.00
Payment from plan	$55.00
Withhold	**$5.00**
Physician's adjustment (write-off)	$30.00

Note: The withhold of $5.00 must be tracked until the end of the year or contract period.

- *Capitation versus fee-for-service plan*—Example 18-6 illustrates the difference in payment between capitation and fee for service.

EXAMPLE 18-6
Capitation versus Fee-for-Service Plan

Capitation plan—A specialist physician group may have 90,000 patients in a capitated plan and the group receives $0.81 per patient. The group receives payment of $72,900 each month for all 90,000 patients whether the patients are seen or not.

versus

Fee-for-service plan—A patient is seen and the physician is paid for each service delivered. Under the fee-for-service system, expenditures increase only if the fees increase and also if more units of service are charged for or more expensive services are substituted for less expensive ones. A physician group may charge for services worth $90,000 for the month and receive $48,000 (80 percent of allowed amount or 80 percent of $60,000) from the insurance company. This requires an adjustment of $30,000 (difference between the charged amount and allowed amount) and the patients pay a portion totaling $12,000 (20 percent of allowed amount or 20 percent of $60,000).

ACCOUNTS PAYABLE

Procedures for verifying invoices and writing checks to pay invoices is another major part of running a business. You must learn to record medical practice expenditures in a **disbursement record** (check register); a separate journal that has many columns used to categorize expenditures (Figure 18-7A-C).

Check Controls

The following guidelines will help maintain safe controls over the office checking account:

- Request that the physician maintain a separate checking account; for income tax purposes, this type of recordkeeping clearly separates business expenses from personal expenditures.

- Do not provide blank checks to anyone; maintain control over the stock of blank checks by keeping them under lock and key.

- Use sequentially numbered checks to be sure that none are missing.

- Determine a time each month to write checks. A weekly, biweekly, or a monthly schedule will depend on the size of the practice, timing of incoming bills, and cash flow.

- Check purchase orders against supplies to verify the price, quantity, condition, and promised discount prior to making payment.

- Prepare checks from invoices or other legitimate documents; review statements from suppliers.

- Monitor and compare monthly utility bills.

- Do not abbreviate names or amounts when writing checks; spell everything out.

- Use roller-ball or felt-tip pens to write checks; ballpoint or permanent ink can be washed out.

- Make notations in the memo area indicating what the check is for.

- Sign all checks yourself; do not use the physician's signature stamps.

- Write or stamp "paid" with the current date, check number, and amount on each invoice that is paid.

- Have someone other than the check writer reconcile the bank accounts.

PAYROLL

Office managers or medical assistants have varying responsibilities for **payroll** records and reports. Payroll refers to all wages and salaries paid to employees, including deductions. Since wages, salaries, and benefits constitute a major portion of a practice's expenses, great care should be taken to be sure these functions are done properly. The OM must be familiar with federal and state requirements for wages and hours of work in order to oversee employees and issue payroll.

Wages and Hours of Work

Minimum wage and overtime standards are covered by the Fair Labor Standards Act (FLSA). This act is administered by the Wage and Hour Division of the Employment Standards Administration (see Resource section at the end of chapter). Rules apply to *nonexempt** employees. An *exempt* employee is one who is exempt from requirements of federal and state wage and hour laws. Administrative medical assistants would be non-exempt; however, office managers may fall into the exempt category since their work is "primarily intellectual, managerial, or creative, and which requires exercise of discretion and independent judgment."

A federal minimum wage amount is set for all employees 21 years in age or older. Youth minimum wage applies to workers under 20 years of age during their first 90 consecutive calendar days of employment. Individual states may have their own minimum wage laws that would supercede federal law and require payment of a higher wage. Special rules cover home workers, child labor, foreign workers, and non-immigrant workers. Although state laws vary, typically a 30 minute mealtime is required (without pay) when an employee works greater than five hours as well as 10 minute break times for every four hours worked.

Overtime

FLSA does not place a limit on the total hours worked; however, it does require that for all covered employees 16 years of age or older, the rate of pay in excess of 40 hours in a workweek be paid at a rate of one and one-half times their hourly wage. Individual states may have laws for employees working in excess of eight hours a day and rules that apply to double time.

Workers earning less than $23,660 per year are considered nonexempt and are granted overtime protection.

RECORD OF CHECKS DRAWN ON _College National Bank_

MONTH OF _June_   20XX   PAGE NO. _1_

CHECK REGISTER

	MEMO	PAID TO	DATE	GROSS AMOUNT	DIS-COUNT		AMOUNT OF CHECK	CHECK NO.
							BALANCE FORWARD ⟶	
1		South Coast Medical	6/2/XX	75 00	7 50		67 50	1423
2		Sargeants	6/2/XX				37 90	1424
3		First Church	6/2/XX				100 00	1425
4		Faulkners	6/2/XX				58 87	1426
5		Mary Wells	6/6/XX				349 50	1427
6		Auto Club	6/6/XX				45 00	1428
7		White Motors	6/6/XX				97 85	1429
8		Professional Building Corp	6/6/XX				2200 00	1430
9		Model Laundry	6/6/XX				74 70	1431
10		Cash-Personal	6/6/XX				1000 00	1432
11	Reception chair	Fairfax Store	6/6/XX				206 85	1433
12		Union Oil	6/8/XX				32 90	1434
13		Love to Travel	6/8/XX				245 75	1435
14	Decorator	H. Cain	6/8/XX				305 00	1436
15	Direct Payment	Woodland Hill Light Co.	6/8/XX				138 90	
16		Petty Cash	6/8/XX				63 50	1437
17		Mary Wells	6/13/XX				349 50	1438
18		Woodland Hills County Collector (o/c)	6/13/XX				218 75	1439
19		American Medical Assn.	6/13/XX				549 20	1440
20		Dinner Dr. & Mrs. Ross	6/13/XX				151 50	1441
21		County Line Florist	6/13/XX				52 75	1442
22		Mary Wells	6/20/XX				349 50	1443
23		General Life Ins. Co.	6/20/XX				415 54	1444
24		Community Fund	6/20/XX				200 00	1445
25		First National Bank	6/20/XX				750 00	1446
26		Comp USA	6/20/XX				1175 00	1447
27		Mary Wells	6/27/XX				349 50	1448
28		Home Federal Bank	6/27/XX					
29	Deposit	Security National Bank	6/30/XX				140 00	1449
30		Bell Telephone	6/30/XX				330 00	1450
TOTAL							10,055 46	

Ⓐ   Ⓑ   Ⓒ

PROOF FORMULAS: 7.50   67.50   75.00

DISBURSEMENTS – COL'S. Ⓑ + Ⓒ = Ⓐ

COL. Ⓐ TOTAL = TOTAL OF COLUMNS USED FOR EXPENSE DISTRIBUTION.

195.77+
511.85+
1,398+
2,200+
468.90+
32+
218.75+
175.75+
74.70+
204.25+
245.75+
140+
1,175+
549.20+
300+
2,165.54
10,055.46*

Figure 18-7A. Completed accounts payable disbursement record (part 1)

MONTH OF _June_   _20XX_

(MEMO) BANK BALANCE	LINE NO	Deposit DATE	Deposit AMOUNT	1 Medical Supplies	2 Office Maint.	3 Salaries	4 Rent Upkeep	5 Utilities	6 Office Supplies	7 Taxes and Licenses	8 Books & Journals	9 Auto Maint.	10 Laundry & Cleaning	11 Promotion & Entertain.
15728 00														
15660 50	1			67 50										
15622 60	2			37 90										
15522 60	3													
15463 73	4			58 87										
1514 23	5					349 50								
15069 23	6											45 00		
14971 38	7											97 85		
12771 38	8						2200 00							
12696 68	9												74 70	
11696 68	10													
11489 83	11				206 85									
11456 93	12											32 90		
11211 18	13													
10906 18	14				305 00									
10767 28	15							138 90						
10703 78	16			31 50					32 00					
10354 28	17					349 50								
10135 53	18									218 75				
9586 33	19													
9434 83	20													151 50
9382 08	21													52 75
9032 58	22					349 50								
8617 04	23													
8417 04	24													
7667 04	25													
6492 04	26													
6142 54	27					349 50								
6365 74	28	6/27/XX	223 20											
6225 74	29													
5895 74	30							330 00						
TOTAL			223 20	195 77	511 85	1398 00	2200 00	468 90	32 00	218 75		175 75	74 70	204 25

PREPARED BY _Marilyn Fordney_

Figure 18-7B. Completed accounts payable disbursement record (part 2)

Posting Requirements

Employers must clearly post specific Federal Labor Law information. Posting of local laws will vary from state to state. Following are key items included in posting requirements:

- Federal Minimum Wage (Fair Labor Standards Act)
- Civil Rights Act of 1964
- Discrimination Acts: Age, Americans with Disabilities, Title VII
- Occupational Safety and Health Act of 1970
- Rehabilitation Act of 1973
- Vietnam Era Veterans Readjustment Assistance Act of 1974
- Employee Polygraph Protection Act of 1988
- Family and Medical Leave Act of 1993 (50 or more employees)
- Workers' Compensation Coverage
- Unemployment Benefits
- Disability Insurance
- Payday Schedule

MONTH OF _June_ 20XX

	12 Business Travel		13 Collections		14 NSF Checks		15 Equip. & Maintenance		16 Prof. Meetings		17 Bus. Insurance		18 Contributions		19		20		21		22		MISCELLANEOUS DESCRIPTION	AMOUNT	
LINE NO.																										
1																										
2																										
3														100	00											
4																										
5																										
6																										
7																										
8																										
9																										
10																								Personal Cash	1000	00
11																										
12																										
13	245	75																								
14																										
15																										
16																										
17																										
18																										
19											549	20														
20																										
21																										
22																										
23																								Life Ins	415	54
24														200	00											
25																								Treasury Notes	750	00
26								1175	00																	
27																										
28																										
29					140	00																				
30																										
TOTAL	245	75			140	00			1175	00	549	20			300	00									2165	54

Figure 18-7C. Completed accounts payable disbursement record (part 3)

Payroll Procedures

Employers must keep records on hours worked, wages, and other information as set forth in the Department of Labor's regulations. Payroll information must be posted on a separate earnings record and employees given an itemized statement with each paycheck. Regular paydays must be set by employers and pay distributed within 10 days of the end of each pay period. If an employee resigns, wages must be paid within 72 hours; if fired or laid off, wages are to be paid immediately.

Practices with five or more employees may hire a bookkeeper or an accountant or utilize payroll software. If the payroll is done by a computer system, it should have the capabilities to calculate deductions and taxes, print forms and year-end reports, and write checks. Small offices may prefer to use a write-it-once payroll journal, which resembles the pegboard bookkeeping system and combines check writing with an itemized account of all deductions. This system is explained in detail at the end of this chapter.

PROCEDURE 18-1

Create Headings and Post Entries in an Accounts Payable System; Write Checks

Objective: To create headings and post entries to an accounts payable disbursement journal.

Equipment/Supplies: Disbursement journal sheets, invoices, checks, and pen.

Directions: Follow these step-by-step procedures, which include rationales, to learn this skill, which is presented in the *Workbook* (Job Skill 18-1) for practice.

1. Fill in the top of the check register and each page with the name of the bank, date, and page number.

2. Create and write in the names of the column headings under which you will record basic check information, such as name of payee, date, gross amount, discount, amount of check, and check number (see Figure 18-7A).

3. Write in the column headings for the bank balance and bank deposit (see Figure 18-7B).

4. Write in the column headings for each type of business expense (see Figure 18-7B). These categories can vary from practice to practice, but some might be medical supplies, office maintenance, salaries, rent and upkeep, utilities, office supplies, taxes and licenses, books and journals, automobile maintenance, laundry and cleaning, promotion and entertainment, business travel, collections, NSF checks, equipment and maintenance, professional meetings, business insurance, contributions, and miscellaneous for personal withdrawal account (see Figures 18-7B and C).

5. Write the check for the expenditure indicating:

    a. written paid amount

    b. name and address of who the check is paid to the order of

    c. current date

    d. gross amount (prior to discount or for payroll)

    e. discount amount (or total of deductions for payroll)

    f. check amount (net amount after discount or deductions)

    g. signature (as it appears on the bank signature card)

6. Complete check stub information and bring balance forward. (Figure 18-8).

7. Record the name of the vendor or supplier, the date paid, the amount of check, and the check number in the appropriate columns. Review the columns for categorizing each expense and list the amount under the appropriate heading. If, for example, in Figure 18-7A the check was written to pay an electricity bill (Woodland Hills Light Company), it should appear in the "Utilities" column. Follow this procedure for each check written during the month. In some instances, a check may be written that must be divided among two or three categories; for example, a check for $63.50 written to "Petty Cash" and used for medical supplies and office supplies would be entered as $63.50 for the amount of the check, then as $31.50 under "Medical Supplies" and $32 under "Office Supplies."

8. Total each disbursement column at the end of the month.

9. Total the column for the amount of checks written. The total of the check column and the sum of all of the disbursement columns should agree (balance).

10. Carry forward each total to the disbursement record (check register) for the next month so the physician can make a comparison of income and expenses by month.

11. Enter all totals on an annual summary sheet that is maintained monthly to be available when tax returns are prepared. This sheet also contains monthly income information, payroll deductions and taxes, and accounts receivable monthly totals.

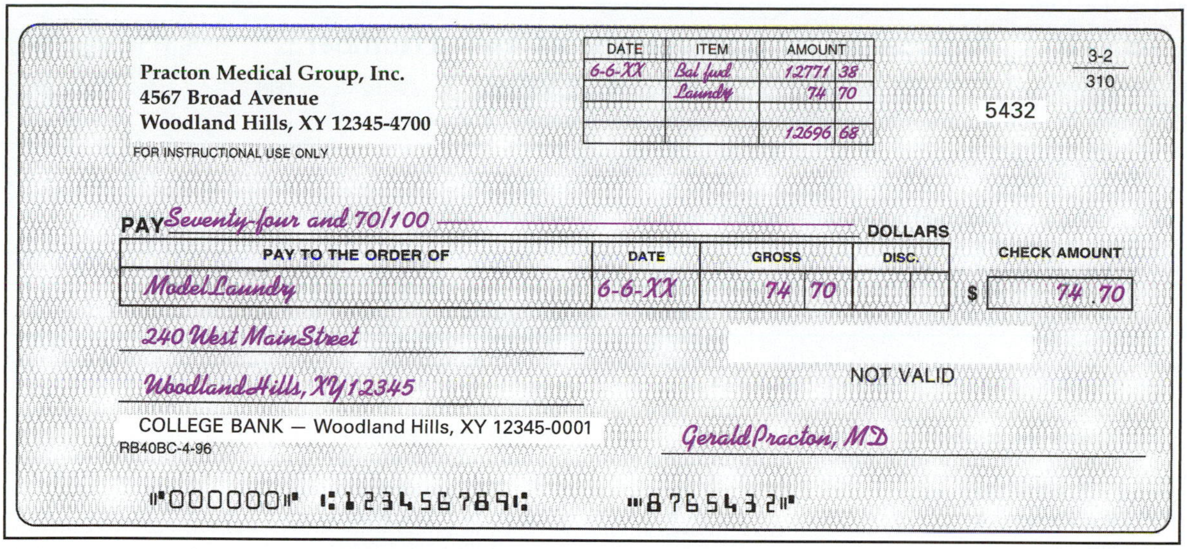
Practon Medical Group, Inc.
4567 Broad Avenue
Woodland Hills, XY 12345-4700
FOR INSTRUCTIONAL USE ONLY

DATE	ITEM	AMOUNT	
6-6-XX	Bal fwd	12771	38
	Laundry	74	70
		12696	68

3-2
310
5432

PAY Seventy-four and 70/100 DOLLARS

PAY TO THE ORDER OF	DATE	GROSS		DISC.		CHECK AMOUNT
Model Laundry	6-6-XX	74	70			$ 74.70

240 West Main Street
Woodland Hills, XY 12345
NOT VALID
COLLEGE BANK — Woodland Hills, XY 12345-0001
RB40BC-4-96
Gerald Practon, MD
⑈000000⑈ ⑆123456789⑆ ⑈8765432⑈

Figure 18-8. Completed pegboard check for a medical practice expenditure

When the office manager or medical assistant is in complete charge of the payroll, responsibilities might include: explaining payroll procedures and policies to new employees, obtaining payroll information, processing payroll checks, and understanding the regulations and forms legislated by the **Federal Insurance Contributions Act (FICA)** (called **Social Security taxes**), the Fair Labor Standards Act, the federal and state unemployment compensation acts, income tax laws, and **state income tax** laws. Quarterly and annual reports must be filed with the Internal Revenue Service (IRS), and in some states reports are also filed with a state agency.

Employer Identification Number

Every physician-employer must have a tax identification number for federal tax accounting purposes. The **employer identification number (EIN)** is a nine-digit number (see Example 18-7).

COMPLIANCE

Complying with payroll mandates and reporting taxes fall under both federal and state laws. Payment that accompanies the monthly Federal Tax Deposit Coupons (Form 8109), as well as the payment that accompanies the quarterly reports, needs to be made in a timely manner. Visit your local tax office annually to obtain brochures so that you will have the latest information.

EXAMPLE 18-7

Employer Identification Number

12-3456789

The physician applies for a number from the Internal Revenue Service, using Form SS-4 (Figure 18-9). In states that require employers' reports, the physician must also apply to the proper state agency. applies for a tax identification number.

Social Security Number

Each person born in the United States is required to obtain a Social Security number by age 2. The card contains a nine-digit tax identification number used by employees and retained for life (Example 18-8).

Application may be made at the nearest Social Security office using Form SS-5. Those who are not born in the United States may obtain a Social Security card by proving age, identity, and status. An original birth certificate, other forms of identification, and documents from the Immigration and Naturalization Service (INS) are needed. The first three digits indicate where the cardholder lived when the card was requested. The middle two numbers follow a pattern known only to government officials and can be used to spot phony cards. The last four numbers are randomly assigned with no two individuals having the same number. When in the process of being hired, each person is required to provide his or her

Form **SS-4**

(Rev. February 2006)
Department of the Treasury
Internal Revenue Service

Application for Employer Identification Number

(For use by employers, corporations, partnerships, trusts, estates, churches, government agencies, Indian tribal entities, certain individuals, and others.)

▶ See separate instructions for each line. ▶ Keep a copy for your records.

OMB No. 1545-0003

EIN

Type or print clearly.

1   Legal name of entity (or individual) for whom the EIN is being requested

2   Trade name of business (if different from name on line 1)

3   Executor, administrator, trustee, "care of" name

4a   Mailing address (room, apt., suite no. and street, or P.O. box)

5a   Street address (if different) (Do not enter a P.O. box.)

4b   City, state, and ZIP code

5b   City, state, and ZIP code

6   County and state where principal business is located

7a   Name of principal officer, general partner, grantor, owner, or trustor

7b   SSN, ITIN, or EIN

8a   Type of entity (check only one box)
☐ Sole proprietor (SSN) _____
☐ Partnership
☐ Corporation (enter form number to be filed) ▶ _____
☐ Personal service corporation
☐ Church or church-controlled organization
☐ Other nonprofit organization (specify) ▶ _____
☐ Other (specify) ▶

☐ Estate (SSN of decedent) _____
☐ Plan administrator (SSN) _____
☐ Trust (SSN of grantor) _____
☐ National Guard   ☐ State/local government
☐ Farmers' cooperative   ☐ Federal government/military
☐ REMIC   ☐ Indian tribal governments/enterprises
☐ Group Exemption Number (GEN) ▶ _____

8b   If a corporation, name the state or foreign country (if applicable) where incorporated

State

Foreign country

9   Reason for applying (check only one box)
☐ Started new business (specify type) ▶ _____
☐ _____
☐ Hired employees (Check the box and see line 12.)
☐ Compliance with IRS withholding regulations
☐ Other (specify) ▶

☐ Banking purpose (specify purpose) ▶ _____
☐ Changed type of organization (specify new type) ▶ _____
☐ Purchased going business
☐ Created a trust (specify type) ▶ _____
☐ Created a pension plan (specify type) ▶ _____

10   Date business started or acquired (month, day, year). See instructions.

11   Closing month of accounting year

12   First date wages or annuities were paid (month, day, year). Note. If applicant is a withholding agent, enter date income will first be paid to nonresident alien, (month, day, year) .... ▶

13   Highest number of employees expected in the next 12 months (enter -0- if none).
Do you expect to have $1,000 or less in employment tax liability for the calendar year?
☐ Yes   ☐ No. (If you expect to pay $4,000 or less in wages, you can mark yes.)

Agricultural	Household	Other

14   Check one box that best describes the principal activity of your business.
☐ Construction   ☐ Rental and leasing   ☐ Transporting & warehousing   ☐ Health care & social assistance   ☐ Wholesale-agent/broker
☐ Real estate   ☐ Manufacturing   ☐ Finance & insurance   ☐ Accomodation & food service   ☐ Wholesale-other   ☐ Retail
☐ Other (specify)

15   Indicate principal line of merchandise sold, specific construction work done, products produced, or services provided.

16a   Has the applicant ever applied for an employer identification number for this or any other business? .... ☐ Yes   ☐ No
Note. If "Yes," please complete lines 16b and 16c.

16b   If you checked "Yes" on line 16a, give applicant's legal name and trade name shown on prior application if different from line 1 or 2 above.
Legal name ▶   Trade name ▶

16c   Approximate date when, and city and state where, the application was filed. Enter previous employer identification number if known.
Approximate date when filed (mo., day, year)   City and state where filed   Previous EIN

Third Party Designee

Complete this section only if you want to authorize the named individual to receive the entity's EIN and answer questions about the completion of this form.

Designee's name

Designee's telephone number (include area code)
(   )

Address and ZIP code

Designee's fax number (include area code)
(   )

Under penalties of perjury, I declare that I have examined this application, and to the best of my knowledge and belief, it is true, correct, and complete.

Name and title (type or print clearly) ▶

Applicant's telephone number (include area code)
(   )

Applicant's fax number (include area code)
(   )

Signature ▶   Date ▶

For Privacy Act and Paperwork Reduction Act Notice, see separate instructions.

Cat. No. 16055N

Form **SS-4** (Rev. 2-2006)

Figure 18-9. Application for employer identification number, Form SS-4

EXAMPLE 18-8

Social Security Number

123-XX-6789

Social Security number and the employer then lists the number on all payroll transactions.

Employment Eligibility Verification

The Immigration and Nationality Act requires employers to verify that all employees hired, citizens and noncitizens, are authorized to work. The Employment Eligibility Verification Form I-9 is completed for each new hire and filed with the INS within three business days of hiring. After the employee completes this form, any documents presented proving the employee's identity and work eligibility need to be examined by the employer for genuineness prior to being recorded.

Employers in all states are able to verify Social Security numbers and work eligibility in the United States electronically. This is through a pilot program that has been extended until November 2008. Verification must be made within three days of hire.

Employee Withholding Allowance Certificate

Because income taxes are deducted on a pay-as-you-go plan, each new employee must complete an **Employee's Withholding Allowance Certificate (Form W-4)**, stating the number of claimed **exemptions** (Figure 18-10). Each employee is entitled to one exemption for himself or herself and one for each person claimed as a dependent. The employee who takes no exemptions, thereby increasing the amount of withheld tax, may qualify for an income tax refund at the end of the year. An employee who paid no tax last year or expects to pay no tax this year can be exempt from any withholding tax.

Generally, by December 1 of each year, the person doing payroll should ask each employee to file a new W-4 form, requesting any changes such as name, address, marital status, and number of exemptions. Make sure employees also report any name changes to the Social Security Administration, and *do not* change payroll records until the employee has obtained a new Social Security card. This can ensure more accurate wage reporting and eliminate earnings being held in a suspense file rather than credited to an employee's earning record.

Cut here and give Form W-4 to your employer. Keep the top part for your records.

Form **W-4** — Department of the Treasury, Internal Revenue Service

Employee's Withholding Allowance Certificate

▶ **Whether you are entitled to claim a certain number of allowances or exemption from withholding is subject to review by the IRS. Your employer may be required to send a copy of this form to the IRS.**

OMB No. 1545-0074 — **2007**

1 Type or print your first name and middle initial: Kevin — Last name: O'Brien

2 Your social security number: 271 : XX : 1963

Home address (number and street or rural route): 2521 Olive Avenue

3 ☒ Single ☐ Married ☐ Married, but withhold at higher Single rate.

Note. If married, but legally separated, or spouse is a nonresident alien, check the "Single" box.

City or town, state, and ZIP code: Woodland Hills, XY 12345-0001

4 **If your last name differs from that shown on your social security card, check here. You must call 1-800-772-1213 for a new card.** ▶ ☐

5 Total number of allowances you are claiming (from line **H** above **or** from the applicable worksheet on page 2) — 5: 1

6 Additional amount, if any, you want withheld from each paycheck — 6: $

7 I claim exemption from withholding for 2006, and I certify that I meet **both** of the following conditions for exemption.

- Last year I had a right to a refund of **all** federal income tax withheld because I had **no** tax liability **and**
- This year I expect a refund of **all** federal income tax withheld because I expect to have **no** tax liability.

If you meet both conditions, write "Exempt" here ▶ 7

Under penalties of perjury, I declare that I have examined this certificate and to the best of my knowledge and belief, it is true, correct, and complete.

Employee's signature (Form is not valid unless you sign it.) ▶ Kevin O'Brien — **Date** ▶ January 2, 20XX

8 Employer's name and address (Employer: Complete lines 8 and 10 only if sending to the IRS.): Practon Medical Group, Inc. 4567 Broad Avenue, Woodland Hills, XY 12345-4700

9 Office code (optional)

10 Employer identification number (EIN): 95 : 36640XX

For Privacy Act and Paperwork Reduction Act Notice, see page 2. Cat. No. 10220Q Form **W-4** (2006)

Figure 18-10. Employee's Withholding Allowance Certificate, Form W-4

Payroll Deductions

Payroll deductions are categorized as before-tax and after-tax deductions. Before-tax deductions include all monies that are exempt from income taxes such as flexible spending accounts, medical insurance, and voluntary tax-deferred retirement contributions (e.g., 401K). After-tax deductions are not exempt from income taxes and FICA. These include long-term disability, union dues, and charitable contributions (e.g., United Way).

Federal Insurance Contributions Act (FICA) Taxes

Under Social Security, there are three separate programs financed from one payroll tax to which employers and employees contribute at a rate specified by law. The retirement program, or Old Age Survivors and Disabilities Insurance (OASDI), provides the elderly with retirement benefits and their surviving dependents with survivors' benefits. The Hospital Insurance (HI) or Medicare program provides hospitalization insurance for the elderly. The public Disability Insurance (DI) program provides workers with insurance if they become disabled during their working years. FICA tax rates for 2006 are listed in Table 18-1.

For example, in 2006, the FICA tax is 7.65 percent and is divided into two rates: a 1.45 percent **payroll tax** that helps finance Medicare's hospital insurance and a 6.2 percent payroll tax that pays for Social Security benefits. Employers pay another 7.65 percent on each worker's wages. In 2006 the wage base for the Social Security tax was $94,200. There was no wage base for the Medicare tax. A **wage base** is the maximum amount of salaries or wages that is subject to tax for the year. The employee's 7.65 percent is

withheld from the salary; the employer's contribution and the employee's withheld amount are paid by the employer in a monthly federal tax deposit or with a quarterly report on March 31, June 30, September 30, and December 31. An optional Social Security program is the Supplemental Medical Insurance (SMI) program for people over the age of 65. Contributions are made by both the retired person and the federal government.

Income Tax Deductions

All physician-employers are required by the federal government to withhold income taxes on employees' earnings. Income tax **deductions** (withholding) can be found in standard tax tables. A penalty is imposed if the tax is underwithheld. The **federal withholding tax (FWT)**, more commonly known as the federal income tax deduction, is paid quarterly to a regional IRS office at the same time FICA taxes are paid. After an employee files Form W-4 stating the number of exemptions claimed, this information plus the employee's **gross income** (amount earned before deductions) for the payroll period determine the amount to be withheld. Tax tables are referred to for weekly, biweekly, semimonthly, monthly, daily, or miscellaneous payroll periods, which appear in Circular E, *Employer's Tax Guide,* available free of charge from the IRS center where the returns are filed. Divorced people are considered single people on federal tax tables and heads of households on state tax tables. The biweekly table is referred to for employees paid every two weeks. The semimonthly tables are used for employees paid twice a month, usually on the 15th and 30th. If an employee is single but qualifies as head of a household, the single table for federal deductions and head of household table for state deductions are used.

Table 18-1. Federal Insurance Contribution Act (FICA), also called Old Age Survivors and Disabilities Income Insurance (OASDI), 2006 Dollar Figures and Percentage Tax Rates Withheld from Salaries

	Employer/Employee Tax Rates**	Self-Employed Tax Rates	Maximum Wage Base
FICA/OASDI*	6.2%	12.4%	$94,200
Medicare	1.45%	2.9%	None
Totals	7.65%	15.3%	$94,200

These dollar figures and percentage rates are subject to change in subsequent years.

***Both the employee and employer pay the same rates.*

Some states and cities require income taxes to be withheld from employees' earnings as advance payment. To determine deductions, reference can be made to state or local city tax tables.

At times there are tax credits offered for employers who hire members of certain targeted groups. Local state job service agencies can provide information on qualified target groups.

Disability Insurance Deductions

As mentioned in Chapter 17, **Unemployment Compensation Disability (UCD)** deductions, also know as **Temporary Disability Insurance (TDI)** or **State Disability Insurance (SDI)**, are mandatory in five states—California, Hawaii, New Jersey, New York, and Rhode Island—and Puerto Rico. It is a form of insurance that is part of an employment security program providing temporary cash benefits for employees suffering a wage loss due to nonindustrial illness or injury. A small percentage, about 1 percent, of the gross pay is deducted from the employee's paycheck each month, although physicians may choose to pay all or part of the cost as a fringe benefit for employees. The money is sent quarterly to the state and put into a special fund. Each state sets a maximum annual amount to be contributed; after the employee has had the maximum amount deducted for the year, no more is deducted.

Optional Payroll Deductions or Benefits

Some physicians provide fringe benefits for their employees consisting of partial or full payment of health insurance, life insurance, pension plans, profit-sharing plans, and stock or savings bonds. When the employee is paying for part or all of such a program, deductions can be made if agreed to by the employee. Such deductions may be canceled by the employee during specified times of the calendar year. Other typical optional deductions are credit union deposits and loan payments. Some employees are given fringe benefits, for example, uniform allowance or automobile expenses, which might include payment for mileage and toll fees. Car expenses are figured into the pay after deductions have been taken.

The dollar amount from a benefit package should be considered along with the wages earned by the employee. The federal and Social Security tax on the dollar value of some benefits may be required by law

to be reported as wages (see the federal publication *Taxable and Nontaxable Income*); examples might be bonuses, sick or vacation pay, and so on. Other items can be considered *practice expenses* instead of taxable wages, such as uniform allowances, professional dues, and job-related education. Good benefit packages will attract new employees and add incentives to present staff if the employee realizes the dollar value (Figure 18-11).

Federal Unemployment Tax

Under the **Federal Unemployment Tax Act (FUTA)**, most employers of one or more people pay a federal tax that is used to pay the administrative costs of the state unemployment programs. Usually, credit is given in an employer's FUTA tax account for amounts paid into a state unemployment fund up to a certain percentage. Deposits are generally made quarterly to a federal reserve bank and are accompanied by Form 508. This form is not shown here, but it is similar to Form 8109-B shown in Figure 18-12. A supply of Forms 508 is sent to the employer after an employer identification number is applied for, or the form may be obtained from an IRS office. The amount to be paid is stated in the federal publication Employer's Tax Guide.

Annual Tax Return

Employers must report payments of federal unemployment taxes under FUTA by filing an annual report on Form 940 (Figures 18-13A and B, see pages 638 and 639). This should be filed by January 31 of the new year following the taxable year, and any tax still due is paid with the return. If all deposits were paid in full, the return is due on February 10.

State Unemployment Tax

Medical offices may also be required to pay into a state unemployment tax program; these funds are used to pay unemployment compensation to unemployed people who are looking for a new job. In some states an unemployment tax is paid by both employee and employer. In some states, an employer with fewer than four employees does not have to pay a state unemployment tax. The date of payment of state unemployment taxes varies from state to state, with a penalty often imposed on employers for late payment. A form is sent to the employer from the unemployment compensation fund stating the rate the employer is required to

EMPLOYEE BENEFITS

Benefit	Employer Pays	Employee Pays
Medical insurance	$ 8,190.00	$ 420.00
Life insurance	$ 210.00	$
Accident insurance	$ 81.00	$
Disability insurance	$	$
Workers' compensation	$	$
Holiday # 7	$ 728.00	$
Vacation # 10	$ 1040.00	$
Sick leave # 6	$ 624.00	$
Personal leave	$	$
Education	$ 100.00	$
Incentive bonus	$	$
Retirement	$	$
Uniforms	$ 420.00	$
Other	$	$
TOTAL BENEFITS	$ 11,393.00	$ 420.00

Wage of employee $ 13/hr

Gross wage for 20X___ $ 24,648.00

Total employment package $ 36,041.00

Employee name: Garth Cartwright   Date: 11/7/XX

Figure 18-11. Example of a summary of employee benefit package

pay. State laws frequently change in regard to coverage, rate of contributions required, eligibility to receive benefits, and amounts of benefits payable.

Tax Reports

All medical practices are required to prepare and file various payroll records for each employee. The physician is not considered an employee unless the prac-

tice is incorporated. If the physician is considered self-employed, neither income taxes nor FICA taxes are withheld from the amounts withdrawn as earnings. However, as a self-employed person, a tax is paid to provide benefits similar to those that employees receive from FICA deductions.

The office manager should carefully read the information that is included on commonly used forms along with directions for completing each form. Refer

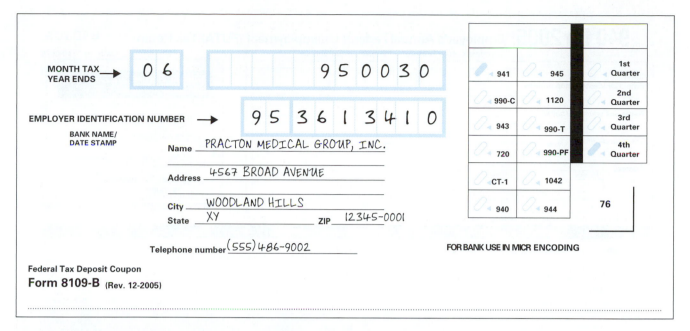

Figure 18-12. Federal Tax Deposit Coupon, Form 8109-B

to Circular E, *Employer's Tax Guide*, which is published by the Department of the Treasury, Internal Revenue Service, for current guidelines and requirements in submitting quarterly reports and for making federal tax deposits and unemployment tax payments. The time of year for submitting each form should be entered on a tickler file, allowing time for completion before each deadline.

Federal Tax Deposits and Receipts

Social Security legislation and the Internal Revenue Code require employers to act as collection agents by obtaining from their employees both the FICA tax and income tax. Each pay period the office manager or medical assistant doing payroll must also handle employer and employee taxes as well as Social Security taxes and income taxes that are being withheld for that time frame. The physician-employer's total liability will determine whether deposits are necessary, and, if so, how often they must be made; frequency of the deposits depends on the amount of taxes involved. The current regulations appear on the reverse side of the Employer's Quarterly Federal Tax Return, Form 941, as shown in Figure 18-14A and B. If payment is made with Form 941, the attached voucher 941V (see Figure 18-15) should be included; deposits should be submitted on Form 8109-B (Figure 18-12). Instructions on when to make a payment instead of a deposit are included on page 3 of Form 941.

Federal tax deposits may be made via an electronic funds transfer system (EFTS) through TAX-LINK instead of writing a paper check. This can be accessed by telephone, computer, or electronic payment with the physician's bank. The physician must sign up for EFTS with the bank.

Employer's Quarterly Federal Tax Return

An **Employer's Quarterly Federal Tax Return**, Form 941, must be filed by the physician-employer on or before April 30, July 31, October 31, and January 31, each covering the preceding three months' activity (see Figure 18-14). The total of the income tax and the FICA tax withheld are stated on the front of the form. The amount payable is figured by subtracting the sum of the amounts paid as monthly federal tax deposits from the total taxes withheld. When Form 941 is sent to the director of the IRS for the district where the employer is located, the balance due must be submitted. The original is for the IRS and the copy is for the physician-employer's file.

Wage and Tax Statement

On or before January 31 of each year or within 30 days after an employee terminates service, the employer is required to give each employee a **Wage and Tax Statement, (Form W-2)** (Figure 18-16). This form is completed, *(text continues on page 642)*

Form **940 for 2006:** Employer's Annual Federal Unemployment (FUTA) Tax Return   850106

Department of the Treasury — Internal Revenue Service   OMB No. 1545-0028

(EIN)
Employer identification number ☐☐ – ☐☐☐☐☐☐☐

Name *(not your trade name)*

Trade name *(if any)*

Address
Number   Street   Suite or room number

City   State   ZIP code

Type of Return
(Check all that apply.)

☐ **a.** Amended

☐ **b.** Successor employer

☐ **c.** No payments to employees in 2006

☐ **d.** Final: Business closed or stopped paying wages

Read the separate instructions before you fill out this form. Please type or print within the boxes.

Part 1: Tell us about your return. If any line does NOT apply, leave it blank.

1 If you were required to pay your state unemployment tax in ...

     1a One state only, write the state abbreviation ....**1a** ☐☐
     - OR -
     1b More than one state (You are a multi-state employer)--------**1b** ☐ Check here. Fill out Schedule A.

2

Part 2: Determine your FUTA tax before adjustments for 2006. If any line does NOT apply, leave it blank.

3 Total payments to all employees ------------------------------- **3** ☐.

4 Payments exempt from FUTA tax ------------- **4** ☐.

     Check all that apply: **4a** ☐ Fringe benefits   **4c** ☐ Retirement/Pension   **4e** ☐ Other
                     4b ☐ Group term life insurance   **4d** ☐ Dependent care

5 Total of payments made to each employee in excess of $7,000 ---**5** ☐.

6 Subtotal (line 4 + line 5 = line 6)-------------------------**6** ☐.

7 Total taxable FUTA wages (line 3 - line 6 = line 7)-----------**7** ☐.

8 FUTA tax before adjustments (line 7 x .008 = line 8)-----------**8** ☐.

Part 3: Determine your adjustments. If any line does NOT apply, leave it blank.

9 If ALL of the taxable FUTA wages you paid were excluded from state unemployment tax, multiply line 7 by .054 (line 7 x .054 = line 9). Then go to line 12 -------------**9** ☐.

10 If SOME of the taxable FUTA wages you paid were excluded from state unemployment tax, OR you paid ANY state unemployment tax late (after the due date for filing Form 940), fill out the worksheet in the instructions. Enter the amount from line 7 of the worksheet onto line10....**10** ☐.

11

Part 4: Determine your FUTA tax and balance due or overpayment for 2006. If any line does NOT apply, leave it blank.

12 Total FUTA tax after adjustments (lines 8 + 9 + 10 = line 12) -------------**12** ☐.

13 FUTA tax deposited for the year, including any payment applied from a prior year ....**13** ☐.

14 Balance due (If line 12 is more than line 13, enter the difference on line 14.)
     • if line 14 is more than $500, you must deposit your tax.
     • If line 14 is $500 or less and you pay by check, make your check payable to the United States Treasury and write your EIN, *Form 940,* and *2006* on the check ----------------------**14** ☐.

15 Overpayment (If line 13 is more than line 12, enter the difference on line 15 and check a box below)---**15** ☐.

                                     Check one ☐ Apply to next return.
                                                 ☐ Send a refund.

▶ You **MUST** fill out both pages of this form and **SIGN** it.

Next ➡

For Privacy Act and Paperwork Reduction Act Notice, see the back of Form 940-V, Payment Voucher.   Cat. No. 112340   Form **940** (2006)

Figure 18-13A. Employer's Annual Federal Unemployment (FUTA) Tax Return, Form 940 (front)

850206

Name (not your trade name)   Employer identification number (EIN)

Part 5: Report your FUTA tax liability by quarter only if line 12 is more than $500. If not, go to Part 6.

16 Report the amount of your FUTA tax liability for each quarter; do NOT enter the amount you deposited. If you had no liability for a quarter, leave the line blank.

16a **1st quarter** (January 1 – March 31)................................16a [____ . __]

16b **2nd quarter** (April 1 – June 30)...................................16b [____ . __]

16c **3rd quarter** (July 1 – September 30)............................16a [____ . __]

16b **4th quarter** (October 1 – December 31)........................16d [____ . __]

17 **Total tax liability for the year** (lines 16a + 16b + 16c + 16d = line 17) 17 [____ . __] Total must equal line 12.

Part 6: May we speak with you third-party designee?

Do you want to allow an employee, a paid tax preparer, or another person to discuss this return with the IRS? See the instructions for details.

☐ **Yes.** Designee's name [_____]

Select a 5-digit Personal Identification Number (PIN) to use when talking to IRS [_][_][_][_][_]

☐ **No.**

Part 7: Sign here.

You MUST fill out both pages of this form and SIGN it.

Under penalties of perjury, I declare that I have examined this return, including accompanying schedules and statements, and to the best of my knowledge and belief, it is true, correct, and complete, and that no part of any payment made to a state unemployment fund claimed as a credit was, **or is to** be, deducted from the payments made to employees.

X **Sign your name here** [_____] Print your name here [_____]

Print your title here [_____]

Date [__/__/__] Best daytime phone (___) ___ – ____

Part 8: For PAID preparers only (optional)

If you were paid to prepare this return and are not an employee of the business that is filing this return, you may choose to fill out Part 8.

Paid Preparer's name [_____] Preparer's SSN/PTIN [_____]

Paid Preparer's signature [_____] Date [__/__/__]

☐ **Check if you are self-employed.**

Firm's name [_____] Firm's EIN [_____]

Street address [_____]

City [_____] State [_____] ZIP code [_____]

Figure 18-13B. Employer's Annual Federal Unemployment (FUTA) Tax Return, Form 940 (back)

Form **941 for 2006**: Employer's QUARTERLY Federal Tax Return

(Rev. January 2006)

Department of the Treasury — Internal Revenue Service

950106

OMB No. 1545-0029

(EIN)
Employer identification number ☐ ☐ — ☐ ☐ ☐ ☐ ☐ ☐ ☐

Name (not your trade name)

Trade name (if any)

Address

Number   Street   Suite or room number

City   State   ZIP code

Report for this Quarter ...
(Check one.)

☐ **1.** January, February, March

☐ **2:** April, May, June

☐ **3:** July, August, September

☐ **4:** October, November, December

Read the separate instructions before you fill out this form. Please type or print within the boxes.

Part 1: Answer these question for this quarter.

1 Number of employees who received wages, tips, or other compensation for the pay period including: *Mar. 12* **(Quarter 1)**, *June 12* **(Quarter 2)**, *Sept. 12* **(Quarter 3)**, *Dec. 12* **(Quarter 4)**   **1** ☐

2 Wages, tips, and other compensation . . . . **2** ☐

3 Total income tax withheld from wages, tips, and other compensation . . . . **3** ☐

4 If no wages, tips, and other compensation are subject to social security or Medicare tax .   ☐ Check and go to line 6.

5 Taxable social security and Medicare wages and tips:

	Column 1		Column 2
5a Taxable social security wages	☐	x .124 =	☐
5b Taxable social security tips	☐	x .124 =	☐
5c Taxable Medicare wages & tips	☐	x .029 =	☐

5d Total social security and Medicare taxes (*Column 2*, lines 5a + 5b + 5c = line 5d) . . **5d** ☐

6 Total taxes before adjustments (lines 3 + 5d = line 6)................................. **6** ☐

7 TAX ADJUSTMENTS (Read the instructions for line 7 before completing lines 7a through 7h.):

7a Current quarter's fractions of cents . . . . ☐

7b Current quarter's sick pay . . . . ☐

7c Current quarter's adjustments for tips and group-term life insurance ☐

7d Current year's income tax withholding (attach Form 941c) . . ☐

7e Prior quarters' social security and Medicare taxes (attach Form 941c) ☐

7f Special additions to federal income tax (attach Form 941c) . . . ☐

7g Special additions to social security and Medicare (attach Form 941 c) ☐

7h TOTAL ADJUSTMENTS (Combine all amounts: lines 7a through 7g.) . . . . **7h** ☐

8 Total taxes after adjustments (Combine lines 6 and 7h.) . . . . **8** ☐

9 Advance earned income credit (EIC) payments made to employees . . . . **9** ☐

10 Total taxes after adjustment for advance EIC (line 8 – line 9 = line 10) . . . . . . **10** ☐

11 Total deposits for this quarter, including overpayment applied from a orior quarter . . . **11** ☐

12 Balance due (If line 10 is more than line 11, write the difference here.) . . . . **12** ☐
Make checks payable to *United States Treasury*.

13 Overpayment (If line 11 is more than line 10, write the difference here.) ☐   Check one ☐ Apply to next return.
  ☐ Send a rfund.

▶ You **MUST** fill out both pages of this form and **SIGN** it.   Next ➡

For Privacy Act and Paperwork Reduction Act Notice, see the back of the Payment Voucher.   Cat. No. 17001Z   Form **940** (Rev. 1-2006)

Figure 18-14A. Employer's Quarterly Federal Tax Return, Form 941 (Part 1)

950206

Name *(not your trade name)*	Employer identification number (EIN)

Part 2: Tell us about your deposit schedule and tax liability for this quarter.

If you are unsure about whether you are a monthly schedule depositor or a semiweekly schedule depositor, see *Pub. 15 (Circular E)*, section 11.

14 ☐ ☐   Write the state abbreviation for the state where you made your deposits OR write "MU" if you made your deposits in multiple states.

15 Check one: ☐   Line 10 is **less** than $2,500. Go to Part 3.

☐   You were a monthly schedule depositor for the entire quarter. Fill out your tax liability for each month. Then go to Part 3.

Tax liability: Month 1 [_____ . __]

Month 2 [_____ . __]

Month 3 [_____ . __]

Total liability for quarter [_____ . __]   Total must equal line 10.

☐   You were a semiweekly schedule depositor for any part of this quarter. Fill out *Schedule B (Form 941): Report of Tax Liability for Semiweekly Schedule Depositors*, and attach it to this form.

Part 3: Tell us about your business. If a question does NOT apply to your business, leave it blank.

16   If your business has closed or you stopped paying wages. . . . . ☐ Check here, and

enter the final date you paid wages   [/ /]

17   If you are a seasonal employer and you do not have to file a return for every quarter of the yea . . . ☐ Check here,

Part 4: May we speak with your third-party designee?

Do you want to allow an employee, a paid tax preparer, or another person to discuss this return with the IRS? See the **instructions** for **details.**

☐ **Yes. Designee's name** [_____]

☐ No.   Phone ( ) –   Personal Identification Number (PIN) ☐☐☐☐☐

Part 5: Sign here. You MUST fill out both sides of this form and SIGN it.

Under penalties of perjury, I declare that I have examined this return, including accompanying schedules and statements, and to the best of \my knowledge and belief, it is true, correct, and complete.

✗ Sign your name here [_____]

Print name and title [_____]

Date [/ /]   Phone ( ) –

Part 6: For PAID preparers only (optional)

Paid Preparer's Signature			
Firm's name			
Address		EIN	
		ZIP code	
Date [/ /] Phone ( ) –		SSN/PTIN	
☐ Check if you are self-employed.			

Form **941** (Rev. 1-2006)

Figure 18-14B. Employer's Quarterly Federal Tax Return, Form 941 (Parts 2–6)

Form **941-V**		Payment Voucher	OMB No. 1545-0029

Department of the Treasury
Internal Revenue Service

▶ Do not staple or attach this voucher to your payment.

2006

1 Enter your employer identification number (EIN).

2 Enter the amount of your payment. ▶ | Dollars | Cents

3 Tax period

○ 1st Quarter   ○ 3rd Quarter

○ 2nd Quarter   ○ 4th Quarter

4 Enter your business name (individual name if sole proprietor).

Enter your address.

Enter your city, state, and ZIP code.

Figure 18-15. Payment Voucher to accompany Form 941, Employer's Quarterly Federal Tax Return

a Control number   2 2 2 2   Void ☐   For Official Use Only ▶   OMB No. 1545-0008

b Employer identification number (EIN)

1 Wages, tips, other compensation   2 Federal income tax withheld

c Employer's name, address, and ZIP code

3 Social security wages   4 Social security tax withheld

5 Medicare wages and tips   6 Medicare tax withheld

7 Social security tips   8 Allocated tips

d Employee's social security number

9 Advance EIC payment   10 Dependent care benefits

e Employee's first name and initial   Last name   Suff.   11 Nonqualified plans   12a See instructions for box 12

13 Statutory employee ☐   Retirement plan ☐   Third-party sick pay ☐   12b

14 Other   12c

12d

f Employee's address and ZIP code

15 State   Employer's state ID number   16 State wages, tips, etc.   17 State income tax   18 Local wages, tips, etc.   19 Local income tax   20 Locality name

Form **W-2**   Wage and Tax Statement   **2006**   Department of the Treasury—Internal Revenue Service

Copy A For Social Security Administration — Send this entire page with Form W-3 to the Social Security Administration; photocopies are **not** acceptable.

For Privacy Act and Paperwork Reduction Act Notice, see back of Copy D.

Cat. No. 10134D

Do Not Cut, Fold, or Staple Forms on This Page — Do Not Cut, Fold, or Staple Forms on This Page

Figure 18-16. Wage and Tax Statement, Form W-2

showing the name and address of the physician-employer with his or her identification number and the employee's name, address, and Social Security number. It shows the FICA taxable wages, FICA tax deducted, Medicare wages and tips, Medicare tax withheld, total wages paid, and federal income tax withheld. Two copies are sent to the employee; one copy is sent to the Social Security Administration; and one copy is retained for the physician-employer's records.

Employers who prepare 20 or fewer W-2s can access blank forms online, fill them in, and submit them. Corrections can be made using Form W-2C online. Employers who report 250 or more W-2s *must* submit reports on magnetic media. More and more businesses are using online electronic reporting via Social Security Administration's telephone bulletin board service. To prevent common errors in reporting W-2 forms and ensure accurate reporting for paper and magnetic media, the following guidelines should be followed:

- Send paper or magnetic media by *Certified Mail* and retain the receipt.

- Verify that the sum of wages on the quarterly Form 941 agrees with the annual total of all W-2 and W-3 forms. (If pensions and annuities are reported, these figures will not agree.)

- Follow Social Security Administration's Software Specifications and Edits for *paper* and *magnetic media.*

- Check the employer identification number (EIN) on forms W-2, W-3, and 941 to see that it is correct, consistent, and is the same number issued by the IRS.

- Put the W-3 on top of the W-2 and mail to the address printed on the W-3.

- If magnetic media is used, *always* make a backup tape.

- When sending magnetic tape or floppy disk, enclose Form 6559, mailing it to the address on the form. Do not enclose paper, for example, Forms W-2 or W-3, in the magnetic package.

Transmittal of Wage and Tax Statements

The physician-employer is required to provide a summary that compares the income taxes withheld and reported on all W-2 forms with the amount of income tax withheld and reported on the four quarterly Forms 941. The **Transmittal of Wage and Tax Statements (Form W-3)** is used for this purpose (Figure 18-17). Form W-3 is used to transmit all W-2 forms attached at the appropriate Social Security office on or before the last day of February each year. The Social Security Administration then furnishes the IRS with the income tax data it needs from those forms.

A summary and schedule for the payroll, tax forms, and tax withholding responsibilities of the office manager appear in Table 18-2.

Employee's Earning Record

A separate financial record is kept for each employee, showing total earnings (gross income), the amounts deducted or withheld from gross income, and **net income**, referred to as take-home pay. The information sheet should contain the employee's name, address, Social Security number, number of exemptions claimed, date of birth, marital status, rate of pay, hours worked, earnings, deductions, net pay, check numbers, and year-to-date earnings (see Figure 18-18 on page 646). If the medical practice is a large one, time cards may be kept for hourly workers and some salaried workers.

Payroll Register

Some medical practices maintain a payroll register, or summary (see Figure 18-19 on page 646), containing information from employees' time cards such as marital status, number of exemptions claimed, pay rates for regular or overtime hours, gross pay, taxable earnings for FICA and unemployment insurance computations, deductions, net pay, and check numbers. All employees who work during a pay period are included.

Payroll via Electronic Banking

As mentioned previously, besides being able to make federal tax deposits via EFTS, if employees wish their monthly paycheck deposited automatically to their bank account, they must give their bank account numbers to the employer. Advantages when using this system are that money is available on the day of deposit, the employee cannot lose a paycheck, and he or she does not have to get to the bank before it closes. Employees receive a record with a notification of the deposit so earnings and deductions can be easily tracked.

Write-It-Once Check Writing and Payroll Journal System

The write-it-once check writing and payroll journal system is implemented as follows:

1. Place the payroll disbursement journal over the pegboard and position a bank of shingled checks on the pegs to align them over the journal on the first open line. Each check contains a carbonized strip on the back.

DO NOT STAPLE

a Control number	33333	For Official Use Only ▶ OMB No. 1545-0008		

b Kind of Payer ▶	941 ☐ CT-1 ☐	Military ☐ Hshld. emp. ☐	943 ☐ Medicare govt. emp. ☐	944 ☐ Third-party sick pay ☐	1 Wages, tips, other compensation	2 Federal income tax withheld

	3 Social security wages	4 Social security tax withheld

c Total number of Forms W-2	d Establishment number	5 Medicare wages and tips	6 Medicare tax withheld

e Employer identification number (EIN)	7 Social security tips	8 Allocated tips

f Employer's name	9 Advance EIC payments	10 Dependent care benefits

	11 Nonqualified plans	12 Deferred compensation

	13 For third-party sick pay use only

	14 Income tax withheld by payer of third-party sick pay

g Employer's address and ZIP code

h Other EIN used this year

15 State Employer's state ID number	16 State wages, tips, etc.	17 State income tax

	18 Local wages, tips, etc.	19 Local income tax

Contact person	Telephone number ( )	For Official Use Only

Email address	Fax number ( )	

Under penalties of perjury, I declare that I have examined this return and accompanying documents, and, to the best of my knowledge and belief, they are true, correct, and complete.

Signature ▶ _____ Title ▶ _____ Date ▶ _____

Form **W-3** Transmittal of Wage and Tax Statements **2006** Department of the Treasury Internal Revenue Service

Send this entire page with the entire Copy A page of Form(s) W-2 to the Social Security Administration. Photocopies are not acceptable.

Do not send any payment (cash, checks, money orders, etc.) with Forms W-2 and W-3.

What's New

New checkbox for box b on Form W-3. Use the "944" checkbox in box b if you file Form 944, Employer's Annual Federal Tax Return. Form 944 for 2006 is a newly developed form.

Magnetic media filing is discontinued. The Social Security Administration (SSA) will no longer accept any magnetic media reporting of Forms W-2.

Reminder

Separate instructions. See the 2006 Instructions for Forms W-2 and W-3 for information on completing this form.

Purpose Of Form

Use Form W-3 to transmit Copy A of Form(s) W-2, Wage and Tax Statement. Make a copy of Form W-3 and keep it with Copy D (For Employer) of Form(s) W-2 for your records. Use Form W-3 for the correct year. File **Form W-3 even if only one Form W-2 is being filed.** If you are filing Form(s) W-2 electronically, do not file Form W-3.

Where To File

File Form W-3 with Copy A of Form(s) W-2 by February 28, 2007.

Where To File

Send this entire page with the entire Copy A page of Form (s) W-2 to:

Social Security Administration Data Operations Center Wilkes-Barre, PA 18769-0001

Note. If you use "Certified Mail" to file, change the ZIP code to "18769-0002." If you use an IRS-approved private delivery service, add "ATTN: W-2 Process, 1150 E. Mountain Dr." to the address and change the ZIP code to "18702-7997." See Publication 15 (Circular E), Employer's Tax Guide, for a list of IRS-approved private delivery services.

For Privacy Act and Paperwork Reduction Act Notice, see back of Copy D of Form W-2.

Cat. No. 10159Y

Figure 18-17. Transmittal of Wage and Tax Statements, Form W-3

Table 18-2. Schedule and Summary of the Medical Assistant's Payroll, Tax Forms, and Tax Withholding Responsibilities*

Apply for physician-employer identification number	*Physician-Employer Identification Number*—If the physician does not already have an employer identification number, fill out a duplicate Form SS-4 and send it to the District Director of IRS.
When new employees are hired	*Income tax withholding*—Ask each new employee to fill out a withholding exemption certification Form W-4 and file it with the District Director of IRS. To strengthen enforcement of court-ordered child support and the judicial collection of other creditor claims, the Personal Responsibility and Work Opportunity Act of 1996 requires that employers report new hires on Form W-4 no later than 20 days after hire or twice a month if reporting electronically or magnetically.
	Social Security (FICA)—Obtain and record the employees' account numbers as shown on the Social Security card. If an employee has no card, file an application using Form SS-5 with any field office of the Social Security administration.
	Immigration and Naturalization Service (INS)—File the Employment Eligibility Verification Form 1-9.
On payment of wages to employees	*Income tax withholding*—Withhold tax from each wage payment according to the exemption certificate and the withholding rate given in Circular E, Employers Tax Guide.
	Federal Insurance Contributions Act (FICA)—Withhold the appropriate percentage from each wage payment; the amount is to be matched by the physician.
By the fifteenth day of each month or semiweekly	*Payroll tax deposit*—The employer's deposit is based on the total tax liability reported on Form 941. There are two deposit schedules. If $50,000 or less was reported in taxes for the lookback period, i.e., beginning July 1 and ending June 30 of the two previous years, a deposit would be made monthly. If more than $50,000 was reported for the lookback period, make the deposit semiweekly. When paying on the monthly schedule, deposit Social Security, Medicare, and income taxes paid during the month by the 15th of the following month using form 941.
On or before April 30, July 31, October 31, and January 31	*Quarterly tax return*—File Form 941 with the District Director of IRS and pay the full amount of taxes due for the previous quarter on both the income tax withheld from wages and from the physician-employer Social Security taxes.
Before December 1 of each year at the end of employment	*If employees have*—any changes in name, address, marital status, or number of exemptions from those recorded the previous year, request that they file a new Form W-4.
On or before January 31 and at the end of employment	*Provide a withholding statement* (Form W-2)—in duplicate to each employee, showing total wages and the amount of income tax withheld as well as the amount of Social Security taxes withheld with the amount of wags subject to this tax.
On or before February 28 of each year	*Income tax withholding*—File Form W-3, Reconciliation of Income Tax Withheld from Wages, together with all District Director's copies of withholding statements provided employees on Form W-2 for the preceding year.
On or before January 31 of each year	*Federal Unemployment Tax Act* (FUTA)—File annual return on Form 940 and remit the tax to the District Director of IRS.

*The employer's income tax return reports are not shown in this table.

EMPLOYEE EARNINGS RECORD FOR

Name __Mary Jo Davis__ Date of Hire __August 1, 20XX__

Address __2200 Sunset Lane__ Date of Birth __11-28-70__

__Woodland Hills, XY 12345__ Position __Administrative Medical Assistant__ PT (FT)

Telephone __(555) 438-0900__ No. of Exemptions __(1) Single__ (S) M

Social Security Number __939-XX-5678__ Rate of Pay __$13/hour__ (hr) wk/mo

| Period Ended | Total Hours Worked | EARNINGS | | | DEDUCTIONS | | | | | | Check No. | NET PAY | Year to Date |
		Reg. Pay	Over-time Pay	Gross Pay	FICA	Fed. Inc. Tax	State Inc. Tax	SDI	Medicare	TOTAL DEDUC.			
								--					
								--					

Figure 18-18. Example of a completed employee earning record

MONTHLY PAYROLL REGISTER FOR PERIOD ENDING: August 31, 20XX

| EMPLOYEE NAME | No. of Exempts | Hours Worked | Hourly Rate | EARNINGS | | | DEDUCTIONS | | | | | | | |
				Reg. Pay	Over-time	Gross Pay	FICA	Fed. Inc. Tax	State Inc. Tax	SDI	Medicare	TOTAL DEDUC.	Check No.	NET PAY
Mary Jo Davis	1-S	168	13.00	2184.00	78.00	2262.00	140.24	243.00	49.06	–	32.80	465.10	554	1796.90
Beverly Woo	0-S	168	Salary	2500.00	–	2500.00	155.00	317.00	73.72	–	36.25	581.97	555	1918.03
Harold Bohrn	2-M	88	12.00	1056.00	–	1056.00	65.47	1.00	0	–	15.31	81.78	556	974.22
Joan Gonzalez	1-M	168	Salary	2300.00	–	2300.00	142.60	176.00	24.41	–	33.35	376.36	557	1923.64

Figure 18-19. Example of a monthly payroll register

2. Slide the employee earnings record between the check and the journal. As the check is written, the data on the check instantly transfer to the employee record and journal, completing three entries in one writing.

3. The check is inserted into a companion double-window envelope. No addressing is necessary.

The physician's name and address show through the upper window and the payee's name and address show through the lower window.

4. At the end of each month, the columns are totaled for the various deductions (withheld taxes) on the payroll disbursement journal.

PROCEDURE 18-2

Create Category Headings, Determine Deductions, Calculate Payroll, and Make Entries to a Payroll Register

Objective: To create category headings, calculate payroll, and post entries to a payroll register (employees' earnings record).

Equipment/Supplies: Monthly payroll register sheets (see Figure 18-19), employees' time cards, W-4 forms, rate of pay, IRS tax tables, checks, check register, and pen.

Directions: Follow these step-by-step procedures to learn this skill, which is presented in the *Workbook* (Job Skill 18-4 and 18-5) for practice.

Set up a monthly payroll register:

1. Insert the names of the three major column headings for the basic payroll check information, such as employee name, earnings, and deductions.

2. Insert the column headings for number of exemptions, hours worked, and hourly rate of pay.

3. Insert the column headings for earnings, such as regular pay, overtime pay, and gross pay.

4. Insert the column headings for the payroll deductions, such as Federal Insurance Contributions Act (FICA) tax, federal income tax, state income tax, state disability insurance (SDI), and Medicare.

5. Insert the column headings for the total deductions, check number, and net pay.

Enter data on a payroll register and calculate pay:

6. Record employee names, number of exemptions, and hours worked from all employees' time cards under the appropriate columns. Enter rate of pay from confidential records.

7. Calculate the total regular pay by multiplying hourly rate by the regular hours worked; for example, 40 hours per week including any paid vacation or paid holidays, if applicable. Enter the totals under the appropriate headings on the payroll register. If an employee is on salary, list the salary in "Regular Pay."

8. Compute the total overtime pay by calculating the pay rate for overtime pay (for example, time and a half or double time) and multiply-ing the number of hours worked overtime by the overtime rate. Enter the totals under the appropriate headings on the payroll register.

9. Add the regular pay and the overtime pay and record the total salary under "Gross Pay" on the payroll register.

10. Determine federal and state tax deductions using IRS and state tax tables and data on the employee earnings record based on the employee's marital status, number of exemptions, and frequency of payroll. Look under the proper heading (single, married, and paid weekly, biweekly, semimonthly, monthly, and so forth). Record the amount of tax under the proper heading.

11. Compute the amount of FICA tax to withhold for Social Security and Medicare. Enter the total amount withheld from all employees for FICA under the headings for Social Security and Medicare. The employer must match these amounts.

12. Follow state procedures to determine the amount of state income taxes (if any) to with-hold based on the employee's marital status, number of exemptions, and frequency of payroll.

13. Calculate the employer's contributions to FUTA and to the state unemployment fund. Post these amounts to the employer's account.

14. Enter any other deductions, such as health insurance or contributions to a 401(k) fund.

15. Total deductions and list the total amount under "Total Deductions."

16. Subtract the total deductions from the gross pay amount and record the total under "Net Pay."

17. Record the deductions on the check stub, if indicated, including the employee's name, date, pay period, gross earnings, deductions, and net pay.

18. Write the payroll check for the "Net Pay" amount and deposit each deduction in a tax liability account.

STOP AND THINK CASE SCENARIO

Prepare an Analysis to Determine the Effectiveness of Capitated Plans

Scenario: Your physician asks you to do an analysis of capitated plans in your office and compare their reimbursement totals with the same population of patients as if they had fee-for-service plans.

Critical Thinking:

1. What information do you need to gather before you can start the analysis?

_____

_____

_____

2. What type of formula will you use to make this determination?

_____

_____

_____

3. What additional information, perhaps covered in previous chapters, can you think of that would have an impact on this analysis?

_____

_____

_____

_____

STOP AND THINK CASE SCENARIO

Determine Payroll Category and Frequency for Deduction

Scenario: You are a married female administrative medical assistant and the physician asks you to take over some bookkeeping duties including the preparation of the office payroll. The office manager is a single woman who gets paid by salary at the beginning of the month. A part-time high school boy does the filing and gets paid an hourly rate each week on Friday. Occasionally, the physician's teenage daughter comes in and helps where needed; she gets paid at the conclusion of her workday. The remaining staff gets paid an hourly rate every other week on Fridays; this includes a married woman who does the insurance billing, a single woman who is the receptionist, a divorced woman who is the clinical medical assistant, and a married man who is the x-ray and laboratory technician.

Critical Thinking: Determine the dates you will be making out payroll for each type of employee for next month and circle them on a calendar. Select where you will look to find the deductions from the following choices that appear on the withholding tables. Write your answers by each staff member: [single person—weekly] [married persons—weekly] [single persons—biweekly] [married persons—biweekly] [single person—semimonthly] [married persons—semimonthly] [single persons—monthly] [married persons—monthly] [single persons—daily or miscellaneous] [married persons—daily or miscellaneous]

1. Office manager: _____
2. Part-time employees: _____
3. Physician's teenage daughter: _____
4. Insurance biller: _____
5. Receptionist: _____
6. Clinical medical assistant: _____
7. X-ray and lab tech: _____

FOCUS   ON CERTIFICATION*

CMA Content Summary

- Medical abbreviations
- Professionalism
- Working as a team member
- Internal Revenue Service forms
- Employment laws
- Personnel records
- Aging accounts receivable
- Write checks
- Employee payroll records
- Calculate wages and taxes
- Prepare payroll checks and earning statements
- Deposit taxes, file, and mail tax reports

RMA Content Summary

- Medical terminology and abbreviations
- Accounting procedures

- Accounts payable
- Disbursement accounts
- Employee payroll procedures
- Payroll withholding and deductions
- Payroll tax forms and deposits
- Payroll calculations

CMAS Content Summary

- Medical and insurance terminology
- Accounting principles
- Financial computations
- Accounts payable
- Check writing
- Employee payroll and reports
- Payroll tax deductions and records

REVIEW   EXAM-STYLE QUESTIONS

1. The most widely used of all computer applications in a medical practice is:

   a. insurance billing

   b. patient statements

   c. financial management

   d. appointment scheduling

   e. word processing

2. If the office manager wanted to find out how effectively the medical assistant was collecting old accounts, he or she would use the following:

   a. accounts receivable minus accounts payable calculation

   b. collection ratio formula

   c. overhead expense formula

   d. cost per procedure formula

   e. capitation versus fee-for-service plan

3. To find out what the cost is to run a medical practice on a monthly basis, the office manager would:

   a. look at the checkbook

   b. analyze the accounts receivable

   c. look at the accounts payable record

   d. use the overhead expense formula

   e. look at the payroll records

---

*This textbook and the accompanying Workbook *meet the entry-level administrative and general competencies for the CMA outlined by the* AAMA Examination Content Outline and Role Delineation Study *and for the RMA and CMAS outlined by the AMT Competencies and Examination Specifications (see Competency Grid in Appendix B).*

4. When comparing yearly managed care revenues against fee-for-service charges, it is important to:

   a. compare capitated amounts per patient with the managed care eligibility list

   b. determine the average number of managed care patients seen each month

   c. total the capitation receipts for one month

   d. divide total capitation revenues by total capitation visits

   e. subtract the write-off amounts that are not collected from fee-for-service charges

5. When paying bills, the office manager would record expenditures in a/an:

   a. disbursement record

   b. accounts receivable ledger

   c. payroll register

   d. bank register

   e. notebook

6. If an employee resigns, wages must be paid within:

   a. 24 hours

   b. 36 hours

   c. 72 hours

   d. 1 week

   e. 2 weeks

7. Both the employee and the employer pay the same tax rate for:

   a. FICA

   b. Medicare tax

   c. Federal income tax

   d. State tax

   e. both a and b

8. An Employer's Quarterly Federal Tax Return, Form 941, must be filed by the physician-employer on or before:

   a. January 1, April 1, July 1, October 1

   b. January 30, April 30, July 30, October 30,

   c. April 30, July 31, October 31, January 31

   d. February 28, May 31, August 31, November 30

   e. March 30, June 30, September 30, December 31

9. When following the medical assistant's payroll and tax schedule, payroll tax deposits in an amount exceeding $50,000 need to be made:

   a. monthly

   b. by the 1st of every month

   c. by the 15th of every month

   d. semimonthly

   e. weekly

10. Information used to calculate pay and record on each employee's payroll register comes from:

    a. the employee's time card

    b. the office checkbook

    c. the employee handbook

    d. the office policy and procedures manual

    e. the employee's resumé

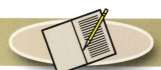

WORKBOOK ASSIGNMENT

To develop competency-based job skills, refer to the *Workbook* and complete the:

- Abbreviation and Spelling Review
- Review Questions

- Critical Thinking Exercises
- Job Skill activities, which are outlined at the beginning of this chapter under "Performance Objectives in the *Workbook*."

Performance Objectives (Job Skills) in the *Workbook*

▍ Complete a job application form (Job Skill 19-1).

▍ Compose a cover letter of introduction (Job Skill 19-2).

▍ Key a resumé (Job Skill 19-3).

▍ Prepare a follow-up thank-you letter (Job Skill 19-4).

OUTLINE ⟩ WITH LECTURE NOTES

Employment Opportunities

_____

_____

_____

_____

Beginning a Job Hunt
Employment Agencies

_____

_____

_____

_____

Classified Advertisements

_____

_____

_____

_____

Other Job Sources

_____

_____

_____

_____

Computerized Search

_____

_____

_____

_____

Application Form

_____

_____

_____

_____

Letter of Introduction

_____

_____

_____

_____

Resumé
Chronological Resumé

_____

_____

_____

_____

Functional Resumé

_____

_____

_____

_____

Combination Resumé

_____

_____

_____

_____

Results-Oriented Resumé

_____

_____

_____

_____

Electronic Resumé

_____

_____

_____

_____

Scannable Resumé

_____
_____
_____
_____

References

_____
_____
_____
_____

The Job Interview
Portfolio

_____
_____
_____
_____

Preparing for an Interview

_____
_____
_____
_____

Interview Guidelines

_____
_____
_____

After the Interview

_____
_____
_____

_____
_____

Preparing for a Performance Evaluation

_____
_____
_____
_____

Negotiating Pay and Asking for a Raise

_____
_____
_____
_____

Tips for Holding the Medical Position

_____
_____
_____
_____

Conclusion

_____
_____
_____
_____

KEY TERMS

blind letter
chronological resumé
combination resumé
cover letter
diplomate
electronic job search
employment agencies

format
functional resumé
human resource department
performance evaluation
portfolio
results-oriented resumé
resumé

HEART OF THE HEALTH CARE PROFESSIONAL

Service

The health care profession offers a multitude of service-oriented positions focused on attending to patient needs. As you have discovered throughout this textbook, patient needs involve more than quality medical care provided by the physician and clinical staff. It involves walking in the patient's shoes from the time of the first telephone call and assisting along the path that they will travel to restore good health or prevent illness and disease. Your ability to care, communicate, and assist provides immeasurable support along the journey that is seldom chosen and frequently difficult.

EMPLOYMENT OPPORTUNITIES

Service-oriented positions in the medical field continue to provide about half the employment opportunities in the United States. In addition to private medical practices (solo and group), hospitals, and clinics, people trained as administrative medical assistants have the opportunity to be employed in a variety of health care facilities, including health insurance companies, pharmacies, laboratories, managed care organizations, diet control centers, mental health agencies, industrial clinics, physical therapy practices, specialty groups, nurse practitioner offices, and medical supply companies. People of all ages and men as well as women train to become medical assistants. Refer to "Employment Opportunities" in Chapter 1 to review job positions available to people trained as administrative medical assistants.

Research studies indicate that even though the job-seeking person has all the skills to do a job, he or she often does not have the skills required to get a job. Therefore, before the job applicant begins actively seeking employment in a medical facility, there are steps to take to prepare for locating and securing the best possible position. First, the job seeker should consider the primary reasons employers give for rejecting job applicants. These include the following:

1. Poorly completed job application form or resumé

2. Unacceptable personal appearance, manners, and mannerisms

3. Little interest or poor reasons for desiring a job

4. Inability to communicate effectively during the interview

5. Immaturity

6. Past history of job hopping

7. Inability to verify previous employment or educational background

8. Poor work record

9. Lack of job-related skills

BEGINNING A JOB HUNT

Preparation for a career in the medical field should begin with an inventory of skills, abilities, and interests and an evaluation of personal traits that will ensure eventual movement to higher career levels. The student can refresh his or her memory by reading through the job duties and responsibilities shown in Chapter 1, Figure 1-3, Generic Job Description for Entry-Level Administrative Medical Assistant. Also review the list of procedures learned that appears in the front matter of this text. Turn to Chapter 2 to review types of medical practice settings and medical specialists (see Table 2-3). After gathering this information determine what you like to do and in what type of practice you would flourish. Think about the job responsibilities, diversity of job duties, growth potential, continuing education opportunities, other staff members, and the type of patient population. Remember to try to match your personality with the type of job you are seeking.

When conducting a search for a position look at the various methods for job hunting and follow through on all possible leads. Job seekers who have recently completed their education might contact school placement personnel and place their names on file and attend medical assistant meetings and workshops open to the public; these are usually announced in local newspapers (Figure 19-1). Because many jobs are never formally advertised, the job candidate should spread the word that he or she is seeking a position and stay in touch with classmates, teachers, school counselors, professional acquaintances, and friends working in medical settings, all of whom might know of openings in medical facilities.

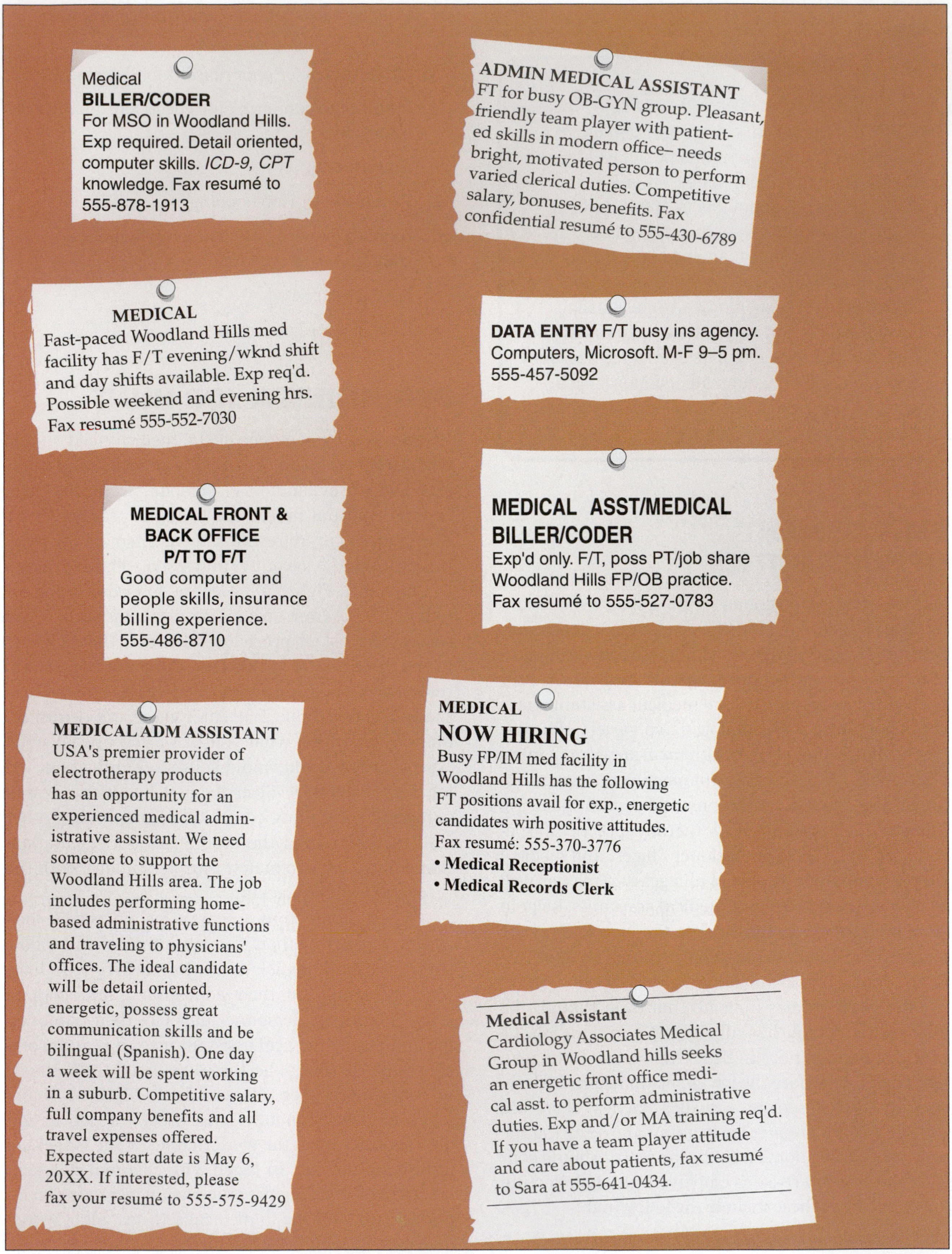

Medical
BILLER/CODER
For MSO in Woodland Hills.
Exp required. Detail oriented,
computer skills. *ICD-9, CPT*
knowledge. Fax resumé to
555-878-1913

ADMIN MEDICAL ASSISTANT
FT for busy OB-GYN group. Pleasant,
friendly team player with patient-
ed skills in modern office– needs
bright, motivated person to perform
varied clerical duties. Competitive
salary, bonuses, benefits. Fax
confidential resumé to 555-430-6789

MEDICAL
Fast-paced Woodland Hills med
facility has F/T evening/wknd shift
and day shifts available. Exp req'd.
Possible weekend and evening hrs.
Fax resumé 555-552-7030

DATA ENTRY F/T busy ins agency.
Computers, Microsoft. M-F 9–5 pm.
555-457-5092

**MEDICAL FRONT &
BACK OFFICE
P/T TO F/T**
Good computer and
people skills, insurance
billing experience.
555-486-8710

**MEDICAL ASST/MEDICAL
BILLER/CODER**
Exp'd only. F/T, poss PT/job share
Woodland Hills FP/OB practice.
Fax resumé to 555-527-0783

MEDICAL ADM ASSISTANT
USA's premier provider of
electrotherapy products
has an opportunity for an
experienced medical administrative assistant. We need
someone to support the
Woodland Hills area. The job
includes performing home-
based administrative functions
and traveling to physicians'
offices. The ideal candidate
will be detail oriented,
energetic, possess great
communication skills and be
bilingual (Spanish). One day
a week will be spent working
in a suburb. Competitive salary,
full company benefits and all
travel expenses offered.
Expected start date is May 6,
20XX. If interested, please
fax your resumé to 555-575-9429

MEDICAL
NOW HIRING
Busy FP/IM med facility in
Woodland Hills has the following
FT positions avail for exp., energetic
candidates wirh positive attitudes.
Fax resumé: 555-370-3776
• **Medical Receptionist**
• **Medical Records Clerk**

Medical Assistant
Cardiology Associates Medical
Group in Woodland hills seeks
an energetic front office medical asst. to perform administrative
duties. Exp and/or MA training req'd.
If you have a team player attitude
and care about patients, fax resumé
to Sara at 555-641-0434.

Figure 19-1. Examples of classified advertisements from a local newspaper

Hiring is often done through a network or grapevine of contacts referred to as the "hidden job market." An employer passes the word of a specific job opening to friends and colleagues, who, in turn, spread the word and refer qualified persons they know. Because 75 percent of job opportunities derive from personal contact, the most important job sources are acquaintances.

Remember, every job search is different and success requires endurance, so plan to be in it for the long haul. Do not set your sights on only one position at one place of employment. If you get a potential offer, do not stop looking. Until a job is landed, keep searching, keep applying, and keep interviewing. To relieve stress and reduce frustration, establish a set number of hours per day or week that you will devote to securing a desired position. Your chances for success will increase if you create a balance in your life, reduce stress, and remain enthusiastic. Do not let fear of the unknown overwhelm you, instead envision yourself in the position you have trained for.

Keep a positive attitude and remember that the traits listed highest by employers are punctuality, following directions, asking for help when needed, accepting responsibility, meeting deadlines, and handling unexpected change.

Employment Agencies

The job seeker should visit public and private employment agencies, including both state and federal government offices. There are agencies that provide opportunities for part-time and full-time work as well as "temp-to-hire" positions; that is, temporary positions that might lead to permanent employment. The local medical society can also provide leads. Professional **employment agencies** operate as referral services and make their money by placing suitable applicants in jobs; they are paid a fee by either the applicant or the employer.

Complete application forms carefully and be prepared to take any required skills tests they administer (Figure 19-2). Any questions about health, disabilities, and past workers' compensation claims are not legal according to the Americans with Disabilities Act of 1990, so they need not be answered.

Often when a job applicant calls an employment agency about an advertised job opportunity, it will already have been filled. However, the agency may suggest a visit to the office to fill out an application,

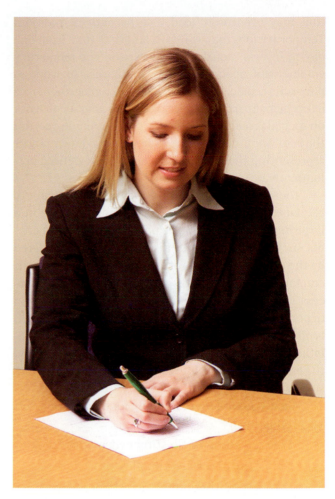

Figure 19-2. This applicant is carefully thinking over information before writing it on the application form to prevent making errors

perform testing, and talk about other openings. Before agreeing to an appointment, the job seeker should find out as much as possible about the other jobs because he or she may already have learned about them from another source or agency (some positions are listed with more than one agency). Make sure the agency handles jobs in the medical field specific to the type you are seeking. Also, before signing a legally binding contract, the job seeker should read it carefully to determine whether the applicant or the employer pays the agency fee and under what conditions it is due and payable.

Temporary Employment

Contracting to work for an agency that places its employees in temporary jobs often provides the prospective full-time job applicant with office experience that may eventually lead to a permanent position. Temporary jobs may range in length of time from one day to several months or even years. The temporary employment agency provides employees to work as part-time replacements, as vacation replacements, as extra help during peak periods of the year, or to work on special projects. The agency pays the employee, not the firm. Some contracts may be made so an employee representing the temporary agency can be hired permanently by an office or firm.

Today it is not uncommon for the job applicant to be placed as a "temporary worker" in a position in a large medical facility and be paid by the agency. Benefits, such as life and health insurance, are often offered by the agency as well as other perks. This relieves the employer of many duties involved in the hiring process and gives both the employer and employee an opportunity to try each other out. If a suitable match is not made, the employer is relieved by law from regulations involved with discharge of the employee, and the employee is reevaluated by the agency for a more suitable position.

A few advantages of working for a temporary service company are:

- Free screening and testing to demonstrate skills
- Obtaining experience in office procedures
- Diversity of work duties; less chance of work becoming boring and repetitive
- Flexible work schedules
- Benefit package offered by agency

To learn the names of companies that feature temporary services, look in the local Yellow Pages section of the telephone book under the heading "Employment, Temporary." Some national companies that might be listed under the heading are Kelly Services; Manpower Incorporated; Western Temporary Service, Incorporated; and Olsten Temporary Services.

Classified Advertisements

The help-wanted ads in the classified section of newspapers are another source of leads. The advertisement explains how to make the initial contact (by telephone, written communication, faxed resumé). To "tune in" to a local job market and respond to advertisements, the job seeker can subscribe to the principal newspaper of a city in which employment is desired. Help-wanted advertisements appearing in newspapers cannot mention a preference for age, sex, and race; but "situations-wanted" ads can.

Other Job Sources

Occasionally, a *cold call* (i.e., unannounced visit) or a **blind letter** to an office where a possible job opportunity is discovered through a friend or where the job seeker would especially like to work will result in a positive response. In such cases, the first impression of the job seeker presented in person or via a letter is of utmost importance. Communicating a strong desire to work at the facility along with a confident approach will enhance your chances of obtaining employment. Be prepared to answer questions during the telephone contact but do not interview over the phone. Be brief and to the point, sound businesslike, and communicate your enthusiasm.

Advance planning is necessary if the job seeker must travel to an unfamiliar geographical area. Nothing is more discouraging to an unemployed person than a prolonged job search in unfamiliar surroundings. Use the Internet to search for directions and download maps (see Resources). A late arrival for completion of a job application, delivery of a resumé, or interview appointment will present a negative first impression and decrease your chance of being hired.

The Yellow Pages of telephone directories provide listings of professional offices, clinics, and hospitals. Chambers of Commerce publications contain membership directories, names of major professional employers in specific areas, and brochures describing regional facts. Some county and state medical societies operate employment agencies or may be able to direct the job seeker to someone who has access to employment opportunities.

Join a chapter of the American Association of Medical Assistants (AAMA) as a student member. This can provide excellent networking opportunities because members are usually the first to know of possible openings. Attend meetings and let members know you are seeking a position. Receive their professional magazines and bulletins to learn of job opportunities. Place a notice in the local chapter newsletter about your job search. Contact the national headquarters of the association for further information about local chapters in the state by referring to Resources at the end of this chapter.

Computerized Job Search

Classified advertisements and printed resumés may become obsolete because of innovative advances in **electronic job search** databases. Cyberspace offers health care job seekers the ability to pursue national

PROCEDURE 19-1

STEP 1 2 3

Answer a Classified Advertisement

Objective: To compose a letter to respond to a classified advertisement in a local newspaper that relays your qualifications and will generate enough interest to arrange an interview.

Equipment/Supplies: Local newspaper classified employment advertisements, 8½ × 11-inch white bond paper, number 10 envelope, computer or typewriter, and pen.

Directions: Follow these step-by-step procedures, which include rationales, to learn this skill.

1. Review letter styles and composition in Chapter 11 and envelope preparation in Chapter 12 to determine and utilize proper format.

2. Compose a rough draft of the letter to include:

   a. Name of newspaper the classified advertisement is listed in

   b. Date of publication

   c. Title of position for which you are applying in case the employer has several advertisements for various positions

   d. Statement communicating your enthusiastic interest and motivation in obtaining the new position

   e. List of qualifications, including job skills relevant to the advertised requirements

   f. Request of a response to your letter by telephone, fax, e-mail, or standard mail so an interview appointment can be made

   g. Information about where you may be contacted if the employer is interested in reaching you

   h. Courteous conclusion with an expression of appreciation for considering your request

3. Reread the letter and reword as necessary to be sure you communicate your interest, intent, enthusiasm, and qualifications in the best possible manner.

4. Proofread the letter on-screen for content, typographical errors, grammar, and punctuation to be sure all important information has been addressed and the letter contains absolutely no errors.

5. Print and proofread the letter again in hard copy, making sure it is perfect.

6. Key a number 10 envelope to the attention of the person responsible for hiring; include your name and return address.

7. Mail promptly after the advertisement is listed.

---

employment opportunities. The Internet is becoming the classified page of the computer age so professionals can market their services nationwide. The main advantage of the Internet is the ability to communicate with individuals in other locations to obtain professional level job listings and career advice. Hundreds of jobs may be found on the Internet's World Wide Web. Go to a Web site with a search engine such as AltaVista, HotBot, Infoseek, Lycos, or Yahoo. Enter a key word or words describing a topic and click "search." A list of related Web sites will appear. Click on an address or the underlined or highlighted words to get to a site. Descriptions of medical practice opportunities are available from America's Job Bank, *Career Magazine*, E-Span Employment Database Search, and so on. Refer to Resources at the end of this chapter for

Web addresses of these and other sites. MedSearch America, another health employment service, posts job advertisements that include hospitals, managed care organizations, and pharmaceutical companies so job seekers can e-mail their resumés for free on-line posting.

Another way to carry out an electronic job search is to subscribe monthly or annually to one or more on-line computer services, such as America Online, Prodigy, or CompuServe. These services have bulletin boards for those interested in medical positions, and a notice or resumé may be posted on them to communicate that a job search is being conducted.

Chat room and discussion groups are available to explore aspects of the work world regarding your current job or career changes.

American Computerized Employment Service in Irvine, California, has also entered the job placement field with a trademarked system called Tele-Recruiting (see Resources). Job candidates register for no charge after completing an extensive profile questionnaire outlining experience, skills, and other job-related factors, such as maximum commuting distance and flextime requirements. This company acts as a liaison between employers and applicants. Employers use a Touch-Tone telephone to access the computer and search for candidates meeting their requirements by annual subscription, pay-per-search, or package searches. Applicants may register under more than one category and may update their data when new skills and additional qualifications have been acquired. Data remain online after a job is obtained, so the service is helpful when advancing in a present career or when seeking a career change.

APPLICATION FORM

The employment application is the employer's first introduction to a job-seeker. It is a tool used to gather information about the prospective employee's background, which can be used as a starting point to ask questions during the interview. If it provides solid information and makes a good first impression, it can lead to an interview.

The job seeker should complete a mock application form and record all dates, names, and addresses of relevant information (Figure 19-3). This can be taken to job sites and used as a reference. Visit the **human resource department** or the *personnel office* of hospitals, clinics, and large medical facilities to check personnel bulletin boards. If no jobs are currently listed, find out if they keep files of potential job applicants, and, if so, complete a questionnaire or application form provided for that purpose.

PROCEDURE 19-2

STEP 1 2 3

Complete a Job Application Form

Objective: To accurately complete a job application. Follow instructions and study each question carefully before answering.

Equipment/Supplies: Job application form, completed mock application (or data containing list of names and addresses, dates of employment and so on), and pen or pencil.

Directions: Follow these step-by-step procedures, which include rationales, to learn this skill, which is presented in the *Workbook* (Job Skill 19-1) for practice.

1. Read the entire application; some instructions might be hidden on the last page or last line.

2. Read the fine print, taking note of such instructions as "please print," "put last name first," or "use pen only." Following instructions precisely indicates an ability to understand and follow directions.

3. Complete the application in ink unless directed to use a pencil.

4. Block print if specified or if handwriting is illegible, and abbreviate words only when there is lack of space.

5. Refer to the completed mock application form or data that you have carried with you and which has been checked for accuracy. Copy information onto each application form, taking time to be neat.

6. Record dates of previous employment; be exact because most employers verify employment history. If the form asks the reason for leaving a position, it may be left blank and discussed during the interview.

7. List job skills relevant to the position and be specific.

8. Enter hourly wage expected or salary amount if a salary is requested. A proper answer might be "negotiable" or "flexible" and further discussion conducted at the interview.

9. Sign and date the application on completion.

EMPLOYMENT APPLICATION FORM

Directions: Answer all questions using black ink (print).

PERSONAL NAME

(LAST) GRANT	(FIRST) SARASUE	(MI) T.	

ADDRESS – STREET 21185 West Amber Street	CITY Encino	STATE CA	ZIP 91316-0002

PHONE NUMBER: (555) 211-8773   SOCIAL SECURITY NUMBER: 201-XX-0731

POSITION DESIRED: Administrative Medical Assistant

EXPECTED SALARY OR HOURLY WAGE: Negotiable

EDUCATION

NAME OF SCHOOL	ADDRESS	DATE(S)	DEGREE/CERTIFICATE
HIGH SCHOOL L.B. Johnson High School	123 West Blvd. Newbury Park, CA	19XX – 20XX	Diploma
COLLEGE Valley College (Vocational/Technical)	421 Dylan Street Woodland Hills, CA	20XX – 20XX	AA Degree
OTHER Externship: Valley Medical Group	1212 Center Street Woodland Hills, CA	June Aug 20XX – 20XX	Certificate

WORK EXPERIENCE – Give present position (or last position held first).

JOB TITLE:	EMPLOYER	ADDRESS	DATES
Part-Time Teacher's Aide	Valley College	421 Dylan Street Woodland Hills, CA	6/XX to 9/XX
DUTIES PERFORMED: Typing, filing, duplicating, Educational materials			

JOB TITLE:	EMPLOYER	ADDRESS	DATES
Part-Time Receptionist and File Clerk	Ames Medical Laboratory	311 Main Street Newbury Park, CA	6/XX to 9/XX
DUTIES PERFORMED: Telephone, filing			

JOB TITLE:	EMPLOYER	ADDRESS	DATES
DUTIES PERFORMED:			

REFERENCES – List three persons (other than relatives) who have known you for at least 2 years

NAME/TITLE	ADDRESS	TELEPHONE NUMBER
Upon Request		

APPLICANT'S SIGNATURE ___*Sarasue T. Grant*___   1-28-XX

Date

Figure 19-3. Example of an employment application form

The application must be neat, accurate, and professional looking. It is important to review the entire form, read and follow all directions, and study each question carefully before answering. The object of a particular question may be to see if the applicant can follow instructions (e.g., print in black ink). Use your best handwriting and stay within the designated area, if possible. Other objectives of the application are to assess handwriting legibility and spelling and evaluate educational requirements, salary expectations, and work experience.

The applicant should furnish as much information as possible, but if an item does not apply or cannot be answered he or she should indicate that the question has not been overlooked by inserting "no," "none," "NA" (not applicable), or "DNA" (does not apply). If the prospective employee's history includes sensitive background information, write "request personal conference," instead of leaving it blank or writing something that misrepresents the truth.

If a visit has been made to an office to pick up an application, the assistant should look for the opportunity to suggest an immediate interview or request a later appointment. An interview is the ultimate goal in the job-seeking process and should be welcomed by the applicant regardless of the time or convenience.

LETTER OF INTRODUCTION

The purpose of a *letter of introduction,* or **cover letter** if a resumé is attached, is to acquaint the prospective physician-employer with you to match your education, experience, or personality traits to the position, and to attract attention to outstanding features so an interview appointment can be subsequently made. The letter of introduction should respond to the ad, be brief and eye-catching, and state in a few, well-chosen words how the applicant learned about the position and how specific assets will qualify the applicant for the job (Figure 19-4). Be sure to include information regarding your certification and/or degrees. Type the letter using a standard, business-letter format and address it to a specific person if possible, not just to the personnel office of a company. Check to make sure the name is properly spelled. If an advertisement provides a post office box number, fax, or telephone number for providing an application, the job seeker should inquire and ask for the name of the personnel supervisor or person most likely to be doing the interviewing so the cover letter can include that person's name. When the name is unknown, the salutation might be "Dear Doctor," "Dear Office Manager," or "Dear Members of the Personnel Committee."

The concluding sentence paves the way for an interview appointment by calling attention to a telephone number or specifying plans to contact the office on a certain date. Since this letter is a preview of the applicant's writing composition skills, it should be free of typographical errors and errors in spelling, punctuation, and grammar; ask one or two persons with excellent English skills to proofread it.

Another type of letter of introduction is a *letter of inquiry.* This is written to inquire about the possibility of a job that has not been advertised. It follows the same guidelines; however, it is written in more general terms to cover many potential job possibilities.

RESUMÉ

The purpose of a **resumé** is to sell job qualifications and to present an in-depth evaluation of those qualifications in a creative, brief, and attractive format so an interview may be obtained. It summarizes the applicant's education, work experience, and vocational skills with emphasis on administrative accomplishments related to the medical field. Do not forget to include school and outside activities as they relate to the job you are seeking. Most people do not see a relationship between the two; however, employers are looking for leadership skills, a strong work ethic, and a sense of responsibility, and involvement, which may be demonstrated by committee attendance, volunteer work, or extracurricular projects. The importance of the resumé as a marketing tool cannot be overstated.

A one- or two-page resumé typed on high-grade 25 pound, wrinkle-free bond paper—white or light color—is appropriate. Similar stationery should be chosen for the resumé, cover letter, and envelope. It should contain as many action words as possible and avoid the personal pronoun (I). If it is impossible to confine the resumé to one page, it can be keyed using a smaller font. Brevity is important, as long as all relevant information is included. Data should be single spaced with double spacing between unrelated items, with balanced spacing on all four margins employing basic principles of graphic design. For example, headings might be keyed using extra large (14 point) or script-style elements. Four **formats** used in the preparation of resumés are *chronological, functional, combination,* and *results-oriented.*

No matter which format is chosen, personal data, such as the applicant's name, address, and telephone number, are outlined briefly in a few lines at the

4721 West Fifth Street
Kearney, NE 68845
June 1, 199x

October 29, 20XX

Robert M. Whitewall, MD
Underhill Clinic
90 East Manhattan Avenue
Lexington, NE 68850

Personalized to the recipient ———→ Dear Dr. Whitewall:

Targets the position and briefly cites credentials using the same key words as in the employment ad; highlights medical background ———→ The position of administrative medical assistant described in your advertisement in the Saturday <u>New Press</u> is an ideal match to my educational background and career objectives.

I know I can be an asset to your office as a Certified Medical Assistant (CMA), having gained practical experience working part-time in several medical facilities these past three years while completing my education.

Polite and positive closing ———→ I would welcome the opportunity to meet with you to further explore your needs and to answer specific questions regarding my qualifications. I can be reached after 3 p.m. daily at 320-1132. I look forward to hearing from you.

Sincerely,

Margaret McGuire

Margaret McGuire, CMA

Notation indicating resumé enclosed if requested; otherwise hand-carry resumé to the interview ———→ Encl.: Resumé

Figure 19-4. Example of a letter of introduction or a cover letter

beginning of the resumé sheet. The Civil Rights Act of 1964, enforced by the Equal Employment Opportunity Commission, states that information concerning height, weight, birthdate, marital status, Social Security number, and physical condition may be excluded, but, sometimes, listing these can enhance getting a job.

When telephoning a prospective employer, inquire if they prefer the resumé e-mailed, faxed, or mailed. In a competitive employment atmosphere where time is important, it is wise to use every advantage possible.

Chronological Resumé

The **chronological resumé** (Figure 19-5) is the most widely accepted and familiar to employers. It provides them with an interview script and is the easiest for

Margarita Gonzales
22 East Eighth Street
New York, NY 10029
Telephone and Fax: 555/298-0840
E-mail: mgonzales@aol.com

WORK EXPERIENCE

19XX–20XX Receptionist: Harbor Medical Center, Ventura, CA (160 Externship Hours) Received patients, physicians, pharmaceutical representatives, and other visitors; answered telephone and directed calls to appropriate person; made appointments; kept reception room tidy

19XX–19XX Part-time file clerk: Woodland Hills Urgent Care Center, Oxnard, CA Transcribed and filed letters and reports

EDUCATION

20XX–20XX Ames College, Oxnard, CA Medical Assisting Diploma Program—Graduate

19XX–20XX Culver City High School Culver City, CA—Graduate

ACTIVITIES Vice President of Secretarial Science Club of Ames College
Treasurer of the Culver City High School Senior Class

SKILLS Professional telephone skills
Computer literate in Word and Medical Manager programs
Accurate computer filing skills
Posting of payments and charges
Bilingual (Spanish)

REFERENCES Available upon request

Figure 19-5. Chronological resumé, emphasizing work experience

the applicant to prepare. Specific dates and employers are listed in chronological order with the most current first. Either work experience or education may be presented first, depending on the area of background to be emphasized. The chronological format stresses a steady employment record, but lack of experience is starkly revealed and skills are not highlighted. To counteract these weaknesses, the applicant can enclose photocopies of certificates in specific areas, such as word processing, transcription, and medical insurance billing.

Functional Resumé

The **functional resumé** also called the *skill focused* or *skill based* resumé (Figure 19-6) is usually the choice of the applicant just finishing high school, trade or vocational school, or college with a spotty employment record. It highlights qualifications and marketable skills but does not list specific job titles or descriptions with dates. Prospective employers can easily access skills and ascertain whether the applicant is qualified for a position.

Norm Mancewicz

1499 West Grand Avenue, Peoria, IL 61600-0001
Telephone: (555) 425-7880 Fax: (555) 920-4661
E-Mail: Norm-mancewicz@sbcglobal.net

CAREER OBJECTIVE

To find a position as an office manager of a medical facility in which I may utilize the following personal attributes and skills.

QUALIFICATIONS/SKILLS

- Nationally Certified Insurance Coding Specialist (NCICS) by the National Center for Competency Testing (20XX)
- Practice management and supervisory experience
- Knowledgeable with HIPAA compliance and CCI edits
- Experience with contract negotiations (managed care and fee-for-service)
- Accounts reconciliation, analysis, and collection experience
- Accounts payable responsibilities
- Payroll distribution
- Computer literate in Medical Manager, MediSoft, MediTech, and accounting programs

WORK EXPERIENCE

- James and Hopper, Inc. A Medical Corporation
  1555 Telegraph Road, Peoria, IL 61600
- Alan Avers, MD, FCCP and Hal Oppen, MD, FCCP
  1313 Montrose Place, Peoria, IL 61600
- John Mueller, CPA
  1900 Bell Air Avenue, Peoria, IL 61600

EDUCATION

- Valley Harmon Career Institute—Graduate: Administrative Medical Assisting
- Glendora Community College—4.0 GPA
  Accounting courses
  Medical terminology
  Anatomy and Physiology
  Medical Insurance Billing and Coding

REFERENCES AVAILABLE UPON REQUEST

Figure 19-6. Functional (skill-based) resumé, highlighting marketable skills

Combination Resumé

The **combination resumé** (Figure 19-7) emphasizes the applicant's work skills and lists employers and dates of employment. The format shows at a glance an applicant's entire work and education background, stressing most relevant medical skills and work experience while minimizing less significant experience. A major weakness is that it tends to become too lengthy.

Results-Oriented Resumé

A **results-oriented resumé** focuses on results, not characteristics. This type of resumé helps prospective employers reduce the risks that are associated with hiring because it shows what the job seeker has accomplished as well as his or her attitude toward work. Cite examples by describing your accomplishments and how you helped previous employers improve their profitability, service to patients, recognition, and vis-

SARASUE T. GRANT
21185 West Amber Street
Encino, CA 91316-0002

Telephone: 555/211-8773
Fax: 555/455-8799
E-mail: Sarasuegrant@hotmail.com

Career Objective	To secure a position as an Administrative Medical Assistant
Attributes	Effective communication skills Self-motivated, enthusiastic, honest, and responsible

Skills	• Keying: 60 wpm on computer
	• Filing: Certificates, alphabetic and numeric
	• Computer: Basic computer operations and trouble-shooting
	     Computer applications in business: Microsoft Word 2000
	     Medical Software: MediSoft 11, accounting and office
	     hours
	• Administrative Skills:
	     Organized and directed meeting of Future Business Leaders
	     of America.
	     Coordinated and set up a volunteer program of Candystripers
	     for College Hospital, Woodland Hills, CA

Education	

20XX-20XX	Graduate of Valley College, Woodland Hills, CA;
	     A.S. Degree with a Certificate of Achievement in
	     Medical Assisting

19XX-20XX	Graduate of L.B. Johnson High School, Newbury Park, CA
	     Named Outstanding Business Student of
	     Senior Class

Medical Assisting Courses	• Bookkeeping • Computer Technology and Word Processing • Filing • Medical Insurance Billing • Medical Office Procedures • Medical Terminology • Medical Transcription • Procedure and Diagnostic Coding
Work Experience	

20XX Summer	• Part-time teacher's aide: Chemistry Department
	  Valley College, Woodland Hills, CA
	  Typing, filing, and duplicating educational materials

20XX Summer	• Part-time receptionist and file clerk: Ames
	  Medical Laboratory, Newbury Park, CA
	  Telephone, filing, receptionist desk

References	Attached

Figure 19-7. Combination resumé, stressing education and skills

ibility. This provides short scenarios indicating how your abilities have been tested and focuses on the needs of the employer rather than your own needs.

Electronic Resumé

Electronic resumés are received faster and processed quicker. They allow the employer to search a database of resumés for key terms and screen potential candidates. They are easy to sort and track and may be passed on electronically. If a resumé is e-mailed, be sure to follow up with a hard copy of the cover letter and resumé. Hard copies offer a more striking format and can be handed out to physicians after being reviewed by the office manager.

Once a medical position has been discovered and an electronic resumé is requested, some basic steps are:

STEP 1 2 3

PROCEDURE 19-3

Prepare a Resumé

Objective: To prepare a resumé listing education, experience, and job skills that will create enough interest in a prospective employer to arrange an interview for employment.

Equipment/Supplies: Summary of education, work experience, and job skills; 8 ½-inch × 11-inch white bond paper; number 10 envelope; computer or typewriter; and pen.

Directions: Follow these step-by-step procedures, which include rationales, to learn this skill, which is presented in the *Workbook* (Job Skill 19-3) for practice.

1. Write down a list of all activities, awards, accomplishments, and experiences on a separate page.

2. Collect your mock application form, which includes your work history and educational background.

3. Gather a list of all the job skills you have learned (refer to the front portion of this textbook).

4. Determine the style of resumé and key or type, never handwrite, data. Format the resumé and use visual "hooks" to grab the eye of the reader, such as boldface fonts, bullets, or indents.

5. Insert a heading that includes contact information: name, address, telephone number, fax number, and e-mail address; this allows the reader to quickly respond if interested.

6. Insert a brief statement of employment goals and career goals for the next 5 or 10 years. Be brief; the purpose of a resumé is to get an interview, not to detail all your hopes and dreams.

7. Assemble education data and arrange in reverse chronologic order. List the most recent schooling first.

8. Indicate the highest education degree or diploma with the name of the college or high school and year of graduation because formal training may be desired for the position.

Provide titles of courses, related conferences or workshops, and list details, such as transcription and typing speeds, computer skills and software applications, coding skills, and expertise in insurance claims completion. List special certificates and scholarship awards as well as the grade average if it was good.

9. Assemble work experience dates and arrange in reverse chronologic order.

10. State previous work experience briefly, listing information that may be valuable to the present job opening. Work experience should include the name and address of the firm or employer, job title, length of time worked, and a brief description of duties or responsibilities. Student externships may also be included. (Previous employers may be contacted about exact employment dates by mailing a stamped, self-addressed envelope with a brief letter including spaces for them to fill in starting and termination dates, position held, and salary.)

11. List job skills obtained both through education and experience.

12. Detail previous job titles and duties if not self-explanatory. Emphasize positive points using action verbs; avoid mention of weaknesses.

13. List professional licenses or certifications, and mention awards, special interests, and activities that relate to the medical profession. This indicates interest in the profession. List them either alphabetically or by order of importance.

14. List volunteer activities and memberships in professional organizations, especially if they are related to the medical field, and if leadership responsibilities were contributed.

15. Indicate that references (with addresses and telephone numbers) are available upon request, or state that they are attached. Prospective employers usually verify the employment history of job applicants; this procedure

(continues)

PROCEDURE 19-3 *continued*

ensures that the records agree. Before an interview, always obtain permission from friends and former employers before listing them as references. This courtesy allows the reference person time to prepare a response before receiving an unexpected telephone call or communication.

16. Avoid mentioning an hourly rate or salary requirement.

17. Proofread the resumé for accuracy of spelling, completeness of content, attractive format, typographical errors, and punctuation; make all corrections and necessary adjustments.

18. Print the resumé on high-quality paper and enlist another set of eyes to proofread it again.

19. Make a copy for your files.

20. Compose a cover letter with an enclosure notation (see Figure 19-4).

21. Key a number 10 envelope with an attention line stating the person's name in charge of hiring; list your return name and address.

22. Use every avenue available to get the resumé into the hands of your target market and the person who does the hiring.

- Compose a computerized resumé and verify spelling with the spell-check feature and then save in a job search file.

- Discard traditional resumé-writing techniques, such as focusing on action verbs. Instead think descriptive nouns, such as medical assistant, education, experience, skills, knowledge, and abilities.

- Avoid decorative graphics and complex typefaces, underlining, or italics.

- Forget the one-page rule; electronic resumés may be three to four pages.

- Use the "copy and paste" feature of the word processing software and copy information from the Word document; then either paste it into an e-mail message or "attach a file" to the message, which may serve as a cover letter.

- It is not necessary to post a letter of introduction when posting a resumé to either an online job-seeking service or a bulletin board.

- To post a resumé online, upload the resumé using a file-transfer feature of the software, following the computer manual directions.

If the file is sent across the Internet, not all browsers and software programs interpret characters and formatting the same way. A format that you print may end up being received as a jumbled mess with odd characters, poor line breaks, and misaligned spacing. In addition, depending on the server it may need to be doctored up in a technical form-encoded by the sender and decoded by the receiver. There are two basic options for electronic resumés: an ASCII version or an HTML version. ASCII stands for American Standard Code for Information Interchange and relates to standard computer characters that do not vary from program to program. HTML stands for hypertext markup language and relates to formatting for the World Wide Web. Generally, an ASCII file may be easily accessible and quickly downloaded by most employers via the Internet.

Scannable Resumé

A *scannable resumé* is a hard-copy document designed to be scanned by an optical character reader (OCR) and put into a computerized database. Then it is screened via computer software for keywords that are in a description posted for a job opening. The resumé that contains more keywords than others will be picked for further evaluation for a personal interview. Thus, it is important to incorporate as many keywords from the medical job described as well as acronyms and abbreviations with spelled-out forms because the software may have been programmed to search for these. Use synonyms to avoid repeating the same keywords.

References

References are usually not included with a resumé but instead the statement "References upon request" is listed as the last line. The list may be attached if the resumé is short. When determining who you will

PROCEDURE 19-4

Prepare a Resumé in ASCII Text

Objective: To prepare a resumé in ASCII text to include education, experience, and job skills that can be posted on the Internet to interest a prospective employer.

Equipment/Supplies: Summary of education, work experience, and job skills and a computer with Internet connection.

Directions: Follow these step-by-step procedures, which include rationales, to learn this skill.

1. Use 10-point Courier font for the entire resumé.

2. Create the message using Word software (or WordPerfect).

3. Set the right margin to 5 inches or less (lines no more than 65 characters in length). Longer lines may break incorrectly on the receiver's screen. Put a space at the beginning of each blank line between paragraphs.

4. Do not justify text; align from the left.

5. Use spaces in place of tabs.

6. Avoid columns.

7. For emphasis, use capital letters for headings and place above paragraphs. Use more white space; do not center text.

8. Avoid italics, bold, and underlined text.

9. Use standard ASCII characters (A–Z in upper- and lowercase, 0–9, and only the following punctuations: ! " # $ & ' () * + , - . / : ; ? _ ` ~).

10. Change long "em" dashes (—) to two hyphens (--) and smart quotes (" ") to straight quotes (" ").

11. Adjust the spacing and characters until they look good; proofread the resumé.

12. Save the files as plain ASCII text (text only with line breaks).

13. To upload the ASCII text to a bulletin board, log onto the board and go to the message Menu following the bulletin board's directions.

14. Select or type "All" or "Resumé posting" from the bulletin board's message Menu for the recipient and subject.

15. Upload the resumé following the software manual's directions for the communications program being used.

16. Depending on the bulletin board, a "Message Edit" menu or the next available line will appear issuing message-editing commands. Customize the resumé by typing in additional information related to the specific job.

---

include as references, make a list of people who know you well, can vouch for your character, and who will speak truthfully. Candidates may be long-time friends who would be able to indicate your ongoing mood, stability, and personality characteristics; former employers (especially supervisors), who could speak favorably about your work ethic, team interaction, organization skills, and job responsibilities; or professionals in prestigious positions who know you well, for example, an attorney, physician, clergy, or administrator. If you do not have a work history, sometimes an instructor is willing to be a reference.

Carefully select the most favorable three to five prospective references and ask each if he or she is willing to speak on your behalf. Explain to your references which skills and experiences you would like them to emphasize and find out exactly what they will say about you. Provide your references with a copy of your cover letter and resume and notify them of all upcoming interviews. Key or type the reference list on the same type of paper used for your resume and take it with you while job hunting. Do not include a date on the reference list but make sure you update it frequently.

Most employers will check references, and a positive reference can be a powerful tool in the decision-making process. When employers call people listed as a reference, they usually ask questions such as: How long you have known the person? What qualities do you like about the applicant? Tell me one strength and one weakness. When calling former employers, questions center around attendance, quantity and quality

PROCEDURE 19-5

Prepare and Format a Scannable Resumé

Objective: To prepare a scannable resumé to include education, experience, and job skills that can be either sent to prospective employers or downloaded from the Internet and scanned by interested prospective employers.

Equipment/Supplies: Summary of education, work experience, and job skills, and a computer.

Directions: Follow these step-by-step procedures, which include rationales, to learn the skill of formatting a scannable resumé.

1. Do not use boldface, italics, underlining, script, bullets, logos, shading, horizontal or vertical lines, or any other graphic devices. Asterisks may be used for emphasis.

2. Do not use columns.

3. Begin at the left margin and do not justify the right margin.

4. Use a laser printer, black ink, and good-quality paper of 20- or 24-pound weight.

5. Limit the resumé to one page. If more than one page, use a paper clip (not a staple) to keep the pages together and use a continuation heading on the second page (name and page number).

6. Center the heading, providing important information so the employer can contact you.

7. List sections with headings, such as Objective, Skills (e.g., administrative, computer), Employment History, Education, and Continuing Education.

8. Include single-spaced data that have as many keywords and synonyms for the key words as possible.

9. Do not fold or crease the resumé; mail it in a large envelope.

---

of work, strengths, and areas of improvement. A common question is: Would the job candidate be eligible for rehire?

THE JOB INTERVIEW

According to the Bureau of National Affairs, the interview is so important in the job search that it most likely will determine whether an applicant will be offered employment. Research studies show that when two applicants have similar skills and education, the decision on which candidate will be hired is based almost entirely on physical appearance at the interview. You will not get a second chance to make a good first impression; and a judgment may be made within the first minute of the interview.

The importance of good grooming in projecting a favorable first impression cannot be overemphasized because prospective employers expect applicants to dress to impress. If the applicant is a woman, a clean tailored suit or dress is usually preferable to wearing pants. Low-heeled pumps, neutral shaded hose, and small handbag are appropriate. A man should wear a clean, dark-toned suit or sport coat, conservative necktie, white shirt, plain slacks, and well-shined shoes.

Men should avoid excessive facial hair, long hair, earrings, and heavy aftershave lotion. Women should style their hair in a conservative and becoming manner and wear jewelry sparingly. They should avoid heavy makeup, lowcut necklines, sleeveless dresses, strong perfume, and dark or bright nail polish. Since looks speak louder than words and reveal inner feelings of personal pride, the applicant who looks his or her best can be more confident and relaxed at the interview (Figure 19-8).

In a survey of job placements across the United States, it was determined that the last person interviewed for a position is more likely to be hired than the first; therefore, choosing the right time for an interview is important. Early morning interviews are discouraged as are late Monday and Friday afternoons between 4:00 p.m. and 5:00 p.m. because Monday is usually a catch-up day that is heavily scheduled and Friday is getaway day.

Portfolio

A **portfolio** displaying pertinent information relevant to job skills and tasks of a medical assistant is becoming the accepted way to demonstrate accomplishments to the prospective employer. Its purpose is

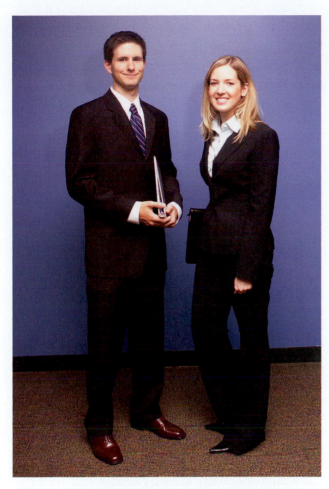

Figure 19-8. Female and male job applicants, emphasizing good grooming and proper attire, preparing for an interview for a medical assisting position

to provide documentation to support information provided in the resume.

An attractive loose-leaf notebook with plastic page covers and typed divider labels corresponding with a table of contents will organize the portfolio for presentation. Items that might be included are:

- Autobiography stressing career goals
- Chronological record with expanded information in addition to that on the resume
- Documentation of skills learned, including an official copy of college transcript(s), workshop certificates, short courses completed, and grade point average if good
- Letters of recommendation from several previous employers, instructors, and medical office or hospital contacts, naming positive characteristics and explaining special skills utilized. These letters should be constantly updated.

- Volunteer and community service exhibits, including newspaper clippings related to leadership positions, special awards and commendations from community organizations, and letters from co-volunteers verifying service.
- Samples of error-free work with instructor's remarks left in, or carefully removed and an explanation of procedures used to prepare each document. Items to include might be a 5-minute timed keyboarding sample certified by the instructor, a completed insurance claim with evidence of coding skills, a completed patient record, a page with posted transactions from a daily journal or ledger, a keyed letter displaying writing ability, a completed appointment page, transcription material with speeds attained, word processing documents, and filing certificates earned.
- Special accomplishments would include magazines and books read that pertain to medical career goals, any evidence of talents or creativity, and a list of outside interests and hobbies.
- Copy of Social Security card
- Extra copies of resume

If you are certified, a copy of the following placed in your portfolio would be helpful to verify your credentials, show the areas you studied, and indicate the multiple skills you have acquired and been tested on:

- CMA—Copy of AAMA membership card, *AAMA Role Delineation Study: Occupational Analysis of the Medical Assistant and AAMA (CMA) Certification Examination Content*
- RMA—Copy of AMT membership card, *Registered Medical Assistant Certification Examination Competencies and Construction Parameters*
- CMAS—Copy of AMT membership card, *American Medical Technologists Certified Medical Administrative Specialist Competencies and Examination Specifications*

Alien Applicants

A job applicant born outside of the United States must show one of the following: a naturalization certificate (citizenship papers), an alien registration receipt card, a temporary resident receipt card, or an employment authorization card. One or more of these items can be in the portfolio available if requested by the prospective employer at the interview.

The employer must have on file for any alien employee a completed Employment Eligibility Verification Form I-9, and it must be kept for at least one year after the person leaves. The Employment Eligibility Verification Form I-9 can be obtained by writing the Immigration and Naturalization Service (INS) at 425 I Street, NW, Washington, DC 20536, within three days of hiring an applicant born outside the United States.

Preparing for an Interview

A number of job seekers go into an interview knowing almost nothing about the medical practice he or she is hoping to be hired by. Researching all prospective employers will first benefit you when deciding where you would like to work and then will be essential if you are asked the question, "What do you know about us?"

Find out as much as possible about the position and the doctor before the interview, particularly if the physician is a specialist. Refer to Chapter 2, Table 2-3 for a listing of medical specialties with descriptions of each. The physician who is certified in a medical specialty must fulfill educational and internship requirements and pass an examination beyond the standard medical degree. When the physician has been certified in a field of *specialization,* he or she is known as a **diplomate**.

Chapter 2, Table 2-4, contains a list of abbreviations for various professional positions in the field of medicine. The applicant for a job of administrative medical assistant should be familiar with these abbreviations, because he or she will use them repeatedly when employed in a medical facility.

The interview appointment may be the only time the office manager or physician will have to make a firsthand evaluation of the applicant's maturity, manners, personality, and verbal skills and to acquire information that does not appear on the resumé. The applicant must therefore take steps to prepare appropriate responses to project the best possible image. Applicants should write down three or four specific items that qualify them for the position so they will be better prepared to relay the information at the interview. Being knowledgeable about the physician's expectations makes it easier to relax and to respond more intelligently to questions. In conversation during the interview, do not be afraid to use words or phrases such as self-starter, ambitious, energetic, hard worker when speaking of yourself, if they are true.

Interview Guidelines

The interview will consist of several stages; the first stage is greeting the interviewer. The second stage, referred to as the warming up period, consists of a few brief moments where the interviewer tries to establish rapport. Be yourself and make a friendly comment to help establish this common ground so the interview conversation will flow smoothly. Next is the fact-finding stage. This is when the employer wants to learn more about you, but it is also a time for you to learn more about the employer. Try to establish the employer's needs so you can explain how you can meet them. Then ask questions, as appropriate. As the interview comes to an end, a summing up period is the final stage, where you will reiterate how you believe things will proceed from this point. At the conclusion, be sure to verbalize whether you are interested in the job and tell the interviewer why you will be a good employee and how you can do an excellent job. Following are some suggestions for the applicant to follow:

1. Arrive alone and promptly for the interview appointment and greet the interviewer by name; let the interviewer initiate a handshake and wait to be seated until the interviewer sits down or directs you to be seated.

2. Listen attentively to each question and ask for clarification if the question can be interpreted in more than one way.

3. Let the interviewer do much of the talking—50 percent of the time should be spent listening.

4. Do not answer questions about your personal life unless the answer will demonstrate an ability to perform the job.

5. Be prepared for the question, "Tell me about yourself."

6. Be discreet in referring to former employers and avoid negative comments.

7. Make responses short, but avoid one-word answers.

8. Demonstrate interest in the position by asking questions about job specifications, continuing education policies, medical benefits, and to whom you will be responsible.

9. Be prepared to reply to a question about salary expectations, having determined average salary levels by reading newspaper advertisements and by talking to people employed in medical offices.

Use the term "negotiable" or "flexible" if you do not want to be specific. In negotiating a salary you may decide to accept a salary that is lower than you want with the understanding that a review of your work and a subsequent increase in pay is forthcoming within a three- to six-month period.

10. Body language such as leaning forward in a chair, nodding in agreement, smiling, and making eye contact are proven methods of showing interest.

11. Be prepared to accept flexible working hours that are utilized by many offices with multiple physicians and increased work schedules.

12. Think before giving an answer; then answer slowly but confidently.

13. If unable to respond to a question, be honest and say, "I'm not able to answer your question." Occasionally, interviewers ask questions they know cannot be answered.

Interview Questions

The Americans with Disabilities Act (ADA) was passed in 1990 to protect disabled workers from discrimination. As long as the disability can be accommodated without "undue hardship" on the employer, the ADA prohibits the employer from denying employment based on the disability.

The job applicant would be wise to prepare responses to the following typical questions a physician or personnel supervisor might ask at a job interview. The focus of most questions will be the job seeker's attitude toward work and people, and matching the personality of the job seeker with the nature of the job. Following are typical questions asked during an interview:

1. Why did you decide on a career as a medical assistant?

2. What courses in school did you take that were related to the medical field and which subject did you enjoy most?

3. What experience have you had that relates to the job applied for?

4. Have you ever done any volunteer work for a medical agency or hospital?

5. Why did you leave your previous job(s)?

6. What do you think your past employers and teachers would say about you?

7. What two or three accomplishments in your life have given you the greatest satisfaction?

8. What do you consider to be your strengths and weaknesses?

9. What rewards do you expect from your career as a medical assistant?

10. Are you able to take the initiative in doing work, or do you need supervision? (List examples.)

11. What types of community and professional activities do you participate in?

12. Which of your past jobs did you like best and least?

13. Would you be interested in and able to attend workshops or seminars to update your medical knowledge and skills?

14. What are your salary expectations?

15. Will you be able to work overtime?

16. Are you sympathetic to people who are ill? If so, how do you demonstrate your sympathy?

17. Can you be trusted to keep a confidence?

18. Are you aware of the legal implications involved in a medical practice? Name some.

19. How would you describe your personality?

20. Do you have any plans to continue your education? What are they?

21. Describe the type of medical position you would most like to have.

22. Why do you want to work for us?

23. Have you ever had to handle an emergency situation? If so, how well did you adapt?

24. Do you like working alone or with people?

25. Do changes and interruptions upset you?

26. What do you read?

27. If you get this position, how will you want me to assist you in your work?

28. How do you work under pressure? Give examples.

29. Describe a crisis you had to deal with and tell me how you coped with it.

30. In your opinion, what are the most important current trends in the health care industry?

31. In your lifetime, what is your greatest failure?

32. What publications would you recommend to remain well informed about the health care industry?

33. What are your pet peeves?

34. Would you rather be part of a team or in charge of a project?

35. What do you expect to be doing in your work life five years from now?

The interviewer may ask hypothetical questions, such as:

- What would you do if a supervisor told you to do something now and another supervisor told you it could wait until later?

- What would you do if someone walked into the office, came straight up to the reception desk, and started yelling at you about their bill?

- What would your response be if a coworker told you that they borrowed $25 from the cash drawer but put it back today, so all is well?

Such questions make the interviewee think quickly and give the interviewer a good idea of the applicant's problem solving skills. Take the opportunity to further demonstrate these skills by indicating to the employer what you can do for them. For example:

- I believe I can save the physician money—because I have excellent collection skills.

- I would like to try to improve the patients' perception of the medical practice—with my friendly and concerned attitude.

- I can reduce your turnover rate—because I am reliable and have a strong work ethic.

- I can make the business operations run smoothly—because I am well trained.

Remember that each person is unique and brings special qualities to a job. Focus on what you can bring to the job that you are interviewing for that would differentiate you from a classmate or another applicant with the same training.

Concluding the interview successfully is almost as important as getting it off to a good start. To indicate the end of the interview, the office manager or physician will probably stand, which is the applicant's cue to stand and prepare to leave, letting the interviewer take the lead in shaking hands at the conclusion of the interview (Figure 19-9). The applicant should ask when he or she might expect to hear if the job is to

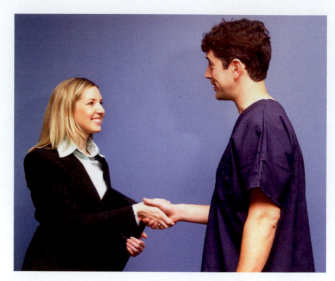

Figure 19-9. MA facing and shaking hands with a job applicant

be offered, then leave with a "thank you" to both the interviewer and the receptionist.

Illegal Questions

Some questions may be asked by the interviewer that legally do not have to be answered unless the information is job related; relevance to the job is the criterion. Jobs are to be offered on the basis of qualifications; therefore, discriminatory questions about an applicant's personal life cannot be asked by a prospective employer.

Personal questions that cannot be asked are:

1. Age, height, weight (However, questions regarding age would be legal if a law regulating a procedure included an age limit.)

2. Birthdate

3. Birthplace

4. Club or organization memberships

5. Credit rating

6. Gender/sex

7. Ethnic background

8. Explanation of employment gaps to determine why time was taken off

9. Physical or emotional defects (But an interviewer can ask whether an applicant has any job-related defects if there is any reason the applicant cannot perform any procedures listed in the job description.)

10. Home and/or automobile ownership

11. Maiden name

12. Marital status

13. Native language

14. Number of dependent children

15. Pregnancy and family planning

16. Provision for child care

17. Religious preference

18. Employment and earnings of spouse

To diffuse discriminatory questions, try to reassure the employer of your competence as a medical assistant. Highlight your qualifications and emphasize your job history. Following are three suggestions for handling the situation if the interviewer asks one or more illegal questions: (1) answer the question and ignore the fact that you know it is illegal; (2) answer with the statement "I think the question is not relevant to the requirements of the medical position"; "I'm not sure what this has to do with my ability to do the job"; and (3) refuse to answer and consider contacting the nearest Equal Employment Opportunity Commission office. This last action probably should be avoided unless the violation is demeaning and you can prove it resulted in your not getting the position. Some employers are not familiar with the code requirements regarding interviews. The second answer is probably the best answer. It may cost you the job but you may not be interested in working in an office with people who are that concerned about your personal life.

Career Fair Interviews

If you are able to visit a job fair that has medical employers you will have direct access to the representatives that do the hiring. Be prepared with an application and resumé in hand and research which clinics, hospitals, and medical groups will be there so you are familiar with their general background information. Look sharp and use the time wisely to sell your accomplishments so that you make a good impression and they will remember your smile and positive attitude.

After the Interview

If a job offer is not initiated at an interview and you have not been contacted within a day or two or around the time you were told to expect a call, it is time to write a follow-up note of thanks (Figure 19-10) or place a call to express continued interest in the position. The object of the thank-you letter is to briefly restate the applicant's assets, add additional information not given at the interview, emphasize any strong feelings he or she may have about obtaining the position, and reiterate the time he or she may be reached by telephone. A follow-up letter generally works to the candidate's advantage by keeping the applicant's name before the potential employer. Even if the position is not offered, the applicant will learn from each interview until able to secure the right job.

Once a position is secured, it is well for the applicant to remember that no matter at what level hired, he or she is still a beginner in that office with much to learn. It is a good idea to ask permission to borrow the office procedure manual to review office routines. Arriving for work the first day with a notebook to take notes for future reference saves the subsequent embarrassment of having to ask how to perform tasks after they have been explained. Taking notes also reinforces office procedures and demonstrates a desire to do the best job possible.

PREPARING FOR A PERFORMANCE EVALUATION

Usually the physician, with the office manager, will review the performance of a new employee after a 90-day probationary period—this has been discussed with the employee before employment and is outlined in the employee handbook (see Chapter 17 for comprehensive information on this topic). This period allows the staff to get to know the new assistant and to observe work habits and behavior. The **performance evaluation** based on an accurately written position description in checklist format used to evaluate job performance, attendance and punctuality, quality and quantity of work, ability to work as a team member as well as the assistant's attitude toward coworkers and patients, technical knowledge, written and oral expression, and appearance. A performance evaluation form is an important communications tool because it indicates not only weaknesses in job performance but also acknowledges work well done (Figure 19-11). For situations where work is unsatisfactory, it may be used to terminate employment.

An office manager and one supervisor or physician separately determine strengths and weaknesses and each make check marks on the form to indicate

234 Marshall Way, Apt. No. 6
San Francisco, CA 94942

July 2, 20XX

Sheehan Hospital
Health Information Management Department
124 North Bay Harbor Way
San Francisco, CA 94966

Attention: Mildred Spencer, RN

Dear Mrs. Spencer:

Thank you for granting me an interview last Friday,
June 28, when I applied for the position of medical
records clerk.

I enjoyed talking to you and learning about the filing
system utilized by the health information management
department and I am very much interested in obtaining
the position. I know I can perform the work to your
satisfaction and am interested in working for such a
prestigious hospital.

If you need additional information to assist you in making
a decision regarding my qualifications for the position,
I can be contacted at (555)725-0991 before 8 a.m. and after
4:30 p.m. on weekdays. I appreciate you considering me for
this position.

Sincerely,

Roberta Trask
Roberta Trask

Figure 19-10. Thank-you letter written to follow-up after an interview

one of five levels of appraisal. This assessment is based on experience with the employee after 90 days of employment compared to other employees with similar duties. Careful and sound judgment in rating the employee must be used and each item should be discussed with the employee. Evaluations are done to develop improved performance in areas of weakness and to determine job satisfaction and job security.

When the medical assistant has been hired on a permanent basis, the file should include the application for employment, government forms (e.g., W-4), a record of wage and salary information, bonuses given, attendance record, and a signed resignation form if employment is terminated. Several states have enacted laws enabling employees to inspect their personnel files once a year on written request.

Negotiating Pay and Asking for a Raise

Whether you are trying to negotiate pay at a job interview or are asking for a raise, tact and timing are critical. Research the current market to find out what the pay is for related positions by looking at classified ads, calling employment agencies, contacting professional friends, and reviewing out online salary surveys. Make sure your physician is experiencing revenue growth and not a downturn of income caused by managed care restraints or decreased Medicare payments. Securing an agreement ahead of time indicating what is required to receive a raise will ensure a positive outcome. Schedule an appointment and give your supervisor reasons why you deserve a raise.

PERFORMANCE EVALUATION

Name of employee   Position

Period of employment form: To:

	Outstanding	Exceeds Expectations	Meets Expectations	Needs Improvement	Unsatisfactory
1. Attendance/ Punctuality					
Comments:					
2. Quantity of Work/ Production					
Comments:					
3. Quality of Work/ Accuracy					
Comments:					
4. Cooperation/ Teamwork					
Comments:					
5. Attitude					
Comments:					
6. Technical Knowledge					
Comments:					
7. Communication					
Comments:					
8. Grooming					
Comments:					

_____ After completing this form and discussing the evaluation with the employee, the 90-day assessment period is satisfactory.

_____ Since several areas require additional supervision and development, there is an extension of the assessment period for _____ additional days.

_____ The employee has not met the job requirements. It is in the best interest of this employee as well as the medical practice to give the employee the option to look elsewhere for a position; therefore he/she is released from the employ of this medical practice on _____

Employee comments: _____

_____   _____

Employee Signature   Date

_____   _____

Signature of first appraiser   Signature of second appraiser

Figure 19-11. Example of a performance evaluation form

PROCEDURE 19-6

STEP 1 2 3

Compose and Send a Thank-You Letter

Objective: To compose an appropriate, professional thank-you letter after a job interview (see Figure 19-10).

Equipment/Supplies: Sheet of 8½-inch × 11-inch white bond paper, number 10 envelope, computer or typewriter, and pen.

Directions: Follow these step-by-step procedures, which include rationales, to learn this skill, which is presented in the *Workbook* (Job Skill 19-4) for practice.

1. Prepare to write a letter within one or two days after the job interview.

2. Review letter styles and letter composition in Chapter 11 and envelope preparation in Chapter 12.

3. Compose a rough draft of the letter addressed to the individual who interviewed you.

4. In the first paragraph, thank the interviewer for granting the interview and taking the time to give information and answer questions.

5. In the second paragraph, state your continued, enthusiastic interest and motivation in obtaining the new position and how you find it challenging. You might state how your skills and qualifications make you ideal for the position.

6. Conclude the letter with an expression of appreciation for considering you for the position and insert information on when and where you can be contacted. Ask for a response to your letter by telephone, fax, e-mail, or standard mail.

7. Proofread the letter on-screen for content, typographical errors, grammar, and punctuation to be sure all important information has been addressed and the letter contains absolutely no errors.

8. Print the letter and proofread it again to make sure it is perfect.

9. Key a number 10 envelope with your return name and address.

Take time to analyze, document, and list the reasons why you merit an increase in pay. Possible reasons include:

- Work ethic of a higher standard than your coworkers

- Skills and knowledge of your job as it relates to this medical practice are valuable assets not easily replaced

- Generated an increased revenue much greater than the raise you are asking for

- Helped the practice create a positive public image and have good rapport with all patients

- Present positive documentation that the compensation you are paid, for the work you do, is below that of other professional associates

- Work is accurate, fast, and exceeds expectations

While presenting the list, indicate that you have achieved the expected outcome measures mentioned when you were hired or at your last evaluation. Consider, in advance how you would respond if the office manager declines your request or presents an unfavorable offer. Direct visual contact combined with a moment or two of silence is often effective, or you could reply, "that is unacceptable." Other options might be to discuss when a raise might be appropriate and get it in writing. Or ask for another review in three months. It is important to remember that a job consists of much more than pay. The work atmosphere, feelings of accomplishment, serving others, and fringe benefits are just a few additional reasons why people state that they like their jobs.

Tips for Holding the Medical Position

In an open job market with many persons competing for one office position, job security is never ensured. Therefore, when the new employee has been hired, it is recommended that he or she be aware of behavior that will help to hold a job:

1. Be punctual upon arrival in the morning, and after lunch and coffee breaks.

2. Avoid unnecessary absences.

3. Wear neat, clean, appropriate clothing.

4. Avoid criticizing staff members.

5. Accept all responsibilities without complaint.

6. Follow instructions given by the physician or office manager.

7. Limit personal telephone calls.

8. Offer to assist other staff members when assigned duties have been completed.

9. Limit social visiting with other employees.

10. Express empathy toward patients.

11. Adjust to new ideas with a learning attitude.

12. Smile! Be courteous and friendly.

CONCLUSION

You have read many scenarios that illustrate the statement, "the medical assistant is the heart of the health care professional." For the administrative medical assistant, being the first contact on the telephone, the first impression at the front desk, scheduling an appointment when the patient calls fearful about a health situation, solving insurance problems, extending understanding when a statement is not paid on time, and being a friendly face and the communicator between the physician or other health care professionals and the patient is a big responsibility. It is also a great privilege that has many rewards. You have learned how a medical practice functions, studied and practiced many job skills, and now have the ability to make this world a better place by serving patients' needs and becoming a vital part of the health care world. Believe in yourself, always do your best, and remember there is no goal you cannot achieve.

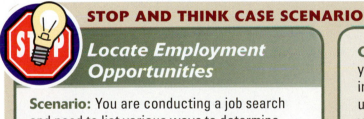

STOP AND THINK CASE SCENARIO

Locate Employment Opportunities

Scenario: You are conducting a job search and need to list various ways to determine employment opportunities in your community.

Critical Thinking: Research job openings in your town or city using suggestions learned in this chapter. State which resources you used and why. List any jobs discovered in your search.

_____

_____

_____

_____

_____

_____

_____

_____

_____

STOP AND THINK CASE SCENARIO

Select a Resumé Style

Scenario: You are preparing for a job search as a medical assistant and need to prepare your resumé.

Critical Thinking: Outline information pertaining to your education, work experience, and skills. Then study the four styles of resumés (chronological, functional, combination, and results-oriented) and decide which style would be most suitable for you. State why you chose a particular format based on the area you would like to emphasize.

_____

_____

_____

_____

STOP AND THINK CASE SCENARIO

Verbalize One Personal Strength and Weakness

Scenario: During an interview, the office manager who is hiring asks you to address one of your strengths and one weakness.

Critical Thinking: If you have not already done so, make a list of your strengths and weaknesses. Then select one of each that may be shared during a job interview. How would you discuss these topics with the individual who is interviewing you for a potential position?

Strength:_____

_____

Weakness: _____

_____

FOCUS ON CERTIFICATION*

CMA Content Summary

- Accept responsibility for own actions
- Resumé and cover letter
- Methods of job searching
- Interviewing
- Professional presentation
- Work as team member
- Adapt communication to level of understanding

_____

* *This textbook and the accompanying Workbook meet the entry-level administrative and general competencies for the CMA outlined by the AAMA Examination Content Outline and Role Delineation Study and for the RMA and CMAS outlined by the AMT Competencies and Examination Specifications (see Competency Grid in Appendix B).*

- Verbal and nonverbal communication
- Using tact, diplomacy, courtesy, and responsibility
- Interviewing
- Fundamental writing skills
- Keyboard, format, proofread data entry
- Word processing

RMA Content Summary

- Medical terminology definitions
- Interpersonal skills

- Oral and written communication
- Business format
- Listening skills

CMAS Content Summary

- Spell medical terms
- Professionalism
- Written and oral communication
- Format business correspondence
- PC-based environment; word processing
- Performance reviews

REVIEW   EXAM-STYLE QUESTIONS

1. When preparing to begin a job search, what is the *first* item of business?

   a. look at the local newspaper classified add section for job openings

   b. determine a resumé style and key a resumé

   c. gather personal data and fill in a mock application form

   d. inventory skills, abilities, interests, and personal traits

   e. ask your instructor whether students in your area are being hired

2. During a job search, what can be done to relieve stress and reduce frustration?

   a. practice yoga and meditation

   b. concentrate on the job search; all other responsibilities should take a lower priority until a job is secured

   c. establish a set number of hours per day or week that you will devote to securing a desired position

   d. go out with friends and forget about not having a job

   e. devote all your time to the job search so you can stay focused

3. What is a "temp-to-hire" position?

   a. a temporary position secured through an employment agency

   b. a temporary position that might lead to a permanent position

   c. a permanent position worked on a temporary basis

   d. a part-time position secured through an employment agency

   e. a permanent position secured through an employment agency

4. What is a "cold call"?

   a. an unannounced visit to an office where a possible job opportunity exists

   b. a visit to a potential job site where the applicant is treated in a "cold" manner

   c. a visit to a potential job site to drop off an employment application

   d. a visit to a potential job site to drop off a resumé

   e. a letter sent to a potential job site requesting an interview

5. What tool is used to typically introduce an employer to a job seeker?

   a. resumé

   b. cover letter

   c. application form

   d. blind letter

   e. telephone call

6. What department would you go to in a large clinic or hospital to obtain an application form?

    a. reception desk of admitting department

    b. health information management department

    c. finance department

    d. human resource department

    e. staffing department

7. What format should be used when preparing a letter of introduction?

    a. special brief-letter format

    b. standard business-letter format

    c. open punctuation

    d. closed punctuation

    e. mixed punctuation

8. The ultimate purpose of a resumé, is to:

    a. sell job qualifications

    b. detail personal information

    c. list work experience

    d. highlight education

    e. obtain an interview

9. A resumé that emphasizes the applicant's work skills and lists employers and dates of employment is called a/an:

    a. chronological resumé

    b. functional resumé

    c. combination resumé

    d. results-oriented resumé

    e. electronic resumé

10. Research studies show that when two applicants have similar skills and education, the decision to hire is based almost entirely on:

    a. where the applicant was educated

    b. testing scores

    c. personality

    d. physical appearance

    e. who the applicant knows

12. The typical probationary period is:

    a. 30 days

    b. 60 days

    c. 90 days

    d. 6 months

    e. 1 year

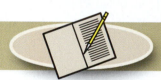

WORKBOOK ASSIGNMENT

To develop competency-based job skills, refer to the *Workbook* and complete the:

- Abbreviation and Spelling Review
- Review Questions

- Critical Thinking Exercises
- Job Skill activities, which are outlined at the beginning of this chapter under "Performance Objectives in the *Workbook*."

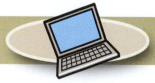

COMPUTER ASSIGNMENT

To review the concepts you have learned in this chapter, insert the *Student Practice* CD-ROM into a computer and work through the *StudyWARE* activities and games. Answer review questions in the practice mode and read the feedback, studying the questions you have missed. Take the chapter quiz until you achieve a minimum score of 90 percent. Successfully completing the *Critical Thinking Challenge* at the end of this course will help you think through scenarios and develop problem solving skills.

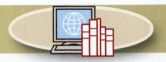

RESOURCES

Refer to Chapter 1, Table 1-2, for resources on certification and registration.

Books

Boost Your Interview IQ: Interview Fitness Training
Carole Martin
Web site: http://www.AllExperts.com

Job Hunting Handbook
Dalstrom and Company
(800) 222-0009
Web Site: http://www.dalstromandcompany.com

Weddle's Directory to Employment Related Internet Sites 2005/06

Weddle's Guide to Employment Web Sites 2005/06
(203) 964-1888
Web site: http://www.weddles.com/recruitcatalogue.htm

Job Sources

American Association of Medical Assistants
20 North Wacker Drive, Suite 1575
Chicago, IL 60606
(800) 228-2262
Web site: http://www.aama-ntl.org

International Association of Administrative Professionals (IAAP)
PO Box 20404
Kansas City, MO 64195-0404
(816) 891-6600
Web site: http://www.iaap-hq.org

Registered Medical Assistant/AMT
710 Higgins Road
Park Ridge, IL 60068
(847) 823-5169
Web site: http://www.amt1.com

If planning to specialize as a transcriptionist, contact:

Association for Healthcare Documentation Integrity
4230 Kiernan Ave., Suite 130
Modesto, CA 95356
(800) 982-2182
Fax: (209) 527-9633
E-mail: ahdi@ahdionline.com
Web site: http://www.ahdionline.com

Medical Transcription Industrial Alliance
Web site: http://www.mtia.com

MT Jobs
Web site: http://www.mtjobs.com

If planning to specialize as an insurance coder or insurance specialist, contact:

American Academy of Professional Coders (for CPT certification information)
PO Box 704004
Salt Lake City, UT 84170
(800) 626-2633
E-mail: info@aapc.com
Web site: http://www.aapc.com

American Health Information Management Association
233 North Michigan Avenue, Suite 2150
Chicago, IL 60601
(800) 335-5535
E-mail: info@ahima.org
Web site: http://www.ahima.org

Internet

Directions and Maps

MapQuest
Web site: http://www.MapQuest.com

Rand McNally
Web site: http://www.randmcnally.com

Yahoo
Web site: http://www.maps.yahoo.com

Employment Agencies

Kelly Services
Web site: http://www.kellyservices.com

Manpower Incorporated
Web site: http://www.manpower.com

Job Descriptions and Salary Information

Business and Legal Reports (BLR)
Web site: http://www.hrnext.com

Office Team
(800) 804-8367
Web site: http://www.officeteam.com

SalaryExpert
Web site: http://www.salaryexpert.com

Job Sources (General)

America's Employers
http://www.americasemployers.com

America's Job Bank
http://www.ajb.dni.us

Career Builder
http://www.careerbuilder.com

Career.Com
http://www.career.com

Career Crafting
http://www.careercraft.com

Career Magazine
http://www.careermag.com/careermag

Career Net
http://www.careernet.com

Forty Plus of Southern California
http://www.40plussocal.org

JobWeb
http://www.jobweb.org

APPENDIX A

CMS-1500 (REVISED 08/05) CLAIM FORM FIELD-BY-FIELD INSTRUCTIONS AND A COMMERCIAL INSURANCE TEMPLATE

The following instructions contain information needed to complete the revised CMS-1500 claim form (08/05) using optical character recognition (OCR) guidelines for commercial payers, Medicare (Medicare/Medicaid, Medicare/Medigap, and Medicare Secondary Payer), and TRICARE programs. Information on specific coverage guidelines, program policies, and practice specialties are not included for conciseness and because guidelines for completing claim forms vary at the state and local levels. Consult your local intermediary or commercial insurance carrier for detailed instructions.

To use these instructions, follow these steps:

1. Locate the field number you need instruction for. Field numbers match those on the CMS-1500 claim form.

2. Identify the type of insurance program you are completing the claim for; titles appear in bold face, color-coded capital letters.

3. Read the instructions for specific field requirements. Guidelines for completing *Workbook* exercises are indented and appear in color when there are optional ways of completing a field.

4. Refer to the section of the CMS-1500 claim form for a visual example. The field being referred to is highlighted in yellow.

5. Screened areas on insurance templates do not apply to the program examples illustrated and should be left blank. See Figure A-1 and Figures 16-3, 16-6, and 16-9 in Chapter 16.

When generating paper claims from a computer, some software programs insert the commercial carrier's name and address in the top right corner of the CMS-1500 claim form; however, new revised guidelines state that this area is to be left blank. When completing a claim form for the *Workbook* exercises, follow this format to indicate where the claim is to be sent.

Program icons and descriptions are as follows:

ALL THIRD-PARTY PAYERS: Guidelines cover all private insurance companies and all federal and state programs.

COMMERCIAL PAYERS: Guidelines cover all private insurance companies.

MEDICARE: Guidelines cover federal Medicare programs as well as Medicare/Medicaid, Medicare/Medigap, and Medicare Secondary Payer (MSP).

TRICARE: Guidelines cover TRICARE Standard (formerly CHAMPUS), TRICARE Prime, and TRICARE Extra programs.

KEY: **R** = Required fields that must always be completed

C = Conditional fields that may need to be completed depending on the circumstances of the insured

1500

HEALTH INSURANCE CLAIM FORM

APPROVED BY NATIONAL UNIFORM CLAIM COMMITTEE 08/05

MIDWEST INSURANCE COMPANY
2515 SOUTH O STREET
LINCOLN NE 68000

CARRIER

| | PICA | | | | | | PICA | |

1. MEDICARE (Medicare #)   MEDICAID (Medicaid #)   TRICARE CHAMPUS (Sponsor's SSN)   CHAMPVA (Member ID#) ☒   GROUP HEALTH PLAN (SSN or ID)   FECA BLK LUNG (SSN)   OTHER (ID)

1a. INSURED'S I.D. NUMBER   (For Program in Item 1)
2984567   **F23**

2. PATIENT'S NAME (Last Name, First Name, Middle Initial)
MITCHELL CALEB S

3. PATIENT'S BIRTH DATE   MM **04** DD **18** YY **1973**   SEX M ☒ F

4. INSURED'S NAME (Last Name, First Name, Middle Initial)
SAME

5. PATIENT'S ADDRESS (No., Street)
444 SHERIDAN WAY

6. PATIENT RELATIONSHIP TO INSURED   Self ☒ Spouse ☐ Child ☐ Other ☐

7. INSURED'S ADDRESS (No., Street)

CITY **WOODLAND HILLS**   STATE **XY**

8. PATIENT STATUS   Single ☒ Married ☐ Other ☐

CITY   STATE

ZIP CODE **12345**   TELEPHONE (Include Area Code) **(555) 486 2233**

Employed ☒ Full-Time Student ☐ Part-Time Student ☐

ZIP CODE   TELEPHONE (Include Area Code) **( )**

9. OTHER INSURED'S NAME (Last Name, First Name, Middle Initial)

10. IS PATIENT'S CONDITION RELATED TO:

11. INSURED'S POLICY GROUP OR FECA NUMBER

a. OTHER INSURED'S POLICY OR GROUP NUMBER

a. EMPLOYMENT? (Current or Previous)   YES ☐ NO ☒

a. INSURED'S DATE OF BIRTH   MM DD YY   SEX M ☐ F ☐

b. OTHER INSURED'S DATE OF BIRTH   MM DD YY   SEX M ☐ F ☐

b. AUTO ACCIDENT?   YES ☐ NO ☒   PLACE (State)

b. EMPLOYER'S NAME OR SCHOOL NAME

c. EMPLOYER'S NAME OR SCHOOL NAME

c. OTHER ACCIDENT?   YES ☐ NO ☒

c. INSURANCE PLAN NAME OR PROGRAM NAME

d. INSURANCE PLAN NAME OR PROGRAM NAME

10d. RESERVED FOR LOCAL USE

d. IS THERE ANOTHER HEALTH BENEFIT PLAN?   YES ☐ NO ☒   If yes, return to and complete item 9 a-d.

READ BACK OF FORM BEFORE COMPLETING & SIGNING THIS FORM.

12. PATIENT'S OR AUTHORIZED PERSON'S SIGNATURE I authorize the release of any medical or other information necessary to process this claim. I also request payment of government benefits either to myself or to the party who accepts assignment below.

SIGNED **Caleb S Mitchell**   DATE **03/20/20XX**

13. INSURED'S OR AUTHORIZED PERSON'S SIGNATURE I authorize payment of medical benefits to the undersigned physician or supplier for services described below.

SIGNED **Caleb S Mitchell**

14. DATE OF CURRENT: ILLNESS (First symptom) OR INJURY (Accident) OR PREGNANCY(LMP)   MM **02** DD **16** YY **20XX**

15. IF PATIENT HAS HAD SAME OR SIMILAR ILLNESS. GIVE FIRST DATE   MM DD YY

16. DATES PATIENT UNABLE TO WORK IN CURRENT OCCUPATION   FROM MM **03** DD **24** YY **20XX** TO MM **04** DD **07** YY **20XX**

17. NAME OF REFERRING PROVIDER OR OTHER SOURCE
THOMAS ROTHSCHILD MD

17a.
17b. NPI **23345678XX**

18. HOSPITALIZATION DATES RELATED TO CURRENT SERVICES   FROM MM **03** DD **24** YY **20XX** TO MM **03** DD **30** YY **20XX**

19. RESERVED FOR LOCAL USE

20. OUTSIDE LAB?   YES ☐ NO ☒ $ CHARGES

21. DIAGNOSIS OR NATURE OF ILLNESS OR INJURY (Relate Items 1, 2, 3 or 4 to Item 24E by Line)
1. **003.0**   3.
2.   4.

22. MEDICAID RESUBMISSION CODE   ORIGINAL REF. NO.

23. PRIOR AUTHORIZATION NUMBER

24. A. DATE(S) OF SERVICE From MM DD YY	To MM DD YY	B. PLACE OF SERVICE	C. EMG	D. PROCEDURES, SERVICES, OR SUPPLIES (Explain Unusual Circumstances) CPT/HCPCS MODIFIER	E. DIAGNOSIS POINTER	F. $ CHARGES	G. DAYS OR UNITS	H. EPSDT Family Plan	I. ID. QUAL.	J. RENDERING PROVIDER ID. #
1 03 24 20XX		21		99223	1	152 98	1		NPI	46278897XX
2 03 25 20XX		21		99233	1	76 97	1		NPI	46278892XX
3 03 26 20XX	03 28 20XX	21		99232	1	166 68	3		NPI	46278897XX
4 03 29 20XX		21		99231	1	37 74	1		NPI	46278897XX
5 03 30 20XX		21		99238	1	65 26	1		NPI	46278892XX
6									NPI	

25. FEDERAL TAX I.D. NUMBER   **78 51342XX**   SSN ☐ EIN ☒

26. PATIENT'S ACCOUNT NO.

27. ACCEPT ASSIGNMENT? (For govt. claims, see back)   YES ☒ NO ☐

28. TOTAL CHARGE $ **499 63**

29. AMOUNT PAID $ **10 00**

30. BALANCE DUE $ **489 63**

31. SIGNATURE OF PHYSICIAN OR SUPPLIER INCLUDING DEGREES OR CREDENTIALS (I certify that the statements on the reverse apply to this bill and are made a part thereof.)
GERALD PRACTON MD
SIGNED **Gerald Practon MD**   DATE **03/30/20XX**

32. SERVICE FACILITY LOCATION INFORMATION
COLLEGE HOSPITAL
4500 BROAD AVENUE
WOODLAND HILLS XY 12345 4700
a. **54378601XX**   b.

33. BILLING PROVIDER INFO & PH # **(555) 486 9002**
PRACTON MEDICAL GROUP
4567 BROAD AVENUE
WOODLAND HILLS XY 12345 4700
a. **36640210XX**   b.

PATIENT AND INSURED INFORMATION / PHYSICIAN OR SUPPLIER INFORMATION

NUCC Instruction Manual available at: www.nucc.org

APPROVED OMB-0938-0999 FORM CMS-1500 (08-05)

Figure A-1.   Commercial payer with no secondary coverage

TOP OF FORM ⓒ

1500

HEALTH INSURANCE CLAIM FORM

APPROVED BY NATIONAL UNIFORM CLAIM COMMITTEE 08/05

MIDWEST INSURANCE COMPANY
2515 SOUTH O STREET
LINCOLN NE 68000

PICA								PICA
1. MEDICARE MEDICAID TRICARE CHAMPUS CHAMPVA GROUP HEALTH PLAN FECA BLK LUNG OTHER							1a. INSURED'S I.D. NUMBER 2984567	(For Program in Item 1) F23
(Medicare #) (Medicaid #) (Sponsor's SSN) (Member ID#) ☒ (Member ID#) (SSN) (ID)								
2. PATIENT'S NAME (Last Name, First Name, Middle Initial) MITCHELL CALEB S			3. PATIENT'S BIRTH DATE MM 04 DD 18 YY 1973 SEX M ☒ F ☐				4. INSURED'S NAME (Last Name, First Name, Middle Initial) SAME	

Insert name and address of insurance company in the top right corner of the insurance form using all capital letters and no punctuation. This format is being used to demonstrate that the student knows where to direct the claim even though some carriers (e.g., Medicare) do not follow this guideline.

FIELD 1 ®

1500

HEALTH INSURANCE CLAIM FORM

APPROVED BY NATIONAL UNIFORM CLAIM COMMITTEE 08/05

MIDWEST INSURANCE COMPANY
2515 SOUTH O STREET
LINCOLN NE 68000

PICA								PICA
1. MEDICARE MEDICAID TRICARE CHAMPUS CHAMPVA GROUP HEALTH PLAN FECA BLK LUNG OTHER							1a. INSURED'S I.D. NUMBER 2984567	(For Program in Item 1) F23
(Medicare #) (Medicaid #) (Sponsor's SSN) (Member ID#) ☒ (Member ID#) (SSN) (ID)								
2. PATIENT'S NAME (Last Name, First Name, Middle Initial) MITCHELL CALEB S			3. PATIENT'S BIRTH DATE MM 04 DD 18 YY 1973 SEX M ☒ F ☐				4. INSURED'S NAME (Last Name, First Name, Middle Initial) SAME	

COMMERCIAL PAYERS

Individual Health Plan: Mark "Other" for an individual covered under an individual policy.

Group Health Plan: Mark this box for those covered under any group contract insurance (e.g., insurance obtained through employment); also for patients who receive services paid by managed care programs (e.g., HMOs, PPOs, IPAs).

> *Workbook* Exercises: If the insured is employed, assume the insurance is through the employer and mark "group" insurance; otherwise, assume it is an individual policy and mark "other."

MEDICARE: Mark this box for patients who receive Medicare benefits.

Medicare/Medicaid: Mark "Medicare" and "Medicaid" if the patient is covered under Medicare and Medicaid programs.

Medicare/Medigap: Mark "Medicare" and, if the patient has group or individual Medigap coverage, mark "Group" or "Other," depending on health plan.

> *Workbook* Exercises: If the insured is employed, assume the insurance is through the employer and mark "group" insurance; otherwise, assume it is an individual policy and mark "other."

MSP: Mark "Group" or "Other" (depending on health plan) and "Medicare" when a Medicare patient has insurance primary to Medicare coverage.

TRICARE: Mark "TRICARE/CHAMPUS" for individual receiving TRICARE benefits.

FIELD 1a ®

1500

HEALTH INSURANCE CLAIM FORM
APPROVED BY NATIONAL UNIFORM CLAIM COMMITTEE 08/05

MIDWEST INSURANCE COMPANY
2515 SOUTH O STREET
LINCOLN NE 68000

	PICA								PICA		
1. MEDICARE	MEDICAID	TRICARE CHAMPUS	CHAMPVA	GROUP HEALTH PLAN	FECA BLK LUNG	OTHER	1a. INSURED'S I.D. NUMBER	(For Program in Item 1)			
(Medicare #)	(Medicaid #)	(Sponsor's SSN)	(Member ID#) ☒	(Member ID#)	(SSN)	(ID)	2984567	F23			
2. PATIENT'S NAME (Last Name, First Name, Middle Initial) MITCHELL CALEB S			3. PATIENT'S BIRTH DATE MM 04 DD 18 YY 1973 SEX M ☒ F ☐				4. INSURED'S NAME (Last Name, First Name, Middle Initial) SAME				

COMMERCIAL PAYERS: Insert the patient's policy (identification or certificate) number in the left portion of the field and the group number, if applicable, in the right portion of the field. Insert the numbers as they appear on the insurance card, *without punctuation.*

MEDICARE: Insert the patient's Medicare Health Insurance Claim (HIC) number from the patient's Medicare card in the left portion of this field, regardless of whether Medicare is the primary or secondary payer.

Medicare/Medicaid: Insert the patient's Medicare number in the left portion of this field.

Medicare/Medigap: Insert the patient's Medicare number in the left portion of this field.

MSP: Insert the patient's Medicare number in the left portion of this field. See Field 11 for primary insurance.

TRICARE: First insert sponsor's Social Security number (SSN) in the left portion of this field. Then, if the patient is a NATO beneficiary, add "NATO" or, if sponsor is a security agent, add "SECURITY." Do not provide the patient's SSN unless the patient and sponsor are the same.

FIELD 2 ®

1500

HEALTH INSURANCE CLAIM FORM
APPROVED BY NATIONAL UNIFORM CLAIM COMMITTEE 08/05

MIDWEST INSURANCE COMPANY
2515 SOUTH O STREET
LINCOLN NE 68000

	PICA								PICA		
1. MEDICARE	MEDICAID	TRICARE CHAMPUS	CHAMPVA	GROUP HEALTH PLAN	FECA BLK LUNG	OTHER	1a. INSURED'S I.D. NUMBER	(For Program in Item 1)			
(Medicare #)	(Medicaid #)	(Sponsor's SSN)	(Member ID#) ☒	(Member ID#)	(SSN)	(ID)	2984567	F23			
2. PATIENT'S NAME (Last Name, First Name, Middle Initial) MITCHELL CALEB S			3. PATIENT'S BIRTH DATE MM 04 DD 18 YY 1973 SEX M ☒ F ☐				4. INSURED'S NAME (Last Name, First Name, Middle Initial) SAME				

ALL THIRD-PARTY PAYERS: Insert the last name, first name, and middle initial of the patient—in that order—as shown on the patient's identification card, even if it is misspelled. Do not use nicknames or abbreviations. Do not use commas. If a name is hyphenated, a hyphen may be used. Some examples follow:

- Hyphenated name: Jones-Brown = JONES-BROWN
- Prefixed name: McDougall = MCDOUGALL
- Seniority name with numeric suffix: James N. Peri, III = PERI III JAMES N

FIELD 3 ®

1500

HEALTH INSURANCE CLAIM FORM
APPROVED BY NATIONAL UNIFORM CLAIM COMMITTEE 08/05

MIDWEST INSURANCE COMPANY
2515 SOUTH O STREET
LINCOLN NE 68000

	PICA								PICA		
1. MEDICARE	MEDICAID	TRICARE CHAMPUS	CHAMPVA	GROUP HEALTH PLAN	FECA BLK LUNG	OTHER	1a. INSURED'S I.D. NUMBER	(For Program in Item 1)			
(Medicare #)	(Medicaid #)	(Sponsor's SSN)	(Member ID#) ☒	(Member ID#)	(SSN)	(ID)	2984567	F23			
2. PATIENT'S NAME (Last Name, First Name, Middle Initial) MITCHELL CALEB S			3. PATIENT'S BIRTH DATE MM 04 DD 18 YY 1973 SEX M ☒ F ☐				4. INSURED'S NAME (Last Name, First Name, Middle Initial) SAME				

ALL THIRD-PARTY PAYERS: Insert the patient's birth date using eight digits (02092004). The patient's age must be as follows to correlate with the diagnosis in Field 21:

- Birth: Newborn diagnosis

- Birth to 17 years: Pediatric diagnosis

- 12 to 55 years: Maternity diagnosis

- 15 to 124 years: Adult diagnosis

Mark the appropriate box for the patient's sex. If left blank, gender field defaults to "female."

FIELD 4 Ⓒ

1500	MIDWEST INSURANCE COMPANY
HEALTH INSURANCE CLAIM FORM	2515 SOUTH O STREET
APPROVED BY NATIONAL UNIFORM CLAIM COMMITTEE 08/05	LINCOLN NE 68000

☐ PICA		PICA ☐
1. MEDICARE MEDICAID TRICARE CHAMPUS CHAMPVA GROUP HEALTH PLAN FECA BLK LUNG OTHER	1a. INSURED'S I.D. NUMBER	(For Program in Item 1)
☐(Medicare #) ☐(Medicaid #) ☐(Sponsor's SSN) ☐(Member ID#) ☒(Member ID#) ☐(SSN) ☐(ID)	2984567	F23
2. PATIENT'S NAME (Last Name, First Name, Middle Initial) MITCHELL CALEB S	3. PATIENT'S BIRTH DATE MM 04 DD 18 YY 1973 SEX M ☒ F ☐	4. INSURED'S NAME (Last Name, First Name, Middle Initial) SAME

COMMERCIAL PAYERS: Insert "SAME" when the insured is also the patient. If the insured is not the patient, insert the name of the insured (last name first).

MEDICARE: Do not fill in if Medicare is primary and the insured is also the patient. Insert the insured's name, if different from the patient's.

Medicare/Medicaid: Follow Medicare guidelines.

Medicare/Medigap: Follow Medicare guidelines.

MSP: Insert the name of the insured (last name first).

TRICARE: Insert the sponsor's last name, first name, and middle initial, not a nickname or abbreviation. Leave blank if "self" is checked in Field 6.

FIELD 5 Ⓡ

5. PATIENT'S ADDRESS (No., Street) 444 SHERIDAN WAY	6. PATIENT RELATIONSHIP TO INSURED Self ☒ Spouse ☐ Child ☐ Other ☐	7. INSURED'S ADDRESS (No., Street)	
CITY WOODLAND HILLS	STATE XY	8. PATIENT STATUS Single ☒ Married ☐ Other ☐	CITY	STATE
ZIP CODE 12345	TELEPHONE (Include Area Code) (555) 486 2233	Employed ☒ Full-Time Student ☐ Part-Time Student ☐	ZIP CODE	TELEPHONE (Include Area Code) ( )

COMMERCIAL PAYERS: Insert the patient's mailing address and residential telephone number.

MEDICARE: Insert the patient's mailing address and residential telephone number. On the first line, enter the street address; on the second line, the city and two-character state code (e.g., CO = Colorado); on the third line, enter the ZIP code and residential telephone number. Punctuation is not necessary (e.g., ST CHARLES, no period after ST).

Medicare/Medicaid: Insert the patient's mailing address and residential telephone number.

Medicare/Medigap: Insert the patient's mailing address and residential telephone number.

MSP: Insert the patient's mailing address and residential telephone number.

TRICARE: Insert the patient's mailing address and residential telephone number. Provide the actual place of residence; do not enter a Post Office box number. If the address contains a rural route number, a rural route box number is required, too. Use an APO/FPO address if the person is residing overseas.

FIELD 6 ⓒ

5. PATIENT'S ADDRESS (No., Street) 444 SHERIDAN WAY		6. PATIENT RELATIONSHIP TO INSURED Self ☒ Spouse ☐ Child ☐ Other ☐	7. INSURED'S ADDRESS (No., Street)	
CITY WOODLAND HILLS	STATE XY	8. PATIENT STATUS Single ☒ Married ☐ Other ☐	CITY	STATE
ZIP CODE 12345	TELEPHONE (Include Area Code) (555) 486 2233	Employed ☒ Full-Time Student ☐ Part-Time Student ☐	ZIP CODE	TELEPHONE (Include Area Code ( )

COMMERCIAL PAYERS: Indicate the patient's relationship to the insured. If the patient is an unmarried "domestic partner," mark "Other."

MEDICARE: Mark the relationship to insured when Field 4 is completed; otherwise, leave blank.

Medicare/Medicaid: Follow Medicare guidelines.

Medicare/Medigap: Follow Medicare guidelines.

MSP: Mark the relationship to insured.

TRICARE: Indicate the patient's relationship to the sponsor. If patient is the sponsor, mark "self" (e.g., retiree). If the patient is a child or stepchild, mark the box for child. If "other" is marked, indicate how the patient is related to the sponsor in Field 19 or on an attachment (e.g., former spouse).

FIELD 7 ⓒ

5. PATIENT'S ADDRESS (No., Street) 444 SHERIDAN WAY		6. PATIENT RELATIONSHIP TO INSURED Self ☒ Spouse ☐ Child ☐ Other ☐	7. INSURED'S ADDRESS (No., Street)	
CITY WOODLAND HILLS	STATE XY	8. PATIENT STATUS Single ☒ Married ☐ Other ☐	CITY	STATE
ZIP CODE 12345	TELEPHONE (Include Area Code) (555) 486 2233	Employed ☒ Full-Time Student ☐ Part-Time Student ☐	ZIP CODE	TELEPHONE (Include Area Code ( )

COMMERCIAL PAYERS: Do not complete if Field 4 indicates "same." Insert "SAME" if Field 4 is filled in and the address is identical to that listed in Field 5. Insert address if different from that listed in Field 5.

MEDICARE: Do not complete if Field 4 is blank. Insert "SAME" if Field 4 is filled in and the address is identical to that listed in Field 5. Insert address if different from that listed in Field 5.

Medicare/Medicaid: Follow Medicare guidelines.

Medicare/Medigap: Follow Medicare guidelines.

MSP: Fill in only when Field 4 is completed. If insured is other than the patient, list insured's address and if the address is the same as in Field 5, insert "SAME."

TRICARE: Insert "SAME" if address is the same as that of the patient listed in Field 5. Insert the sponsor's address (e.g., an APO/FPO address or active duty sponsor's duty station or the retiree's mailing address) if different from the patient's address.

FIELD 8 Ⓡ/ⓒ

5. PATIENT'S ADDRESS (No., Street) 444 SHERIDAN WAY		6. PATIENT RELATIONSHIP TO INSURED Self ☒ Spouse ☐ Child ☐ Other ☐	7. INSURED'S ADDRESS (No., Street)	
CITY WOODLAND HILLS	STATE XY	8. PATIENT STATUS Single ☒ Married ☐ Other ☐	CITY	STATE
ZIP CODE 12345	TELEPHONE (Include Area Code) (555) 486 2233	Employed ☒ Full-Time Student ☐ Part-Time Student ☐	ZIP CODE	TELEPHONE (Include Area Code ( )

COMMERCIAL PAYERS: Mark the appropriate box for the patient's marital status and whether employed or a student. Mark "other" when a patient is covered under his or her children's health insurance plan or for a domestic partner.

MEDICARE: Mark the appropriate box or boxes for the patient's marital status and whether employed or a student (e.g., a beneficiary may be employed, a student, and married). Indicate "single" if widowed or divorced. In some locales, this field is not required by Medicare.

Medicare/Medicaid: Check the appropriate box for the patient's marital status and whether employed or a student. Check "single" if widowed or divorced.

Medicare/Medigap: Mark the appropriate box for the patient's marital status and whether employed or a student. Indicate "single" if widowed or divorced.

MSP: Mark the appropriate box for the patient's marital status and whether employed or a student. Indicate "single" if widowed or divorced.

TRICARE: Mark the appropriate box for the patient's marital status and whether employed or a student.

FIELD 9 Ⓒ

9. OTHER INSURED'S NAME (Last Name, First Name, Middle Initial)	10. IS PATIENT'S CONDITION RELATED TO:	11. INSURED'S POLICY GROUP OR FECA NUMBER
a. OTHER INSURED'S POLICY OR GROUP NUMBER	a. EMPLOYMENT? (Current or Previous) ☐ YES ☒ NO	a. INSURED'S DATE OF BIRTH MM DD YY SEX M ☐ F ☐
b. OTHER INSURED'S DATE OF BIRTH MM DD YY SEX M ☐ F ☐	b. AUTO ACCIDENT? PLACE (State) ☐ YES ☒ NO	b. EMPLOYER'S NAME OR SCHOOL NAME
c. EMPLOYER'S NAME OR SCHOOL NAME	c. OTHER ACCIDENT? ☐ YES ☒ NO	c. INSURANCE PLAN NAME OR PROGRAM NAME
d. INSURANCE PLAN NAME OR PROGRAM NAME	10d. RESERVED FOR LOCAL USE	d. IS THERE ANOTHER HEALTH BENEFIT PLAN? ☐ YES ☒ NO *If yes*, return to and complete item 9 a-d.

COMMERCIAL PAYERS: For primary insurance submission, do not fill in. For secondary insurance submission, insert patient's full name in last name, first name, and middle initial sequence.

MEDICARE: Do not complete for primary insurance. Do not list Medicare supplemental coverage (private, not Medigap) on the primary Medicare claim. File a separate claim.

Medicare/Medicaid: Insert Medicaid patient's full name in last name, first name, and middle initial sequence.

Medicare/Medigap: Insert the last name, first name, and middle initial of the Medigap enrollee if it dif-fers from that in Field 2; otherwise, insert "SAME." Only Medicare participating physicians and suppliers should complete Field 9 and its subdivisions, and only when the beneficiary wishes to assign his or her benefits under a Medigap policy to the participating physician or supplier. Do not complete if no Medigap benefits are assigned.

MSP: Do not fill in.

TRICARE: Do not fill in for primary insurance. For secondary insurance held by someone other than the patient, insert the name of the insured. Fields 11a–d should be used to report other health insurance held by the patient.

FIELD 9a Ⓒ

COMMERCIAL PAYERS: Insert the policy and/or group number of the other (secondary) insured's insurance coverage.

MEDICARE: Follow appropriate secondary coverage guidelines.

Medicare/Medicaid: Insert Medicaid policy number here or in Field 10d. Check with your local fiscal intermediary for individual state guidelines.

Workbook Exercises: Enter the Medicaid policy number in Field 10d.

Medicare/Medigap: Insert the policy and/or group number of the Medigap enrollee preceded by the word "MEDIGAP," "MG," or "MGAP." If a patient has a third insurance (i.e., employer-supplemental), all information for the third insurance should be submitted on an attachment.

Workbook Exercises: Enter the word "MEDIGAP."

MSP: Leave blank.

TRICARE: Insert the policy or group number of the secondary insurance policy.

FIELD 9b Ⓒ

COMMERCIAL PAYERS: Insert the other insured's date of birth and gender.

MEDICARE: Follow appropriate secondary coverage guidelines.

Medicare/Medicaid: Insert the Medicaid enrollee's birth date, using eight digits (e.g., 02092004), and gender. Do not fill in if same as patient's.

Medicare/Medigap: Insert the Medigap enrollee's birth date, using eight digits (e.g., 02092004), and gender. Do not fill in if same as patient's.

MSP: Do not fill in.

TRICARE: For secondary coverage held by someone other than the patient, insert the other insured's date of birth and check the appropriate box for gender.

FIELD 9c Ⓒ

COMMERCIAL PAYERS: Insert employer's name when patient has secondary coverage.

MEDICARE: Follow appropriate secondary coverage guidelines.

Medicare/Medicaid: Do not fill in.

Medicare/Medigap: Insert the Medigap insurer's claim processing address. Ignore "employer's name or school name." Abbreviate the street address to fit in this field by deleting the city, and using the two-letter state postal code and ZIP code. For example, 264 Oak Drive, Santa Barbara, California 93105 would be typed "264 OAK DR CA 93105." *Note: If a carrier-assigned unique identifier (sometimes called "Other Carrier Name and Address," or OCNA) for a Medigap insurer appears in Field 9d, then Field 9c may be left blank.*

MSP: Do not fill in.

TRICARE: For secondary coverage held by someone other than the patient, insert the name of the other insured's employer or name of school.

FIELD 9d Ⓒ

COMMERCIAL PAYERS: Insert name of secondary insurance plan or program.

MEDICARE: Follow appropriate secondary coverage guidelines.

Medicare/Medicaid: Do not fill in.

Medicare/Medigap: Insert the Medigap insurer's nine-digit alphanumeric PAYERID number if known (often called the OCNA key), and Field 9c may be left blank. If not known, insert the name of the Medigap enrollee's insurance company. For participating providers, all of the information in Fields 9 through 9d must be complete and correct or the Medicare carrier cannot electronically forward the claim information to the Medigap insurer. For multiple insurance information, enter "ATTACHMENT" in Field 10d and provide information on an attached sheet.

MSP: Do not fill in.

TRICARE: For secondary coverage held by someone other than the patient, enter name of insured's other health insurance program. On an attached sheet, provide a complete mailing address for all other insurance information and insert the word "ATTACHMENT" in Field 10d. If the patient is covered by a health maintenance organization, attach a copy of the document indicating that the service is not covered by the HMO.

FIELD 10a Ⓡ

9. OTHER INSURED'S NAME (Last Name, First Name, Middle Initial)	10. IS PATIENT'S CONDITION RELATED TO:	11. INSURED'S POLICY GROUP OR FECA NUMBER
a. OTHER INSURED'S POLICY OR GROUP NUMBER	a. EMPLOYMENT? (Current or Previous) ☐ YES ☒ NO	a. INSURED'S DATE OF BIRTH MM DD YY SEX M ☐ F ☐
b. OTHER INSURED'S DATE OF BIRTH MM DD YY SEX M ☐ F ☐	b. AUTO ACCIDENT? ☐ YES ☒ NO PLACE (State)	b. EMPLOYER'S NAME OR SCHOOL NAME
c. EMPLOYER'S NAME OR SCHOOL NAME	c. OTHER ACCIDENT? ☐ YES ☒ NO	c. INSURANCE PLAN NAME OR PROGRAM NAME
d. INSURANCE PLAN NAME OR PROGRAM NAME	10d. RESERVED FOR LOCAL USE	d. IS THERE ANOTHER HEALTH BENEFIT PLAN? ☐ YES ☒ NO *If yes, return to and complete item 9 a-d.*

ALL THIRD-PARTY PAYERS: Mark "yes" or "no" to indicate whether patient's diagnosis described in Field 21 is the result of an accident or injury that occurred on the job or an industrial illness.

FIELD 10b Ⓡ

COMMERCIAL PAYERS: Mark "yes" in Field 10b to indicate a third-party liability case and file the claim with the other liability insurance or automobile insurance company. Enter the abbreviation of the state in which the accident took place (e.g., VA for Virginia).

MEDICARE: Mark "no." If "yes" applies, bill the liability insurance as primary insurance and Medicare as secondary.

Medicare/Medicaid: Follow Medicare guidelines.

Medicare/Medigap: Follow Medicare guidelines.

MSP: Follow Medicare guidelines.

TRICARE: Mark "yes" or "no" to indicate whether automobile liability applies to one or more of the services described in Field 24. If "yes," provide information concerning potential third-party liability. If a third party is involved in the accident, the beneficiary must complete Form DD 2527 (Statement of Personal Injury—Possible Third-Party Liability) and attach it to the claim.

FIELD 10c Ⓡ

COMMERCIAL PAYERS: Mark "yes" or "no" to indicate whether the patient's condition is related to an accident other than automobile or employment. Verify primary insurance.

MEDICARE: Mark "yes" or "no" to indicate whether the patient's condition is related to an accident other than automobile or employment. Verify primary insurance.

Medicare/Medicaid: Follow Medicare guidelines.

Medicare/Medigap: Follow Medicare guidelines.

MSP: Follow Medicare guidelines.

TRICARE: Mark "yes" or "no" to indicate whether another accident (not automobile or work related) applies to one or more of the services described in Field 24. If so, provide information concerning potential third-party liability. If third party is involved in the accident, the beneficiary must complete Form DD 2527 (Statement of Personal Injury—Possible Third-Party Liability) and attach it to the claim.

FIELD 10d Ⓒ

COMMERCIAL PAYERS: Do not complete.

MEDICARE: Do not complete.

Medicare/Medicaid: Insert the patient's Medicaid (MCD) number preceded by the abbreviation "MCD."

Medicare/Medigap: Do not complete.

MSP: Do not complete.

TRICARE: Generally, do not complete unless regional fiscal intermediary gives special guidelines. However, if Field 11d is checked "yes," the mailing address of the insurance carrier must be attached to the claim form, and in this block enter "ATTACHMENT."

Workbook Exercises: Leave blank.

FIELD 11 Ⓒ

9. OTHER INSURED'S NAME (Last Name, First Name, Middle Initial)	10. IS PATIENT'S CONDITION RELATED TO:	11. INSURED'S POLICY GROUP OR FECA NUMBER
a. OTHER INSURED'S POLICY OR GROUP NUMBER	a. EMPLOYMENT? (Current or Previous) ☐ YES ☒ NO	a. INSURED'S DATE OF BIRTH MM DD YY SEX M ☐ F ☐
b. OTHER INSURED'S DATE OF BIRTH SEX MM DD YY M ☐ F ☐	b. AUTO ACCIDENT? PLACE (State) ☐ YES ☒ NO ___	b. EMPLOYER'S NAME OR SCHOOL NAME
c. EMPLOYER'S NAME OR SCHOOL NAME	c. OTHER ACCIDENT? ☐ YES ☒ NO	c. INSURANCE PLAN NAME OR PROGRAM NAME
d. INSURANCE PLAN NAME OR PROGRAM NAME	10d. RESERVED FOR LOCAL USE	d. IS THERE ANOTHER HEALTH BENEFIT PLAN? ☐ YES ☒ NO *If yes, return to and complete item 9 a-d.*

COMMERCIAL PAYERS: Do not complete Fields 11 through 11c if no private secondary coverage. If secondary insurance, see Fields 9–9d.

MEDICARE: Enter "NONE" if other insurance is not primary to Medicare and go to Field 12. Field 11 must be completed by the physician/supplier to acknowledge that a good faith effort has been made to determine whether Medicare is the primary or secondary payer.

Medicare/Medicaid: Follow Medicare guidelines.

Medicare/Medigap: Follow Medicare guidelines.

MSP: Enter the insured's policy and/or group number only when insurance is primary to Medicare and complete Fields 11a through 11c.

TRICARE: Do not complete.

FIELD 11a C

COMMERCIAL PAYERS: Do not complete.

MEDICARE: Do not complete.

Medicare/Medicaid: Do not complete.

Medicare/Medigap: Do not complete.

MSP: Insert the insured's eight-digit date of birth (02092004) and gender if different from that listed in Field 3; otherwise leave blank.

TRICARE: Insert the sponsor's date of birth and indicate gender, if different from that listed in Field 3; otherwise leave blank.

FIELD 11b C

COMMERCIAL PAYERS: For secondary insurance, enter the name of the employer, school, or organization if primary policy is a group plan; otherwise, leave blank.

MEDICARE: Do not complete.

Medicare/Medicaid: Do not complete.

Medicare/Medigap: Do not complete.

MSP: Insert the employer's name of primary insurance. Also use this field to indicate a change in the insured's insurance status (e.g., "RETIRED" and the eight-digit retirement date). Submit paper claims with a copy of the primary payer's Remittance Advice (RA) document to be considered for Medicare Secondary Payer benefits. Instances when Medicare may be secondary include the following:

1. Group coverage
   - Disability (large group health plan)
   - End-stage renal disease
   - Working aged
2. Liability coverage
   - Automobile
   - Commercial
   - Homeowner
3. Work-related illness/injury
   - Black lung
   - Veterans' benefits
   - Workers' compensation

TRICARE: Insert sponsor's branch of service, using abbreviations (e.g., United States Air Force = USAF).

FIELD 11c C

COMMERCIAL PAYERS: For secondary insurance, insert the name of the primary insurance plan; otherwise, leave blank.

MEDICARE: Do not complete.

Medicare/Medicaid: Do not complete.

Medicare/Medigap: Do not complete.

MSP: Insert the complete name of the insurance plan or program that is primary to Medicare. Include the primary payer's claim processing address directly on the EOB.

TRICARE: Insert TRICARE.

FIELD 11d ⒞

COMMERCIAL PAYERS: Mark "yes" or "no" to indicate whether there is another health plan. If "yes," Fields 9a through 9d must be completed.

MEDICARE: Do not complete.

Medicare/Medicaid: Do not complete.

Medicare/Medigap: Do not complete.

MSP: Do not complete.

TRICARE: Mark "yes" or "no" to indicate if there is another health plan. If "yes," Fields 9a through 9d must be completed.

FIELD 12 ⓡ

READ BACK OF FORM BEFORE COMPLETING & SIGNING THIS FORM.	
12. PATIENT'S OR AUTHORIZED PERSON'S SIGNATURE I authorize the release of any medical or other information necessary to process this claim. I also request payment of government benefits either to myself or to the party who accepts assignment below.	13. INSURED'S OR AUTHORIZED PERSON'S SIGNATURE I authorize payment of medical benefits to the undersigned physician or supplier for services described below.
SIGNED _Caleb S Mitchell_ DATE _03/20/20xx_	SIGNED _Caleb S Mitchell_

or

READ BACK OF FORM BEFORE COMPLETING & SIGNING THIS FORM.	
12. PATIENT'S OR AUTHORIZED PERSON'S SIGNATURE I authorize the release of any medical or other information necessary to process this claim. I also request payment of government benefits either to myself or to the party who accepts assignment below.	13. INSURED'S OR AUTHORIZED PERSON'S SIGNATURE I authorize payment of medical benefits to the undersigned physician or supplier for services described below.
SIGNED _SIGNATURE ON FILE_ DATE	SIGNED _SIGNATURE ON FILE_

COMMERCIAL PAYERS: Release of medical information for claims processing is indicated by a signature here. Have the patient or the authorized representative sign and date this field. If the patient has signed a consent form, "Signature on File" can be entered here. Some carriers accept the acronym "SOF." The consent form must be current, may be lifetime, and must be in the physician's file. When the patient's representative signs, the relationship to the patient must be indicated. If the signature is indicated by a mark (X), a witness must sign his or her name and insert the address next to the mark.

Workbook Exercises: The abbreviation "SOF" can be used.

MEDICARE: Payment of benefits to the physician (if the physician accepts assignment) *and* release of medical information for claims processing is indicated by a signature here. Have the patient or the authorized representative sign and date this field. If the patient has signed a consent form, "Signature on File" can be typed here. Be sure the form includes both authorizations just mentioned. The form must be current, may be lifetime, and must be in the physician's file. When the patient's representative signs, the relationship to

the patient **must** be indicated. If the signature is by mark (X), a witness must sign his or her name and enter the address next to the mark.

Medicare/Medicaid: Follow Medicare guidelines.

Medicare/Medigap: Follow Medicare guidelines.

MSP: Follow Medicare guidelines.

TRICARE: Authorization of payment of benefits to the physician (if the physician accepts assignment) and release of medical information for claims processing is indicated by a signature here. Have the patient or the authorized representative sign and date this field. If the patient has signed a consent form, "Signature on File" or "SOF" can be inserted here. Be sure the form includes both authorizations just mentioned. The form must be current, may be lifetime, and must be in the physician's file. When the patient's representative signs, the relationship to the patient **must** be indicated. If the signature is by mark (X), a witness must sign his or her name and enter the address next to the mark.

Workbook Exercises: The abbreviation "SOF" can be used.

FIELD 13 C

READ BACK OF FORM BEFORE COMPLETING & SIGNING THIS FORM.	13. INSURED'S OR AUTHORIZED PERSON'S SIGNATURE I authorize payment of medical benefits to the undersigned physician or supplier for services described below.
12. PATIENT'S OR AUTHORIZED PERSON'S SIGNATURE I authorize the release of any medical or other information necessary to process this claim. I also request payment of government benefits either to myself or to the party who accepts assignment below.	
SIGNED Caleb S Mitchell DATE 03/20/20XX	SIGNED Caleb S Mitchell

or

READ BACK OF FORM BEFORE COMPLETING & SIGNING THIS FORM.	13. INSURED'S OR AUTHORIZED PERSON'S SIGNATURE I authorize payment of medical benefits to the undersigned physician or supplier for services described below.
12. PATIENT'S OR AUTHORIZED PERSON'S SIGNATURE I authorize the release of any medical or other information necessary to process this claim. I also request payment of government benefits either to myself or to the party who accepts assignment below.	
SIGNED SIGNATURE ON FILE DATE	SIGNED SIGNATURE ON FILE

COMMERCIAL PAYERS: Insert patient's signature when benefits are assigned. The abbreviation "SOF" may be used if the patient's signature is on file.

MEDICARE: Do not complete.

Medicare/Medicaid: Do not complete.

Medicare/Medigap: Participating providers should obtain a signature to authorize payment of "mandated" Medigap benefits when required Medigap information is included in Fields 9 through 9d. Insert the signature of the patient or authorized representative, or insert "Signature on File" if the signature is on file as a separate Medigap authorization.

MSP: The signature of the patient or authorized representative should appear in this block or insert "SOF" if the signature is on file for benefits assigned from the primary carrier.

TRICARE: Do not complete.

FIELD 14 C

14. DATE OF CURRENT: ILLNESS (First symptom) OR INJURY (Accident) OR PREGNANCY(LMP) MM DD YY 02 16 20XX	15. IF PATIENT HAS HAD SAME OR SIMILAR ILLNESS. GIVE FIRST DATE MM DD YY	16. DATES PATIENT UNABLE TO WORK IN CURRENT OCCUPATION FROM 03 24 20XX TO 04 07 20XX
17. NAME OF REFERRING PROVIDER OR OTHER SOURCE THOMAS ROTHSCHILD MD	17a. / 17b. NPI 23345678XX	18. HOSPITALIZATION DATES RELATED TO CURRENT SERVICES FROM 03 24 20XX TO 03 30 20XX
19. RESERVED FOR LOCAL USE		20. OUTSIDE LAB? ☐ YES ☒ NO $ CHARGES

COMMERCIAL PAYERS: Insert the eight-digit date the patient's first symptoms occurred from the current illness, if stated in the medical record; date of injury or accident; or for pregnancy, first day of last menstrual period. For chiropractic treatment, enter the eight-digit date that treatment began.

MEDICARE: Insert the eight-digit date the patient's first symptoms occurred from the current illness, if stated in the medical record; date of injury or accident; or for pregnancy, first day of last menstrual period. For chiropractic treatment, insert the eight-digit date that treatment began.

Medicare/Medicaid: Follow Medicare guidelines.

Medicare/Medigap: Follow Medicare guidelines.

MSP: Follow Medicare guidelines.

TRICARE: Insert the eight-digit date the patient's first symptoms occurred from the current illness, if stated in the medical record; date of injury or accident; or for pregnancy, first day of last menstrual period. For chiropractic treatment, insert the eight-digit date that treatment began.

FIELD 15 C

14. DATE OF CURRENT: ILLNESS (First symptom) OR INJURY (Accident) OR PREGNANCY(LMP) MM DD YY 02 16 20XX	15. IF PATIENT HAS HAD SAME OR SIMILAR ILLNESS. GIVE FIRST DATE MM DD YY	16. DATES PATIENT UNABLE TO WORK IN CURRENT OCCUPATION FROM 03 24 20XX TO 04 07 20XX
17. NAME OF REFERRING PROVIDER OR OTHER SOURCE THOMAS ROTHSCHILD MD	17a. / 17b. NPI 23345678XX	18. HOSPITALIZATION DATES RELATED TO CURRENT SERVICES FROM 03 24 20XX TO 03 30 20XX
19. RESERVED FOR LOCAL USE		20. OUTSIDE LAB? ☐ YES ☒ NO $ CHARGES

COMMERCIAL PAYERS: Insert eight-digit date when patient had same or similar illness, if applicable, and documented in the medical record.

MEDICARE: Do not complete.

Medicare/Medicaid: Do not complete.

Medicare/Medigap: Do not complete.

MSP: Do not complete.

TRICARE: Insert eight-digit date when patient had same or similar illness, if applicable, and documented in the medical record.

FIELD 16 ©

14. DATE OF CURRENT: MM DD YY 02 16 20XX	ILLNESS (First symptom) OR INJURY (Accident) OR PREGNANCY(LMP)	15. IF PATIENT HAS HAD SAME OR SIMILAR ILLNESS. GIVE FIRST DATE MM DD YY	16. DATES PATIENT UNABLE TO WORK IN CURRENT OCCUPATION MM DD YY MM DD YY FROM 03 24 20XX TO 04 07 20XX
17. NAME OF REFERRING PROVIDER OR OTHER SOURCE THOMAS ROTHSCHILD MD	17a. 17b. NPI 23345678XX		18. HOSPITALIZATION DATES RELATED TO CURRENT SERVICES MM DD YY MM DD YY FROM 03 24 20XX TO 03 30 20XX
19. RESERVED FOR LOCAL USE			20. OUTSIDE LAB? ☐ YES ☒ NO $ CHARGES

COMMERCIAL PAYERS: Insert eight-digit dates patient is employed but cannot work in current occupation. *From:* Enter first *full* day patient was unable to perform job duties. *To:* Enter last day patient was disabled before returning to work.

MEDICARE: Insert six- or eight-digit dates patient is employed but cannot work in current occupation. *From:* Enter first *full* day patient was unable to perform job duties. *To:* Enter last day patient was disabled before returning to work.

Medicare/Medicaid: Follow Medicare guidelines.

Medicare/Medigap: Follow Medicare guidelines.

MSP: Follow Medicare guidelines.

TRICARE: Follow commercial guidelines.

FIELD 17 ©

14. DATE OF CURRENT: MM DD YY 02 16 20XX	ILLNESS (First symptom) OR INJURY (Accident) OR PREGNANCY(LMP)	15. IF PATIENT HAS HAD SAME OR SIMILAR ILLNESS. GIVE FIRST DATE MM DD YY	16. DATES PATIENT UNABLE TO WORK IN CURRENT OCCUPATION MM DD YY MM DD YY FROM 03 24 20XX TO 04 07 20XX
17. NAME OF REFERRING PROVIDER OR OTHER SOURCE THOMAS ROTHSCHILD MD	17a. 17b. NPI 23345678XX		18. HOSPITALIZATION DATES RELATED TO CURRENT SERVICES MM DD YY MM DD YY FROM 03 24 20XX TO 03 30 20XX
19. RESERVED FOR LOCAL USE			20. OUTSIDE LAB? ☐ YES ☒ NO $ CHARGES

COMMERCIAL PAYERS: Insert complete name and degree of referring physician, when applicable. Do not list other referrals (i.e., friends or family).

MEDICARE: Insert the name and degree of referring or ordering physician on all claims for Medicare-covered services and items resulting from a physician's order or referral. Use a separate claim form for each referring and/or ordering physician.

Surgeon: All surgeons must complete this block for Medicare claims. Insert the primary surgeon's name if the patient has not been referred and on an assistant's surgeon's claim.

Referring physician: When a physician refers a patient to another physician for a service, insert the referring physician's name. When a physician extender (e.g., nurse practitioner) refers a patient for a consultation, enter the name of the physician supervising the physician extender.

Ordering physician: A physician who orders non-physician services for the patient, such as diagnostic radiology, laboratory, pathology tests; pharmaceutical services; durable medical equipment (DME); parenteral and enteral nutrition; immunosuppressive drugs.

When the ordering physician is also the performing physician (e.g., the physician who actually performs the in-office laboratory tests), the performing physician's name and assigned NPI number must appear in Fields 17 and 17b.

When a patient is referred to a physician who also orders and performs a diagnostic service, *a separate claim* form is required for the diagnostic service.

- Insert the original referring physician's name and NPI in Fields 17 and 17b of the first claim form.

- Insert the ordering (performing) physician's name and NPI in Fields 17 and 17b of the second claim form.

Medicare/Medicaid: Follow Medicare guidelines.

Medicare/Medigap: Follow Medicare guidelines.

MSP: Follow Medicare guidelines.

TRICARE: Insert name, degree, and address (optional) of referring provider for all consultation claims. If the patient was referred from a military treatment facility (MTF), insert the name of the MTF and attach DD Form 2161 or SF 513, "Referral for Civilian Medical Care."

FIELD 17a **C**

14. DATE OF CURRENT: ILLNESS (First symptom) OR INJURY (Accident) OR PREGNANCY(LMP) MM 02 DD 16 YY 20XX	15. IF PATIENT HAS HAD SAME OR SIMILAR ILLNESS. GIVE FIRST DATE MM DD YY	16. DATES PATIENT UNABLE TO WORK IN CURRENT OCCUPATION MM DD YY MM DD YY FROM 03 24 20XX TO 04 07 20XX
17. NAME OF REFERRING PROVIDER OR OTHER SOURCE THOMAS ROTHSCHILD MD	17a. 17b. NPI 23345678XX	18. HOSPITALIZATION DATES RELATED TO CURRENT SERVICES MM DD YY MM DD YY FROM 03 24 20XX TO 03 30 20XX
19. RESERVED FOR LOCAL USE		20. OUTSIDE LAB? YES ☒ NO $ CHARGES

ALL THIRD PARTY PAYERS: Effective 5/23/07 the UPIN is no longer accepted in this field; the NPI must be submitted in Field 17b.

FIELD 17b **C**

14. DATE OF CURRENT: ILLNESS (First symptom) OR INJURY (Accident) OR PREGNANCY(LMP) MM 02 DD 16 YY 20XX	15. IF PATIENT HAS HAD SAME OR SIMILAR ILLNESS. GIVE FIRST DATE MM DD YY	16. DATES PATIENT UNABLE TO WORK IN CURRENT OCCUPATION MM DD YY MM DD YY FROM 03 24 20XX TO 04 07 20XX
17. NAME OF REFERRING PROVIDER OR OTHER SOURCE THOMAS ROTHSCHILD MD	17a. 17b. NPI 23345678XX	18. HOSPITALIZATION DATES RELATED TO CURRENT SERVICES MM DD YY MM DD YY FROM 03 24 20XX TO 03 30 20XX
19. RESERVED FOR LOCAL USE		20. OUTSIDE LAB? YES ☒ NO $ CHARGES

COMMERCIAL PAYERS: Insert the referring physician's NPI number.

MEDICARE: Insert the CMS-assigned NPI number of the referring or ordering physician (or the supervising physician for a physician extender) as detailed in Medicare Field 17.

Medicare/Medicaid: Follow Medicare guidelines.

Medicare/Medigap: Follow Medicare guidelines.

MSP: Follow Medicare guidelines.

TRICARE: Insert the referring physician's state license number. Leave blank if the patient is referred from a military treatment facility.

FIELD 18 **C**

14. DATE OF CURRENT: ILLNESS (First symptom) OR INJURY (Accident) OR PREGNANCY(LMP) MM 02 DD 16 YY 20XX	15. IF PATIENT HAS HAD SAME OR SIMILAR ILLNESS. GIVE FIRST DATE MM DD YY	16. DATES PATIENT UNABLE TO WORK IN CURRENT OCCUPATION MM DD YY MM DD YY FROM 03 24 20XX TO 04 07 20XX
17. NAME OF REFERRING PROVIDER OR OTHER SOURCE THOMAS ROTHSCHILD MD	17a. 17b. NPI 23345678XX	18. HOSPITALIZATION DATES RELATED TO CURRENT SERVICES MM DD YY MM DD YY FROM 03 24 20XX TO 03 30 20XX
19. RESERVED FOR LOCAL USE		20. OUTSIDE LAB? YES ☒ NO $ CHARGES

ALL THIRD-PARTY PAYERS: Insert six or eight-digit admitting and discharge dates in this field when a medical service is furnished as a result of, or subsequent to, a related (inpatient) hospitalization, skilled nursing facility, or nursing home visit. Do not complete for outpatient hospital services, ambulatory surgery, or emergency department services. If the patient is still hospitalized at the time of the billing, enter eight zeros in the "TO" field.

FIELD 19 ©

14. DATE OF CURRENT:		ILLNESS (First symptom) OR INJURY (Accident) OR PREGNANCY(LMP)	15. IF PATIENT HAS HAD SAME OR SIMILAR ILLNESS. GIVE FIRST DATE MM DD YY	16. DATES PATIENT UNABLE TO WORK IN CURRENT OCCUPATION
MM DD YY 02 16 20XX				FROM 03 24 20XX TO 04 07 20XX

17. NAME OF REFERRING PROVIDER OR OTHER SOURCE	17a.		18. HOSPITALIZATION DATES RELATED TO CURRENT SERVICES
THOMAS ROTHSCHILD MD	17b. NPI	23345678XX	FROM 03 24 20XX TO 03 30 20XX

19. RESERVED FOR LOCAL USE	20. OUTSIDE LAB? ☐ YES ☒ NO $ CHARGES

COMMERCIAL PAYERS: Depending on commercial carrier guidelines this field may be completed in a number of different ways. Some examples are:

- Insert the word "ATTACHMENT" when an operative report, discharge summary, invoice, or other attachment is included.

- Insert an explanation regarding unusual services or unlisted services.

- Insert all applicable modifiers when modifier -99 is used in Field 24D (see Example A-1). If -99 appears with more than one procedure code, list the line number (24-1, 2, 3, and so on) for each -99 listed.

- Insert the drug name and dosage when submitting a claim for not otherwise (NOC) classified drugs. Enter the word "ATTACHMENT" and attach the invoice.

- List the supply when the code 99070 is used.

- Insert the x-ray date for chiropractic treatment.

MEDICARE: CMS guidelines state this field may be completed in a number of different ways depending on the circumstances of the services provided to the patient. This field can only contain up to three conditions per claim. Some common uses are:

- When submitting a claim for not otherwise classified (NOC) drugs, enter the drug's name and dosage. Enter the word "ATTACHMENT" and include a copy of the invoice.

- For *unlisted procedures* include a description. If there is not sufficient room in this field, send an attachment.

- When modifier -99 is used in Field 24D (e.g., 99–80 51), enter all applicable modifiers. If -99 appears with more than one procedure code, list the line number (1, 2, 3, and so on) for each -99 listed.

- When an independent laboratory renders an electrocardiogram or collects a specimen from a patient who is homebound or institutionalized enter, "Homebound."

- When a Medicare beneficiary refuses to assign benefits to a participating provider, enter the statement "Patient refuses to assign benefits." No payment to the physician will be made on the claim in this case.

- When submitting a claim to obtain an intentional denial from Medicare as the primary payer for hearing aid testing and a secondary payer is involved, enter "Testing for hearing aid."

- When a dental examination is being performed, enter the name of the specific dental surgery.

- When billing for low osmolar contrast material for which there is no Level 2 HCPCS code, enter the name and dosage.

- When providers share postoperative care for global surgery claims, enter either a six- or eight-digit assumed and relinquished dates of care for each provider.

- When a physician gives service to a hospice patient but the hospice in which the patient resides does not employ the physician, enter the statement "Attending physician, not hospice employee."

- When a purchased interpretation of a diagnostic test is performed, enter the NPI of the performing physician.

Medicare/Medicaid: Follow Medicare guidelines.

Medicare/Medigap: Follow Medicare guidelines.

MSP: Follow Medicare guidelines.

TRICARE: This block is typically reserved for local use (e.g., to indicate referral authorization number or enter x-ray date for chiropractic treatment).

FIELD 20 Ⓒ

14. DATE OF CURRENT:	ILLNESS (First symptom) OR INJURY (Accident) OR PREGNANCY(LMP)	15. IF PATIENT HAS HAD SAME OR SIMILAR ILLNESS. GIVE FIRST DATE MM | DD | YY	16. DATES PATIENT UNABLE TO WORK IN CURRENT OCCUPATION
MM 02 | DD 16 | YY 20XX			FROM 03 | 24 | 20XX TO 04 | 07 | 20XX
17. NAME OF REFERRING PROVIDER OR OTHER SOURCE THOMAS ROTHSCHILD MD	17a. 17b. NPI 23345678XX		18. HOSPITALIZATION DATES RELATED TO CURRENT SERVICES FROM 03 | 24 | 20XX TO 03 | 30 | 20XX
19. RESERVED FOR LOCAL USE			20. OUTSIDE LAB? ☐ YES ☒ NO $ CHARGES

COMMERCIAL PAYERS: Insert "yes" when billing for diagnostic laboratory tests that were performed *outside* the physician's office. Typically "No" is inserted, which means the tests were performed by the billing physician in the office laboratory. If "yes," enter purchase price of the test in the Charges portion of this field and complete Field 32.

MEDICARE: Complete this field ONLY when billing purchased diagnostic laboratory tests. Typically "No" is inserted, which means the tests were performed by the billing physician/laboratory. "Yes" means that the laboratory test was performed *outside* of the physician's office and that the physician is billing for the laboratory service. If "yes," enter purchase price of the test in the Charges portion of this field and complete Field 32. *Note: All clinical laboratory services must be billed to Medicare on an assigned basis.*

Medicare/Medicaid: Follow Medicare guidelines.

Medicare/Medigap: Follow Medicare guidelines.

MSP: Follow Medicare guidelines.

TRICARE: Follow commercial guidelines.

FIELD 21 ⬤R

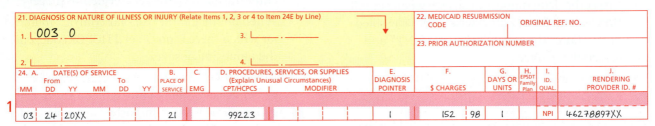

ALL THIRD-PARTY PAYERS: Insert up to four diagnostic codes in priority order, with the primary diagnosis in the first position. Codes must be carried out to their highest degree of specificity. Do not use decimal points or add any code narratives. Attach descriptions of unlisted codes. Code only the conditions or problems that the physician is actively treating and that relate directly to the services billed. *Note: Effective 7/1/07, Medicare accepts up to a maximum of 8 diagnostic codes on both paper and electronic claims. Codes not accommodated in Field 21 may be entered in Field 19. Check with private and other governmental programs to verify their guidelines regarding this.*

FIELD 22 Ⓒ

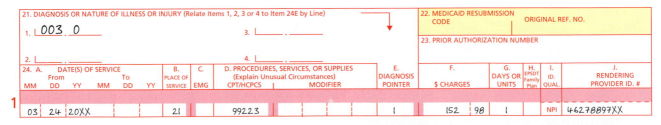

COMMERCIAL PAYERS: Do not complete.

MEDICARE: Do not complete.

Medicare/Medicaid: Do not complete.

Medicare/Medigap: Do not complete.

MSP: Do not complete.

TRICARE: Do not complete.

FIELD 23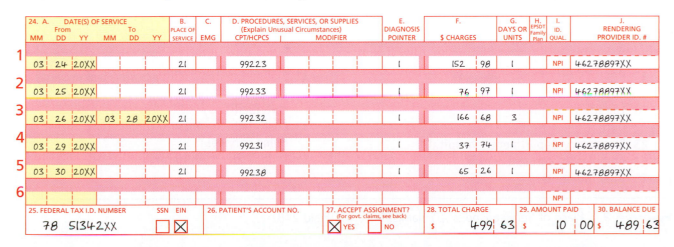

21. DIAGNOSIS OR NATURE OF ILLNESS OR INJURY (Relate Items 1, 2, 3 or 4 to Item 24E by Line)				22. MEDICAID RESUBMISSION CODE	ORIGINAL REF. NO.
1. 003 . 0	3. ___ . ___				
2. ___ . ___	4. ___ . ___			23. PRIOR AUTHORIZATION NUMBER	

24. A. DATE(S) OF SERVICE						B. PLACE OF SERVICE	C. EMG	D. PROCEDURES, SERVICES, OR SUPPLIES (Explain Unusual Circumstances) CPT/HCPCS	MODIFIER	E. DIAGNOSIS POINTER	F. $ CHARGES	G. DAYS OR UNITS	H. EPSDT Family Plan	I. ID. QUAL.	J. RENDERING PROVIDER ID. #
From MM	DD	YY	To MM	DD	YY										
03	24	20XX				21		99223		1	152 98	1		NPI	46278897XX

COMMERCIAL PAYERS: Insert the quality improvement-organization (QIO) professional or 10-digit prior authorization number when applicable.

MEDICARE: CMS guidelines state this field may be completed in a number of different ways depending on the circumstances of the services provided to the patient. Some common uses are:

- Insert the 10-digit prior authorization or pre-certification number for procedures requiring PRO prior approval.
- Insert the investigational device exemption (IDE) number if billing for an investigational device.
- Insert the 10-digit CLIA (Clinical Laboratory Improvement Amendments) federal certification number when billing for laboratory services billed by a physician office laboratory.
- Insert the 6-digit Medicare provider number of the hospice or home health agency (HHA) when billing for care plan oversight services.

Medicare/Medicaid: Follow Medicare guidelines.

Medicare/Medigap: Follow Medicare guidelines.

MSP: Follow Medicare guidelines.

TRICARE: Insert the professional (peer) review organization (PRO) 10-digit prior authorization or precertification number for procedures requiring PRO prior approval. Enter the investigational device exemption (IDE) number when billing for an investigational device. Attach a copy of the authorization.

FIELDS 24A–24J

Each of the six lines in **Fields 24A through J** have been divided horizontally to accommodate submission of both the NPI and legacy identifier number during the NPI transition period, which has passed. The shaded areas may not be used to bill 12 lines of service. Additional information must be entered on a separate claim form if the case requires more than six detail lines; treat it as an independent claim totaling all charges on each claim. Claims cannot be "continued" from one to another. Do not list a procedure on the claim form for which there is no charge. Use the top portion (shaded area) to report supplemental information for all carriers except Medicare. Use the bottom portion to enter data, i.e., dates of service, place of service, *CPT* codes and so forth for each field being used.

24. A. DATE(S) OF SERVICE						B. PLACE OF SERVICE	C. EMG	D. PROCEDURES, SERVICES, OR SUPPLIES (Explain Unusual Circumstances) CPT/HCPCS	MODIFIER	E. DIAGNOSIS POINTER	F. $ CHARGES	G. DAYS OR UNITS	H. EPSDT Family Plan	I. ID. QUAL.	J. RENDERING PROVIDER ID. #
From MM	DD	YY	To MM	DD	YY										
03	24	20XX				21		99223		1	152 98	1		NPI	46278897XX
03	25	20XX				21		99233		1	76 97	1		NPI	46278897XX
03	26	20XX	03	28	20XX	21		99232		1	166 68	3		NPI	46278897XX
03	29	20XX				21		99231		1	37 74	1		NPI	46278897XX
03	30	20XX				21		99238		1	65 26	1		NPI	46278897XX
														NPI	

25. FEDERAL TAX I.D. NUMBER	SSN	EIN	26. PATIENT'S ACCOUNT NO.	27. ACCEPT ASSIGNMENT? (For govt. claims, see back)	28. TOTAL CHARGE	29. AMOUNT PAID	30. BALANCE DUE
78 51342XX	☐	☒		☒ YES ☐ NO	$ 499 63	$ 10 00	$ 489 63

COMMERCIAL PAYERS: Insert the month, day, and year (eight digits with no spaces) for each procedure, service, or supply reported in Field 24D. Make sure the dates shown are no earlier than the date of the current illness if listed in Field 14. If the "from" and "to" dates are the same, enter only the "from" date. Enter the "to" date when reporting a consecutive range of dates for the same procedure code. Use a separate line for each month and a separate claim form for a different year.

MEDICARE: Insert the month, day, and year (six or eight digits with no spaces) for each procedure, service, or supply reported in Field 24D. Make sure the dates shown are no earlier than the date of the current illness if listed in Field 14. If the "from" and "to" dates are the same, enter only the "from" date. Enter the "to" date when reporting a consecutive range of dates for the same procedure code. Use a separate line

for each month except when reporting weekly radiation therapy, durable medical equipment, or oxygen rental. Use a separate claim form for a new year.

Medicare/Medicaid: Follow Medicare guidelines.

Medicare/Medigap: Follow Medicare guidelines.

MSP: Follow Medicare guidelines.

TRICARE: Insert the month, day, and year (eight digits with no spaces) for each procedure, service, or supply reported in Field 24D. Make sure the dates shown are no earlier than the date of the current illness if listed in Field 14. If the "from" and "to" dates are the same, enter only the "from" date. Insert the "to" date when reporting a consecutive range of dates for the same procedure code. Use a separate line for each month and a separate claim for each year.

FIELD 24B ®

24. A. DATE(S) OF SERVICE						B. PLACE OF SERVICE	C. EMG	D. PROCEDURES, SERVICES, OR SUPPLIES (Explain Unusual Circumstances) CPT/HCPCS	MODIFIER	E. DIAGNOSIS POINTER	F. $ CHARGES		G. DAYS OR UNITS	H. EPSDT Family Plan	I. ID. QUAL.	J. RENDERING PROVIDER ID. #
MM	DD	YY	MM	DD	YY											
1 03	24	20XX				21		99223		1	152	98	1		NPI	46278897XX
2 03	25	20XX				21		99233		1	76	97	1		NPI	46278897XX
3 03	26	20XX	03	28	20XX	21		99232		1	166	68	3		NPI	46278897XX
4 03	29	20XX				21		99231		1	37	74	1		NPI	46278897XX
5 03	30	20XX				21		99238		1	65	26	1		NPI	46278897XX
6															NPI	

25. FEDERAL TAX I.D. NUMBER	SSN	EIN	26. PATIENT'S ACCOUNT NO.	27. ACCEPT ASSIGNMENT? (For govt. claims, see back)	28. TOTAL CHARGE	29. AMOUNT PAID	30. BALANCE DUE
78 51342XX	☐	☒		☒ YES ☐ NO	$ 499 63	$ 10 00	$ 489 63

ALL THIRD-PARTY PAYERS: Insert the appropriate "Place of Service" code shown in Figure A-2. Identify by location where the service was performed or an item was used. Use the inpatient hospital code only when a service is provided to a patient admitted to the hospital for an overnight stay. Enter the name, address, and provider number of the hospital in Field 32.

11 Doctor's Office	31 Skilled nursing facility (swing bed visits)
12 Patient's Home	32 Nursing facility (intermediate/long-term care facilities)
21 Inpatient hospital	33 Custodial care facility (domiciliary or rest home services)
22 Outpatient hospital	
23 Emergency Department—hospital	81 Independent laboratory
24 Ambulatory surgical center	
25 Birthing center	

Figure A-2. Place of Service Codes; partial list (insert in Field 24B)

FIELD 24C C

24. A. DATE(S) OF SERVICE From / To						B. PLACE OF SERVICE	C. EMG	D. PROCEDURES, SERVICES, OR SUPPLIES (Explain Unusual Circumstances) CPT/HCPCS / MODIFIER		E. DIAGNOSIS POINTER	F. $ CHARGES		G. DAYS OR UNITS	H. EPSDT Family Plan	I. ID. QUAL.	J. RENDERING PROVIDER ID. #
MM	DD	YY	MM	DD	YY											
1	03	24	20XX				21		99223		1	152	98	1		NPI	46278897XX
2	03	25	20XX				21		99233		1	76	97	1		NPI	46278897XX
3	03	26	20XX	03	28	20XX	21		99232		1	166	68	3		NPI	46278897XX
4	03	29	20XX				21		99231		1	37	74	1		NPI	46278897XX
5	03	30	20XX				21		99238		1	65	26	1		NPI	46278897XX
6															NPI	

25. FEDERAL TAX I.D. NUMBER	SSN	EIN	26. PATIENT'S ACCOUNT NO.	27. ACCEPT ASSIGNMENT? (For govt. claims, see back)	28. TOTAL CHARGE	29. AMOUNT PAID	30. BALANCE DUE
78 51342XX	☐	☒		☒ YES ☐ NO	$ 499 63	$ 10 00	$ 489 63

COMMERCIAL PAYERS: Do not complete.

MEDICARE: Do not complete.

Medicare/Medicaid: Do not complete.

Medicare/Medigap: Do not complete.

MSP: Do not complete.

TRICARE: Insert "Y" (yes) in the bottom unshaded area of this field to indicate the service was provided in a hospital emergency department; leave blank if it does not apply.

FIELD 24D R

24. A. DATE(S) OF SERVICE From / To						B. PLACE OF SERVICE	C. EMG	D. PROCEDURES, SERVICES, OR SUPPLIES (Explain Unusual Circumstances) CPT/HCPCS / MODIFIER		E. DIAGNOSIS POINTER	F. $ CHARGES		G. DAYS OR UNITS	H. EPSDT Family Plan	I. ID. QUAL.	J. RENDERING PROVIDER ID. #
MM	DD	YY	MM	DD	YY											
1	03	24	20XX				21		99223		1	152	98	1		NPI	46278897XX
2	03	25	20XX				21		99233		1	76	97	1		NPI	46278897XX
3	03	26	20XX	03	28	20XX	21		99232		1	166	68	3		NPI	46278897XX
4	03	29	20XX				21		99231		1	37	74	1		NPI	46278897XX
5	03	30	20XX				21		99238		1	65	26	1		NPI	46278897XX
6															NPI	

25. FEDERAL TAX I.D. NUMBER	SSN	EIN	26. PATIENT'S ACCOUNT NO.	27. ACCEPT ASSIGNMENT? (For govt. claims, see back)	28. TOTAL CHARGE	29. AMOUNT PAID	30. BALANCE DUE
78 51342XX	☐	☒		☒ YES ☐ NO	$ 499 63	$ 10 00	$ 489 63

COMMERCIAL PAYERS: Insert the appropriate *CPT/ HCPCS* code for each procedure, service, or supply and applicable modifier without a hyphen. Up to four modifiers may be placed per line of service. Some carriers may still accept use of multiple modifier -99 with the modifiers listed in Field 19.

MEDICARE: Insert one *CPT/HCPCS* code and applicable modifiers (up to four) for each line of service representing a procedure, service, or supply. Do not include a hyphen or narrative description. When procedure codes do not require modifiers, leave modifier area blank. List the procedure with the highest fee first for multiple surgical procedures. For unlisted procedure codes a narrative description to support the billed service may be listed in the shaded portion of Field 24D, or it may be listed in Field 19 (e.g., 99499, "Unlisted Evaluation and Management Service"). If information does not fit in this area, include an attachment. Submit an operative note as a claim attachment when inserting an unlisted surgery code.

Medicare/Medicaid: Follow Medicare guidelines.

Medicare/Medigap: Follow Medicare guidelines.

MSP: Follow Medicare guidelines.

TRICARE: Insert the appropriate *CPT/HCPCS* code for each procedure, service, or supply and applicable mod-ifier without a hyphen. When not otherwise classified (NOC) codes are submitted (e.g., supplies and injections), provide a narrative of the service in the shaded portion of Field 24D, in Field 19, or on an attachment.

FIELD 24E ®

21. DIAGNOSIS OR NATURE OF ILLNESS OR INJURY (Relate Items 1, 2, 3 or 4 to Item 24E by Line)							22. MEDICAID RESUBMISSION CODE / ORIGINAL REF. NO.

1. | 003 . 0 | 3. |_____._____| 23. PRIOR AUTHORIZATION NUMBER

2. |_____._____| 4. |_____._____|

24. A. DATE(S) OF SERVICE From MM DD YY — To MM DD YY	B. PLACE OF SERVICE	C. EMG	D. PROCEDURES, SERVICES, OR SUPPLIES (Explain Unusual Circumstances) CPT/HCPCS | MODIFIER	E. DIAGNOSIS POINTER	F. $ CHARGES	G. DAYS OR UNITS	H. EPSDT Family Plan	I. ID. QUAL.	J. RENDERING PROVIDER ID. #
1	03 24 20XX	21		99223	1	152 | 98	1		NPI	46278897XX
2	03 25 20XX	21		99233	1	76 | 97	1		NPI	46278897XX
3	03 26 20XX 03 28 20XX	21		99232	1	166 | 68	3		NPI	46278897XX
4	03 29 20XX	21		99231	1	37 | 74	1		NPI	46278897XX
5	03 30 20XX	21		99238	1	65 | 26	1		NPI	46278897XX
6									NPI	

25. FEDERAL TAX I.D. NUMBER SSN EIN	26. PATIENT'S ACCOUNT NO.	27. ACCEPT ASSIGNMENT? (For govt. claims, see back)	28. TOTAL CHARGE	29. AMOUNT PAID	30. BALANCE DUE
78 51342XX ☐ ☒		☒ YES ☐ NO	$ 499 | 63	$ 10 | 00	$ 489 | 63

COMMERCIAL PAYERS: Insert only one diagnosis code reference "pointer" number per line item (unless you have verified that independent carriers allow more than one) linking the diagnostic code listed in Field 21. When multiple services are performed, insert the corresponding diagnostic reference number for each service (e.g., 1, 2, 3, or 4). DO NOT USE ACTUAL *ICD-9-CM* CODES IN THIS FIELD.

Workbook Exercises: More than one diagnosis reference "pointer" number per line item may be used, leaving one space between numbers.

MEDICARE: Insert only one diagnosis code reference "pointer" number per line item linking the diagnostic codes listed in Field 21. DO NOT USE ACTUAL *ICD-9-CM* CODES IN THIS FIELD. When multiple services are performed, enter the corresponding diagnostic reference number for each service (e.g., 1, 2, 3, or 4). Up to four additional diagnosis codes may be listed in Field 19 and will be considered, if needed during claims processing.

Medicare/Medicaid: Follow Medicare guidelines.

Medicare/Medigap: Follow Medicare guidelines.

MSP: Follow Medicare guidelines.

TRICARE: Insert the diagnosis reference number (i.e., indicating up to four *ICD-9-CM* codes) as shown in Field 21 to relate the date of service and the procedures performed to the appropriate diagnosis. If multiple procedures are performed, enter the diagnosis code reference number for each service with one space in between (e.g., 1 2).

FIELD 24F ®

21. DIAGNOSIS OR NATURE OF ILLNESS OR INJURY (Relate Items 1, 2, 3 or 4 to Item 24E by Line)							22. MEDICAID RESUBMISSION CODE	ORIGINAL REF. NO.

1. | 003 . 0 | 3. | ___ . ___ |

23. PRIOR AUTHORIZATION NUMBER

2. | ___ . ___ | 4. | ___ . ___ |

| 24. A. DATE(S) OF SERVICE | | | | | | B. PLACE OF SERVICE | C. EMG | D. PROCEDURES, SERVICES, OR SUPPLIES (Explain Unusual Circumstances) CPT/HCPCS \| MODIFIER | E. DIAGNOSIS POINTER | F. $ CHARGES | | G. DAYS OR UNITS | H. EPSDT Family Plan | I. ID. QUAL. | J. RENDERING PROVIDER ID. # |
From MM	DD	YY	To MM	DD	YY										
1	03	24	20XX				21		99223		1	152	98	1		NPI	46278897XX
2	03	25	20XX				21		99233		1	76	97	1		NPI	46278897XX
3	03	26	20XX	03	28	20XX	21		99232		1	166	68	3		NPI	46278897XX
4	03	29	20XX				21		99231		1	37	74	1		NPI	46278897XX
5	03	30	20XX				21		99238		1	65	26	1		NPI	46278897XX
6															NPI	

25. FEDERAL TAX I.D. NUMBER	SSN	EIN	26. PATIENT'S ACCOUNT NO.	27. ACCEPT ASSIGNMENT? (For govt. claims, see back)	28. TOTAL CHARGE	29. AMOUNT PAID	30. BALANCE DUE
78 51342XX	☐	☒		☒ YES ☐ NO	$ 499 63	$ 10 00	$ 489 63

ALL THIRD-PARTY PAYERS: Insert the fee for each listed service from the appropriate fee schedule. *Do not enter dollar signs or decimal points. Always include cents.* If the same service is performed on consecutive days (see Field 24, line 3), multiply the fee for a single service by the number of times it was performed and enter the total for this line of service (e.g., 55.56 × 3 = 166.68).

Workbook Exercises: For private and TRICARE cases, use the **Mock Fee.** For Medicare participating provider cases, use **the Participating Provider Fee.** For nonparticipating provider cases, use the **Limiting Charge.**

FIELD 24G ®

21. DIAGNOSIS OR NATURE OF ILLNESS OR INJURY (Relate Items 1, 2, 3 or 4 to Item 24E by Line)							22. MEDICAID RESUBMISSION CODE	ORIGINAL REF. NO.

1. | 003 . 0 | 3. | ___ . ___ |

23. PRIOR AUTHORIZATION NUMBER

2. | ___ . ___ | 4. | ___ . ___ |

| 24. A. DATE(S) OF SERVICE | | | | | | B. PLACE OF SERVICE | C. EMG | D. PROCEDURES, SERVICES, OR SUPPLIES (Explain Unusual Circumstances) CPT/HCPCS \| MODIFIER | E. DIAGNOSIS POINTER | F. $ CHARGES | | G. DAYS OR UNITS | H. EPSDT Family Plan | I. ID. QUAL. | J. RENDERING PROVIDER ID. # |
From MM	DD	YY	To MM	DD	YY										
1	03	24	20XX				21		99223		1	152	98	1		NPI	46278897XX
2	03	25	20XX				21		99233		1	76	97	1		NPI	46278897XX
3	03	26	20XX	03	28	20XX	21		99232		1	166	68	3		NPI	46278897XX
4	03	29	20XX				21		99231		1	37	74	1		NPI	46278897XX
5	03	30	20XX				21		99238		1	65	26	1		NPI	46278897XX
6															NPI	

25. FEDERAL TAX I.D. NUMBER	SSN	EIN	26. PATIENT'S ACCOUNT NO.	27. ACCEPT ASSIGNMENT? (For govt. claims, see back)	28. TOTAL CHARGE	29. AMOUNT PAID	30. BALANCE DUE
78 51342XX	☐	☒		☒ YES ☐ NO	$ 499 63	$ 10 00	$ 489 63

COMMERCIAL PAYERS: Insert the number of days or units that apply to each line of service. This field is important for calculating multiple visits, anesthesia minutes, or oxygen volume.

MEDICARE: Insert the number of days or units that apply to each line of service. This field is important for calculating multiple visits, number of miles, units of supplies, drugs, anesthesia minutes, or oxygen volume. For example, when a physician reports consecutive hospital care services using *CPT* code number 99232 on March 26, 27, and 28, it would be listed and totaled as shown in the example.

Medicare/Medicaid: Follow Medicare guidelines.

Medicare/Medigap: Follow Medicare guidelines.

MSP: Follow Medicare guidelines.

TRICARE: Follow Medicare guidelines.

FIELD 24H C

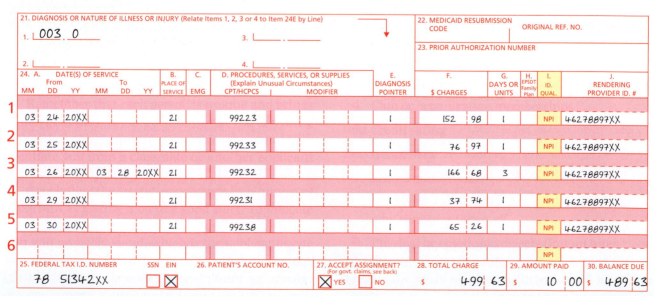

COMMERCIAL PAYERS: Do not complete.

MEDICARE: Do not complete.

Medicare/Medicaid: Do not complete.

Medicare/Medigap: Do not complete.

MSP: Do not complete.

TRICARE: Do not complete. *Note: This field is used for the Medicaid program.*

FIELD 24I C

COMMERCIAL PAYERS: Do not complete.

MEDICARE: Do not complete.

Medicare/Medicaid: Do not complete.

Medicare/Medigap: Do not complete.

MSP: Do not complete.

TRICARE: Do not complete.

FIELD 24J C

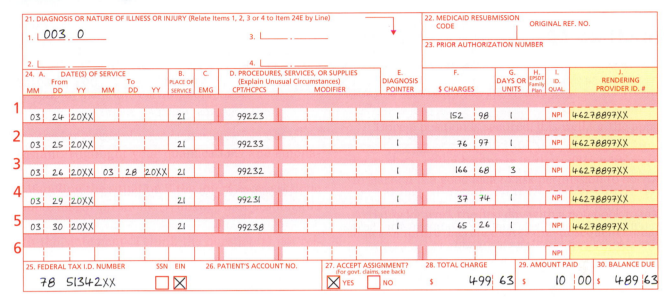

21. DIAGNOSIS OR NATURE OF ILLNESS OR INJURY (Relate Items 1, 2, 3 or 4 to Item 24E by Line)		22. MEDICAID RESUBMISSION CODE	ORIGINAL REF. NO.
1. 003.0	3.		
2.	4.	23. PRIOR AUTHORIZATION NUMBER	

24. A. DATE(S) OF SERVICE From MM DD YY	To MM DD YY	B. PLACE OF SERVICE	C. EMG	D. PROCEDURES, SERVICES, OR SUPPLIES (Explain Unusual Circumstances) CPT/HCPCS / MODIFIER	E. DIAGNOSIS POINTER	F. $ CHARGES	G. DAYS OR UNITS	H. EPSDT Family Plan	I. ID. QUAL.	J. RENDERING PROVIDER ID. #
1 03 24 20XX		21		99223	1	152 98	1		NPI	46278897XX
2 03 25 20XX		21		99233	1	76 97	1		NPI	46278897XX
3 03 26 20XX	03 28 20XX	21		99232	1	166 68	3		NPI	46278897XX
4 03 29 20XX		21		99231	1	37 74	1		NPI	46278897XX
5 03 30 20XX		21		99238	1	65 26	1		NPI	46278897XX
6									NPI	

25. FEDERAL TAX I.D. NUMBER SSN EIN	26. PATIENT'S ACCOUNT NO.	27. ACCEPT ASSIGNMENT? (For govt. claims, see back)	28. TOTAL CHARGE	29. AMOUNT PAID	30. BALANCE DUE
78 51342XX ☐ ☒		☒ YES ☐ NO	$ 499 63	$ 10 00	$ 489 63

COMMERCIAL PAYERS: Effective May 23, 2007, insert the rendering provider's NPI number in the lower, non-shaded portion of the field. For "incident to" services, if the person who ordered the service is not supervising, insert the NPI of the supervisor. Prior to May 23, 2007, the upper, shaded portion was used for non-NPI numbers.

MEDICARE: Effective May 23, 2007, insert the rendering Medicare provider's NPI number in the lower, non-shaded portion of the field. For "incident to" services, if the person who ordered the service is not supervising, enter the NPI of the supervisor. Prior to May 23, 2007, the upper, shaded portion was used for PIN numbers.

Medicare/Medicaid: Follow Medicare guidelines.

Medicare/Medigap: Follow Medicare guidelines.

MSP: Follow Medicare guidelines.

TRICARE: Insert the attending physician's state license number in the lower, non-shaded portion of the field. The state license number is an alpha character followed by six numeric digits. If there are not six digits, enter appropriate number of zero(s) after the alpha character (i.e., Z9876 would be Z009876).

FIELD 24K

This field was deleted on the revised CMS-1500 (08/05) claim form.

FIELD 25 R

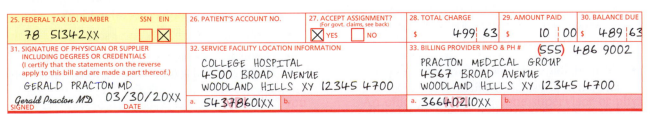

25. FEDERAL TAX I.D. NUMBER SSN EIN	26. PATIENT'S ACCOUNT NO.	27. ACCEPT ASSIGNMENT? (For govt. claims, see back)	28. TOTAL CHARGE	29. AMOUNT PAID	30. BALANCE DUE
78 51342XX ☐ ☒		☒ YES ☐ NO	$ 499 63	$ 10 00	$ 489 63
31. SIGNATURE OF PHYSICIAN OR SUPPLIER INCLUDING DEGREES OR CREDENTIALS (I certify that the statements on the reverse apply to this bill and are made a part thereof.) GERALD PRACTON MD *Gerald Practon MD* 03/30/20XX SIGNED DATE	32. SERVICE FACILITY LOCATION INFORMATION COLLEGE HOSPITAL 4500 BROAD AVENUE WOODLAND HILLS XY 12345 4700 a. 54378601XX b.		33. BILLING PROVIDER INFO & PH # (555) 486 9002 PRACTON MEDICAL GROUP 4567 BROAD AVENUE WOODLAND HILLS XY 12345 4700 a. 36640210XX b.		

ALL THIRD-PARTY PAYERS: Insert the physician/supplier's federal tax I.D. number. This may be the Employer Identification Number (EIN) or Social Security Number (SSN). Mark the corresponding box.

- For Medicaid, check individual state guidelines for this requirement.

- For Medicare/Medigap, the physician's federal tax I.D. number is required for transfer of the Medigap claim.

Workbook Exercises: Enter the physician's Tax I.D. number and mark EIN.

FIELD 26 Ⓒ

25. FEDERAL TAX I.D. NUMBER	SSN	EIN	26. PATIENT'S ACCOUNT NO.	27. ACCEPT ASSIGNMENT? (For govt. claims, see back)	28. TOTAL CHARGE	29. AMOUNT PAID	30. BALANCE DUE
78 51342XX	☐	☒		☒ YES ☐ NO	$ 499 63	$ 10 00	$ 489 63

31. SIGNATURE OF PHYSICIAN OR SUPPLIER INCLUDING DEGREES OR CREDENTIALS (I certify that the statements on the reverse apply to this bill and are made a part thereof.)	32. SERVICE FACILITY LOCATION INFORMATION	33. BILLING PROVIDER INFO & PH # (555) 486 9002
GERALD PRACTON MD *Gerald Practon MD* 03/30/20XX SIGNED DATE	COLLEGE HOSPITAL 4500 BROAD AVENUE WOODLAND HILLS XY 12345 4700 a. 5437860IXX b.	PRACTON MEDICAL GROUP 4567 BROAD AVENUE WOODLAND HILLS XY 12345 4700 a. 36640210XX b.

ALL THIRD-PARTY PAYERS: Insert the patient's account number assigned by the physician's computer system. Do not use punctuation. Complete this field when Medicare is billed electronically.

Workbook Exercises: List the patient account number when provided.

FIELD 27 Ⓡ

25. FEDERAL TAX I.D. NUMBER	SSN	EIN	26. PATIENT'S ACCOUNT NO.	27. ACCEPT ASSIGNMENT? (For govt. claims, see back)	28. TOTAL CHARGE	29. AMOUNT PAID	30. BALANCE DUE
78 51342XX	☐	☒		☒ YES ☐ NO	$ 499 63	$ 10 00	$ 489 63

31. SIGNATURE OF PHYSICIAN OR SUPPLIER INCLUDING DEGREES OR CREDENTIALS (I certify that the statements on the reverse apply to this bill and are made a part thereof.)	32. SERVICE FACILITY LOCATION INFORMATION	33. BILLING PROVIDER INFO & PH # (555) 486 9002
GERALD PRACTON MD *Gerald Practon MD* 03/30/20XX SIGNED DATE	COLLEGE HOSPITAL 4500 BROAD AVENUE WOODLAND HILLS XY 12345 4700 a. 5437860IXX b.	PRACTON MEDICAL GROUP 4567 BROAD AVENUE WOODLAND HILLS XY 12345 4700 a. 36640210XX b.

COMMERCIAL PAYERS: Mark "yes" or "no" to indicate whether the physician accepts assignment of benefits. If yes, then the physician agrees to accept the allowed amount paid by the third party as payment in full plus any copayment and/or deductible.

Workbook Exercises: Mark "yes."

MEDICARE: Mark "yes" or "no" to indicate whether the physician accepts assignment of benefits. If yes, then the physician agrees to accept the allowed amount paid by the third party as payment in full plus any copayment or deductible. If this field is left blank, "no" is assumed, and a participating physician's claim will be denied. The following provider/supplier must file claims on an assignment basis:

- Clinical diagnostic laboratory services performed in physician's office.

- Physicians may accept assignment on clinical laboratory services but not other ser-

vices but should submit two separate claims, one "assigned" for laboratory and one "nonassigned" for other services. Submit all charges on a nonassigned claim, indicating "no" in Field 27, and write "I accept assignment for the clinical laboratory tests" in the shaded portion of Field 24.

- Participating physician and supplier services.

- Medicare/Medicaid physician's services.

- Services of physician assistants, nurse practitioners, clinical nurse specialists, nurse midwives, certified registered nurse anesthetists, clinical psychologists, clinical social workers.

- Ambulatory surgical center services.

- Home dialysis supplies and equipment paid under Method II (monthly capitation payment).

Medicare/Medicaid: Mark "yes."

Medicare/Medigap: Mark "yes."

MSP: Mark "yes" or "no" to indicate whether the physician accepts assignment of benefits for primary insurance and Medicare.

Workbook Exercises: Mark "yes."

TRICARE: Follow Medicare guidelines. Note: participation in TRICARE may be made on a case-by-case basis.

FIELD 28 Ⓡ

25. FEDERAL TAX I.D. NUMBER	SSN	EIN	26. PATIENT'S ACCOUNT NO.	27. ACCEPT ASSIGNMENT? (For govt. claims, see back)	28. TOTAL CHARGE	29. AMOUNT PAID	30. BALANCE DUE
78 5I342XX	☐	☒		☒ YES ☐ NO	$ 499 63	$ 10 00	$ 489 63

| 31. SIGNATURE OF PHYSICIAN OR SUPPLIER INCLUDING DEGREES OR CREDENTIALS (I certify that the statements on the reverse apply to this bill and are made a part thereof.) GERALD PRACTON MD *Gerald Practon MD* 03/30/20XX SIGNED DATE | 32. SERVICE FACILITY LOCATION INFORMATION COLLEGE HOSPITAL 4500 BROAD AVENUE WOODLAND HILLS XY 12345 4700 a. 5437860IXX b. | 33. BILLING PROVIDER INFO & PH # (555) 486 9002 PRACTON MEDICAL GROUP 4567 BROAD AVENUE WOODLAND HILLS XY 12345 4700 a. 366402I0XX b. |

ALL THIRD-PARTY PAYERS: Insert total charges, including cents, for services listed in Field(s) 24F. If more than one unit is listed in Field 24G, multiply the number of units by the charge and list the total amount in 24F. Do not enter dollar signs or decimal points.

FIELD 29 Ⓒ

25. FEDERAL TAX I.D. NUMBER	SSN	EIN	26. PATIENT'S ACCOUNT NO.	27. ACCEPT ASSIGNMENT? (For govt. claims, see back)	28. TOTAL CHARGE	29. AMOUNT PAID	30. BALANCE DUE
78 5I342XX	☐	☒		☒ YES ☐ NO	$ 499 63	$ 10 00	$ 489 63

| 31. SIGNATURE OF PHYSICIAN OR SUPPLIER INCLUDING DEGREES OR CREDENTIALS (I certify that the statements on the reverse apply to this bill and are made a part thereof.) GERALD PRACTON MD *Gerald Practon MD* 03/30/20XX SIGNED DATE | 32. SERVICE FACILITY LOCATION INFORMATION COLLEGE HOSPITAL 4500 BROAD AVENUE WOODLAND HILLS XY 12345 4700 a. 5437860IXX b. | 33. BILLING PROVIDER INFO & PH # (555) 486 9002 PRACTON MEDICAL GROUP 4567 BROAD AVENUE WOODLAND HILLS XY 12345 4700 a. 366402I0XX b. |

COMMERCIAL PAYERS: Insert only the amount paid for the charges listed on the claim.

MEDICARE: Insert only the amount paid for the charges listed on the claim.

Medicare/Medicaid: Follow Medicare guidelines.

Medicare/Medigap: Insert only the amount paid for charges listed on the claim.

MSP: Insert only the amount paid for charges listed on the claim. It is mandatory to enter amount paid by primary carrier and attach an explanation of benefits document when billing Medicare.

TRICARE: Insert only amount paid by other carrier for the charges listed on the claim. If the amount includes payment by any other health insurances, the other health insurance explanation of benefits, other documents, or denial showing the amounts paid must be attached to the claim. Payment from the beneficiary should not be included.

FIELD 30 Ⓒ

25. FEDERAL TAX I.D. NUMBER	SSN	EIN	26. PATIENT'S ACCOUNT NO.	27. ACCEPT ASSIGNMENT? (For govt. claims, see back)	28. TOTAL CHARGE	29. AMOUNT PAID	30. BALANCE DUE
78 5I342XX	☐	☒		☒ YES ☐ NO	$ 499 63	$ 10 00	$ 489 63

| 31. SIGNATURE OF PHYSICIAN OR SUPPLIER INCLUDING DEGREES OR CREDENTIALS (I certify that the statements on the reverse apply to this bill and are made a part thereof.) GERALD PRACTON MD *Gerald Practon MD* 03/30/20XX SIGNED DATE | 32. SERVICE FACILITY LOCATION INFORMATION COLLEGE HOSPITAL 4500 BROAD AVENUE WOODLAND HILLS XY 12345 4700 a. 5437860IXX b. | 33. BILLING PROVIDER INFO & PH # (555) 486 9002 PRACTON MEDICAL GROUP 4567 BROAD AVENUE WOODLAND HILLS XY 12345 4700 a. 366402I0XX b. |

COMMERCIAL PAYERS: Insert balance due on claim (Figures in Field 28 less Field 29).

MEDICARE: Do not complete.

Medicare/Medicaid: Do not complete.

Medicare/Medigap: Do not complete.

MSP: Do not complete.

TRICARE: Insert balance due on claim (Figures in Field 28 less Field 29).

FIELD 31 ®

25. FEDERAL TAX I.D. NUMBER SSN EIN	26. PATIENT'S ACCOUNT NO.	27. ACCEPT ASSIGNMENT? (For govt. claims, see back)	28. TOTAL CHARGE	29. AMOUNT PAID	30. BALANCE DUE
78 51342XX ☐ ☒		☒ YES ☐ NO	$ 499 63	$ 10 00	$ 489 63

31. SIGNATURE OF PHYSICIAN OR SUPPLIER INCLUDING DEGREES OR CREDENTIALS (I certify that the statements on the reverse apply to this bill and are made a part thereof.)	32. SERVICE FACILITY LOCATION INFORMATION	33. BILLING PROVIDER INFO & PH # (555) 486 9002
GERALD PRACTON MD *Gerald Practon MD* 03/30/20XX SIGNED DATE	COLLEGE HOSPITAL 4500 BROAD AVENUE WOODLAND HILLS XY 12345 4700 a. 54378601XX b.	PRACTON MEDICAL GROUP 4567 BROAD AVENUE WOODLAND HILLS XY 12345 4700 a. 36640210XX b.

ALL THIRD-PARTY PAYERS: Type the provider's name and show the signature of the physician or the physician's representative above or below the name. Enter the six- or eight-digit date the form was prepared. Many insurance carriers will accept a stamped signature, but the stamp must be completely inside the block. Do not type the name of the association or corporation. A signature on file may be accepted by some carriers. Guidelines for nonphysician practitioners may vary. See Medicare's Web site, http://www.cms.gov, for Medicare requirements.

FIELD 32 ©

25. FEDERAL TAX I.D. NUMBER SSN EIN	26. PATIENT'S ACCOUNT NO.	27. ACCEPT ASSIGNMENT? (For govt. claims, see back)	28. TOTAL CHARGE	29. AMOUNT PAID	30. BALANCE DUE
78 51342XX ☐ ☒		☒ YES ☐ NO	$ 499 63	$ 10 00	$ 489 63

31. SIGNATURE OF PHYSICIAN OR SUPPLIER INCLUDING DEGREES OR CREDENTIALS (I certify that the statements on the reverse apply to this bill and are made a part thereof.)	32. SERVICE FACILITY LOCATION INFORMATION	33. BILLING PROVIDER INFO & PH # (555) 486 9002
GERALD PRACTON MD *Gerald Practon MD* 03/30/20XX SIGNED DATE	COLLEGE HOSPITAL 4500 BROAD AVENUE WOODLAND HILLS XY 12345 4700 a. 54378601XX b.	PRACTON MEDICAL GROUP 4567 BROAD AVENUE WOODLAND HILLS XY 12345 4700 a. 36640210XX b.

COMMERCIAL PAYERS: Do not complete if the facility furnishing services is the same as that of the biller listed in Field 33. *If other* than home or office, enter the name and address of the facility (e.g., hospital name for physician's hospital services). For durable medical equipment, enter the *location* where the *order is taken.* When billing for purchased diagnostic tests performed outside the physician's office but billed by the physician, insert the facility's name, address, and ZIP code.

MEDICARE: Insert the name and address including ZIP code if the facility furnishing services is other than the patient's home (12). When billing for purchased diagnostic tests performed outside the physician's office but billed by the physician, insert the facility's name and address.

Medicare/Medicaid: Follow Medicare guidelines.

Medicare/Medigap: Follow Medicare guidelines.

MSP: Follow Medicare guidelines.

TRICARE: Follow commercial guidelines. For partnership providers, indicate the name of the military treatment facility.

FIELD 32a Ⓒ

25. FEDERAL TAX I.D. NUMBER	SSN EIN	26. PATIENT'S ACCOUNT NO.	27. ACCEPT ASSIGNMENT? (For govt. claims, see back)	28. TOTAL CHARGE	29. AMOUNT PAID	30. BALANCE DUE
78 51342XX	☐ ☒		☒ YES ☐ NO	$ 499 63	$ 10 00	$ 489 63

31. SIGNATURE OF PHYSICIAN OR SUPPLIER INCLUDING DEGREES OR CREDENTIALS (I certify that the statements on the reverse apply to this bill and are made a part thereof.)	32. SERVICE FACILITY LOCATION INFORMATION	33. BILLING PROVIDER INFO & PH # (555) 486 9002
GERALD PRACTON MD Gerald Practon MD 03/30/20XX SIGNED DATE	COLLEGE HOSPITAL 4500 BROAD AVENUE WOODLAND HILLS XY 12345 4700 a. 54378601XX b.	PRACTON MEDICAL GROUP 4567 BROAD AVENUE WOODLAND HILLS XY 12345 4700 a. 36640210XX b.

ALL THIRD-PARTY PAYERS: If a service facility is listed in Field 32, insert the NPI.

FIELD 32b Ⓒ

25. FEDERAL TAX I.D. NUMBER	SSN EIN	26. PATIENT'S ACCOUNT NO.	27. ACCEPT ASSIGNMENT? (For govt. claims, see back)	28. TOTAL CHARGE	29. AMOUNT PAID	30. BALANCE DUE
78 51342XX	☐ ☒		☒ YES ☐ NO	$ 499 63	$ 10 00	$ 489 63

31. SIGNATURE OF PHYSICIAN OR SUPPLIER INCLUDING DEGREES OR CREDENTIALS (I certify that the statements on the reverse apply to this bill and are made a part thereof.)	32. SERVICE FACILITY LOCATION INFORMATION	33. BILLING PROVIDER INFO & PH # (555) 486 9002
GERALD PRACTON MD Gerald Practon MD 03/30/20XX SIGNED DATE	COLLEGE HOSPITAL 4500 BROAD AVENUE WOODLAND HILLS XY 12345 4700 a. 54378601XX b.	PRACTON MEDICAL GROUP 4567 BROAD AVENUE WOODLAND HILLS XY 12345 4700 a. 36640210XX b.

ALL THIRD-PARTY PAYERS: This field was provided to report other ID numbers. For purchased diagnostic tests, insert the supplier's PIN. For certified mammography screening centers, insert the 6-digit FDA approved certification number. For durable medical, orthotic, and prosthetic claims, insert the PIN of the location where the order was accepted if the name and address were not provided in Field 32.

FIELD 33 Ⓡ

25. FEDERAL TAX I.D. NUMBER	SSN EIN	26. PATIENT'S ACCOUNT NO.	27. ACCEPT ASSIGNMENT? (For govt. claims, see back)	28. TOTAL CHARGE	29. AMOUNT PAID	30. BALANCE DUE
78 51342XX	☐ ☒		☒ YES ☐ NO	$ 499 63	$ 10 00	$ 489 63

31. SIGNATURE OF PHYSICIAN OR SUPPLIER INCLUDING DEGREES OR CREDENTIALS (I certify that the statements on the reverse apply to this bill and are made a part thereof.)	32. SERVICE FACILITY LOCATION INFORMATION	33. BILLING PROVIDER INFO & PH # (555) 486 9002
GERALD PRACTON MD Gerald Practon MD 03/30/20XX SIGNED DATE	COLLEGE HOSPITAL 4500 BROAD AVENUE WOODLAND HILLS XY 12345 4700 a. 54378601XX b.	PRACTON MEDICAL GROUP 4567 BROAD AVENUE WOODLAND HILLS XY 12345 4700 a. 36640210XX b.

COMMERCIAL PAYERS: Follow Medicare guidelines.

MEDICARE: Insert the name, address and 9-digit ZIP code for the physician, clinic, or supplier billing for services.

Medicare/Medicaid: Follow Medicare guidelines.

Medicare/Medigap: Follow Medicare guidelines.

MSP: Follow Medicare guidelines.

TRICARE: Insert the name and address for the physician, clinic, or supplier billing for services. Radiologists, pathologists, and anesthesiologists may use their billing address if they have no *physical address*.

FIELD 33a Ⓡ

25. FEDERAL TAX I.D. NUMBER	SSN EIN	26. PATIENT'S ACCOUNT NO.	27. ACCEPT ASSIGNMENT? (For govt. claims, see back)	28. TOTAL CHARGE	29. AMOUNT PAID	30. BALANCE DUE
78 51342XX	☐ ☒		☒ YES ☐ NO	$ 499 63	$ 10 00	$ 489 63

31. SIGNATURE OF PHYSICIAN OR SUPPLIER INCLUDING DEGREES OR CREDENTIALS (I certify that the statements on the reverse apply to this bill and are made a part thereof.)	32. SERVICE FACILITY LOCATION INFORMATION	33. BILLING PROVIDER INFO & PH # (555) 486 9002
GERALD PRACTON MD Gerald Practon MD 03/30/20XX SIGNED DATE	COLLEGE HOSPITAL 4500 BROAD AVENUE WOODLAND HILLS XY 12345 4700 a. 54378601XX b.	PRACTON MEDICAL GROUP 4567 BROAD AVENUE WOODLAND HILLS XY 12345 4700 a. 36640210XX b.

COMMERCIAL PAYERS: Follow Medicare guidelines.

MEDICARE: Insert the individual physician or group NPI.

Medicare/Medicaid: Follow Medicare guidelines.

Medicare/Medigap: Follow Medicare guidelines.

MSP: Follow Medicare guidelines.

TRICARE: Insert the physician's Tax Identification Number.

FIELD 33b

Effective May 23, 2007, this field is not reported.

BOTTOM OF FORM

Enter insurance billing specialist's reference initials in lower left corner of the insurance claim form.

APPENDIX B

COMPETENCY GRIDS WITH REFERENCE NUMBERS CORRELATING TEXT AND ASSIGNMENTS BY CHAPTER

- CAAHEP Curriculum Competencies
- ABHES Curriculum Competencies
- CMA Certification Examination Content
- RMA Certification Examination Competencies
- CMAS Examination Specifications
- AAMA Role Delineation Study

CAAHEP CURRICULUM COMPETENCIES

The Commission on Accreditation and Allied Health Education Programs (CAAHEP) have established standards and guidelines for medical assisting educational programs. The 2003 minimum curriculum standards have been adopted by the American Association of Medical Assistants (AAMA) and used in the accreditation process for programs who train individuals to enter the medical assisting profession. Following are entry-level competencies for medical assistants.* These are cross-referenced in a chapter-by-chapter grid (see Table B-1) to help locate them in the *Administrative Medical Assisting* textbook and *Workbook*.

III.C.3.a. ADMINISTRATIVE COMPETENCIES
(1) Perform Clerical Functions
- (1)(a) Schedule and manage appointments
- (1)(b) Schedule inpatient and outpatient admissions and procedures
- (1)(c) Organize a patient's medical records
- (1)(d) File medical records

(2) Perform Bookkeeping Procedures
- (2)(a) Prepare a bank deposit
- (2)(b) Post entries on a daysheet
- (2)(c) Perform accounts receivable procedures
- (2)(d) Perform billing and collection procedures
- (2)(e) Post adjustments
- (2)(f) Process credit balance
- (2)(g) Process refunds
- (2)(h) Post NSF checks
- (2)(i) Post collection agency payments

(3) Process Insurance Claims
- (3)(a) Apply managed care policies and procedures
- (3)(b) Apply third-party guidelines
- (3)(c) Perform procedural coding
- (3)(d) Perform diagnostic coding
- (3)(e) Complete insurance claim forms

III.C.3.b. CLINICAL COMPETENCIES†
(1) Fundamental Procedures
- (1)(d) Dispose of biohazardous materials

(4) Patient Care
- (4)(c) Obtain and record patient history
- (4)(h) Maintain medication and immunization records

III.C.3.c GENERAL COMPETENCIES
(1) Professional Communications
- (1)(a) Respond to and initiate written communications
- (1)(b) Recognize and respond to verbal communications
- (1)(c) Recognize and respond to nonverbal communications
- (1)(d) Demonstrate telephone techniques

(2) Legal Concepts
- (2)(a) Identify and respond to issues of confidentiality
- (2)(b) Perform within legal and ethical boundaries
- (2)(c) Establish and maintain the medical record
- (2)(e) Document appropriately
- (2)(f) Demonstrate knowledge of federal and state health care legislation and regulations

(3) Patient Instruction
- (3)(a) Explain general office policies
- (3)(b) Instruct individuals according to their needs
- (3)(c) Provide instruction for health maintenance and disease prevention
- (3)(d) Identify community resources

(4) Operational Functions
- (4)(a) Perform an inventory of supplies and equipment
- (4)(b) Perform routine maintenance of administrative and clinical equipment
- (4)(c) Utilize computer software to maintain office systems
- (4)(d) Use methods of quality control

The competencies are reprinted with permission from the Commission on Accreditation for Allied Health Programs.

†*Only those clinical competencies that apply to this text are listed.*

Table B-1. Commission on Accreditation of Allied Health Education Programs (CAAHEP) Standards and Guidelines for Medical Assisting Educational Programs, 2003

		III.C.3.a. ADMINISTRATIVE COMPETENCIES			III.C.3.b. CLINICAL COMPETENCIES	III.C.3.c. GENERAL COMPETENCIES			
Ch	Title	1. Perform Clerical Functions	2. Perform Bookkeeping Procedures	3. Process Insurance Claims	Clinical	1. Professional Communication	2. Legal Concepts	3. Patient Instruction	4. Operational Functions
1	A Career As an Administrative Medical Assistant	a, b, c, d	e	b			a	a, b, c, d	c
2	The Health Care Environment: Past, Present, and Future	a, b, c, d					d	b	
3	Medicolegal and Ethical Responsibilities	✓					a, b, d, e		c
4	The Art of Communication					b, c	a	b	
5	The Receptionist	a, d					a, d	a, b, c, d	
6	Telephone Procedures	c, d, e				b, d, e			
7	Appointments	a, b				a, b, d	d	a	
8	Filing Procedures	c, d	a, c						
9	Medical Records	c, d	c, e				b, c, d		
10	Drug and Prescription Records				(1)e, (4)c, h		d	b	
11	Written Correspondence					a			
12	Processing Mail and Telecommunications	✓				a			c
13	Fees, Credit, and Collection	✓	c, d, e, f, g, h, i			a, b			
14	Banking	✓	a, e–i						
15	Bookkeeping	✓	b, c, e–i						
16	Health Insurance Systems			a, b, c, d, e					
17	Office Managerial Responsibilities	✓		a		a	e		a, b, d
18	Financial Management of the Medical Practice	✓	a, b				e		
19	Seeking a Position As an Administrative Medical Assistant	✓				a, b, c	b		

ABHES CURRICULUM COMPETENCIES

The Accrediting Bureau of Health Education Schools (ABHES) is a nationally recognized, independent, non-profit accrediting agency of institutions and educational programs that predominantly provide allied health education. Policies, procedures and standards have been developed for the accreditation of medical assisting programs and the 2006 entry-level competencies required for successful completion are outlined as follows.* These are cross-referenced in a chapter-by-chapter grid (see Table B-2) to help locate them in the *Administrative Medical Assisting* textbook and *Workbook*.

VI.B.1.a.1. PROFESSIONALISM

- 1(a)   Project a positive attitude
- 1(b)   Maintain confidentiality at all times
- 1(c)   Be a "team player"
- 1(d)   Be cognizant of ethical boundaries
- 1(e)   Exhibit initiative
- 1(f)   Adapt to change
- 1(g)   Evidence a responsible attitude
- 1(h)   Be courteous and diplomatic
- 1(i)   Conduct work within scope of education, training, and ability

VI.B.1.a.2. COMMUNICATION

- 2(a)   Be attentive, listen, and learn
- 2(b)   Be impartial and show empathy when dealing with patients
- 2(c)   Adapt what is said to the recipient's level of comprehension
- 2(d)   Serve as liaison between physician and others
- 2(e)   Use proper telephone techniques
- 2(f)   Interview effectively
- 2(g)   Use appropriate medical terminology
- 2(h)   Receive, organize, prioritize, and transmit information expediently
- 2(i)   Recognize and respond to verbal and non-verbal communication
- 2(j)   Use correct grammar, spelling, and formatting techniques in written works
- 2(k)   Use principles of verbal and nonverbal communication
- 2(l)   (duplicate i)
- 2(m)   Adapt to individualized needs
- 2(n)   Apply electronic technology
- 2(o)   Use fundamental writing skills
- 2(p)   Exhibit professional components
- 2(q)   Understand allied health professions and credentialing

VI.B.1.a.3. ADMINISTRATIVE DUTIES

- 3(a)   Perform basic secretarial skills
- 3(b)   Prepare and maintain medical records
- 3(c)   Schedule and monitor appointments
- 3(d)   Apply computer concepts for office procedures
- 3(e)   Perform medical transcription
- 3(f)   Locate resources and information for patients and employers
- 3(g)   Manage physicians' professional schedule and travel
- 3(h)   Schedule inpatient and outpatient admissions
- 3(i)   File medical records
- 3(j)   Prepare a bank statement and deposit record
- 3(k)   Reconcile a bank statement
- 3(l)   Post entries on a day sheet
- 3(m)   Perform billing and collection procedures
- 3(n)   Prepare a check
- 3(o)   Establish and maintain a petty cash fund
- 3(p)   Post adjustments
- 3(q)   Process credit balance
- 3(r)   Process refunds
- 3(s)   Post NSF checks
- 3(t)   Post collection agency payments
- 3(u)   Apply managed care policies and procedures
- 3(v)   Obtain managed care referrals and pre-certification
- 3(w)   Perform diagnostic coding
- 3(x)   Complete insurance claim forms
- 3(y)   Use physician fee schedule

VI.B.1.a.4. CLINICAL DUTIES†

- 4(a)   Interview and record patient history
- 4(e)   Recognize emergencies
- 4(l)   Screen and follow up patient test results

The competencies are reprinted with permission from the Accrediting Bureau of Health Education Schools.

†*Only those clinical competencies that apply to this text are listed.*

4(n) Maintain medication and immunization records

4(q) Dispose of biohazardous materials

4(r) Practice standard precautions

VI.B.1.a.5. LEGAL CONCEPTS

5(a) Determine needs for documentation and reporting

5(b) Document accurately

5(c) Use appropriate guidelines when releasing records or information

5(d) Follow established policy in initiating or terminating medical treatment

5(e) Dispose of controlled substances in compliance with government regulations

5(f) Maintain licenses and accreditation

5(g) Monitor legislation related to current healthcare issues and practices

5(h) Perform risk management procedures

VI.B.1.a.6. OFFICE MANAGEMENT

6(a) Maintain physical plant

6(b) Operate and maintain facilities and perform routine maintenance

of administrative and clinical equipment safely

6(c) Inventory equipment and supplies

6(d) Evaluate and recommend equipment and supplies for practice

6(e) Maintain liability coverage

6(f) Exercise efficient time management

VI.B.1.a.7. INSTRUCTION

7(a) Orient patients to office policies and procedures

7(b) Instruct patients with special needs

7(c) Teach patients methods of health promotion and disease prevention

7(d) Orient and train personnel

VI.B.1.a.8. FINANCIAL MANAGEMENT

8(a) Use manual and computerized bookkeeping systems

8(b) Implement current procedural terminology and *ICD-9* coding

8(c) Analyze and use current third-party guidelines for reimbursement

8(d) Manage accounts payable and receivable

8(e) Maintain records for accounting and banking purposes

8(f) Process employee payroll

Table B-2. Accrediting Bureau of Health Education Schools (ABHES) Competencies for Medical Assisting Programs, 2006

		VI.B.1.a.1.	VI.B.1.a.2.	VI.B.1.a.3.	VI.B.1.a.4.	VI.B.1.a.5.	VI.B.1.a.6.	VI.B.1.a.7.	VI.B.1.a.8.
Administrative Medical Assisting, 6ed.		Profession-alism	Commun-ication	Adminis-trative Duties	Clinical Duties	Legal Concepts	Office Management	Instruction	Financial Management
Ch	Title								
1	A Career As an Administrative Medical Assistant	a, b, d, e, f, g, h, i	b, d, g, h, j, m, n, o, p, q	a, d, f		f		a, b, c	
2	The Health Care Environment: Past, Present, and Future	c	a, c, d, g	e, u	a	g		b	
3	Medicolegal and Ethical Responsibilities	a, d	j, n		a, d		b, c, d, g, h		
4	The Art of Communication	a, b, h	a, b, c, d, f, g, h, i, k, l, m, p				a, b		
5	The Receptionist	a, b, c, h	e, f, g, m	a, f	e	g	a, b, c		
6	Telephone Procedures	b, h	a, e, h, j, k	a	e	b			
7	Appointments	h	a, d, g, h, j, n	a, c, d, g, h	e	a		a	
8	Filing Procedures		h	b, i		c			
9	Medical Records		g, i, j, n, o	b, e, i	a	a, b, c			
10	Drug and Prescription Records		g, j	b, f, j	n, q	b, e, f	c	c	
11	Written Correspondence		g, j, n, o	a, d, e					
12	Processing Mail and Telecommunications		g, h, j, o	a					
13	Fees, Credit, and Collection		a, b, d, g, i, j, k, o	a, m, p, q, r, s, t, y				a	
14	Banking			a, j, k, n, p, q, r, s, t					d, e
15	Bookkeeping		n	a, j, l, o–t, y					a, d, e
16	Health Insurance Systems			u, v, w, x, y					b, c
17	Office Managerial Responsibilities		o	g	q, r	g, h	a–f	a, d	
18	Financial Management of the Medical Practice	h		d, j, k, o, n, u		g	✓		d, e, f
19	Seeking a Position As an Administrative Medical Assistant	a, c, d, e, g, h	a, c, i, j, k, o, p	a					

CMA CERTIFICATION EXAMINATION CONTENT

The American Association of Medical Assistants (AAMA) has developed a content outline for the Certified Medical Assistant (CMA) certification examination as follows.* These are cross-referenced in a chapter-by-chapter grid (see Table B-3) to help locate them in the *Administrative Medical Assisting* textbook and *Workbook*.

I. **GENERAL**
  A. Medical Terminology
    1. Word building and definitions
      a. Basic structure
        (1) roots or stems
        (2) prefixes
        (3) suffixes
        (4) plurals
        (5) abbreviations
        (6) symbols
      b. Surgical procedures
      c. Diagnostic procedures
      d. Medial specialties
      e. Common diseases and pathology
    2. Uses of technology
      a. Spelling and pronunciation
      b. Selection and use
      c. Reference sources
  B. Anatomy and Physiology[†]
    1. Body as a whole, including multiple systems
    2. Systems, including structure, function, related conditions and diseases
  C. Psychology
    1. Basic principles
      a. Meaning of individual self-worth
      b. Understanding human behavior-Maslow's hierarchy of needs
      c. Social needs of people
      d. Understanding emotional behavior
    2. Developmental stages of the life cycle
      a. Developmental theories used to explain behavior and development
      b. Human growth and development
    3. Hereditary, cultural, and environmental influences on behavior
      a. Helping patients adjust to illness
      b. Cultural influences on behavior
      c. Importance of recognizing cultural differences and attitudes toward the health care system
      d. Recognizing social and environmental influences on behavior
    4. Defense mechanisms
      a. Recognition
      b. Management
  D. Professionalism
    1. Displaying professional attitude
      a. Supporting professional organization
      b. Accepting responsibility for own actions
    2. Job readiness and seeking employment
      a. Resumé and cover letter
      b. Methods of job searching
      c. Interviewing as a job candidate
      d. Professional presentation
    3. Performing within ethical boundaries
      a. Ethical standards
        (1) AAMA Code of Ethics
        (2) AMA Code of Ethics
      b. Patient rights
      c. Current issues in medical bioethics
    4. Maintaining confidentiality
      a. Agent of physician
        (1) patient rights
        (2) releasing patient information
      b. Intentional tort
        (1) invasion of privacy
        (2) slander and libel
    5. Working as a team member to achieve goals
      a. Member responsibility
      b. Promoting competent patient care
      c. Utilizing principles of group dynamics
  E. Communication
    1. Adapting communication to an individual's ability to understand
      a. Blind
      b. Deaf
      c. Elderly
      d. Children
      e. Seriously ill
      f. Mentally impaired
      g. Illiterate
      h. Non-English-speaking

The competencies are reprinted with permission from the American Association of Medical Assistants.
†*Only those anatomy and physiology competencies that apply to this text are listed.*

    i.   Anxious
    j.   Angry/Distraught
    k.   Motor impaired

2. Recognizing and responding to verbal and nonverbal communication
   a. Positive body language
   b. Listening skills
   c. Eye contact
   d. Barriers to effective communication
   e. Identifying needs of others

3. Patient instructions
   a. Explaining general office policies
   b. Instructing individuals according to their needs
   c. Instruction and demonstrating the use and care of patient equipment
   d. Providing instruction for health maintenance and disease prevention
   e. Identifying community resources

4. Professional communication and behavior
   a. Professional situations
      (1) tact
      (2) diplomacy
      (3) courtesy
      (4) responsibility
   b. Therapeutic relationships
      (1) impartial behavior
      (2) effective responses to cultural differences
      (3) empathy

5. Evaluating and understanding communication
   a. Observation
   b. Active listening
   c. Feedback

6. Interviewing techniques
   a. Guiding, controlling, and ending interviews
   b. Using questions
   c. Specific interviews
      (1) interviewee
      (2) setting
   d. Legal restrictions

7. Receiving, organizing, prioritizing, and transmitting information
   a. Modalities for incoming and outgoing data
   b. Prioritizing incoming and outgoing data

8. Telephone techniques
   a. Incoming calls management criteria
      (1) screening
      (2) effective conversation
      (3) maintaining confidentiality
      (4) gathering data
      (5) multiple-line competency
      (6) transferring appropriate calls
      (7) screening and referral
      (8) identifying caller, office, and self
      (9) taking messages
      (10) ending calls
   b. Monitoring special calls
      (1) problem calls
      (2) emergency calls

9. Fundamental writing skills
   a. Sentence structure
   b. Grammar
   c. Punctuation
   d. Spelling

F. Medicolegal Guidelines and Requirements
   1. Licenses and accreditation
      a. Medical practice acts
      b. Renewal of license
      c. Revocation/suspension of license
         (1) criminal/unprofessional conduct
         (2) professional/personal incapacity
      d. Facility accreditation
         (1) state requirements (certificate of need/laboratory registration)
         (2) federal requirements (ambulatory surgical center/physician office laboratory)
   2. Legislation
      a. State compliance
         (1) personnel standards, hiring, and termination
         (2) Medicare/Medicaid reimbursement policies
         (3) acts (living wills/anatomical gifts)
         (4) reportable incidences (public health statutes/criminal acts)
      b. Federal compliance
         (1) OSHA
         (2) right to privacy
         (3) controlled substances
         (4) Medicare/Medicaid regulations
         (5) Clinical Laboratory Improvement Act
         (6) Americans with Disabilities Act
         (7) Health Insurance Portability and Accountability Act

3. Documentation/reporting
    a. Sources of information
    b. Drug Enforcement Administration
    c. Internal Revenue Service
    d. Employment laws
    e. Personal injury occurrences
    f. Workers' compensation
    g. Medical records
        (1) patient activity
        (2) patient care
        (3) patient confidentiality
        (4) ownership
    h. Personnel records
        (1) evaluation
        (2) privacy
4. Releasing medical information
    a. Consent
        (1) patient written authorization
        (2) state and federal codes
    b. Rescinding authorization for release
5. Physician-patient relationship
    a. Contract
        (1) legal obligations
        (2) consequences for
        noncompliance
    b. Responsibility and rights
        (1) patient
        (2) physician
        (3) medical assistant
    c. Guidelines for third-party
        agreements
    d. Professional liability
        (1) current standard of care
        (2) current legal standards
        (3) informed consent
    e. Arbitration agreements
    f. Affirmative defenses
        (1) statute of limitations
        (2) comparative/contributory
        negligence
        (3) assumption of risk
    g. Termination of medical care
        (1) establishing policy
        (2) elements for withdrawal
        (3) patient notification and
            documentation

II. **ADMINISTRATIVE**
    G. Data Entry
        1. Keyboard fundamentals and functions
            a. Alpha, numeric, and symbol keys
            b. Spacing and margins

c. Horizontal and vertical centering
d. Tabulation
2. Formats
    a. Letters
    b. Memos
    c. Reports
    d. Manuscripts
    e. Envelopes
    f. Chart notes
    g. Templates
3. Proofreading
    a. Proofreader's marks
    b. Making corrections from rough
        draft
H. Equipment
    1. Equipment operation
        a. Calculator
        b. Photocopier
        c. Computer/Word processor
        d. Fax machine
        e. Telephone services and use
            (1) multi-button telephone
            (2) types of calls
            (3) features
        f. Scanners
    2. Maintenance and repairs
        a. Contents of instruction material
        b. Routine maintenance
            (1) agreements
            (2) warranty
            (3) repair service
I. Computer Concepts
    1. Computer components
        a. Terminology
        b. Central processing unit, monitor,
            keyboard
        c. Scanner
        d. Printers
        e. Disk drive
        f. Storage devices
        g. Operating systems
        h. Basic commands*
    2. Care and maintenance of computer
        a. Main unit and components
        b. Protection/safety
        c. Maintenance agreements
        d. Support
        e. Leasing
    3. Computer applications
        a. Word processing
        b. Database
        c. Spreadsheets, graphics
        d. Electronic mail

Only those computer basic command competencies that apply to this text are listed.

e. Networks
f. Multi-user/Multi-task system
g. Security/Password
h. Training programs
i. Medical management software
   (1) file maintenance
   (2) new patient entry
   (3) diagnostic and procedural code entry
   (4) payment/entry transaction
   (5) electronic claims
   (6) routine billing (superbill/itemized statements to third parties/monthly statements)
   (7) report generation (monthly revenue/accounts receivable)
   (8) utilities
4. Internet services

J. Records Management
1. Needs, purposes, and terminology of filing systems
  a. Basic filing systems
   (1) alphabetic
   (2) numeric
   (3) geographic
   (4) subject
  b. Special filing systems
   (1) color-code
   (2) tickler file
   (3) electronic data processing files
   (4) cross-reference/master file
2. Process for filing documents
3. Organization of patient's medical record
4. Filing guidelines
  a. Storing
  b. Protecting/safekeeping
  c. Transferring
  d. Retaining
  e. Purging
  f. Destroying
5. Medical records
  a. Types
   (1) problem oriented
   (2) source oriented
  b. Collecting information
  c. Making corrections
  d. Retaining and purging
   (1) statute of limitations
   (2) deceased patients

K. Screening and Processing Mail
1. US Postal Service
  a. Regulations
  b. Classifications
  c. Types of mail services
  d. Tracing mail
  e. Recalling mail
2. Private services
  a. Alternate delivery
  b. Fax services
3. Postal machine/meter
4. Processing incoming mail
5. Preparing outgoing mail
  a. Labels
  b. Optical Character Reader guidelines

L. Scheduling and Monitoring Appointments
1. Utilizing appointment schedules/types
  a. Stream
  b. Wave
  c. Modified wave
  d. Open booking
  e. Categorization
2. Appointment guidelines
  a. Legal aspects
  b. New/Established patient
  c. Patient needs/preference
  d. Physician preference/habits
  e. Facilities/equipment requirements
3. Appointment protocol
  a. Follow-up visits
   (1) routine
   (2) urgent
  b. Emergency/Acutely ill
  c. Physician referrals
  d. Cancellations/No-shows
  e. Physician delay/unavailability
  f. Outside services
  g. Reminders/Recalls
   (1) appointment cards
   (2) tickler file

M. Resource Information and Community Services
1. Services available
2. Appropriate referrals
3. Follow-up
4. Patient advocate

N. Managing Physician's Professional Schedule and Travel
1. Arranging meetings
2. Scheduling travel
3. Integrating meetings and travel with office schedule
  a. Matrix appointment schedule
  b. Arranging professional coverage
  c. Return schedule requirements

O. Managing the Office
1. Maintaining the physical plant
  a. Office environment
  b. Personnel
   (1) recruiting

(2) interviewing
(3) hiring
(4) evaluating performance
(5) disciplining
(5) termination
(7) documenting
c. Facilities and equipment
  (1) maintenance and repair
  (2) safety regulations (OSHA/ CDC/ADA/fire/security)
2. Equipment and supply inventory
  a. Inventory control
  b. Storage and security
  c. Purchasing
3. Maintaining liability coverage
  a. Types of coverage
  b. Recordkeeping
4. Time management
  a. Establishing priorities
  b. Managing routine duties

P. Office Policies and Procedures
1. Patient information booklet
2. Patient education
3. Instructions for patients with special needs
4. Personnel manual
5. Policy and procedures manuals/protocols
6. Compliance plan

Q. Managing Practice Finances
1. Bookkeeping systems
  a. Demographic data
  b. Day sheets, charge slips, receipts, ledgers, etc.
    (1) charges, payments, and adjustments
    (2) transactions
    (3) identifying and correcting errors
  c. Petty cash
2. Coding systems
  a. Types
    (1) *Current Procedure Terminology (CPT)*
    (2) *International Classification of Diseases, Clinical Modification (ICD-CM)*
    (3) *Healthcare Financing Common Procedural Coding Systems (HCPCS Level II)*
  b. Relationship between procedures and diagnostic codes
3. Third-party billing
  a. Types
    (1) capitated plans

(2) commercial carriers
(3) government plans (Medicare/ Medicaid/TRICARE/CAMPVA)
(4) prepaid HMO, PPO, POS
(5) workers' compensation
b. Processing claims
  (1) manual and electronic preparation of claims
  (2) tracing claims
  (3) sequence of filing
  (4) reconciling payments/ rejections
  (5) inquiry and appeal process
c. Applying managed care policies and procedures
  (1) referrals
  (2) precertification
  (3) contracts and fees
d. Fee schedules
  (1) methods for establishing fees (RVS/RBRVS/DRG)
  (2) updating fee schedules
4. Accounting and banking procedures
  a. Accounts receivable
    (1) collecting/updating demographic data
    (2) billing procedures (itemization/billing cycles)
    (3) aging/controlling accounts receivable
    (4) collection procedures (analysis/office efforts/ agencies/consumer protection acts)
  b. Accounts payable
    (1) ordering goods and services
    (2) monitoring invoices
    (3) tracking merchandise
    (4) paying accounts
    (5) writing checks
  c. Banking procedures
    (1) processing accounts receivable
    (2) preparing bank deposits
    (3) electronic banking
    (4) reconciling bank statement
    (5) maintaining financial records
5. Employee payroll
  a. Maintaining payroll records
  b. Calculating wages and taxes
  c. Preparing payroll checks and earning statements
  d. Depositing taxes
  e. Filing and mailing tax reports

III. **CLINICAL***
    R. Principles of Infection Control
        3. Disposal of biohazardous material
    S. Treatment Area
        3. Restocking supplies
    U. Patient History Interview
        1. Components of patient history
            a. Personal data
            b. Chief complaint
            c. Past, present, family and social history
            d. Review of systems
        2. Documentation guidelines
    W. Preparing and Administering Medications
        1. Pharmacology
            a. Classes of drugs
            b. Drug forms
            c. Drug action/uses
            d. Side effects/adverse reactions
            e. Emergency use
            f. Substance abuse
            g. Calculation of dosage
            h. Immunizations
        3. Prescriptions
            a. Prescription parts
            b. Safekeeping
            c. Recordkeeping
            d. Reordering
            e. Controlled substances
        4. Maintaining medication and immunization records
        5. Medication disposal
    X. Emergencies
        1. Preplanned action
            a. Policies and procedures

Only those clinical competencies that apply to this text are listed.

Table B-3. American Association of Medical Assistants (AAMA) Certified Medical Assistant (CMA) Examination Content Outline

Administrative Medical Assisting, 6ed.				I. GENERAL		
Ch Title	A. Medical Terminology	B. A & P	C. Psychology	D. Professionalism	E. Communication	F. Medicolegal Guidelines & Requirements
1 A Career As an Administrative Medical Assistant	1a5, 2a	1, 2	1a, 1d, 2, 3a	1, 2d	2e, 3, 4a, 4b3	1b
2 The Health Care Environment: Past, Present, and Future	1a5, 1d, 2			5		
3 Medicolegal and Ethical Responsibilities	1a5, 2			3, 4		1a; 2b2/7; 4, 5
4 The Art of Communication	1a5, 2a, b		1, 2b, 3, 4	1b	1, 2, 3a, b, 4, 5, 6b	
5 The Receptionist	1a5, 2a		3d	1, 4, 5b	3a, b, d, e, 4a, 6c1, 7a, b	3g3
6 Telephone Procedures	1a5			1, 4a2	3a, b, 4, 6a, b, c2, 7a, 8a1–10, b1–2	3g1–3, 4
7 Appointments	1a5, 7, 1e, 2b				2, 3a, 7a, 8	
8 Filing Procedures	1a5			4a2	7b	4
9 Medical Records	1a5	2a–j		4a2		2a3a, 3g
10 Drug and Prescription Records	1a5					1d, 2b3, 3b
11 Written Correspondence	1a5, 2a					
12 Processing Mail and Telecommunications	1a5				7a, b	
13 Fees, Credit, and Collection	1a5				8	
14 Banking	1a5					
15 Bookkeeping	1a5					
16 Health Insurance Systems	1a5					2a2, 2b4, 7, 3e, f
17 Office Managerial Responsibilities	1a5			1a, 5c	3a, 4a1–4, 4b1–3, 6a, c, d	2a1, 2b1, 6, 7, 3d
18 Financial Management of the Medical Practice	1a5			1, 5		3c, d
19 Seeking a Position As an Administrative Medical Assistant				1b, 2a–d, 5	1, 2, 4a1–4, 6d, 9a–d	

						II. ADMINISTRATIVE						III. CLINICAL
G. Data Entry	H. Equipment	I. Computer Concepts	J. Records Management	K. Screening and Processing Mail	L. Scheduling and Monitoring Appointments	M. Resource Information & Community Services	N. Managing Physicians' Professional Schedule and Travel	O. Managing the Office	P. Office Policies and Procedures	Q. Managing Practice Finances	R–Z Clinical
2c	1c	3a, 4						2, 3			
						2				3a–4	
									6		
	1b, c, d, e	3e, i2, i6a	1a1		3b, e	1, 5			2, 5	1b	
	1e1–3								1, 2, 4		
	1c, e	3i–2			1, 2, 3		3a		2		
		3i1	1a, b, 2, 3, 4a–f, 5d1–2								
2f, g	1f		3, 5a, c								U1, 2
		3b									R3, S3, W1a, b, c, d, f, 3, 4, 5
1a–d, 2a, b, e		1d, f, 3a, b									
2e	1b, d	3d, g		1a–d, 2a–b, 3, 4, 5a–b							
										1b1–2, 4a1, 2, 3, 4	
	1a									4c1–5	
	1a									1a, b1–3, 4a, b5	
										2a1–3, 2b, 3a1–3, 3a4, 5, 3b1–5, 3c1–3, 3d1a–c, 2d2	
	2a, b1–3	2a–d, 3, 7					1–3	1a–c, 1c2d, e 2a–c, 3a–b, 4a–b	1, 4, 5, 6	4b1–4	W-4, X-1
								4a3, 5a–e			
1, 2, 3	3a										

RMA CERTIFICATION EXAMINATION COMPETENCIES

The American Medical Technologists (AMT) have established (2005) competencies and construction parameters for the Registered Medical Assistant (RMA) certification examination as follows.* These are cross-referenced in a chapter-by-chapter grid (see Table B-4) to help locate them in the *Administrative Medical Assisting* textbook and *Workbook*.

I. **GENERAL MEDICAL ASSISTING KNOWLEDGE**
   A. Anatomy and Physiology†
      1. Body systems
         a. Skeletal
         b. Muscular
         c. Endocrine
         d. Urinary
         e. Reproductive
         f. Gastrointestinal
         g. Nervous
         h. Respiratory
         i. Cardiovascular
         j. Integumentary
         k. Special senses
   B. Medical Terminology
      1. Word parts
         a. Identify word parts: root, prefixes, and suffixes
      2. Definitions
         a. Define medical terms
      3. Common abbreviations and symbols
         a. Identify and understand utilization of medical abbreviations and symbols
      4. Spelling
         a. Spell medical terms accurately
   C. Medical Law
      1. Medical Law
         a. Types of consent used in medical practice
         b. Disclosure laws and regulations
         c. Laws, regulations, and acts pertaining to the practice of medicine
         d. Scope of practice acts regarding medical assisting
         e. Patient Bill of Rights legislation
      2. Licensure, certification, and registration

         a. Identify credentialing requirements of medical professional
         b. Understand the application of the Clinical Laboratory Improvement Amendments of 1988
      3. Terminology
         a. Define terminology associated with medical law
   D. Medical Ethics
      1. Principles of medical ethics and ethical conduct
         a. Identify and employ proper ethics in practice as a medical assistant
         b. Identify the principles of ethics established by the American Medical Association
         c. Identify and understand the application of the AMA Patient Bill of Rights
         d. Recognize unethical practices and identify the proper response
         e. Recognize the importance of professional development through continuing education
   E. Human Relations
      1. Patient relations
         a. Identify age-group specific responses and support
         b. Identify and employ professional conduct in all aspects of patient care
         c. Understand and properly apply communication methods
      2. Interpersonal relations
         a. Employ appropriate interpersonal skills with:
            (1) employer/administration
            (2) co-workers
            (3) vendors
            (4) business associates
         b. Observe and respect cultural diversity in the workplace
   F. Patient Education
      1. Patient instruction
         a. Health and wellness
         b. Nutrition
         c. Hygiene
         d. Treatment and medications
         e. Pre- and post-operative care
         f. Body mechanics
         g. Personal and physical safety
      2. Patient resource materials

The competencies are reprinted with permission from the American Medical Technologists.

†*Only those anatomy and physiology competencies that apply to this text are listed.*

a. Develop, assemble, and maintain appropriate patient brochures and informational material

3. Documentation

a. Understand and utilize proper documentation of patient encounters and instruction

II. ADMINISTRATIVE MEDICAL ASSISTING

A. Insurance

1. Terminology

a. Identify and define terminology associated with various insurance types in the medical office

2. Plans

a. Identify and understand the application of medical, disability, and accident insurance plans

b. Identify and appropriately apply plan policies and regulations for programs including

(1) HMO, PPO, EPO, indemnity, open, etc.

(2) short-term and long-term disability

(3) Family Medical Leave Act (FMLA)

(4) workers' compensation (first report/follow-up reports)

(5) Medicare (including Advance Beneficiary Notice [ABN])

(6) Medicaid

(7) CHAMPUS/TRICARE

3. Claims

a. Complete and file insurance claims

(1) file claims for paper and Electronic Data Interchange

(2) understand and adhere to HIPAA Security and Uniformity Regulations

b. Evaluate claims response

(1) understand and evaluate explanation of benefits

(2) evaluate claims rejection and utilize proper follow-up procedures

4. Coding

a. Identify HIPAA-mandated coding systems

(1) *ICD-9-CM*

(2) *CPT*

(3) *HCPCS*

b. Properly apply diagnosis and procedure codes to insurance claims

5. Insurance finance applications

a. Identify and comply with contractual requirements of insurance plans

b. Process insurance payments and contractual write-off amounts

c. Track unpaid claims

d. Generate aging reports

B. Financial Bookkeeping

1. Terminology

a. Understand terminology associated with medical financial bookkeeping

2. Patient billing

a. Maintain and explain physician's fee schedules

b. Collect and post payments

c. Manage patient ledgers and accounts

d. Understand and prepare Truth in Lending Statements

e. Prepare and mail itemized statements

f. Understand and employ available billing methods

g. Understand and employ billing cycles

3. Collections

a. Prepare aging reports and identify delinquent accounts

b. Perform skip tracing

c. Understand application of the Fair Debt Collection Practices Act

d. Identify and understand bankruptcy and small claims procedures

e. Understand and perform appropriate collection procedures

4. Fundamental medical office accounting procedures

a. Employ appropriate accounting procedures

(1) pegboard/double entry bookkeeping

(2) computerized

b. Perform daily balancing procedures

c. Prepare monthly trial balance

d. Apply accounts receivable and payable principles

5. Banking procedures

a. Understand and manage petty cash account

b. Prepare and make bank deposits

c. Maintain checking accounts

d. Reconcile bank statements

e. Understand check processing procedures and requirements

(1) non-sufficient funds

(2) endorsements

f. Process payables and practice obligations

g. Understand and maintain disbursement accounts

6. Employee payroll

a. Prepare employee payroll

(1) understand hourly and salary payroll procedures

(2) understand and apply payroll withholding and deductions

b. Understand and maintain payroll records

(1) prepare and maintain payroll tax deduction records

(2) prepare employee tax forms

(3) prepare quarterly tax forms and deposits

c. Understand terminology pertaining to payroll and payroll tax

7. Financial mathematics

a. Understand and perform appropriate calculations related to patient and practice accounts

C. Medical Receptionist/Secretarial/Clerical

1. Terminology

a. Understand and correctly apply terminology associated with medical receptionist and secretarial duties

2. Reception

a. Employ appropriate communication skills when receiving and greeting patients

b. Understand basic emergency triage in coordinating patient arrivals

c. Screen visitors and sales persons arriving at the office

d. Obtain patient demographics and information

e. Understand and maintain patient confidentiality during check-in procedures

f. Prepare patient record

g. Assist patients into examination rooms

3. Scheduling

a. Employ appointment scheduling system

(1) identify and employ various scheduling styles

b. Employ proper procedures for cancellations and missed appointments

c. Understand referral and authorization process

d. Understand and manage patient recall system

e. Schedule non-office appointments

4. Oral and written communication

a. Employ appropriate telephone etiquette

b. Perform appropriate telephone procedures

c. Instruct patients via telephone

d. Inform patients of test results per physician instruction

e. Receive, process, and document results received from outside provider

f. Compose correspondence employing acceptable business format

g. Employ effective written communication skills adhering to ethics and laws of confidentiality

h. Employ active listening skills

5. Records and chart management

a. Manage patient medical record system

b. Record diagnostic test results in patient chart

c. File patient and physician communication in chart

d. File materials according to proper system

(1) chronological

(2) alphabetical

(3) problem-oriented medical records

(4) subject

e. Protect, store, and retain medical records according to proper conventions and HIPAA privacy regulations

f. Prepare and release private health information as required, adhering to state and Federal guidelines

g. Chart information

6. Transcription and dictation

a. Transcribe notes from dictation system

b. Transcribe letter or notes from direct dictation

7. Supplies and equipment management

a. Maintain inventory of medical office supplies and equipment

b. Coordinate maintenance and repair of office equipment

    c. Maintain equipment maintenance logs according to OSHA regulations

8. Computer applications
    a. Identify and understand hardware components
    b. Identify and understand application of basic software and operating systems
    c. Recognize software application for patient record maintenance, bookkeeping, patient accounting system
    d. Employ procedures for integrity of information and compliance with HIPAA Security and Privacy regulations
       (1) encryption
       (2) firewall software and hardware
       (3) personnel passwords
       (4) access restrictions
       (5) activity logs

9. Office safety
    a. Maintain office sanitation and comfort
    b. Develop and maintain office safety manual *
    c. Develop emergency procedures and policies
    d. Employ procedures in compliance with Occupational Safety and Health Administration guidelines and regulations
       (1) hazard communication
       (2) engineering and work practice controls
       (3) employee training program
       (4) standard precautions
    e. Maintain records of biohazardous waste and chemical disposal

III. CLINICAL MEDICAL ASSISTING†

  E. Physical Examinations
    1. Medical history
      a. Obtain patient history employing appropriate terminology and abbreviations

      b. Differentiate between subjective and objective information
      c. Understand and employ SOAP charting system for recording information
    3. Methods of examination
      a. Define methods of examination
        (1) auscultation
        (2) palpation
        (3) mensuration
        (4) percussion
      b. Understand use of each examination method

  F. Clinical Pharmacology
    3. Prescriptions
      a. Identify and define drug schedules and legal prescription requirements for each
      b. Understand procedures for completing prescriptions and authorization of medical refills
      c. Identify and perform proper documentation of medication transactions
    4. Drugs
      a. Identify Drug Enforcement Agency regulations for ordering, dispensing, prescribing, storing, and documenting regulated drugs
      b. Identify and define drug categories
      c. Identify commonly used drugs
      d. Identify and describe routes of medication administration
        (1) parenteral
        (2) rectal
        (3) topical
        (4) vaginal
        (5) sublingual
        (6) oral
        (7) inhalation
        (8) installation
      e. Demonstrate ability to use drug references (*Physician's Desk Reference*)

---

*Denotes advanced skills

†Only those clinical competenies that apply to this text are listed.

Table B-4. American Medical Technologists (AMT) Competencies and Construction Parameters for the Registered Medical Assistant (RMA) Examination

Administrative Medical Assisting, 6ed.		I. GENERAL MEDICAL ASSISTING KNOWLEDGE						II. ADMINISTRATIVE MEDICAL ASSISTING			III. CLINICAL
Ch	Title	A. A & P	B. Medical Termi-nology	C. Medical Law	D. Med-ical Ethics	E. Human Rela-tions	F. Patient Educa-tion	A. Insurance	B. Financial Bookkeeping	C. Medical Receptionist, Secretarial, Clerical	A.–K
1	A Career As an Administrative Medical Assistant	1	1, 2, 3, 4	1d, 2a	1a, 1e	1b, 2a	1a–g				
2	The Health Care Environment: Past, Present, and Future		1, 2, 3, 4				1, 3	2b(1)			
3	Medicolegal and Ethical Responsibilities		1, 2, 3, 4	1a, b, c, e, 3a	1a, b, c, d		1			2e, 4g, 5f	
4	The Art of Communication		1, 2, 3, 4			1, 2				2a, 4h	
5	The Receptionist		1, 2, 3, 4			1b, c	2a, 3a			1a, 2a, b, c, d, e, f, g	
6	Telephone Procedures		1, 2, 3, 4	1b		1c	1, 3a			1a, 4a, b, c, g, h, 5g	
7	Appointments		3a			2a(3), (4)	1, 3a			1a, 3a(1), 4a, b, c	
8	Filing Procedures		1							5a–g	
9	Medical Records	1a–k	1, 3				3a			2d, 4h, 5a, c, d(1–4), e, f, g, 6a, 8d(1), (3)	E1, 3
10	Drug and Prescription Records		1, 2, 3, 4				1, 3a			5g, 6a	F3a, b, c, 4a, b, d, e
11	Written Correspondence		1, 2, 3, 4							4f, g, 6a, b, 8b	
12	Processing Mail and Telecommunications		2, 3							4f, 8d(1–3)	
13	Fees, Credit, and Collection		2, 3					5b, d	2a–g, 3a–e		
14	Banking		2, 3						2b, c, 5b–f		
15	Bookkeeping		2, 3						2a, b, 4a(1–2), b, c, d, 5a, b, 7a		
16	Health Insurance Systems		2, 3					1a, 2a, b(1–7), 3a(1–2), 3b(1–2), 4a(1–3), 4b, 5a, c		3c	
17	Office Managerial Responsibilities		2, 3	1b, c	e	2a(1–4)	2a	2b(3)	7a	7a, c, 8, 9a–e	A2, I1c
18	Financial Management of the Medical Practice		2, 3						1a, 4a, d, 5g, 6a(1–2), b(1–3), c, 7a		
19	Seeking a Position As an Administrative Medical Assistant		2			2a(1)				4f, h	

CMAS EXAMINATION SPECIFICATIONS

The American Medical Technologists (AMT) have developed (2003) competencies and examination specifications for the Certified Medical Administrative Specialist (CMAS) as follows.* These are cross-referenced in a chapter-by-chapter grid (see Table B-5) to help locate them in the *Administrative Medical Assisting* textbook and *Workbook*.

I. MEDICAL ASSISTING FOUNDATIONS

A. Medical Terminology
 1. Use and spell basic medical terms appropriately
 2. Identify root words, prefixes, and suffixes
 3. Define basic medical terms

B. Anatomy and Physiology
 1. Know basic structures and functions of body systems
 2. Know various disorders of the body

C. Legal and Ethical Considerations
 1. Apply principles of medical law and ethics to the health care setting
 2. Recognize legal responsibilities of, and know scope of practice for the medical administrative specialist
 3. Know basic laws pertaining to medical practice
 4. Know and observe disclosure laws
 5. Know the principles of medical ethics established by the AMA
 6. Recognize unethical practices and identify ethical responses for situations in the medical office

D. Professionalism
 1. Employ human relations skills appropriate to the health care setting
 2. Display behaviors of a professional medical administrative specialist
 3. Participate in appropriate continuing education

II. BASIC CLINICAL MEDICAL OFFICE ASSISTING

A. Basic Health History Interview
 1. Obtain preliminary health histories from patients

B. Basic Charting
 1. Chart patient information

C. Vital Signs and Measurements
 1. Measure vital signs
 2. Obtain other vital measurements (weight, height)

D. Asepsis in the medical office
 1. Understand concepts of asepsis, sanitization, disinfection, and sterilization
 2. Understand prevention of disease transmission
 3. Observe standard precautions

E. Examination Preparation
 1. Prepare patients for clinical examinations

F. Medical Office Emergencies
 1. Recognize and respond to medical emergencies
 2. Employ first aid and CPR appropriately
 3. Report emergencies as required by law

G. Pharmacology
 1. Understand basic pharmacological concepts and terminology

III. MEDICAL OFFICE CLERICAL ASSISTING

A. Appointment Management and Scheduling
 1. Schedule and monitor patient and visitor appointments
 2. Address cancellations and missed appointments
 3. Prepare information for referrals and preauthorizations
 4. Arrange hospital admissions and surgery, and schedule patients for outpatient diagnostic tests
 5. Manage recall system and file

B. Reception
 1. Receive and process patients and visitors
 2. Screen visitors and vendors requesting to see physician
 3. Coordinate patient flow into examining rooms

C. Communication
 1. Employ effective written and oral communication
 2. Address and process incoming telephone calls from outside providers, pharmacies, and vendors
 3. Employ appropriate telephone etiquette when screening patient calls and addressing office business
 4. Recognize and employ proper protocols for telephone emergencies

The competencies are reprinted with permission from the American Medical Technologists.

5. Format business documents and correspondence appropriately
6. Process incoming and outgoing mail

D. Patient Information and Community Resources
    1. Order and organize patient informational materials
    2. Maintain list of community referral resources

IV. MEDICAL RECORDS MANAGEMENT
A. Systems
    1. Demonstrate knowledge of, and manage patient medical records systems
    2. Manage documents and patient charts using paper methods
    3. Manage documents and patient charts using computerized methods
B. Procedures
    1. File records alphabetically, numerically, by subject, and by color
    2. Employ rules of indexing
    3. Arrange contents of patient charts in appropriate order
    4. Document and file laboratory results and patient communication in charts
    5. Perform corrections and additions to records
    6. Store, protect, retain, and destroy records appropriately
    7. Transfer files
    8. Perform daily chart management
    9. Prepare charts for external review and audits
C. Confidentiality
    1. Observe and maintain confidentiality of records, charts, and test results
    2. Observe special regulations regarding the confidentiality of protected information

V. HEALTH CARE INSURANCE PROCESSING, CODING, AND BILLING
A. Insurance Processing
    1. Understand private/commercial health care insurance plans (PPO, HMO, traditional indemnity)
    2. Understand government health care insurance plans (Medicare, Medicaid, Veteran's Administration, CHAMPUS, TRICARE, use of Advance Beneficiary Notices)

3. Process patient claims using appropriate forms and time frames
4. Process workers' compensation/disability reports and forms
5. Submit claims for third-party reimbursements including the use of electronic transmission methods

B. Coding
    1. Understand procedure and diagnosis coding
    2. Employ *Current Procedural Terminology (CPT)* and Evaluation and Management codes appropriately
    3. Employ *International Classification of Diagnostic (ICD-9-CM)* codes appropriately
    4. Employ *Health Care Financing Administration Common Procedure Coding System (HCPCS)* codes appropriately

C. Insurance Billing and Finances
    1. Understand health care insurance terminology
    2. Understand billing requirements for health care insurance plans
    3. Process insurance payments
    4. Track unpaid claims and file and track appeals
    5. Understand fraud and abuse regulations

VI. MEDICAL OFFICE FINANCIAL MANAGEMENT
A. Fundamental Financial Management
    1. Understand basic principles of accounting
    2. Perform bookkeeping procedures including balancing accounts
    3. Perform financial computations
    4. Manage accounts payable
    5. Manage accounts receivable
    6. Prepare monthly trial balance reports
    7. Understand basic audit controls
    8. Understand professional fee structures
    9. Understand physician/practice owner compensation provisions
    10. Understand credit arrangements
    11. Manage other financial aspects of office management
B. Patient Accounts
    1. Manage patient accounts/ledgers
    2. Manage patient billing
    3. Manage collections in compliance with state and federal regulations
C. Banking

1. Understand banking services and procedures
2. Manage petty cash

D. Payroll
1. Prepare employee payroll and reports
2. Maintain payroll tax deduction procedures and records

VII. MEDICAL OFFICE INFORMATION PROCESSING

A. Fundamentals of Computing
1. Possess fundamental knowledge of computing in the medical office including keyboarding, data entry, and retrieval
2. Possess fundamental knowledge of PC-based environment
3. Possess fundamental knowledge of word processing, spreadsheet, database, and presentation graphics applications
4. Employ procedures for ensuring the integrity and confidence of computer-stored information

B. Medical Office Computer Applications
1. Employ medical office software applications
2. Use computer for billing and financial transactions
3. Employ e-mail applications

VIII. MEDICAL OFFICE MANAGEMENT

A. Office Communications *
1. Facilitate staff meetings and in-service, and ensure communication of essential information to staff

B. Business Organization Management *
1. Manage medical office business functions

2. Manage office mailing and shipping services
3. Manage outside vendors and supplies
4. Manage contracts and relationships with associated health care providers
5. Comply with licensure and accreditation requirements

C. Human resources *
1. Manage/supervise medical office staff
2. Conduct performance reviews and disciplinary action
3. Maintain office policy manual
4. Manage staff payroll and scheduling
5. Manage staff recruiting in compliance with state and federal laws
6. Orient and train new staff
7. Manage employee benefits

D. Safety
1. Maintain office safety, maintain office safety manual, and post emergency instructions
2. Observe emergency safety requirements
3. Maintain records of biohazardous waste, hazardous chemicals, and safety conditions
4. Comply with Occupational Safety and Health Act guidelines and regulations

E. Supplies and Equipment
1. Manage medical and office supply inventories and order supplies
2. Maintain office equipment and arrange for equipment maintenance and repair

F. Physical Office Plant
1. Maintain office facilities and environment

G. Risk Management and Quality Assurance
1. Understand and employ risk management and quality assurance concepts

---

Job functions may or may not be entry-level; however, the competent specialist should have sound knowledge of these management functions at certification level.

Table B-5. American Medical Technologists (AMT) Competencies and Examination Specifications for the Certified Medical Administrative Specialist (CMAS) Examination

Administrative Medical Assisting, 6ed.

Ch	Title	I. Medical Assisting Foundation	II. Basic Clinical Medical Office Assisting	III. Medical Office Clerical Assisting	IV. Medical Records Management	V. Health Care Insurance Processing, Coding, and Billing	VI. Medical Office Financial Management	VII. Medical Office Information Processing	VIII. Medical Office Management
1	A Career As an Administrative Medical Assistant	A, B1, D1, 2, 3	B-1	D2				A1, A2	B-5
2	The Health Care Environment: Past, Present, and Future	A1, 3	C-2	A3		A1			
3	Medicolegal and Ethical Responsibilities	A1, 3, C1, 3, 4, 5, 6			C-2				G-1
4	The Art of Communication	A1, 3, D1, 4		C1					
5	The Receptionist	A1, 3, C4, D1, 2	A1, F1	B, D	B8, C			A4, B3	D2, 3, F1
6	Telephone Procedures	A1, D1	B, F1	C1, 3, 4	A2, C1				
7	Appointments	A1, D1	B1, F1	A1, 2, 3, 4, 5, B2-3, C3	A2			B1	
8	Filing Procedures				A1-3, B1-4, 6-8, C1-2				
9	Medical Records	A1, B1-2	A1, B1		A1-3, B3, 5, 9, C1			A4	
10	Drug and Prescription Records	A1	B1, G1		A2, 3, B8				
11	Written Correspondence	A1	C1, 5					A1, 2, 3, B1	
12	Processing Mail and Telecommunications	A1		C1, 6	C2			A4, B1, 3	B2
13	Fees, Credit, and Collection	A1					A5, 8, 10, B1-3		
14	Banking	A1					A3-5, B1, C1		
15	Bookkeeping	A1					A1-7, B1, C2	B1, 2	
16	Health Insurance Systems	A1				A1-5, B1-4, C1-4			
17	Office Managerial Responsibilities	A1, D3	D2, F	D1					A1, B1-3, C1-3, 6, 7, D1-7, E1-2, F1
18	Financial Management of the Medical Practice	A1					A1, 3, 4, C1, D1, 2		
19	Seeking a Position As an Administrative Medical Assistant	A1, D2		C1, 5				A2	C2

AAMA ROLE DELINEATION STUDY

Competencies required to practice medical assisting were first described in the American Association of Medical Assistants' 1979 DACUM (**D**eveloping **A** Curricul**UM**). In 1996 and 1997 the AAMA began to do a major occupational analysis of the practice of medical assisting, titled the Role Delineation Study (2003). Content of the information from the study was categorized into the following areas of competency for entry-level medical assistants. These are cross-referenced in a chapter-by-chapter grid (see Table B-6) to help locate them in the *Administrative Medical Assisting* textbook and *Workbook*.

In addition, the books meet the requirements and standards set forth by the National Health Care Skill Standards Project for multiskilling and multitasking for the Information Services Cluster for the occupation of medical assisting.

I. ADMINISTRATIVE
A. Administrative Procedures
   1. Perform basic administrative medical assisting functions
   2. Schedule, coordinate and monitor appointments
   3. Schedule inpatient/outpatient admissions and procedures
   4. Understand and apply third-party guidelines
   5. Obtain reimbursement through accurate claims submission
   6. Monitor third-party reimbursement
   7. Understand and adhere to managed care policies and procedures
   8. Negotiate managed care contracts *
B. Practice Finances
   1. Perform procedural and diagnostic coding
   2. Apply bookkeeping principles
   3. Mange accounts receivable
   4. Mange accounts payable *
   5. Process payroll *
   6. Document and maintain accounting and banking records *
   7. Develop and maintain fee schedules *

   8. Manage renewals of business and professional insurance policies *
   9. Manage personnel benefits and maintain records *
   10. Perform marketing, financial, and strategic planning *

III. CLINICAL [†]
C. Patient Care
   7. Maintain medication and immunization records
   8. Recognize and respond to emergencies
   9. Coordinate patient care information with other health care providers

III. GENERAL
A. Professionalism
   1. Display a professional manner and image
   2. Demonstrate initiative and responsibility
   3. Work as a member of the health care team
   4. Prioritize and perform multiple tasks
   5. Adapt to change
   6. Promote the CMA credential
   7. Enhance skills through continuing education
   8. Treat all patients with compassion and empathy
   9. Promote and practice through positive public relations
B. Communication Skills
   1. Recognize and respect cultural diversity
   2. Adapt communications to individual's ability to understand
   3. Use a professional telephone technique
   4. Recognize and respond effectively to verbal, nonverbal, and written communications
   5. Use medical terminology appropriately
   6. Utilize electronic technology to receive, organize, prioritize, and transmit information
   7. Serve as liaison
C. Legal Concepts
   1. Perform within legal and ethical boundaries
   2. Prepare and maintain medical records
   3. Document accurately
   4. Follow employer's established policies dealing with the health care contract

*Denotes advanced skills

[†]Only those clinical competenies that apply to this text are listed.

5. Implement and maintain federal and state health care legislation and regulations
6. Comply with established risk management and safety procedures
7. Recognize professional credentialing criteria
8. Develop and maintain personnel, policy, and procedure manuals

D. Instruction
1. Instruct individuals according to their needs
2. Explain office policies and procedures
3. Teach methods of health promotion and disease prevention
4. Locate community resources and disseminate information

5. Develop educational materials *
6. Conduct continuing education activities *

E. Operational Functions
1. Perform inventory of supplies and equipment
2. Perform routine maintenance of administrative and clinical equipment
3. Apply computer techniques to support office operations
4. Perform personnel management functions *
5. Negotiate leases and prices for equipment and supply contracts*

*Denotes advanced skills

Table B-6. American Association of Medical Assistants (AAMA) Role Delineation Study
Developed to provide a current analysis of the profession in the workplace (updated 2002)

Administrative Medical Assisting, 6ed.		I. ADMINISTRATIVE		II. CLINICAL	III. GENERAL				
Ch	Title	A. Administrative Procedures	B. Practice Finances	A. B. C. Clinical	A. Professionalism	B. Communication Skills	C. Legal Concepts	D. Instruction	E. Operational Functions
1	A Career As an Administrative Medical Assistant	1		C1-9	1, 2, 4, 5, 6, 7, 8, 9	2, 5, 7	1, 7	1, 2, 3, 4	
2	The Health Care Environment: Past, Present, and Future	1, 7			3	5	3	1	
3	Medicolegal and Ethical Responsibilities	1				5	1, 5, 6	1	
4	The Art of Communication	1			4, 8, 9	1, 2, 4, 5, 7	4	4	
5	The Receptionist	1, 7		C8	1, 3, 4, 5, 8, 9	5, 6, 7	2, 4, 5, 6	2, 3, 4	
6	Telephone Procedures	1		C8	4, 8, 9	2, 3, 4, 5, 6	2, 3	1, 2	
7	Appointments	1, 2, 3		C8, 9		3, 5, 6, 7	2, 3	1, 2	
8	Filing Procedures	1				5, 6	2, 3		
9	Medical Records	1		C2, 7		5, 6	2, 3		3
10	Drug and Prescription Records	1		C7		5, 6	1, 2, 3, 6, 7	1, 2	1
11	Written Correspondence	1				4, 5			
12	Processing Mail and Telecommunications	1				4, 5, 6			3
13	Fees, Credit, and Collection	1	2, 3, 7			5			3
14	Banking	1	2, 3, 4, 6						
15	Bookkeeping	1	2, 3, 4, 7						3
16	Health Insurance Systems	1, 4, 5, 6, 7	1			6			
17	Office Managerial Responsibilities	1	8, 9, 10	C7	1, 2, 3, 7, 9	1, 5, 6, 7	1, 5, 8	1, 2, 5, 6	1, 2, 4, 5
18	Financial Management of the Medical Practice	1, 8	2, 4, 5, 6		1, 3, 4	5, 7	1, 5		3, 4
19	Seeking a Position As an Administrative Medical Assistant	1			1, 2, 3, 9	2, 4, 5, 6			3

GLOSSARY

The number in parentheses after each term is the chapter in which the term is discussed in depth.

ABA number (14)   Coding system developed by the American Bankers Association and used on checks to identify the location of the bank; also called bank number or transit

abstract (9)   In the context of handling a medical record, to extract, or take out, specific information or to summarize from documentation in a patient's chart; often done for insurance purposes

account (15)   Formal record of all transactions made on an individual's financial record, listing debits, credits, and balance; may be computerized. In a medical practice using a manual bookkeeping system, this term is referred to as a ledger or ledger card

account receivable (A/R) (13)   Total amount of money owed for services rendered by all parties

accounts payable (A/P) ledger (15)   Record book that lists detailed amounts owed to creditors for the operation of a business, such as supplies and equipment, services rendered, or facility expenses

accounts receivable (A/R) ledger (15)   Record book that lists all patients' outstanding accounts showing how much each one owes for services rendered

accreditation (1)   Process of meeting a state standard or being evaluated and recognized by a national organization as meeting predetermined standards

active listening (4)   Giving the speaker your undivided attention, resisting urges to respond verbally, mentally focusing and concentrating on the message being relayed

adjudicate (16)   To settle judicially as in a determination of payment for an insurance claim

adjuster (16)   Employee of an insurance carrier with whom a case is assigned and who follows the case until it is adjusted, or settled; grants verbal authorization in workers' compensation cases for testing, procedures, surgeries, and referrals

adjustment (15)   Credit entry made on an account or ledger to decrease a balance that may be due to professional discounts, courtesy adjustments (write-offs), disallowances by insurance companies, or to correct bookkeeping errors

administrative medical assistant (1)   Office personnel whose responsibilities include a variety of secretarial and clerical duties. In a physician's office, works in the front-office and may perform managerial and supervisory functions, manage office personnel, and participate in service activities aimed at improving the health of the community

advance directive (3)   Document stating an individual's preference about treatment if the person becomes incompetent or unable to communicate with medical personnel. It may instruct physicians to withhold or withdraw life-sustaining procedures, or it may contain a request to receive all available treatment. Two types of advance directives are a living will and health care (durable) power of attorney.

agenda (17)   List of items to be discussed at a staff meeting

aggressive (1)   One whose behavior is belligerent, confrontational, pushy, forward, or overbearing

aging accounts (13)   Analysis of accounts receivable indicating 30, 60, 90, and 120 days delinquency

alphabetic filing (8)   Arrangement of names in alphabetic sequence according to filing units

American Association of Medical Assistants (AAMA) (1)   National association of medical assistants, medical assisting students, and medical assisting educators with both state and local chapters; recognized by the American Medical Association

American Medical Technologists (AMT) (1)   Association that features a registered medical assistant (RMA) and certified medical administrative specialist (CMAS) program and examination for certification as well as student membership

annotate (12)   To make explanatory notation in the margins on correspondence so that actions can be taken

answering service (6)   Business that specializes in taking and relaying telephone messages when offices are closed

appointment abbreviations (7)   Shortened words or coded numbers indicating types of appointments, types of patients, types of insurance, and reasons for appointments

appointment block (7)   Segment of time set aside in the appointment schedule for a specific patient type or procedure

appointment book (7)   Set of sheets used to schedule and record time set aside for patients to see health care practitioners for procedures and services

appointment card (7)   Small card preprinted with the physician's name, address, and telephone number showing the day, date, and time of an appointment; given to the patient to serve as a reminder

appointment schedule (7)   List designating chronological fixed times for patients to meet with the physician and/or receive medical services

assertive (1)   One who appears confident and is self-assured

assets (15)   Any possessions, either physical objects (tangible) or resources (intangible) having money value. Tangible assets include cash, inventory, furniture, fixtures, and equipment; intangible assets may be a service, trademark, or goodwill.

assignment (16)   Agreement by which a patient assigns to another party (e.g., a physician) the right to receive payment from a third party (e.g., insurance plan or program) for the service the patient has received

associate practice (2)   Two or more physicians operating as solo practitioners billing under separate tax identification numbers, sharing office expenses, employees, and the on-call schedule

Association of Records Managers and Administrators, Inc. (ARMA International) (8)   Nonprofit records management association organized to promote research and provide standardized filing guidelines

attending physician (9)   Medical staff member who is legally responsible for the care and treatment given to a patient

audit (9)   Periodic examination or review of patient records to verify recordkeeping, documentation for level of service billed, and proper medical care

authorization form (3)   Document for use and disclosure of protected health information not included in a consent form that delineates the purpose for which the health care information is to be used and disclosed

automated files (8)   Electronic equipment that brings records automatically to the operator; used in hospitals, clinics, and large practices

automated teller machine (ATM) (14)   Computerized terminal that enables a customer to deposit, withdraw, or transfer funds, or obtain other bank services

automatic transfer of funds (14)   Withdrawal of funds from one account and transfer to another, in specific amounts, at specified times, and according to a prior written agreement

back ordered (B/0) (17)   Invoice notation indicating that an ordered item will be sent as soon as it is made available to the supplier

backup (8)   Duplicate data file; equipment designed to complete or redo an operation if primary equipment fails

balance (15)   Amount owed on a credit transaction after payments and adjustments have been recorded; also known as outstanding, running, or unpaid balance

balance sheet (18)   Systematic statement of the assets, liabilities, and capital of a business on a specified date

bank by mail (14)   Bank service whereby deposits are mailed by the customer to the bank and credited to the customer's account

bank statement (14)   Monthly itemization of all transactions of a checking account, showing checks paid, deposits made, service charges, and beginning and ending balances; may be accompanied by canceled checks, photocopies of checks, or recorded on microfiche; contains a *bank reconciliation* form to be completed by the payer

bankruptcy (13)   State of being legally unable to pay one's debts

bar code sorter (BCS) (12)   Code imprinted on first-class mail to speed sorting and delivery

bearer (14)   Person delivering an item for payment

bias (4)   To prejudge or have a one-sided opinion that influences your judgment negatively

bill (13)   Statement of fees owed for services rendered

binder file folder (8)   Document container with clamps for securing data

bioethics (3)   Branch of ethics concerning moral issues, questions, and problems that arise in the practice of medicine and in biomedical research

biohazard (5)   Material that is potentially harmful to humans, such as body fluid

blind letter (19)   Communication expressing an interest in a job should one become available

bonding (3)   Obligation of an insurance company or bonding agency to protect an employer against financial loss caused by the acts or omissions of employees

bookkeeping (15)   Process used for analyzing and recording business transactions for the purpose of collecting amounts due and reporting the financial condition of the business at a future date

brand name (10)   Proprietary or trade name of a drug as copyrighted by the manufacturer

burnout (1)   Condition of severe or chronic mental, physical, and/or emotional stress characterized by a specific set of symptoms, which is brought on by working too long and too hard

caduceus (2)   Symbol of the medical profession. The winged, snake-entwined staff carried by Mercury depicting Hermes, the Greek god of science, commerce, eloquence, invention, cunning, and guide of departed souls to Hades

calculator (13)   Machine used to perform basic arithmetic functions

callbacks (6)   Term indicating that a return telephone call is necessary

capital (15)   Physician's share in a business plus operating profit; also known as *owner's equity* or *net worth*

capitation (2, 16)   Method of payment for health services by which a health group is prepaid a fixed, per capita amount for each patient served, without considering the actual amount of service provided to each patient

caption (8)   Name or number used in a filing system under which records are filed

case history (9)   Past and current information used in the evaluation process by the physician; part of the medical record

cash (15)   Money (currency and coins) and negotiable checks, for example, cashier's checks and money orders

cellular telephone (6) Wireless telephone that communicates through cell sites (antenna towers) placed in sections of a city. The caller/receiver is automatically transferred from cell to cell as he or she moves around

certification (1) Statement issued by a board or association that verifies that a person meets professional standards

Certified Mail (12) Service of the U.S. Postal Service that provides, for a fee, a receipt to the sender of First-Class Mail and a record of its delivery

Certified Medical Administrative Specialist (CMAS) (1) Title received after appropriate training in administrative procedures and passing a certification examination administered by the American Medical Technologists (AMT)

Certified Medical Assistant (CMA [AAMA]) (1) Title received after appropriate training and passing a certification examination administered by the American Association of Medical Assistants

charge (13) Amount billed (price) for professional services rendered; "fees" is the preferred term in current usage; a debit to an account

charge-out system (8) Procedure in a filing system provided to account for items removed from the files

check (CK) (14) Order to pay; the most common form of money exchange, with the exception of cash

checking account (14) Account on which interest may be paid depending on the balance. Monies are deposited into the account, and the bank will accept valid orders (e.g., checks) to pay funds to designated recipients

CHEDDAR (9) Abbreviation for *chief complaint, history, examination, details of complaints, drugs* and *dosage, assessment,* and *return visit*; used as a format for charting

chemical name (10) Name, usually long and often complicated, describing the main chemical content of a drug

chronological resumé (19) Data sheet that outlines experience and education by dates

civil law (3) Statute that enforces private rights and liabilities, as differentiated from criminal law

claim (16) Request for payment under an insurance contract or bond

clearinghouse (16) Centralized location where claims are received, edited, and distributed electronically to insurance companies

clinic (2) Establishment where patients undergo physical examination and treatment by a group of health care professionals practicing medicine together; may include several physicians of the same or different specialties; is sometimes limited to serving poor or public patients; and is sometimes limited to facilities for graduate or undergraduate medical education

clinical medical assistant (1) Back-office medical assistant who performs clinical and laboratory duties

closed accounts (18) Accounts with a zero balance or accounts at the end of the year when the final posting is completed

clustering (7) Act of scheduling patients with similar ailments in group sequence

coding (8) Prefiling process of marking correspondence with the caption or number under which it will be stored

coinsurance (16) Cost-sharing requirement under a health insurance policy that stipulates the insured assumes a percentage of the costs of covered services

collection ratio (13) Proportion of money owed to money collected on accounts receivable

colloquialisms (4) Slang or informal language

combination resumé (19) Data sheet that combines specific dates of work experience with education and skills

commercial filing system (8) Customized guides and folders manufactured for professional office use

communicate (4) Transfer information from one party to another

communication cycle (4) Basic elements needed to communicate: (1) *sender*, person who has an idea or information and wants to convey it, (2) *message*, content that needs to be communicated, (3) *channel*, method of sending the message to the receiver, (4) *receiver*, recipient getting the message and interpreting it, and (5) *feedback*, response from the receiver used to decide if clarification is necessary

complaint (3) First pleading (court document) of one who initiates action in a civil case

compliance plan (3) Written protocol outlining practice standards that include federal and state mandates

conference call (6) Telephone call linking several persons at different geographic locations in one conversation; teleconferencing

consent form (3, 16) One-time signed document required *before* physicians use or disclose personally identifiable health information for treatment, payment, or routine health care operations

consulting physician (9) Provider whose opinion or advice regarding evaluation or management of a specific problem is requested by another physician

continuing education unit (CEU(s)) (2) Credit for course hours that an individual receives for attending or taking part in an educational program. State and organization requirements vary when renewing a professional license or certification; also known as continuing education credit (CEC); documented in time (e.g., 1.0 CEU = 10 hours).

conversion privilege (16) Clause in a group insurance policy that allows the insured to continue the same or lesser coverage under an individual policy

coordination of benefits (COB) (16) Provisions and procedures used by insurers to avoid duplicate payment for losses insured under more than one insurance policy

copayment (copay) (16) Type of cost-sharing (flat fee) whereby the insured pays a specified amount per unit of service and the insurer pays the rest of the cost

cover letter (19) In job seeking, a letter of introduction prepared to accompany a resumé

credit (13, 14) From the Latin *credere*, "to believe" or "to trust"; trust in regard to financial obligations; in banking, a deposit or addition to a bank account

credits (15) Bookkeeping entries reflecting a decrease in the account balance; includes payments by debtors (patients) of a sum received on their account or an adjustment (write-off); such amounts are entered on the right-hand side of an account or ledger. A credit increases an income account and decreases an expense account.

currency (14) Paper money in circulation, issued by the government through an act of law

cut (8) Term used in filing to describe the size of the tab on the back of a file folder; usually expressed as a fraction, for example, *one-half cut*

cycle billing (13) Sending itemized statements to portions of the accounts receivable at certain times of the month; can be divided by alphabet, account number, insurance type, or by calendar day of first visit

databases (8) Collection of data (information) stored electronically

daysheet (15) Register for recording all daily business transactions; also known as daybook, daily journal sheet, daily record sheet, or general ledger

debit (14) In banking, a withdrawal from or charge to a bank account

debit card (13) Card used by bank customers to either withdraw cash from any affiliated automated teller machine (ATM) or make electronic transfers of cash from a customer's bank account to a merchant's account; AKA *bank card*

debits (15) Bookkeeping entries reflecting money owed; the increase of an asset or a business expense or the decrease of a liability of an owner's equity; such amounts are entered on the left-hand side of an account

deductible (deduc) (16) Amount the insured must pay in a calendar or fiscal year before policy benefits begin

deductions (18) Amounts withheld from an employee's gross income for income tax purposes

defendant (3) Person sued (defending or denying action); usually the physician in a malpractice case

defensive (4) A response to protect oneself from a perceived threat; usually unconscious. The threat may stem from anxiety, guilt, loss of self-esteem, or an injured ego.

demeanor (4) How a person appears, their expressions and body language

dependents (16) Under an insurance contract, the spouse and children of the insured; in some cases, domestic partners

deposit record (14) Printed receipt for a deposit issued by the bank

deposit slip (14) Form, also known as a *deposit ticket*, provided by banks to itemize monies placed in a savings or checking account

deposits (14) Funds given to a bank to be credited to an account

DHL WorldWide Express (12) National and international letter and package delivery service

diagnosis (9, 16) Determination of the nature of a disease or injury

diagnostic file (8) Information based on the characteristics of a disease or illness learned from patient case histories and filed for reference

diplomate (19) Physician certified by a medical board in a field of specialization

direct deposit service (14) Process by which a check's issuer transmits the check directly to the payee's program or service bank for credit to the latter's account

disbursement record (18) Chronological register of monthly business expenditures and yearly totals

discrimination (4) To unfairly treat an individual or group based on age, culture, gender, race, religion, life style, or sexual orientation

displaced anger (4) Anger that is completely unrelated to the event that is presently occurring; it may be built up or held in from another event and released at an inappropriate time

domestic mail (12) Mail delivered in the United States, Canada, and Mexico

double-entry accounting (15) Bookkeeping system of financial records used in business, whereby equal accounting debits and credits are recorded for each transaction

download (8) Process of transferring data (file or program) from a central computer to a remote computer

downtime (8) Period during which a computer is malfunctioning or not operating correctly

Drug Enforcement Administration (DEA) (10) Federal agency whose mission is to enforce the Controlled Substances laws and regulations of the United States and to bring to justice those organizations involved in the growing, manufacturing, or distribution of controlled substances; issues narcotic and hypnotic licenses to physicians

dun (13) Message or phrase used on the billing statement to remind a person about a delinquent payment

edit (11) Revisions, alterations, and refinements made to documents before final printing

electronic files (8) Collection of related data stored under a single title in a computerized system

electronic funds transfer system (EFTS) (14) Paperless computerized system, which enables funds to be debited, credited, or transferred. For paying bills, a claim is made by electronic notification and a transfer of funds is simultaneously effected; in other words, one computer transfers information to another computer, eliminating the need for personal handling of bills, checks, or similar documents.

electronic health record (EHR) (9) Computerized medical record, also referred to as an electronic medical record (EMR), that has the capability to capture and store data in electronic form and to be transmitted to other health care locations.

electronic job search (19) Locate and investigate job sites and employment opportunities by using the Internet

electronic mail (12) Process of sending, receiving, storing, and forwarding messages and memos in digital form over the Internet; also called e-mail

elimination period (16) Period of time after the onset of a disability for which no benefits will be paid

elite (E) type (11) Type size measuring 12 characters to the horizontal inch

emancipated minors (3) Children of any age who fall outside the jurisdiction and custody of their parents or guardians and who may make financial and medical decisions

emergency care (6) Medical care given for a serious medical condition resulting from injury or illness that if not given immediately puts a person's life in danger

empathy (1) Pertaining to projection of one's own consciousness into another person's situation

employee handbook (17) Written procedures for general personnel policies

Employee Withholding Allowance Certificate (Form W-4) (18) Document completed yearly by new and existing employees to indicate exemptions claimed for tax withholding purposes

employer identification number (EIN) (18) Nine-digit number issued by the Internal Revenue Service to identify tax accounts of employers; also called *tax identification number (TIN)*

Employer's Quarterly Federal Tax Return (18) Schedule of financial information (Form 841) required four times a year by governmental bodies

employment agencies (19) Business organizations that contract with employers to locate, test, and refer qualified job applicants to potential employers

enclosure (enc) (12) Supplemental item contained in an envelope with a written communication

encryption (8) Encoding of computer data for security purposes, making data appear like gibberish to unauthorized computer users

endorsement (14) Approval signature on the reverse side of a check that indicates liability for payment of funds disbursed in the case of default or nonpayment; on an item payable to the order of the endorser, it acknowledges receipt of the funds

enunciate (4) Vocalize, speak, pronounce, articulate

ergonomics (11) Science and technology that seek to fit the anatomical and physical needs of the worker to the workplace

established patient (7) Individual who has received professional health care services from the physician or another physician of the same specialty who belongs to the same group practice within the past three years

ethics (3) Standards of conduct generally accepted as a moral guide for behavior

ethnic (4) A group of society defined by origin or race

etiquette (3) Customary code of conduct, courtesy, and manners

exclusions (16) Specific hazards, perils, or conditions listed in an insurance policy for which the policy will not pay

exclusive provider organization (EPO) (2) Managed care plan operating with a limited network of physicians and a designated primary care physician for each subscriber; governed by state health insurance laws

exemptions (18) Deductions from gross income allowed a taxpayer that reduce the amount of income on which the individual is taxed

expert testimony (3) Statement given concerning a scientific, technical, or professional matter by a person with authority regarding the matter, such as a physician

explanation of benefits (EOB) (16) Recap sheet that accompanies an insurance check from a private payer or managed care plan, showing the breakdown of payment determination on a claim. In the Medicare program, this document is called a Remittance Advice (RA) for physicians and a Medicare Summary Notice (MSN) for patients; in the Medicaid program, this document is called a Remittance Advice (RA); and in the TRICARE program, this document is called a Summary Payment Voucher.

extend (15) To carry forward the balance of an individual account or ledger

face sheet (5) Portion of hospital intake record that provides identifying data

facsimile (fax) communication (12) Electronic process for transmitting written communications over telecommunication lines

Federal Express (FedEx) (12) National and international letter and package delivery service

Federal Insurance Contributions Act (FICA) (18) Law that sets amounts for Social Security taxes and benefits; most frequently termed *Social Security tax*

Federal Unemployment Tax Act (FUTA) (18) Law that provides for taxes to be collected at the federal level to help subsidize individual states' administration of their unemployment compensation programs

federal withholding tax (FWT) (18) Deduction from an employee's gross income determined by the number of withholding exemptions and amount earned for a pay period; also referred to as *federal income tax deduction*

fee-for-service (FFS) (2, 13, 16) Method of payment; the patient or insurance company pays the physician for professional services according to a specific schedule of fees

fee schedule (13) List of medical procedures and services with amounts charged

feedback (4) Oral or nonverbal response such as repeating, restatement, paraphrasing, examples, questions, or summaries

fiscal intermediary (16) Contractor that processes and pays provider claims on behalf of state or federal agencies or insurance companies; also called *fiscal agent*

fixed interval (7) See *stream schedule*

flextime (1) System that allows employees to choose their own times for starting and finishing work within a broad range of available hours

flow sheet (9) One-page lists, charts, and graphs that allow the physician to quickly find medical information and perform comparative evaluations; used for medical data that is hard to track in narrative progress notes

folder (8) Folded cover or container that holds records

forgery (14) Fraudulent signature on document

form letter (11) Standardized communication that may be personalized by the insertion of variable information

format (19) General composition or style (e.g., shape, size, spacing) of a letter, report, or document

full block letter style (11) Typed communication, also known as block style, formatted with all lines flush with the left margin

functional resumé (19) Data sheet that highlights qualifications and skills

garnishment (13) To attach a debtor's property or wages for payment of a debt

general ledger (15) Record that contains all of the financial transactions of all accounts; it has equal debits and credits as evidenced by a trial balance; see *daysheet*

generic name (10) Established, official, or nonproprietary name by which a drug is known as an isolated substance irrespective of its manufacturer

given name (8) Individual's first name

grace period (16) Specified time interval after a premium payment is due, in which the policyholder may make such payment, and during which the protection of the policy continues

grievance committee (3) Impartial panel established to listen to and investigate patients' complaints about medical care or excessive fees

gross income (18) Revenues before deductions

group practice (2) Three or more physicians sharing office space, expenses, employees, income, and using one tax identification number and billing claims under a group name

guide (8) Pressboard sheet or metal divider used in a filing system to guide the eye to a section of a file and to provide support for records

hazardous waste (5) A substance that is dangerous and potentially damaging to humans and the environment

health care power of attorney (3) Document that names another individual as a decision-maker for the patient when the patient is terminally ill or comatose. It may be used for medical decisions including life-prolonging treatment; also known as *durable power of attorney for health care*.

health information management (HIM) (9) (1) A profession that concentrates on health care data and the management of health care information; (2) department of a hospital or large clinic that stores and manages medical records; previously called *medical records department*; (3) health care professional who collects, integrates, analyzes, and codes health care data

Health Insurance Portability and Accountability Act (HIPAA) (3) Provides a standardized framework within which all insurance companies and providers work to enhance the portability of health care coverage; increase accuracy of data; protect private health information and the rights of patients; reduce fraud, abuse, and waste in the health care delivery system; upgrade efficiency and financial management; expedite claim processing; lower administrative costs and simplify implementation; promote Medical Saving Accounts; provide better access to long-term care coverage; and improve customer satisfaction to restore trust in the health care system

health maintenance organization (HMO) (2, 16) Managed care plan offering prepaid health care for a fixed fee to subscribers in a designated geographic area; enrollees receive benefits when they obtain services provided or authorized by selected providers, generally with a primary care physician (gatekeeper)

hospice (1) National program that offers medical care and support to patients and family members dealing with a terminal illness and the loss of a loved one

hospital (2) Facility that provides 24-hour acute care and treatment for the sick and injured

human resource department (19) Organizational unit in a business that has the functional responsibility to ensure that personnel policies are implemented legally and proactively, and to recruit, screen, test, hire, train, counsel, and promote workers; synonymous with *personnel department*

implied contract (3) Agreement, derived by implication or the situation, general language, or conduct of the patient

independent practice association (IPA) (2, 16) Group of individual health care providers who contract with managed care plans to provide care at a discounted rate in their own office setting

indexing unit (8) Parts of a patient's name, which has been separated into these components (units) to be considered when filing

infectious waste (5) Something that has come in contact with body fluids that can potentially transmit infection

inscription (10) Section appearing on a prescription showing the name of the drug, quantity of ingredients, and dose strength

insurance agent (16)   Representative of an insurance company licensed by the state who solicits, negotiates, or effects contracts of insurance and services the policyholder for the insurer

insurance application (16)   Signed statement of facts requested by an insurance company on the basis of which it decides whether or not to issue an insurance policy; it becomes part of the health insurance contract if a policy is issued

insured (16)   Individual or organization who contracts for a policy of insurance and is protected in case of loss of property, life, or health under the terms of the insurance policy

interoffice memorandum (11)   Written informal communication circulated within an organization or office

interpersonal skills (1)   Exemplary personality characteristics that relate to the interactions between individuals, e.g., dedication, commitment, integrity, consideration, respect, friendliness, openness, sensitivity, positive attitude, responsibility, and displaying a sense of warmth and genuineness

inventory cards (17)   Forms that indicate pertinent data on a specific item to facilitate reordering

invoice (17)   Itemized statement of merchandise ordered from a supplier stating quantity, shipping date, price, and other charges

itinerary (17)   Detailed outline for a trip

job descriptions (17)   Written statements outlining work requirements for a particular position

label (8)   Sticker used in filing that attaches to the file folder tab or other part of a folder; it may carry a caption or color code

laboratory (2)   Facility where research, experimentation, and the physical and clinical analysis of specimens are performed

laboratory report (9)   Clinical record of the findings of physical and chemical analysis of specimens

lateral file (8)   Cabinet in which records are stored perpendicular to the opening of the file; also called *vertical file*

ledger card (13, 15)   Individual financial record indicating charges, payments, adjustments, and balances owed

liabilities (15)   Legal obligations of one person to another; debts

licensure (1)   Credentialing sanctioned by state legislature (the government), which passes laws making it illegal for an individual who is not licensed to engage in activities of a licensed occupation

limitations (16)   Provision of an insurance policy that lists exceptions or reductions to specific coverage

litigation (3)   Lawsuit

living will (3)   Document, not legally binding, stating the desires of an individual should he or she become incompetent because of injury or illness when death is imminent

mail classifications (12)   Categories of mail service determined by size, contents, weight, frequency of mailing, destination, and speed of delivery

major medical (16)   Insurance policy especially designed to offset heavy medical expenses resulting from catastrophic or prolonged illness or injury

managed care organization (MCO) (2)   Health care delivery plan that strives to manage the cost, quality, and delivery of health care by emphasizing preventive medicine, reviewing the utilization of services, and contracting with a network of providers; payment is by capitation with some fee-for-service

master patient index (MPI) (8)   Computerized card file that contains information on all patients treated at a health care facility; filed alphabetically

medical assistant (2)   Multiskilled allied health professional whose practitioners work primarily in ambulatory settings such as medical offices and clinics. Medical assistants function as members of the health care delivery team and perform administrative and clinical procedures

medical center (2)   Facility offering medical services at sites other than a hospital setting

medical record (9)   Written or graphic information documenting facts and events during the rendering of patient care

medical report (9)   Permanent, legal document in letter or report format formally stating the elements performed and results of an examination and treatment of a patient

Medicare Summary Notice (MSN) (16)   See *explanation of benefits*

MinuteClinic (2)   Found in small-scale chain stores and generally staffed by physician assistants or nurse practitioners; offers a limited range of basic tests and treatments at a lower cost than most doctor's offices

mixed punctuation (11)   Style of letter punctuation in which a colon or a comma is placed after the salutation and complimentary close

modified block letter style (11)   Typed communication with a more balanced appearance, formatted with date, closing, and writer's information aligned starting at the center; all other lines are flush with the left margin

modified wave (7)   System used to schedule appointments in which patients are allocated appointment times in the first half of each hour, with the second half of each hour left open for work-ins and emergencies

money order (14)   Instrument (similar to a check) purchased for face value (plus a fee) at a bank, post office, or other place of business. It is signed by and issued according to the purchaser's instructions.

multipurpose billing form (13)   All-encompassing tracking device typically containing procedures and services, diagnoses, fees, next appointment, and other information; also called *charge slip, communicator, encounter form, fee ticket, patient service slip, routing form, superbill,* and *transaction slip*; it may be used when a patient submits an insurance claim or to extract information for insurance billing

multiskilled health practitioner (MSHP)* (1)
Persons cross-trained to provide more than one function, often in more than one discipline. These combined functions can be found in a broad spectrum of health-related jobs, ranging in complexity from the nonprofessional to the professional level, including both clinical and administrative functions. The additional functions (skills) added to the original health care worker's job may be of a higher, lower, or parallel level. The terms *multi-skilled*, *multicompetent*, and *cross-trained* can be used interchangeably.

multispecialty practice (2) Group of physicians at the same location, each specializing in a different field of medicine

National Center for Competency Testing (NCCT) (1) An independent certifying agency that validates the competence of a person's knowledge in different areas of the medical profession through examination

National Certified Medical Assistant (NCMA) (1)
One who is a high school graduate or equivalent, a graduate of an approved course of study in the area of certification, or who has two years work experience, and passes a competency examination in the administrative and clinical areas

National Certified Medical Office Assistant (NCMOA) (1) One who is a high school graduate or equivalent, a graduate of an approved course of study in the area of certification, or who has one year work experience, and passes a competency examination in the administrative area

National Provider Identifier (NPI) (16) Ten-digit number, mandated by HIPAA and issued on a lifetime basis as a standard unique health identifier for health-care providers, clearinghouses, and plans who conduct electronic transactions (may be used on paper claims); used by Medicare, Medicaid, TRICARE, CHAMPVA, and may be adopted by private insurance carriers

negotiable instrument (14) Written order to promise to pay a specified sum of money on a specified date to the order of a specific payer or to the bearer

net income (18) Employee's income after deductions have been made

new patient (7) Individual who has not received any professional services from the physician or another physician of the same specialty who belongs to the same group practice within the past three years

noncompliant (4) In a medical setting, refusing to obey the doctor's treatment plan

nonparticipating physician (nonpar) (16)
Physician who decides not to accept the determined allowable charge from an insurance plan as the full fee for professional services rendered; in the Medicare program, a nonparticipating provider is one who does not accept assignment—payment goes directly to the patient, and the patient is responsible to pay the bill in full.

However, a nonparticipating physician has two options of either not accepting assignment for all services or accepting assignment for some services and not accepting assignment for others.

nonsufficient funds (NSF) (14) Term indicating a check drawn against an account in excess of the account balance, in which case, the check is marked with the notation "NSF" or "refer to maker" and returned, unpaid, to the presenter; sometimes referred to as a "bounced check." The customer's account is assessed a fee of several dollars for each NSF check regardless of whether the bank pays it or not.

nonverbal communication (4) Communication without words, expressed through body posture, hand movements, manner of walking, and facial expressions; also called *body language*

no-show (7) Patient who does not keep a scheduled appointment and does not notify the office to cancel

notes (14) Documents indicating an obligation to pay funds, including promissory notes, collateral notes, and installment notes

numeric filing (8) Arrangement of records in number sequence

objective (9) In a medical context, facts that are apparent to the observer; descriptive of findings that can be seen, heard, felt, or measured such as swelling, bleeding, blood pressure, heart sounds, a lump, or laboratory test values

office manager (OM) (17) Individual who has administrative responsibilities for the control or direction of employees

office policies and procedures manual (17) Written guide describing office routines and practices

official name (10) Name of a drug established by the Food and Drug Administration; also known as *generic name* or *established name*

open accounts (13, 15) Accounts that are open to charges made from time to time; also known as *open-book accounts*. Physicians' patient accounts are usually open-book accounts. Record of business transactions on the books that represents an unsecured account receivable where credit has been extended without a formal written contract; payment is expected within a specified period.

open punctuation (11) Style of letter punctuation in which no punctuation mark is placed after the salutation or complimentary close

open-ended questions (4) Questions that allow the person to formulate a response and elaborate

open-shelf files (8) Cabinets with horizontal shelves for record storage

optical character recognition (OCR) (12) Computer device that can read printed or typed characters and then digitally convert them into text or numeric data

*This definition was adopted by the National Multiskilled Health Practitioner Clearinghouse (NMHPC) advisory panel.

ordering physician (9) Physician requesting nonphysician services for a patient (e.g., diagnostic laboratory tests, pharmaceutical drugs, or durable medical equipment)

outguide (8) Manila sheet or folder inserted when a file is taken from a file drawer or cabinet to signal that it has been removed from the file; a substitution card

overdraft (14) Charge against an account in excess of the account balance

pager (6) Small one-way receiver that sounds or vibrates on activation by a caller. Some pagers also display small alphanumeric messages.

partial disability (16) Illness or injury that prevents a person from performing one or more of the functions of a regular job; may be temporary or permanent

participating physician (par) (16) A physician who agrees to accept an insurance plan's preestablished fee or reasonable charge as the maximum amount collected for services rendered, also called *member physician*; in the Medicare program, a participating provider is one who accepts assignment, agrees to the approved amount based on the Medicare fee schedule as the full charge for services rendered, and receives the payment check. Patients must pay cost share and/or deductible or both for services rendered.

partnership (2) Two or more physicians associated in the practice of medicine under a legal partnership agreement

password (8) Secret word, phrase, code, or symbol input for security purposes to identify the authorized computer user who wishes to gain access to the computer system

patient instruction form (5) Checklist of topics and fill-in sheet used by the physician summarizing a patient's office visit and outlining instructions and treatment plan

practice information brochure (9) Printed material explaining office policies and procedures

payee (14) Person named on a draft or check as the recipient of the amount shown; also known as *bearer*

payer (14) Party responsible for payment of the amount owed as shown on a check or note

payroll (18) Wages or salary paid in return for goods or services; list of employees and their compensation

payroll tax (18) Charge levied by government authority on salaries and wages

perceptions (4) Assumptions that people make based on their awareness; individual discernment

performance evaluation (19) Summary of an employee's work habits, behaviors, efficiency, and effectiveness on the job

permanent disability (PD) (16) Illness or injury that is not resolved and prevents an insured person from performing all the functions of a regular job

personal digital assistant (PDA) (17) Small, handheld, computerized portable device, easily accessed, that can capture, store, and manipulate a variety of data

petty cash fund (15) Small amount of monies readily available for minor office expenses

pharmaceutical (10) Relating to pharmacy, drugs, and medicine

pharmaceutical representative (10) Professional salesperson who represents a pharmaceutical firm and offers information on drugs and other products; called a "detail rep" or "detail person"

pharmacist (10) Person skilled in the art or practice of preparing, preserving, compounding, and dispensing drugs; a druggist; an apothecary

photocopy (11) Term designating all the processes employed in producing multiple copies

photocopy machine (11) Duplicating machine that reproduces graphic matter onto paper in a few seconds

physician's profile (16) Compilation kept by each insurance carrier of a physician's charges and payments made through the years for each professional service rendered to a patient; as charges are increased, so are payments, and the profile is then updated through the use of computer data

Physicians' Desk Reference (PDR) (10) Reference book used by physicians and medical assistants to find information about prescription drugs; it contains those drugs submitted to the publisher by drug companies

pica (P) type (11) Type size measuring 10 characters to the horizontal inch

plaintiff (3) One who institutes a lawsuit or action

point-of-service (POS) plan (2, 16) Managed care plan that contracts with independent providers at a discounted rate. Members have the choice at the time services are needed (i.e., at the point-of-service) of receiving services from an HMO, PPO, or fee-for-service plan; sometimes referred to as *open-ended HMOs, swing-out HMOs, self-referral options, flex plans,* or *multiple option plans.* A patient can self-refer himself or herself to a specialist or see a nonnetwork provider for a higher coinsurance payment.

POMR (9) Abbreviation for problem-oriented medical record, a form of recordkeeping

portfolio (19) Compilation of items that represents a job applicant's skills and accomplishments

post (15) To record or transfer financial entries, debits or credits, to an account, for example, daysheet, account or ledger, bank deposit slip, check register, or journal

postdated check (14) Check dated for deposit at a future date; cannot be considered valid or payable until that date

preauthorization (16) Process of requesting permission to render a service/procedure to the patient in which the insurance plan determines the medical necessity and appropriateness of the service; also called *prior authorization* or *prior approval*

precertification (16) To determine whether services (surgery, tests, hospitalization) are covered under a patient's health insurance policy

predetermination (16) Finding out the maximum dollar amount that will be paid for specific services and procedures; also called *preestimate of cost* or *pretreatment estimate*

preexisting condition (16) An injury that occurred, a disease that was contracted, or a physical condition that existed before the issuance of a health insurance policy

preferred provider organization (PPO) (2, 16) Type of health program in which enrollees receive the highest level of benefits when obtaining services from a physician, hospital, or other health care provider called "preferred providers"; enrollees may receive substantial but reduced benefits when obtaining care from a provider of their own choice that is not a "preferred provider"

prejudice (4) Judgment formed prior to gathering all facts

premium (16) Payment made periodically to keep an insurance policy in force

prescriptions (10) Medical preparations compounded according to directions written by a physician to a pharmacist and consisting of four parts: *superscription, inscription, subscription,* and *signature*

primary care physician (PCP) (2) Physician who assumes the ongoing responsibility for the overall treatment of a patient; usually a general or family practitioner, internist, gynecologist, or pediatrician. PCPs also are referred to as *gatekeepers* in managed care plans.

privileged information (3) Data or confidential exchange between a professional (e.g., physician, attorney) and a client or patient, related to the treatment and progress of the patient, that may be released or disclosed only when written authorization of the patient or guardian is obtained

professional corporation (2) Entity unto itself with a legal and business status that is independent of its shareholders

professional courtesy (13) Discount or discharge of a debt granted to certain individuals at the discretion of the physician rendering the service

professionalism (1) Conduct, aspirations, and qualities characteristic of a profession

prognosis (9) Forecast of the outcome of a disease or injury

program (7) See *software*

progress report (9) Written observations made at examinations of a patient subsequent to an initial examination

proofreading (11) Reading a document and locating and marking the corrections as needed

proprietorship (15) Owner's net worth; that is, that which is equal to the assets of the business minus the liabilities of the business; also known as *owner's equity* or *capital*

protected health information (PHI) (3) Information about the patient's past, present, or future health condition that contains personal identifying data

protocol (6) Set of instructions used for reference prescribing strict adherence to correct etiquette and preference

provider (16) Person or institution that gives medical care

purge (8) Procedure used in filing to remove outdated files or items from files, folders, or computer disks

quantum merit (13) Latin for "as much as he deserves"; a common-law principle that means the patient promises to pay the physician as much as he or she deserves for labor

receipt (13) Written acknowledgment of individual payment; generally used for cash

reception room (5) Outer office provided for patients who are awaiting appointments

reconciliation (14) Act of proving the accuracy of all transactions that have occurred on a checking account by performing mathematical computations and comparing the bank's records with those of the customer

recycle (8) Using saved material (e.g., wastepaper) and processing it for reuse

referral (7) Procedure followed when a primary care physician recommends and sends the patient to another physician for further medical treatment

referring physician (9) Physician sending a patient to another physician for the transfer of total or partial medical care. This term is also used loosely for a physician who sends a patient to a specialist for a consultation or for a diagnostic test.

reflective listening (4) To think about, dwell on, mull over, and study or weigh what has been said

Registered Mail (12) First-Class Mail service that provides, for a fee, a record that mail has been delivered and guarantees an indemnity if it is not received

Registered Medical Assistant (RMA) (1) Title received after appropriate training in administrative and clinical areas and passing a certification examination administered by the American Medical Technologists (AMT)

registration form (5) Questionnaire designed to provide identifying data

Remittance Advice (RA) (16) See *explanation of benefits*

respondeat superior (3) Latin for "Let the master answer." A physician's responsibility for any actions performed by his or her employees in the course of their work, including ones that may injure or harm another individual; also known as *vicarious liability*

results-oriented resumé (18) Summary of work experience that focuses on results, not characteristics. This type of resumé helps prospective employers reduce the risks that are associated with hiring because it shows what the job seeker has accomplished as well as his or her attitude toward work.

resumé (18) Summary of education, skills, and work experience, usually in outline form

savings account (14) Money deposited in a bank or similar institution where it earns interest and has been set aside for future use

scores (8) Creases along the lower front flap of a file folder that unfold to allow the folder to expand

screening (6) Process of asking good questions to evaluate and determine the action to be taken on a telephone call or to determine the person who should receive the telephone call

service charges (14) Fees assessed on a bank account for processing transactions and for account maintenance

service endorsement (12) Notification to the Postal Service on the envelope stating what is to be done with undelivered mail

sharps containers (17) Medical waste containers to dispose of sharp objects (e.g., needles) made of rigid puncture-resistant material that, when sealed, are leak resistant and cannot be reopened without great difficulty

shelf life (10) Length of time a drug may be kept before it begins to deteriorate

sign (9) Indication of the presence or existence of a disease or body function disorder; objective evidence or observable physical phenomenon typically associated with a given condition

signature (10) Section of a prescription that gives instructions to the patient on how to take or apply the medication; also known as *transcription*

signature card (14) Document required by banks to identify those authorized to act on (sign) an account or safe deposit box; signing indicates acknowledgment to handle the account according to existing bank laws

simplified letter style (11) Written communication typed without a salutation or complimentary close

single-entry accounting (15) Type of accounting where each transaction is entered only once in the account books. It is not self-balancing; in other words, it does not rely on equal debits or credits.

skip (13) Debtor who has moved and left no forwarding address

SOAP (9) Abbreviation for *subjective* complaints, *objective* findings, *assessment* of status to obtain diagnosis and implement a treatment *plan*; a method of structuring progress or chart notes

Social Security (FICA) taxes (18) Charges levied by the federal government on employers and employees, which provide funds to pay retired people or their survivors who are entitled to receive such payments, either because they paid Social Security taxes themselves or because Congress declared them eligible

software (7) Computer instructions permanently stored in or temporarily programmed into hardware

solo physician practice (2) One physician working alone whose charges are based on a fee-for-service arrangement

speakerphone (6) Telephone with a microphone designed for hands-free communication

specialized care center (2) Facility where a team of specialists treats patients who have similar medical conditions

staff meetings (17) Scheduled gatherings of office personnel for the purpose of informing, training, problem solving, and exchanging of ideas

stale check (14) Check that is previously dated and so old when presented for payment that it is no longer valid; time limit can vary from 90 days to 6 months, and such information is noted on the face of the check; also called a *stale dated check*

State Disability Insurance (SDI) (18) Insurance program that covers off-the-job injury or illness and is paid for by deductions from employee paychecks; similar programs are TDI and UCD

state income tax (18) Charge levied by a state government on employers and employees that provides funds for state use; amounts determined by individual states

stereotype (4) Generalized or oversimplified conception concerning an individual, group, or form of behavior

stop payment orders (14) Written orders by a signer on the account revoking a check before the bank issues payment. A fee may be assessed for stop payment requests, which are typically carried out if there is loss of a check, a disagreement about a purchase, or a disagreement about a payment; it may not be instituted if a check guarantee card was used in the money transaction.

stream (7) System of advance appointment scheduling in which patients are allocated specific periods of time for office visits and procedures; also called *fixed interval*

stress (1) Natural reaction of the body to any physical, psychological, or emotional demand (pleasant or unpleasant) placed upon it either internally or externally

subject filing (8) Alphabetic arrangement of records filed by topic or grouped under a main theme

subjective (9) In a medical context, any information that the patient provides to the physician describing symptoms that cannot be seen, heard, felt, or measured such as pain, lightheadedness, or nausea

subpoena (3) Latin for "under penalty"; a writ that commands a witness to appear at a trial or other proceeding and give testimony, the disobedience to which may be punishable as a contempt of court

***subpoena duces tecum* (3)** Latin for "under penalty in his possession"; a subpoena that requires a witness to appear in court with his or her records, although the judge may permit mailing of records so that the physician is not required to appear in court, which is the typical scenario experienced in many medical practices

subscription (10) Section of a prescription giving directions to the pharmacist on the total quantity of the drug to be given and the form of the medication (e.g., capsules, tablets)

superscription (10) First element imprinted on a prescription; shown as a symbol (Rx), which stands for the word "recipe" (Latin for "take")

surname (8) Individual's last name

sympathy (1) Pertaining to concern for another person's feelings, thoughts, and experiences

symptom (9) Any indication of disease or disorder that is perceived or experienced by the patient; usually described in subjective terms, for example, depressed, confused, experiencing pain, or tired

tab (8) Projection above the body of a folder or guide; used for labeling

telecommunication (6) Transmission of voice or data over a distance

telephone decision grid (6) Record of types of incoming calls identifying the action to be taken

telephone log (6) Written, dated record of all incoming telephone calls noting the reason for the call and action taken

telephone reference aid (6) Alphabetic list of frequently called telephone numbers

template (7) A preset format or pattern, used as a guide. An appointment template designates various time frames for specific appointment types.

temporary disability (TD) (16) Illness or injury that temporarily prevents an injured person from performing the functions of a regular job

Temporary Disability Insurance (TDI) (18) Insurance program that covers off-the-job injury or illness and is paid for by deductions from employee paychecks; similar programs are SDI and UCD

thesaurus (11) Reference book of alphabetized words with their synonyms and antonyms; also found in word processing software

third-party payer (16) Party (insurance carrier or medical assistance program) other than the physician or patient who intervenes to pay hospital or medical expenses; also known as *third-party carrier*

tickler file (8) Chronological file system that calls attention to future dates of appointments or business matters; a follow-up file that "tickles" the memory

time limit (16) Period of time in which a notice of claim or proof of loss must be filed

toll call (6) Telephone call within a large metropolitan area charged at a unit rate

tort (3) Wrongful act or injury to a person that is grounds for legal civil action

total disability (16) Illness or injury that prevents a person from performing the duties of his or her occupation, or from engaging in any other type of work for remuneration

transcription (10) See *Signature*

transcriptionist (11) Person who converts voice-recorded dictation to hard copy

Transmittal of Wage and Tax Statement (Form W-3) (18) Summary comparing income taxes with-held and reported on W-2 forms and the amount of income tax withheld and reported on the four quarterly 941 forms

treating or performing physician (9) Provider who renders a service to a patient or completes a test

triage (6) System of decision making, i.e., selection of patients for allocation of treatment according to the seriousness of their ailment

true wave (7) System of appointment scheduling that allows for variables and flexibility and assumes the time allowed for appointments will average out each hour

Unemployment Compensation Disability (UCD) (18) Insurance program that covers off-the-job injury and illness and is paid for by deductions from employee paychecks; similar programs are SDI and TDI

United Parcel Service (UPS) (12) National and international letter and package delivery service

United States Postal Service (USPS) (12) Domestic and international mail delivery service

universal precautions (5) Standard policies and procedures established by the Centers for Disease Control and Prevention (CDC) and used by all health care workers for protection from infectious diseases

urgent care (6) Treatment of injuries or conditions that need prompt medical attention within 24 hours to prevent serious deterioration of a patient's health, but is not life threatening; also known as *after-hours care*

urgent care centers (2) Private, for-profit facilities offering extended hours that employ salaried physicians who provide primary and urgent care; also known as *freestanding emergency centers* or *ambulatory centers*

usual, customary, and reasonable (UCR) (16) A usual fee is one that an individual physician normally charges for a given professional service to a private patient; a customary fee is in the range of usual fees charged by providers of similar training and experience in a geographic area; a reasonable fee meets the two previous criteria or is justifiable by responsible medical opinion considering the special circumstances of the case

utilization review (2) Evaluation process performed by qualified health care professionals to determine the quality, appropriateness, and medical necessity of medical care

verbal communication (4) The use of language or spoken words to transmit messages

virus (8) Hidden program that enters a computer by means of an outside source, such as software, disks, or online services; can be harmless (flashing an on-screen message), or harmful (replicating itself throughout disk and memory, using up or wiping out data or memory and eventually causing the system to crash)

visa (17) Written permission to enter a foreign country, issued by that country

voice mail (6) Storing and forwarding of one-way messages combining elements of the telephone, the computer, and a recording device

voucher (14, 15)   1. Receipt stating details (as evidence) of a disbursement of cash. 2. Part of the check that has no negotiable value and that remains in the checkbook after a check is written and removed. It is used to itemize or to specify the purpose for which a check is drawn; also called a *check stub* or *check register*. 3. In insurance, a payment check.

Wage and Tax Statement (Form W-2) (18)   Tax form identifying employer and employee that shows gross earnings and deductions for federal, state, FICA, Medicare, and local income taxes. Form is sent by the employer to the IRS and to each employee annually; a copy is attached by the employee to his or her tax return.

wage base (18)   Annual maximum amount of monies earned on which certain taxes are levied

waiting period (w/p) (16)   Time that must elapse before a benefit is paid; also known as *excepted period*

waiver (16)   Attachment to an insurance policy that excludes certain illnesses or disabilities that would otherwise be covered

warrant (14)   Check that is not considered negotiable but can be converted into a negotiable instrument or cash

withdrawal (14)   Removal of funds from a checking account by writing a check or using an ATM; from a savings account, a withdrawal slip may be completed or an ATM may be used

word processing (11)   Communications system using computerized and text-editing equipment to produce printed letters, reports, and other office documents; includes memory

word processing log (11)   Record of incoming and outgoing word processing documents used for accessing written communications quickly and easily

x-ray report (9)   Written findings of an examination of a radiographic study on film

zone improvement plan (ZIP + 4) (12)   Numerical codes, which consist of five or nine digits, written or keyed on envelopes to facilitate the sorting and delivery of mail

INDEX